Pediatric and Congenital Cardiac Care

Paul R. Barach • Jeffery P. Jacobs
Steven E. Lipshultz • Peter C. Laussen
Editors

Pediatric and Congenital Cardiac Care

Volume 2: Quality Improvement and Patient Safety

Springer

Editors
Paul R. Barach
School of Medicine
University of Oslo
Oslo
Norway

Jeffery P. Jacobs
Division of Cardiac Surgery
Department of Surgery
Johns Hopkins All Children's Heart Institute, All Children's Hospital and Florida Hospital for Children
Johns Hopkins University
Saint Petersburg, Tampa and Orlando, FL
USA

Division of Cardiac Surgery
Department of Surgery
Johns Hopkins University
Baltimore, MD
USA

Steven E. Lipshultz
Wayne State University
Detroit, MI
USA

Peter C. Laussen
The Hospital for Sick Children
Toronto, ON
Canada

ISBN 978-1-4471-6565-1 ISBN 978-1-4471-6566-8 (eBook)
DOI 10.1007/978-1-4471-6566-8
Springer London Heidelberg New York Dordrecht

Library of Congress Control Number: 2014955604

Printed on acid-free paper

Springer is part of Springer Science+Business Media (www.springer.com)

We would like to dedicate this book to all patients receiving pediatric and congenital cardiac care and their families. Each of the Editors would like to make the following additional dedications:

To Elijah, to Tore, to Harrison, and to the love of my life, Julie, who makes it all possible.

Paul R. Barach

To my parents David and Marilyn Jacobs for giving me the opportunity, to my wife Stacy for supporting and loving me, to my children Jessica and Joshua for making me proud and motivated, and to my patients, who represent the rationale for this initiative.

Jeffery P. Jacobs

To my wife Tracie and our children Hannah, Zach, Emma, and Sarah, who have always inspired me to do everything possible to improve the health of children. Their motivation has guided me, in the words of others, to "treat every child and family I have the privilege to care for as if they were my first and every day that I am entrusted with their care as if it was my last." These volumes are part of the covenant I have made with many patients and their families to do our very best for them and those who follow. This has been made possible by the wisdom and collaboration of my cherished colleagues and mentors.

Steven E. Lipshultz

To Julia and Joan for their wisdom, guidance, and love. To my children and precious Emery, an inspiration for the future. To the patients I care for and who teach me every day.

Peter C. Laussen

Foreword

A parent taking a child into hospital for diagnosis and treatment hopes for a cure and the restoration of a normal quality of life in the future. They fear many things, ranging from the worst—the death of the child—through their pain and suffering to uncertainty about how to manage the complexity of their own lives, which have so suddenly been disturbed. What they have a right to expect is that the people treating their child know what they are doing, are well trained, and particularly will put the needs of the their child at the center of their decision making.

They are handing over their precious bundle of joy to strangers to care for, aware that that very care might actually threaten the life of that child as well as offer treatment. They are *loaning* their child to these professionals. It demands an enormous amount of trust to do that. As professionals, we need to be able to recognise that level of trust and repay it. Trust is a two-way thing.

The remarkable fall in the mortality for repair of congenital heart defects over the last 60 years could lead to complacency. But we must not forget that mortality is only one outcome measure and cannot reflect all the issues which concern parents. Medicine is dangerous. Many readers will have seen the famous diagram which charts the relative risk of accidents affecting users of organisations, which shows that there are high-reliability organisations like European railroads, western airlines and the nuclear industry but that medicine is about as safe as bungee jumping. This is due to errors that we make, problems we fail to address, complications we fail to tackle. There is no room for complacency if we want to deserve the trust of the parents who have loaned us their child.

If it were my child being treated, this is what I expect:

- I *expect* that my child will be cared for safely in a modern hospital.
- I *expect* my child to be looked after by a well-functioning multi-disciplinary team.
- I *expect* the staff will know the results of the treatment they propose not just in the literature but in their own hands.
- I *expect* the staff to know the complication rates in their hospital and put in place ways to reduce them.
- I *expect* that they will be collecting complete and validated data on all they do and that they will share those data openly with other professionals and the public.

- I *expect* the staff will do all they can to mitigate the certain human error that will occur, by putting in place systems which limit both risk and harm.
- I *expect* that the staff will be honest, open and transparent in all their dealings with me and that if they don't know something, they will say so and let me get a second opinion.
- I *expect* to be involved in decisions about the care of my child and to have my views respected.
- I *expect* that any harmful incident will be fully, openly and honestly investigated as quickly as possible and that learning from the incident will spread widely so that no one else can suffer.
- I *expect* that the team will be interested in the long-term outcome of treatment, not just in hospital, and that they will have mechanisms in place to gather the relevant information.
- I *expect* the truth and to be treated as if I were a friend, with warmth and empathy.

The Editors of this timely book have gathered an array of experts to give guidance as to how these expectations should be met. They give valuable insight into methods and use their own experience to highlight what we can do to be better. Being better, continuous improvement is what it is all about. Our speciality has done well with a relentless pursuit of excellence and is further advanced than many in being open about its results. Yet, it has much to learn from other disciplines, particularly oncology, about the benefits of collaboration over competition. Our discipline was built on the drive and energy of highly competitive alpha males and the disruptive technology of cardiopulmonary bypass. A second wave of disruption has followed the introduction of trans-catheter interventions. But this too has resulted in the same kind of rush to glory that we saw in the 1970s with surgical heart valve implementation and design. We need good studies, strong data and multi-center collaboration if we want to give the best care as quickly as possible.

This book exemplifies the move to collaboration and the drive towards openness and transparency. All our patients and their families are now 'digital natives'. They access the collective memory of Google just as we do. They expect to see our results and can quickly find their way around PubMed. We have a duty to give them insight into the facts they can read. The information provided in this text will help units realise both the importance of good data but also the methods by which it can be used, evaluated, interpreted and reported.

Don't forget, your duty is to keep the child safe and make it as well as you can. This book will help.

London, UK Martin Elliott, MD, FRCS

Preface

The idea that clinical data could be analyzed by multiple congenital heart centers was shared by many enlightened individuals who foresaw the utility of such an organizational structure in the early 1980s. Discussions led to ideas that resulted in primitive data collection systems that catalogued diagnoses, procedures, complications, and survival statistics. The difficulty with these systems was that the nomenclature was not uniform and the challenge of comparing diagnoses and procedures prevented accurate analysis. In short, nomenclature categories were diverse owing to substantial and justified differences of opinion by many leading anatomists. Parallel publications by surgeons and cardiologists resulted in more uniform parochial nomenclature systems, but still there were significant differences between the two that challenged future collaborative efforts. The call to arms was answered by concerned clinicians and anatomists and resulted in a computer mapping strategy that was successful in categorizing diagnoses and procedures by what is actually described and performed and not by what it is called. As a result, the types of ventricular septal defects, atrial septal defects, truncus arteriosus, and the like now had a computer number and not a name. It was revolutionary in concept and comprehensive in scope. It was as if the world had one language even if the cultures varied. Before long, North and South America, Europe, Asia, and Africa were using the standard nomenclature.

This was just the beginning. Data were collected, analyzed, and interpreted to reveal or contradict theretofore clinical assumptions, biases, and largely undocumented hearsay conclusions. Data verification strategies by professional volunteers were planned, and audit visits were instituted. Concurrently, participating center data were to be assessed and compared with the combined experience of the participating centers. This allowed the possibility of program assessment and quality improvement. Complexity scores were developed based on Delphian principles until the time that enough data were collected to allow data-driven risk stratification.

The subsequent analysis of the databases and the developed nomenclature became exponential. Government agencies accepted the documents and instituted registries based on the developed principles. Long-term outcome analyses became a reality with database linking to both the Department of Health and Human Services Centers for Medicare and Medicaid Services Database and the Social Security Death Master File. Ethical issues were being discussed and used to clarify rules and regulations. In addition to these innovations, database documentation of complications has been used to guide the clinician to perform more extensive data-driven informed consent. In an interesting twist of phrases, the database was used to inform the informed consent process.

The benefits of the database systems and the supporting nomenclature were simply too much to document in an expanded treatise. It could only have been accomplished by a book, the like of which is offered in this informative and excellent text. The reader will enjoy this book not only for the rich references that accompany the prose but also for the enjoyable historical account of what some people refer to as simply unbelievable.

Orlando, FL, USA Constantine Mavroudis, MD

Acknowledgments

The Editors of *Pediatric and Congenital Cardiac Care: Volume 1 – Outcomes Analysis and Volume 2 – Quality Improvement and Patient Safety,* Paul R. Barach, Jeffrey P. Jacobs, Peter C. Laussen, and Steven E. Lipshultz, would like to thank all the authors of chapters in this two-volume set of textbooks, the families of these authors, our administrative staff, and our Editorial and Publishing team.

- Our authors represent an international community of scholarship, with chapters written by luminaries and cutting-edge thinkers.
- All the family members of these authors are indeed owed a debt of gratitude because writing chapters markedly decreases the time available with them.
- Finally, this set of textbooks is possible only because of the tremendous efforts of our administrative staff and the Editorial and Publishing team, and we especially acknowledge the coordination throughout this project by Mitzi Wilkinson and the hundreds of hours devoted to this project by Flora Kim and Grant Weston.

Contents

Contributors

J. Elaine-Marie Albert, MD, MHA Pediatric Intensive Care Unit, Department of Pediatric Critical Care Medicine, Seattle Children's Hospital, Seattle, WA, USA

Catherine K. Allan, MD Division of Cardiac Intensive Care, Department of Cardiology, Boston Children's Hospital, Boston, MA, USA

Melvin C. Almodovar, MD Division of Cardiac Intensive Care, Department of Cardiology, Boston Children's Hospital, Boston, MA, USA

René Amalberti, MD, PhD HAS, Saint-Denis La Plaine, France

Jeffrey B. Anderson, MD, MPH Cincinnati Children's Hospital Medical Center, The Heart Institute, Cincinnati, OH, USA

Erle H. Austin III, MD Department of Surgery, Kosair Children's Hospital, Louisville, KY, USA

Department Cardiothoracic Surgery, University of Louisville, Louisville, KY, USA

Emile Bacha, MD Division of Cardiothoracic and Vascular Surgery, Department of Surgery, Columbia University Medical Center, Columbia/NewYork-Presbyterian, New York, NY, USA

Orkun Baloglu, MD Department of Pediatric Critical Care Medicine, Children's Hospital of Wisconsin/Medical College of Wisconsin, Milwaukee, WI, USA

Paul R. Barach, BSc, MD, MPH Department of Health Management and Health Economics, University of Oslo, Oslo, Norway

Dimitar Baronov, PhD Etiometry LLC, Allston, MA, USA

Robert H. Beekman III, MD Cincinnati Children's Hospital Medical Center, The Heart Institute, Cincinnati, OH, USA

Robert A. Berg, MD Department of Critical Care Medicine, The Children's Hospital of Philadelphia, Philadelphia, PA, USA

Sanjay M. Bhananker, MD Department of Anesthesiology, Harborview Medical Center, Seattle, WA, USA

Evan Butler, MS Etiometry LLC, Allston, MA, USA

Robert Campbell, MD Department of Pediatrics, Emory University School of Medicine, Children's Healthcare of Atlanta Sibley Heart Center, Atlanta, GA, USA

Ken Catchpole, BSc, PhD Department of Surgery, Cedars-Sinai Medical Center, Los Angeles, CA, USA

Jonathan M. Chen, MD Department of Pediatric Cardiac Surgery, Congenital Cardiac Surgery, University of Washington School of Medicine, Seattle, WA, USA

Heart Center, Seattle Children's Hospital, Seattle, WA, USA

David S. Cooper, MD, MPH The Heart Institute, Cincinnati Children's Hospital Medical Center, University of Cincinnati College of Medicine, Cincinnati, OH, USA

Peter H. Cosman, BA, MB, BS, PhD, MAICD, FRACS Department of Surgery, St. George Private Hospital, Kogarah, NSW, Australia

Pat Croskerry, MD, PhD, FRCP (Edin) Critical Thinking Program, Division of Medical Education, Faculty of Medicine, Department of Emergency Medicine, QE – Health Sciences Centre, Halifax Infirmary, Dalhousie University, Halifax, NS, Canada

Karen B. Domino, MD, MPH Department of Anesthesiology and Pain Medicine, University of Washington School of Medicine, Seattle, WA, USA

Martin Elliott, MD, FRCS Paediatric Cardiothoracic Surgery, University College London, Gresham College, London, UK

The Great Ormond Street Hospital for Children NHS Foundation Trust, Gresham College, London, UK

Timothy F. Feltes, MD Department of Pediatrics, Nationwide Children's Hospital, The Ohio State University, Columbus, OH, USA

Heather Freeman, RN, MS, CNS, NNP-BC Performance Improvement, Lucile Packard Children's Hospital at Stanford, Palo Alto, CA, USA

Danielle Gottlieb, MS, MD, MPH Department of Pediatric Cardiac Surgery, Columbia University Medical Center, Morgan Stanley Children's Hospital, New York, NY, USA

Nathaniel H. Greene, MD Department of Anesthesiology and Pediatrics, Duke University School of Medicine, Durham, NC, USA

Karen Harrington, MDCM, MSc Departments of Pediatrics and Critical Care, CHU Ste Justine, Montreal, QC, Canada

Silvia M. Hartmann, MD Department of Critical Care Medicine, Seattle Children's Hospital, Seattle, WA, USA

Edward J. Hickey Division of Cardiac Surgery, The Hospital for Sick Children, Toronto, ON, USA

Gerald B. Hickson, MD Department of Quality, Safety & Risk Prevention, Center for Patient and Professional Advocacy, Vanderbilt University Medical Center, Nashville, TN, USA

Jeffrey P. Jacobs, MD, FACS, FACC, FCCP Professor of Surgery, Johns Hopkins University; Director, Andrews/Daicoff Cardiovascular Program, and Surgical Director of Heart Transplantation and Extracorporeal Life Support Programs, Johns Hopkins All Children's Heart Institute; Division of Cardiac Surgery, Department of Surgery, Johns Hopkins All Children's Heart Institute, All Children's Hospital and Florida Hospital for Children, Johns Hopkins University, Saint Petersburg, Tampa and Orlando, FL, USA

Division of Cardiac Surgery, Department of Surgery, Johns Hopkins University, Baltimore, MD, USA

Howard E. Jeffries, MD, MBA Department of Pediatric Critical Care, Seattle Children's Hospital, Seattle, WA, USA

Julie K. Johnson Department of Surgery, Center for Healthcare Studies, Institute for Public Health and Medicine, Feinberg School of Medicine, Northwestern University, Chicago, IL, USA

Brian F. Joy, MD Department of Pediatrics, Nationwide Children's Hospital, The Ohio State University, Columbus, OH, USA

David Kalfa, MD, PhD Department of Pediatric Cardiac Surgery, Morgan Stanley Children's Hospital – New York Presbyterian Hospital, New York, NY, USA

Amanda L. King, MSN, RN Department of Pediatric Critical Care Medicine, Medical College of Wisconsin, Milwaukee, WI, USA

Angela J. Kinstler Department of Patient Services, Cincinnati Children's Hospital Medical Center, Cincinnati, OH, USA

Darren Klugman Divisions of Critical Care Medicine and Cardiology, Children's National Health System, The George Washington University Medical Center, Washington, DC, USA

Carole Lannon Cincinnati Children's Hospital Medical Center, The James M. Anderson Center for Health Systems Excellence, Cincinnati, OH, USA

Matthew M. Large, BSc, MBBS, FRANZCP Department of Mental Health Services, The Prince of Wales Hospitals, Randwick, NSW, Australia

University of New South Wales, Sydney, NSW, Australia

Peter C. Laussen, MBBS, FCICM Department of Critical Care Medicine, The Hospital for Sick Children, Toronto, ON, Canada

Department of Anaesthesia, University of Toronto, Toronto, ON, Canada

Steven E. Lipshultz, MD, FAAP, FAHA Schotanus Family Endowed Chair of Pediatrics, Professor and Chair, Carman and Ann Adams Department of Pediatrics, Professor of Medicine (Cardiology), Oncology, Obstetrics and Gynecology, Molecular Biology and Genetics, Family Medicine and Public Health Sciences, and Pharmacology, Wayne State University School of Medicine, President, University Pediatricians, Pediatrician-in-Chief, Children's Hospital of Michigan, Specialist-in-Chief, Pediatrics, Detroit Medical Center, Interim Director, Children's Research Center of Michigan, Detroit, MI, USA

Jesse Lock, MD, PhD Etiometry LLC, Allston, MA, USA

Leo Lopez, MD, FASE, FACC, FAAP Department of Pediatrics, Albert Einstein College of Medicine, Children's Hospital at Montefiore, Bronx, NY, USA

Gerard R. Martin, MD Division of Cardiology, Center for Heart, Lung and Kidney Disease, Children's National Medical Center, Washington, DC, USA

John E. Mayer Jr., MD Department of Anesthesiology and Critical Care Medicine, The Children's Hospital of Philadelphia, University of Pennsylvania, Philadelphia, PA, USA

Peter A. Meaney, MD, MPH Department of Anesthesiology and Critical Care, University of Pennsylvania, The Children's Hospital of Philadelphia, Philadelphia, PA, USA

Paul V. Miles, MD Quality Improvement and Assessment Programs in Pediatric Practice, American Board of Pediatrics, Chapel Hill, NC, USA

Brian S. Mittman, PhD Department of Research and Evaluation, Kaiser Permanente Southern California, Pasadena, CA, USA

Implementation and Improvement Science Initiative, Clinical and Translational Science Institute, University of California Los Angeles, Los Angeles, CA, USA

VA Center for Implementation Practice and Research Support, US Department of Veterans Affairs Greater Los Angeles Healthcare System, Sepulveda, CA, USA

Larry Mohl, BS EE, MS EE Performance Inspired, Inc., Jamstir Inc., John's Creek, GA, USA

Brigitta U. Mueller, MD, MHCM Pediatrics, All Children's Hospital, Johns Hopkins University, St. Petersburg, FL, USA

Stephen Muething The James M. Anderson Center for Health Systems Excellence, Cincinnati Children's Hospital Medical Center, Cincinnati, OH, USA

Vinay M. Nadkarni, MD, MS Department of Critical Care Medicine, The Children's Hospital of Philadelphia, Philadelphia, PA, USA

David P. Nelson The Heart Institute, Cincinnati Children's Hospital Medical Center, University of Cincinnati School of Medicine, Cincinnati, OH, USA

Dana E. Niles, MS Department of Anesthesiology and Critical Care Medicine, The Children's Hospital of Philadelphia, Philadelphia, PA, USA

Akira Nishisaki, MD, MSCE Department of Anesthesiology and Critical Care Medicine, The Children's Hospital of Philadelphia, Philadelphia, PA, USA

Ingrid Philibert, PhD, MBA Department of Field Activities, Accreditation Council for Graduate Medical Education, Chicago, IL, USA

Sam Phillips, MEng Arcadia Solutions, Burlington, MA, USA

James W. Pichert, PhD Department of Medical Education and Administration, Center for Patient and Professional Advocacy, Vanderbilt University Medical Center, Nashville, TN, USA

Karen L. Posner, PhD Department of Anesthesiology and Pain Medicine, University of Washington School of Medicine, Seattle, WA, USA

Shakeel A. Qureshi, MBCHB, FRCP Department of Congenital Heart Disease, Evelina London Children's Hospital, London, UK

Douglas G. Ririe Pediatric Cardiac Anesthesiology, Department of Anesthesiology, Brenner Children's Hospital at Wake Forest University, Winston Salem, NC, USA

Bill Rostenberg Architecture for Advanced Medicine, Greenbrae, CA, USA

Matthew C. Scanlon, MD, CPPS Departments of Pediatrics and Critical Care, Medical College of Wisconsin, Milwaukee, WI, USA

Andrew Young Shin, MD Cardiovascular Intensive Care, Division of Pediatric Cardiology, Department of Pediatrics, Lucile Packard Children's Hospital, Stanford University Medical Center, Palo Alto, CA, USA

Robert M. Sutton, MD, MSCE Department of Anesthesiology and Critical Care Medicine, The Children's Hospital of Philadelphia, Philadelphia, PA, USA

Alexis Topjian, MD, MSCE Department of Anesthesiology and Critical Care Medicine, The Children's Hospital of Philadelphia, Philadelphia, PA, USA

Jamie Dickey Ungerleider Psychiatry and Behavioral Medicine, Wake Forest School of Medicine, Winston Salem, NC, USA

Ross M. Ungerleider Pediatric Cardiac Surgery, Department of Surgery, Brenner Children's Hospital at Wake Forest University, Winston Salem, NC, USA

Rudolph P. Valentini, MD Pediatric Nephrology, Children's Hospital of Michigan, Wayne State University School of Medicine, Detroit, MI, USA

Glen S. Van Arsdell Division of Cardiac Surgery, The Hospital for Sick Children, University of Toronto, Toronto, ON, Canada

George R. Verghese Pediatric Cardiology, Department of Pediatrics, Brenner Children's Hospital at Wake Forest University, Winston Salem, NC, USA

Peter Weinstock Division of Critical Care Medicine, Department of Anesthesiology, Perioperative and Pain Medicine, Boston Children's Hospital, Harvard Medical School, Boston, MA, USA

David S. Winlaw, MBBS (Hons), MD, FRACS Paediatric Cardiac Surgery, Heart Centre for Children, The Children's Hospital at Westmead, Sydney, NSW, Australia

Sydney Medical School, University of Sydney, Sydney, NSW, Australia

Thomas Witter, RN (Child) Department of Congenital Heart Disease, Evelina London Children's Hospital, Guy's and St Thomas' NHS Foundation Trust, London, UK

Heather A. Wolfe, MD Department of Anesthesiology and Critical Care Medicine, The Children's Hospital of Philadelphia, Philadelphia, PA, USA

Jerry J. Zimmerman, MD, PhD Pediatric Critical Care Medicine, Department of Pediatrics, Seattle Children's Hospital, University of Washington School of Medicine, Seattle, WA, USA

Introduction

1

Paul R. Barach, Jeffrey P. Jacobs, Peter C. Laussen, and Steven E. Lipshultz

Keywords

Patient safety • quality • patient care • high reliability organizations • culture of safety • team work • outcomes • health reform

This book, entitled "***Pediatric and Congenital Cardiac Care: Volume 2: Quality Improvement, and Patient Safety***," is Volume 2 of one of a two volume textbook. The focus of Volume 1 is outcomes analysis. The focus of Volume 2 is quality improvement and patient safety. Leading work has been undertaken in pediatric cardiac care to understand and measure how to establish collaborative definitions and tools of measurement, and to determine robust benchmarks and methodologies to analyze outcomes. The book highlights best practices for measuring outcomes of pediatric cardiac care. The first volume of this textbook concentrated on measurement and analysis of outcomes. Volume 2 focuses on implementation science in terms of continuous quality improvement and safety science and systems.

Meaningful multi-institutional analyses of outcomes requires a database that can incorporate the following seven essential elements: (1) Use of a common language and nomenclature, (2) Use of a database with an established uniform core dataset for collection of information, (3) Incorporation of a mechanism for evaluating case complexity, (4) Availability of a mechanism to assure and verify the completeness and accuracy

P.R. Barach, BSc, MD, MPH (✉)
Department of Health Management and Health Economics, University of Oslo, Oslo, Norway
e-mail: pbarach@gmail.com

J.P. Jacobs, MD, FACS, FACC, FCCP
Division of Cardiac Surgery, Department of Surgery, Johns Hopkins All Children's Heart Institute, All Children's Hospital and Florida Hospital for Children, Johns Hopkins University, Saint Petersburg, Tampa and Orlando, FL, USA

Division of Cardiac Surgery, Department of Surgery, Johns Hopkins University, Baltimore, MD, USA
e-mail: jeffjacobs@msn.com; jeffjacobs@jhmi.edu

P.C. Laussen, MBBS, FCICM
Department of Critical Care Medicine, The Hospital for Sick Children, Toronto, ON, Canada

Department of Anaesthesia, University of Toronto, 555 University Avenue, Toronto, ON M5G 1X8, Canada
e-mail: peter.laussen@sickkids.ca

S.E. Lipshultz, MD, FAAP, FAHA
Department of Pediatrics, Wayne State University School of Medicine, Children's Hospital of Michigan, Detroit, MI 48201-2196, USA
e-mail: slipshultz@med.wayne.edu

P.R. Barach, J.P. Jacobs, S.E. Lipshultz, P.C. Laussen (eds.), *Pediatric and Congenital Cardiac Care: Volume 2: Quality Improvement and Patient Safety*, DOI 10.1007/978-1-4471-6566-8_1, © Springer-Verlag London 2015

of the data collected, (5) Collaboration between a variety of stakeholders including medical and surgical subspecialties, (6) Standardization of protocols for life-long follow-up, and (7) Incorporation of strategies for quality assessment and quality improvement. Volume 1 of this textbook focused on these seven essential areas. This volume, Volume 2 covers both Implementation Science: Continuous Quality Improvement and Safety Science and Systems.

The fields of pediatric cardiology and cardiac surgery have grown and developed faster than most other fields in medicine. Although the fundamental biological substrates contributing to congenital heart disease are far from understood, and there are great variations in the complexity of congenital cardiac defects, there are nevertheless well established treatment options for correction and palliation of most defects. It seems, however, that despite unprecedented levels of spending on pediatric cardiac care, preventable medical errors have not been reduced, uncoordinated care continues to frustrate patients, parents and providers, and healthcare costs continue to rise [1]. The US Institute of Medicine estimates that 100 patients die each day in the United States from iatrogenic causes. There are of course many possible factors related to this unexpected circumstance, including the introduction of new technology that alters rather than improves systems for care, the lack of engagement of front line staff in decision making and change, and of course, the changing quality and safety metrics.

Delivering pediatric cardiac care is complex and complicated. It is also multidisciplinary, How we organize as teams, the systems of care we develop, and the means by which we collaborate and share information are crucial for delivering safe and cost effective care [2]. In the early days of pediatric cardiac surgery, mortality rates were very high. During the past three decades, survival among children born with even the most complex cardiac defects has increased substantially so that from 2005 to 2009, the discharge mortality of index cardiac operations was 4.0 % (3,418/86,297) in the Congenital Heart Surgery Database of the Society of Thoracic Surgeons (85 centers from the United States and Canada) [3, 4]. Across the world, mortality figures have declined, and this outcome variable is perhaps no longer the only metric by which programs can be evaluated. However, the mortality rates between institutions continues to vary up to sixfold depending on the complexity of the diagnosis and procedure, suggesting there is still many modifiable factors related to case volume, experience, and practice variability [5]. Morbidity and preventable adverse events are better metrics for the evaluation of performance and competence, but are difficult to measure, vary between and by systems of care, and are very dependent on the socio-technical interactions of the care we provide and decisions we make [6]. Complications and adverse events result in higher morbidity, and the potential for longer-term disability and decreased quality of life. Indeed, from a societal perspective, the quality of life achieved by our patients following the care we deliver is arguably the most important outcome metric for pediatric cardiac care.

Rapid advancements that followed from improved diagnostic modalities (2D echocardiography among others), improved technology in cardiopulmonary bypass, and the creative solutions and techniques developed including new management paradigms and prostaglandin E1 infusions to maintain patency of the arterial duct, have all contributed to the remarkable successes in treating these children. Despite remarkable advances, there still remains a relatively high rate of early and late adverse events (mortality and morbidity), particularly in newborns and infants. The frequency of events and the focused patient population means that providers caring for children with congenital and pediatric cardiac disease have a compelling model for investigating resilient systems, human errors, and their impact on patient safety [2].

This first of a kind cross-disciplinary collaboration from four clinician editors from disparate medical disciplines (cardiac surgery, cardiology, anesthesia, and critical care), has pulled together an international community of scholarship with articles by luminaries and cutting edge thinkers on the current and future status of pediatric and congenital cardiac care. It is imperative, however, that we understand and measure what we do collectively, that we share common nomenclature, and that we risk-adjust appropriately to enable effective clinical outcome and management.

Intense scrutiny and measurement of clinical outcomes is increasing at a rapid rate, beyond institutions, regions, and borders. Simultaneously, evolution continues in the domains of public reporting, new regulations, and penalties when reported outcomes do not meet expectations. We believe that in many respects, the current multidisciplinary approaches in pediatric cardiac care can provide a collaborative road map for other disciplines and fields in healthcare such as medicine, surgery and general practice. Proscriptive rules, guidelines, and checklists are helping to raise awareness and prevent harm. However, to provide an ultra-safe system for patients and their families, we need to better understand how our system work, understand systems, redesign our work practices, and develop resilience to not only recover from adverse events but to predict them in the first place [2].

Although the field of pediatric and congenital cardiac care has received worldwide recognition as a leader in outcomes analysis, quality improvement, and patient safety and has advocated for system-wide changes in organizational culture, opportunities remain to lower costs, reduce risks, and improve performance. The field has many complex procedures that depend on a sophisticated organizational structure, the coordinated efforts of a team of individuals, and high levels of cognitive and technical performance. In this regard, the field shares many properties with high-technology systems in which performance and outcomes depend on complex individual, technical, and organizational factors and the interactions among them [6]. These shared properties include the specific context of complex team based care, the acquisition and maintenance of individual skills, the role and reliance on technology, and the impact of working conditions on team performance.

Several factors have been linked to poor outcomes in pediatric cardiac care, including institutional and surgeon- or operator-specific volumes, case complexity, team coordination and collaboration, and systems failures [7]. Safety and resilience in these organizations are ultimately understood as a characteristic of the system—the sum of all its parts plus their interactions. Further, many regulatory and government agencies are examining more closely the utility, management of risk, relationships of programmatic volume, and outcomes in the field.

Interventions to improve quality and strategies to implement change should be directed to improve and reduce variations in outcomes. It is imperative that there be an appreciation of the impact of human factors in the field, including an understanding of the complexity of the interactions between:

- the technical task,
- the stresses of the treatment settings,
- the consequences of rigid hierarchies within the staff,
- the equipment and physical architecture,
- the lack of time to brief and debrief, and
- cultural norms that resist change.

Technical skills are fundamental to good outcomes, but non-technical skills—coordination, followership, cooperation, listening, negotiating, and so on—also markedly influence the performance of individuals and teams and the outcomes of treatment [8].

Pediatric cardiac surgical care has been the subject of well publicized inquiries. A consistent theme from the reports of these inquiries is that many staff, patients, and managers had raised concerns about the standard of care provided to their patients before the sentinel event. The events surrounding the Bristol Royal Infirmary [9], the Manitoba Healthcare [10], and the Mid Staffordshire [11] inquiries highlight the importance of engaged leaders and clinicians who appreciate the impact of human factors and

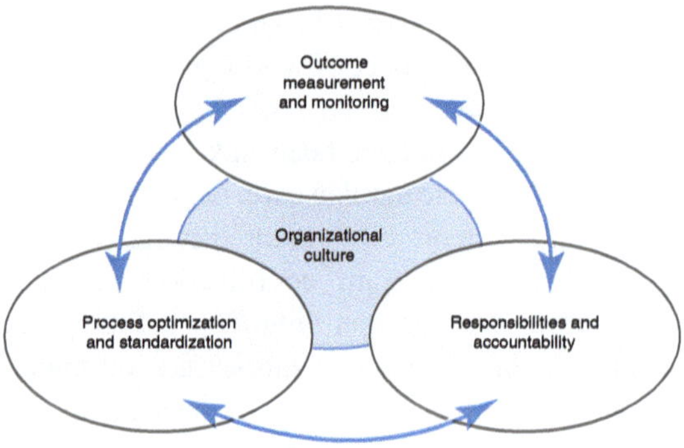

Fig. 1.1 High reliability organizations and their organizational culture (Reproduced with permission from Berg [23])

systems improvement in improving outcomes in pediatric cardiac surgery.

The accidents and adverse events that still occur within systems that possess a wide variety of technical and procedural safeguards (such as operating rooms and intensive care units) have been termed organizational accidents [11, 12]. These are mishaps that arise not from single errors or isolated component breakdowns, but from the accumulation of delayed action failures lying mainly within system flaws that set up good people to fail [13]. People often find ways of getting around processes which seem to be unnecessary or which impede the workflow (called work arounds). This concept is known as normalization of deviance. This accumulated and excepted acceptance of cutting corners or making work-arounds over time poses a great danger to patients and their providers. Similar findings have been described in other investigations into major episodes of clinical failure, and healthcare systems need to heed the lessons of other industries [14, 15]. This concept is shown schematically in Fig 1.1.

The study of human factors is fundamentally about appreciating the nature of socio-technical systems and optimizing the relationship between people, tasks, and dynamic environments [16]. Although a particular human action or omission may be the immediate or suspected cause of an incident, closer analysis in pediatric care usually reveals a preceding series of events and departures from safe practice, potentially influenced by the working environment and the wider organizational context [17]. An organizational accident model proposes that adverse incidents be examined both from an [18]:

- organizational perspective that incorporates the concept of active and latent conditions, and
- individual perspective that considers the cascading nature of human error.

Improving patient outcomes requires that, we create the conditions, resources, and culture in which clinicians can strive to create safe outcomes. Leaders in our field must create and support an organizational climate that allows people to acknowledge mistakes and encourages the clinicians to innovate. There is a very tight coupling and complexity of care across pediatric cardiac care, and the ability of the team to recognize and respond quickly and appropriately to errors and threats is essential to minimize the consequences and ensure recovery [19, 20].

High reliability—or consistent performance at high levels of safety over prolonged periods— is a hallmark for non-health-related, high-risk industries, such as aviation and nuclear power generation [21]. High reliability is centered on supporting and building a culture of trust, transparency, and psychological safety [22]. In the face of health reform and increased competition in the market, moving to high reliability requires adopting and supporting a culture that appreciates the relationships among a variety of organizational risk factors and their effect on patient harm and procedural inefficiency. Improving safety and quality, and providing true value in pediatric cardiac care, will require clinicians to acknowledge their primary responsibility in the care of their patients and their families, as well as managing processes for optimization, standardization, continuous measuring and monitoring of outcomes [23].

Finally, trust and collaboration within teams, between institutions, and across institutional and jurisdictional borders are essential elements in pediatric cardiac care to ensure robust collection of data collection and mechanisms of reporting about possible hazards or unsafe conditions [24–26]. Teams perform more effectively than individuals and their discussions can promote opportunities to detect and correct errors. The real challenge going forward is learning how best to identify and use the data to drive care, give meaningful feedback to providers, promote alignment and efficiency, and assure improvements.

This book came about from a long standing friendship and camaraderie of the editors who collectively believe that we should and can continuously do much better for our patients, and their families, in delivering safer, higher value, and patient centered pediatric cardiac care. The book evolved from two successful special issues of Progress in Pediatric Cardiology [27, 28]. The editor's feel strongly that no one repository exists for the growing wisdom and practices in the rapidly moving field of pediatric cardiac care in the three inter-related domains of outcomes analysis, quality improvement, and patient safety.

We believe that innovation in patient care is best designed in concert with those on the front lines of healthcare delivery—patients and clinicians — and incorporating relevant knowledge from other scientific disciplines such as operations research, organizational behavior, industrial engineering, and human factors psychology. In order to best engage with medical staff, the focus of improvement efforts should be in bringing even more scientific discipline and measurement to the design of healthcare delivery. The need exists to develop innovative models of care that lower the complexity and cost of delivering health care, while simultaneously improving clinical outcomes and the patient experience. In this era of acute health care reform with serious financial constraints, the quality, safety, management of risk, and costs of delivering pediatric cardiac care are vital considerations for patients, families, and clinicians.

The editors are indebted to the wonderful contributions from leaders across the world from a wealth of disciplines with expertise in pediatric cardiac care. The authors are all "thought leaders", have lead important change, and are visionaries. We hope this book provides readers with a roadmap and a common reference source of current initiatives in outcomes analysis, quality improvement, and patient safety in the field of pediatric and congenital cardiac care. Moreover, we hope the content and the authors of this text will inspire readers, and foster engagement, and that through collaboration and sharing, pediatric cardiac care will be enriched and improved.

References

1. Committee on Quality of Health Care in America, Institute of Medicine. To err is human: building a safer health system. Washington, DC: National Academy Press; 1999.
2. Amalberti R, Auroy Y, Berwick DM, Barach P. Five system barriers to achieving ultra-safe health care. Ann Intern Med. 2005;142(9):756–64.
3. Jacobs JP, O'Brien SM, Pasquali SK, Jacobs ML, Lacour-Gayet FG, Tchervenkov CI, Austin 3rd EH, Pizarro C, Pourmoghadam KK, Scholl FG, Welke KF, Mavroudis C. Variation in outcomes for benchmark operations: an analysis of the Society of Thoracic Surgeons Congenital Heart Surgery database. Ann Thorac Surg. 2011;92(6):2184–92.
4. Jacobs JP, O'Brien SM, Pasquali SK, Jacobs ML, Lacour-Gayet FG, Tchervenkov CI, Austin 3rd EH, Pizarro C, Pourmoghadam KK, Scholl FG, Welke KF, Gaynor JW, Clarke DR, Mayer Jr JE, Mavroudis C. Variation in outcomes for risk-stratified pediatric cardiac surgical operations: an analysis of the STS Congenital Heart Surgery database. Ann Thorac Surg. 2012;94(2):564–72.
5. Jacobs JP, Jacobs ML, Austin EH, Mavroudis M, Pasquali SK, Lacour–Gayet FG, Tchervenkov CI, Walters III HW, Bacha EA, del Nido PJ, Fraser CD, Gaynor JW, Hirsch JC, Morales DLS, Pourmoghadam KK, Tweddell JT, Prager RL, Mayer JE. Quality measures for congenital and pediatric cardiac surgery. World J Pediatr Congenit Heart Surg. 2012;3(1):32–47.
6. de Leval MR, Carthey J, Wright DJ, Farewell VT, Reason JT. Human factors and cardiac surgery: a multi-center study. J Thorac Cardiovasc Surg. 2000;119:551–672.
7. Schraagen JM, Schouten T, Smit M, et al. A prospective study of paediatric cardiac surgical microsystems: assessing the relationships between non-routine events, teamwork and patient outcomes. BMJ Qual Saf. 2011. doi:10.1136/bmjqs.2010.048983.
8. Catchpole KR, Mishra A, Handa A, et al. Teamwork and error in the operating room: analysis of skills and roles. Ann Surg. 2008;247:699–706.
9. Kennedy I. Learning from Bristol: the report of the public inquiry into children's heart surgery at the Bristol Royal Infirmary 1984–1995. Department of Health, London: Crown Copyright; 2001.
10. Manitoba Pediatric Cardiac Surgery Inquest Report. http://www.pediatriccardiacinquest.mb.ca/pdf/pcir_intro.pdf. Accessed 10 Aug 2011.

11. Francis R, QC (6 February 2013). Report of the Mid Staffordshire NHS Foundation Trust Public Inquiry (Report). House of Commons. ISBN 9780102981476. Retrieved 17 Mar 2014.
12. Cover-up over hospital scandal. Daily Telegraph, 20 June 2013.
13. Rasmussen J. The role of error in organizing behavior. Ergonomics. 1990;33:1185–99.
14. Norman D. The psychology of everyday things. New York: Basic Books; 1988.
15. Reason J. Managing the risks of organizational accidents. Aldershot: Ashgate; 1997.
16. Sagan SD. The limits of safety: organizations, accidents, and nuclear weapons. Princeton: Princeton University Press; 1994.
17. Catchpole KR, Giddings AE, de Leval MR, Peek GJ, Godden PJ, Utley M, Gallivan S, Hirst G, Dale T. Identification of systems failures in successful paediatric cardiac surgery. Ergonomics. 2006;49:567–88.
18. Cassin B, Barach P. Making sense of root cause analysis investigations of surgery-related adverse events. Surg Clin North Am. 2012;92:101–15. doi:10.1016/j.suc.2011.12.008.
19. Westrum R. Organizational and inter-organizational thought: World Bank workshop on safety control and risk management, Washington, DC, 1988.
20. Perrow C. Normal accidents: living with high-risk technologies. New York: Basic Books; 1984.
21. Weick K, Sutcliffe K, Obstfeld D. Organizing for high reliability: processes of collective mindfulness. In: Boin A, editor. Crisis management. Thousand Oaks: Sage Press; 2008. p. 31–67.
22. Edmondson A. Psychological safety and learning behaviours in work teams. Adm Sci Q. 1999;44(2): 350–83.
23. The more I know, the less I sleep, Global perspectives on clinical governance. KPMG Global Health Practice. 2013.
24. Langer EG. Mindfulness. Boston: Da Capo Press; 1990. ISBN 9780201523416.
25. Bognar A, Barach P, Johnson J, Duncan R, Woods D, Holl J, Birnbach D, Bacha E. Errors and the burden of errors: attitudes, perceptions and the culture of safety in pediatric cardiac surgical teams. Ann Thorac Surg. 2008;85(4):1374–81.
26. Barach P, Small DS. Reporting and preventing medical mishaps: lessons from non-medical near miss reporting systems. BMJ. 2000;320:753–63.
27. Lipshultz S, Barach P, Jacobs J, Laussen P, editors. Quality and safety in pediatric cardiovascular care. Prog Pediatr Cardiol. 2011;1:1–102.
28. Lipshultz S, Barach P, Jacobs J, Laussen P, editors. Quality and safety in pediatric cardiovascular care. Prog Pediatr Cardiol. 2011;2:103–184.

Part I

Implementation Science: Continuous Quality Improvement

Selection, Training and Mentoring of Cardiac Surgeons

2

Ross M. Ungerleider, George R. Verghese, Douglas G. Ririie, and Jamie Dickey Ungerleider

Abstract

This chapter explores the unique challenges of selecting, training and mentoring those who will become the next generation of pediatric cardiac care professionals. In addition to the published literature on selection, training and mentoring, we provide new data from the Congenital Heart Surgeons Society and the European Association for Congenital Heart Surgery elucidating the elements deemed most important to the training and professional development of healthcare providers devoted to pediatric cardiac care.

Keywords

Training • Mentoring • Education

R.M. Ungerleider (✉)
Pediatric Cardiac Surgery, Department of Surgery, Brenner Children's Hospital at Wake Forest University, Winston Salem, NC, USA
e-mail: ungerlei@mac.com

G.R. Verghese
Pediatric Cardiology, Department of Pediatrics, Brenner Children's Hospital at Wake Forest University, Winston Salem, NC, USA
e-mail: gverghes@wakehealth.edu

D.G. Ririe
Pediatric Cardiac Anesthesiology, Department of Anesthesiology, Brenner Children's Hospital at Wake Forest University, Winston Salem, NC, USA
e-mail: dririe@wakehealth.edu

J.D. Ungerleider
Psychiatry and Behavioral Medicine, Wake Forest School of Medicine, Winston Salem, NC, USA
e-mail: jungerle@wakehealth.edu

Introduction

There once was a very wise, old woman who lived in a small town. The people in the town would visit her when they needed advice and her influence reached far and wide. Her reputation was irksome for a group of young boys in the town, who felt that she received far more attention and acclaim than warranted and they wanted to show how she was not nearly as smart as was claimed.

The oldest of the boys developed a plan. He would capture a small bird—one that was tiny and fragile enough that it would fit into his cupped hands. He would then approach the old woman, with the bird cupped in his hands, and he would ask the woman: "This bird in my hands… is it alive or is it dead?" The plan was diabolical and certain to succeed. If the old woman said the bird was alive, he would squeeze his hands,

P.R. Barach, J.P. Jacobs, S.E. Lipshultz, P.C. Laussen (eds.),
Pediatric and Congenital Cardiac Care: Volume 2: Quality Improvement and Patient Safety,
DOI 10.1007/978-1-4471-6566-8_2, © Springer-Verlag London 2015

extinguishing the life from the bird, before opening his hands to show it was actually dead. If she claimed that the bird was dead, he would simply open his hands and let the bird fly away. Either way, they would show that she was not nearly as wise as was claimed. The plan could not fail.

On the selected day, with their appointment to see the old woman secured, and widely advertised to the townspeople, the boys approached the old woman. The leader of the boys had the tiny bird in his hands and he asked the woman: "This bird in my hands…is it alive or is it dead?"

The old woman gazed at them and at the hands that held the bird for a long time. The boys didn't move and the leader of the boys, the one with the bird enclosed in his fateful hands, began to become a bit anxious. Perhaps there was some truth to what was said about this woman. Perhaps she was indeed wise and knew what they were up to. No, that couldn't be. Their plot was perfect.

Finally the woman spoke. She looked at the lead boy and she said:

> About that bird. You ask me if it is alive or if it is dead. It is in your hands.

We are like those boys. We want to know what will become of our profession [1]. It is a profession that is at its greatest. The information in this textbook will illustrate how well we do and how far we have come. We hold the future in our hands.

If we are to see quality and outcomes continue to improve, then our responsibility is to attract those who are most promising. If quality and outcomes are going to improve, we have to find ways to train our successors to be better than we were, despite the challenges that we continuously encounter that alter the training environment—less exposure to cardiac surgery during early years of surgical training, work hour limitations and restrictions for all accredited residency and fellowship training programs, and with diminishing center volumes and emphasis for more "high level" involvement, fewer opportunities for patient management or interventional procedures of any type. If quality and outcomes are going to improve, we need to provide the positive connection to mentors.

Background

This chapter will address each of these challenges: Selection of those who will "follow", training to create a future of excellence, and mentoring to keep providers connected and meaningful to those who will define that future. Our comments will be founded in literature from education, business, psychology, medicine and interpersonal neurobiology and will also be connected to new data acquired for this chapter from two important pediatric cardiac surgical organizations. We will attempt to generalize our information to the challenges encountered across the spectrum of specialties that comprise the profession of pediatric cardiac care, and we will anchor many of our remarks in data obtained from experts in the field of pediatric cardiac surgery.

We've chosen surgery as an anchor for two reasons: first, we have data from this group (and we believe the data can be extrapolated to help us understand challenges that confront each of the other subspecialties) and secondly, we believe that some of the issues facing surgery are unique and require particular attention (although as such, they do appear to some degree in other specialties)—and these will be emphasized where appropriate.

Data Acquisition

In order to better understand what has worked in the past, we surveyed the members of the Congenital Heart Surgeons Society (CHSS) as well as the members of the European Congenital Heart Surgeons Association (ECHSA). Both of these organizations elect members based on merit and are therefore comprised of dedicated congenital heart surgeons who are considered, by their peers, to be successful contributors to our field. We surveyed the members of these two organizations as *surrogates* for the type of individual who has proven success in our field. We could not identify, at this time, a comparable, well-defined group of experts in pediatric cardiology or pediatric cardiac anesthesiology/intensive care; but we believe much of the information provided by our surgical experts is applicable across specialties. In total, 189 surveys were distributed (152 to current active or past CHSS members and 37 to ECHSA members). We received 71 responses (compliance of 38 %; which provides data reliability at a level of 95 % ± 10 %) [2]. However, we believe the response rate is actually higher since many emails were likely sent to retired or inactive members who no longer participate as active members. Of those receiving surveys, 104 were actually "opened" and this yields a response rate of 68 % (reliability of 95 % ± 5 %) for those who actually "received" the survey. Regardless, research on surveys [3–5] suggests that the response rate to surveys from a fairly homogeneous group of respondents who all perform the same activity provides accurate information at response rates greater that 20 %. Our response rate was 2–3 times higher than this and the engagement of the participants (as reflected by numerous "free field" comments) is also a published indicator of survey validity.

The survey questions were created to help us better understand our educational challenges for the future. We are grateful to the members of these two elite organizations who took the time to respond candidly and thoughtfully to this survey.

Selection

Selection begins with rapture.

> When I (RMU) was 8 years old (Mid-late 1950's), I visited a museum in Chicago, Illinois (The Roosevelt Museum of Science and Industry) and there was an exhibit about the "emerging" field of heart surgery. The heart lung machine was becoming an established (although new) technology, and surgeons were beginning to imagine ways to enter the heart of children born with congenital heart lesions and repair these defects. There was a large model of a heart that museum visitors could walk through (in an anatomically correct path from right atrium, to right ventricle, to pulmonary arteries/veins, to left atrium and finally left ventricle). All of this was done to a background of sound. As the lub-dub of the heartbeat influenced the cadence of my steps, I became entranced. There were exhibits of what surgeons might be able to do in order to repair a variety of congenital heart defects. Heart surgery as an extension of thoracic surgery was a new and exciting field (Denton Cooley called the heart lung machine the "can opener for the largest picnic thoracic surgeons will ever know") [6] and I was enraptured.

Of course, it is a natural for us to think of selection from our perspective in the field, but it is not just we who select those whom we choose to train—it is also we (as a field and as individuals) being selected by those who wish to follow our career path as one worth pursuing. (Ironically, training and mentoring reflects this same duality—how many of us have learned from those we train, and how often do we find that friendships extend over decades as our students become our teachers?!). In this chapter, we explore each element: selection, training and mentoring from two perspectives—*ours* as selectors, trainers and mentors; and *the professional literature* on this topic, as it relates to what future trainees are looking for when they select training programs; what they need in order to "train to competence" in their respective fields; and how we can best fulfill our roles as mentors for their future.

First, whom do we choose? How do we excite the imagination and begin to fan the flames of passion for those who want to share with us in our extraordinary field? And how do we ensure that those whom we select will help take our field to new heights?

Current methods of selection (both for medical school and for residency training) seem to be driven most by objective indices of performance—primarily grades and performance on standardized tests (such as MCATs, USMLE, and In-Training Exams). Many medical schools and residency programs are concerned that the students they select perform well on standardized exams. Ultimately, this will be important so that the trainee can pass the exams required to become board certified in their specialty. There are data that link ability to perform well on board certifying exams (or other standardized exams) to past performance on standardized exams, such that students with high scores on MCATs, USMLE, or In-Training Exams (ITE) are most likely to perform well on subsequent qualifying exams [7–11]. No wonder these candidates seem to be most attractive to medical schools or training programs. However, there is growing concern that while they may perform well on standardized exams, they may not have the qualities required to succeed in some specialized fields of healthcare [12–14]—that is, a good test taker might not become a great surgeon, anesthesiologist or cardiologist. Furthermore, test taking ability does not measure ability to communicate effectively in complex teams, nor does it reflect on decision making or physical performance under stressful situations. A good test taker will, however, most likely be a good test taker and continue to pass qualifying exams. A poor test taker of the USMLE exams may simply be someone who would benefit from special supervision or assistance [15].

There is increasing understanding that the skill sets necessary for success are variable and that good test taking only reflects one skill set—although an important one, since good performance on USMLE Step 1 and Step 2 is undeniably related to mastery of applied basic and clinical science knowledge. If program directors consider a solid foundation in these domains to be important measures of readiness for growth and development during graduate medical education, then it is reasonable for them to use USMLE scores as a key factor in their consideration of applicants [7, 16]. This emphasis on USMLE scores for selection into residency programs, however, neglects the numerous other talents and skills required for expertise as a physician. Some correlation studies have suggested that performance on USMLE Step 2 (clinical science) is a better predictor of success in residency than USMLE Step 1 (basic science) [13], whereas other studies have shown that Step 1 scores are only useful in students who had prior clinical experience before taking Step 1 [14]. Other studies have suggested that the abilities that are not measured by USMLE exams (such as self awareness, stress management, leadership, humility, teamwork and other "soft skills" are most predictive of how a resident will perform, particularly in interventional team endeavors such as surgery [17]. Furthermore, although gross motor skills do seem to correlate with academic performance such as class rank and USMLE scores, fine motor dexterity—such as that necessary for certain interventional pediatric cardiac subspecialties—does not correlate with academic performance or class rank [18]. The use of standardized scores as a predictor of ultimate clinical performance for a physician and as a professional has come under increasing scrutiny [19, 20]. Longitudinal studies document better correlation between clinical performance and non-standardized measures such as academic performance on clinical clerkships [21], faculty recommendations [19], election to AOA [21], and numerous other factors related to performance not currently measured by standardized exams [8, 10, 11, 13, 14, 17–19, 22].

The selection of a candidate who will be successful and who will both contribute to the profession, as well as receive a lifetime of joy and stimulation from the profession is the goal of every training program. Our expert survey provides significant insight into the factors that might best predict success for those we choose.

Results

By the nature of the membership process, members of the CHSS and ECHSA have achieved excellence as both clinicians and scientists. For this group, prior academic achievement seems to be a hallmark—2/3 (66.2 %) responded that they were in the top 10 % of their college (undergraduate) class and 87.3 % were in the top 20 % of their undergraduate class (Fig. 2.1).

This ability to perform well academically followed them through medical school where 33.8 % were in the top 5 % of their medical school class, over half (51.2 %) were in the top 10 % of their medical school class and ¾ (76 %) were in the top 25 % of their class (Fig. 2.2).

In fact, when ranking overall medical school performance (grades, recommendations, test scores), 87.3 % were considered to be excellent students (top 25 % of their medical school class) (Fig. 2.3).

For the most part, our responders were highly regarded and successful students through college and medical school. We suspect the same is true for those who have become experts in cardiology,

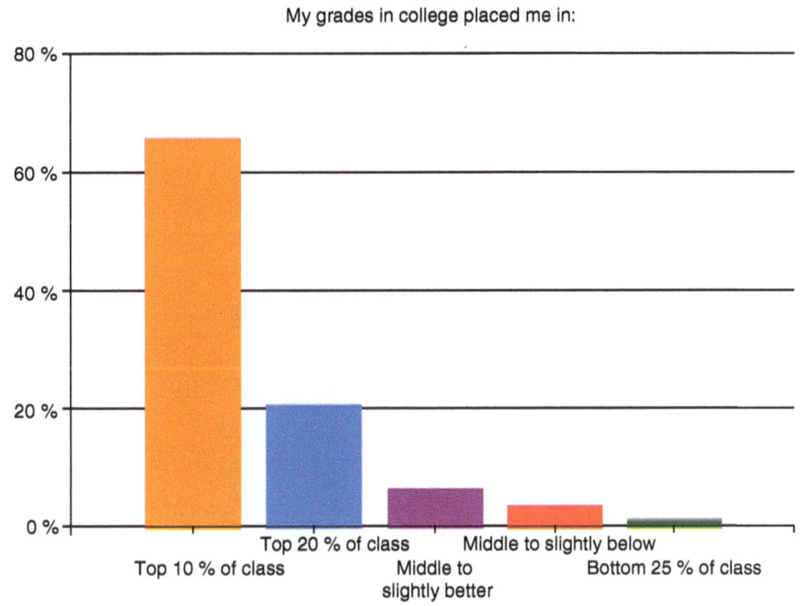

Fig. 2.1 College grades for congenital heart surgeons who are now members of the CHSS (Congenital Heart Surgeons Society) or EACHS (European Association of Congenital Heart Surgeons)

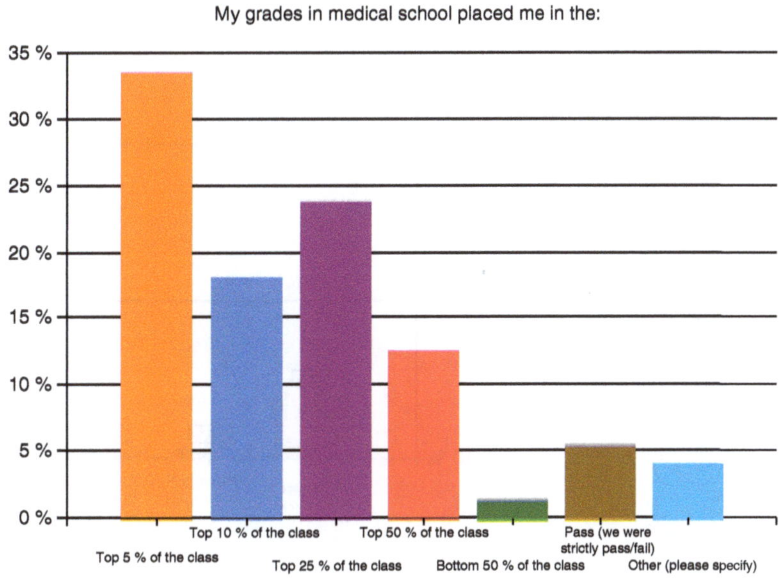

Fig. 2.2 Medical School grades and class rank for congenital heart surgeons who are now members of the CHSS or EACHS

anesthesiology and critical care medicine. For students trained in US medical schools, almost half of our "experts" (45.3 %) were elected to the Alpha Omega Alpha society.

Most of the respondents to this survey had been in practice for over 11 years (84.5 %; and in fact, 40.8 % had been in practice for over 20 years). Over half of today's pediatric cardiac surgeons (53.5 %) decided to pursue congenital heart surgery as a career while they were in their surgical residency (Fig. 2.4). With diminished exposure to cardiac surgery in today's residency programs (Wake Forest University, for example, as is true for numerous other excellent general surgery training programs, does not have general surgery residents rotate onto cardiac surgery services) it may become less likely that surgical residents will become interested in (much less "enraptured by")

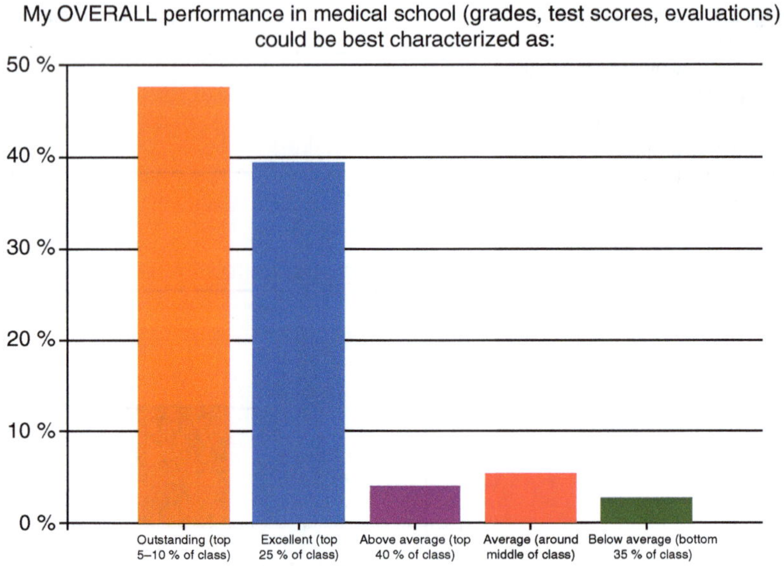

Fig. 2.3 Overall performance rank in medical school for congenital heart surgeons who are now members of the CHSS or EACHS

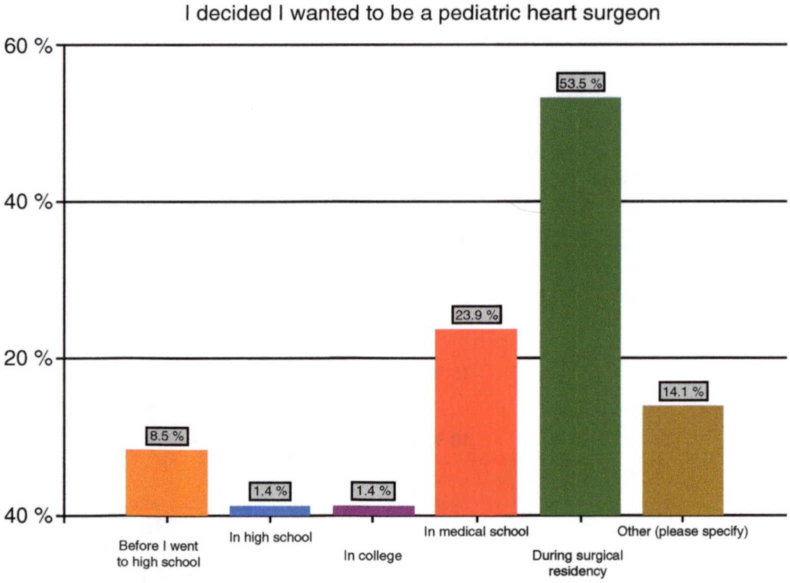

Fig. 2.4 Time period when congenital heart surgeons who are now members of the CHSS or EACHS decided they wanted a career in congenital heart surgery

cardiac surgery. Limited exposure to cardiac surgery during residency, less contact with cardiac surgical faculty mentors who can share their excitement in cardiac surgery and a commitment to mentoring interested residents, and emphasis on the different skill sets of general versus cardiac surgery will likely diminish this previously important pool of residents who will choose to pursue careers in cardiac surgery. Only one fourth (23.9 %) of our respondents decided they wanted to be pediatric heart surgeons in medical school, with another 10 % deciding prior to attending medical school (before high school—8.5 %; in high school—1.4 %; in college—1.4 %).

As the exposure to cardiac surgery becomes less available (at least in surgical residency), and exposure to pediatric cardiac surgery becomes less available during CT residency (most of those in the 14.1 % "other" category decided on pediatric cardiac surgery during their CT residency) our field may not be able to cultivate the kind of excitement and allure—rapture—that was possible in the past; unless we change our expectations of how and when we will attract (and expose) our future colleagues.

With the emergence of a variety of challenges–economic limitations for personal reimbursement; competition amongst centers which diminish individual case volumes; decreasing jobs (at this time) for some specialties like pediatric interventional cardiology and congenital heart surgery; perceived competition between pediatric and adult cardiologists as well as between cardiologists and surgeons for certain procedures; less (sometimes no) exposure to cardiac surgery in many general surgery training programs as well as limited exposure to cardiology and cardiac critical care in even some of the largest pediatric training programs; reluctance of some general surgery program directors to train individuals interested in cardiac surgery; and the lifestyle attractions of alternative career choices–it might be presumed that students in the top 20 % of their classes would not be attracted to a career in pediatric cardiac specialties, and requirements for additional training. But this doesn't take into account the power of rapture.

Educational programs have been changing. In the US, integrated 6 year training programs (I-6) for cardiac surgeons, which not only save time over the traditional programs of general surgery followed by cardiac surgery, but also offer more exposure to cardiac and thoracic surgery to the interested residents throughout the training years [23, 24], have become extremely popular and are attracting highly successful and talented students [25]. It appears (based on our own experience) that extremely talented and exceptional students are interested in and attracted to a career in pediatric cardiac surgery, cardiology and anesthesiology/critical care medicine, despite the perceived challenges mentioned above. There are still several who select this career path later in training, so it will be valuable to maintain some traditional pathways [26].

Selection in a past era revolved around grades, academic performance and an abundance of qualified applicants. The applicant pools to the current I-6 training programs demonstrate that there are still numerous qualified applicants—in fact more than there are current spots to accommodate them [27]. The increased interest of outstanding and qualified medical students to apply for integrated training that can increase their exposure to cardiac surgery is clear [25, 27]. If these opportunities are not available to the medical school applicants, then they might be forced to enter the alternative track of general surgery training programs, which have changed considerably in their content and exposure to cardiac surgery, as well as in their attitudes towards training prospective cardiac surgeons. Although the data from our survey suggest many trainees selected cardiac surgery through their experiences while undertaking general surgery residency, the enormous changes to general surgery training, along with the lifestyle and demands of additional training may make pursuing a cardiac surgery career seem unattractive and undesirable once general surgery training begins. The integrated 6-year training programs provide a "pre-emptive" invitation to enter training in our field. Our options to deal with this challenge might include a more active involvement in medical school curricula, and encouragement of more programs to develop an integrated 6 year training model (as well as support from the Residency Review Committee (RRC) of the ACGME to approve and encourage development of more of these programs) [23], so that we can nurture the interest of those who choose our field by being involved with their training from the time they choose it. It is not as likely that we will be part of the types of surgical training curricula that will be inviting and enticing to residents in general surgery programs—they simply are not having the opportunities in the current programs to be exposed to, much less encouraged to consider a career in, cardiac surgery. Therefore, the previous conventional pathway through general surgery may become less optimal and conventional tracks to cardiac surgery training may disappear, particularly as avenues for the best, brightest and most highly motivated.

Given the multiple competing demands for resident's time in pediatric training programs, even some of the most competitive programs have limited exposure to subspecialties like cardiology (to as little as a 1 month rotation over the 3 years of the training program). A choice by a student to pursue a career in pediatric cardiology or in cardiac anesthesiology/critical care requires selection to a pediatric or anesthesiology training program, followed by

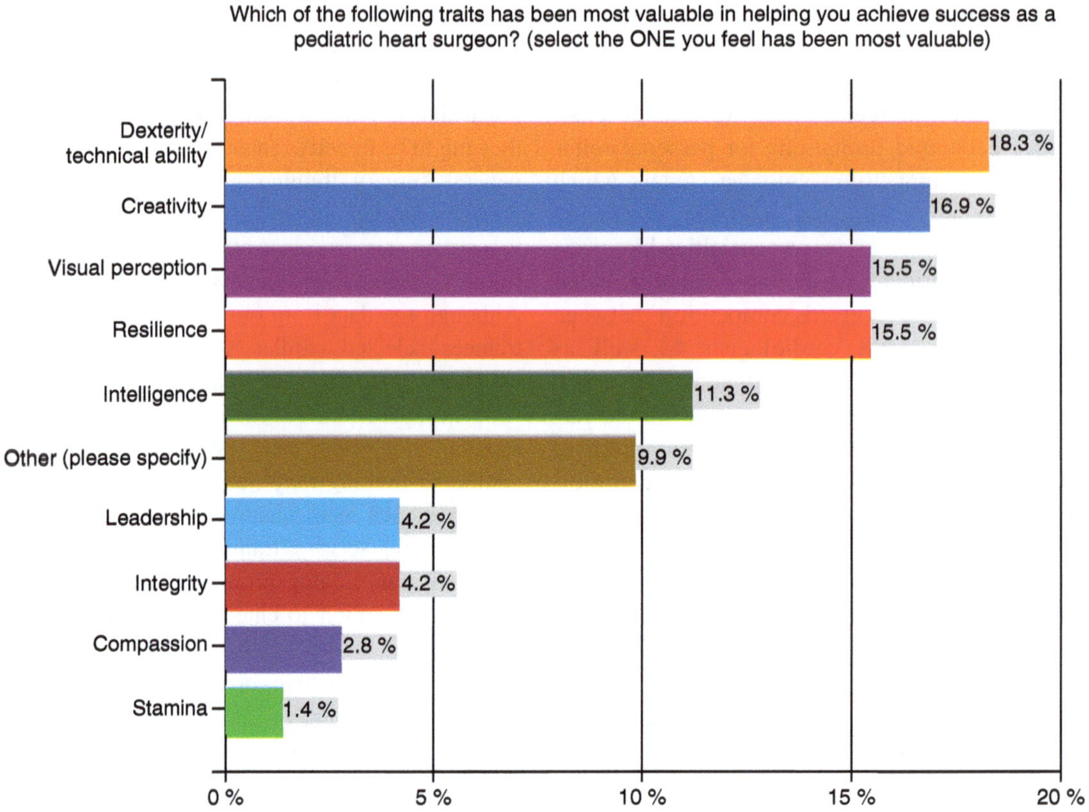

Fig. 2.5 Importance of certain traits deemed by congenital heart surgeons who are now members of the CHSS or EACHS to be valuable to success. The scale demonstrates a degree of importance with the longer bars being considered more valuable

selection into one or more specialty training fellowships.. Recently, a combined pediatric and anesthesiology residency has been developed leading to certification in both specialties. Entry into this type of program involves early selection and may result in development of novel skill sets and permit greater exposure to pediatric cardiac and critical care [28]. Despite this novel integration of training, there are currently no integrated training programs that can "fast-track" the experience and provide increased exposure to congenital heart care to the interested trainee in these specialties. Some have argued that pediatric cardiologists may not require three full years of general pediatrics training to be an academic subspecialist cardiologist [29].

Another consideration in the selection process is the identification of the qualities that are consistent with success in the field of cardiac surgery (and these can certainly be extrapolated to all disciplines). When asked to choose from an extensive list of traits that they felt were most correlated with helping them become successful congenital heart surgeons, the following traits were chosen by more than 10 % of respondents—Dexterity/technical ability (18.3 %); Creativity (16.9 %); Resilience (15.5 %); Visual Perception (15.5 %) and Intelligence (11.3 %) (Fig. 2.5). Many in the "other" group mentioned persistence and commitment—tenacity. As we talk to program directors, many are focused on how to identify and cultivate technical ability and dexterity. We find it fascinating that, on reflection, many of today's most successful surgeons feel that (while technical ability, dexterity and visual perception are certainly important) other traits such as resilience, creativity and tenacity are also extremely valuable. How we identify and select for these traits may be important in how we select those who will follow.

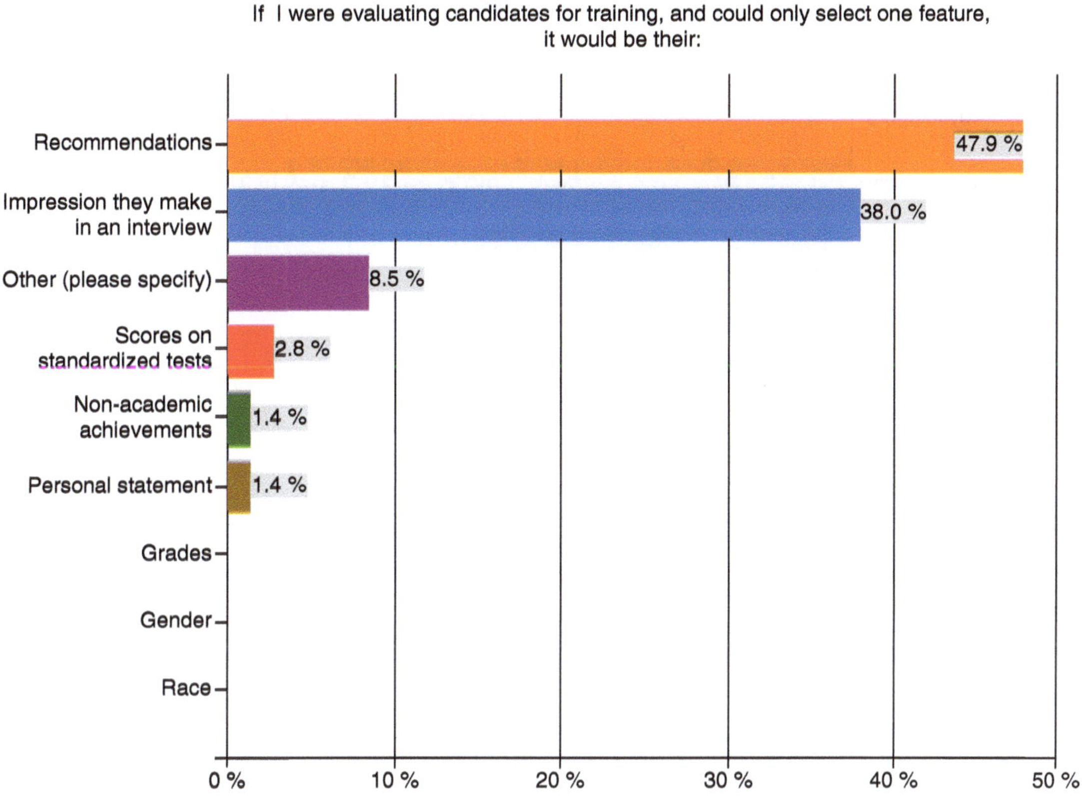

Fig. 2.6 Factors considered to be most valuable when evaluating future congenital heart surgeons, as indicated by surgeons who are now members of the CHSS or EACHS

When asked what factors were most useful in evaluating applicants for training, responses were fairly emphatic—evaluators were looking for passion (rapture), and this was often expressed (as they indicated in separate comments) by "work ethic", resilience, perseverance, determination and motivation to be a successful contributor to the field.

Evaluators were also looking beyond grades and standardized test scores and numerous responders indicated that they were looking for a past history of success (31 %) and outstanding personal values (29.6 %) demonstrated as: emotional intelligence, humility, honesty and ability to listen (also expressed directly as commentary). The importance of this will be discussed in the section under training, but it is clear that in choosing those we wish to train, grades and test scores are no longer adequate as a barometer. More and more experts desire that the applicant possess some cultivation of their personal growth. This is consistent with the research of Goleman [30–32], and others [17, 33–42], who have demonstrated that emotional intelligence (driven by self-awareness and self-management) correlates more with long term success than intellectual intelligence; and both are likely important and necessary to be successful in the practice of high quality pediatric cardiac surgery. Of the experts surveyed, 0 % used grades to evaluate applicants and only 2.8 % used standardized test scores to guide their selection process. Many evaluators believe that they can best assess for these additional qualities through recommendations (47.9 % of responders—and even more so if the recommendations were from people they knew and trusted—stated most frequently in the "other" responses) or by the impression that the candidate makes in an interview (38 %) (Fig. 2.6).

Of particular interest was that when asked which quality (from a long list) (Fig. 2.7) was the

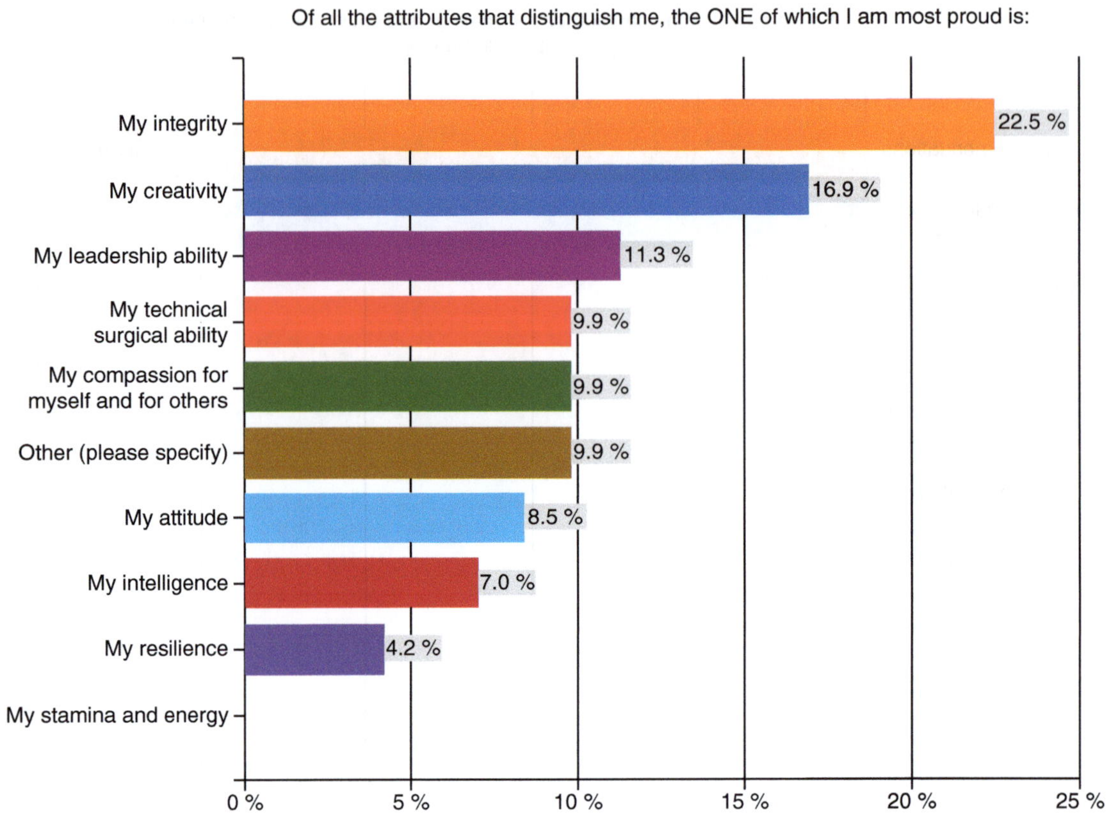

Fig. 2.7 Attributes considered most distinguishing of them as surgeons by members of the CHSS or EACHS. The bars demonstrate a scale of frequency, with the longer bars indicating a trait valued by the highest number of surgeons

ONE that they felt most distinguished them and of which they were most proud, over half indicated their integrity (22.5 %), their creativity (16.9 %) or their leadership ability (11.3 %). No other attributes (including technical abilities or intelligence) were selected by more than 10 % of responders (although compassion for families and others was highly rated). Since these are qualities that are difficult to measure outside of an interview or a recommendation, it is not surprising that these two factors (recommendations and interviews) were rated so highly.

At this time, the majority of applicants for residency training in cardiac surgery in the US are coming through the traditional track of general surgery, as opposed to an integrated 6-year (I-6) training program. Therefore the applicant pool for CT surgery is largely comprised of those who enter general surgery training as a gateway to CT training. An unintentional consequence of this is that we are left to ultimately choose from applicants who meet the criteria set forth by the general surgery programs, which often rely heavily on grades and standardized test scores. By virtue of emphasizing different selection criteria, these general surgery programs may be denying access to the types of applicants who we might find most attractive to select for training in cardiac surgery, particularly pediatric cardiac surgery. This same problem exists in many specialties. In anesthesiology, residency selection has been highly correlated with scores and grades [43]. Unfortunately, academic endeavors such as research and publication history, which may be indicative of "work ethic", seem to have no significant influence. Thus, exceptional candidates who could possibly be outstanding contributors to our field might never have an opportunity to be selected, and they end up pursuing other career options. At least one residency program has addressed this by essentially making the interview process 24 h including meals to permit further interrogation of the "softer" qualities that may be valuable to the success of our professions.

There is another side of selection, which revolves around how we, as a profession, are "chosen." Excellent students are still attracted to cardiac surgery (as well as to related fields in cardiac care) and want us, as educational leaders, to provide them with the kind of training programs that will help them achieve their dreams of contributing to and making our field better. With the significant changes that are occurring in general surgery residency training programs (less exposure to cardiac and thoracic surgery, diminished expressed enthusiasm for cardiac and thoracic surgery as a career option—some general surgery training programs are actually disinclined to take residents with that potential interest, and transition of training to skills that are less comparable to the ones needed for pediatric cardiac surgery in particular), we can imagine that there will be declining interest from general surgery residents to enter the field of cardiac and thoracic surgery, much less pediatric cardiac surgery. The same may likely be happening in pediatrics and in anesthesiology, where training in the field of eventual interest is not available during the initial years of internship and residency. This in part is attributable to the knowledge base and experience required to achieve proficiency in the general principles of each specialty and then the complexity of each subspecialty area further limiting exposure. Prospective candidates may simply become discouraged by the layers that precede the exposure to the training they really want, and in some cases, may choose other fields entirely.

This will be a challenge that we will confront in the future—how do we respond to a pool of potential applicants to our profession that is created by our lack of ability to provide them with exposure to the fields they are most interested in? Once an applicant chooses us, and we choose them, our attention turns to how we can best train them to become successful.

Training

Our ability to train our future has been significantly influenced by changes imposed over the past decade by the ACGME. Accredited training in all specialties is now regulated by rigid duty hour restrictions, which not only limit the number of hours that trainees can work per week, but also regulate how much time they can spend in the hospital on call and how much time they are required to be off (and out of the hospital) between shifts. Although the intent of this work hour limitation is to create a more balanced, healthy and productive health care worker; and to limit errors related to fatigue and stress, the ramifications on training have been enormous, particularly in certain fields (such as surgery or interventional cardiology) where hands-on experience is a vital component of excellence.

There are conflicting reports regarding the affect of duty hour restriction on operative volume in surgical training programs, although for the most part, surgical volumes have decreased in subspecialty training programs [44–49]. Where operative surgical volumes have been maintained, there is legitimate concern that this has been at the expense of residents sacrificing other important experiences, such as outpatient clinic evaluation [49] for preoperative evaluation or postoperative follow up of surgical patients, as well as in-hospital care of convalescing patients [50]. Nevertheless, surgical trainees report spending less time in the operating room [44], and it is not evident that there is less likelihood for medical errors since the result of the duty-hour limitation is increased transitions of care (or cross covering of care), as well as a reduced sense of "ownership" by trainees of the patients they are caring for [44]. In some settings, such as the ICU, there is a national perception of decreased patient safety [51].

Hospital systems have adapted by having much of the work that used to be time consuming delegated to other health care providers, and the multidisciplinary approach has now encouraged a more collaborative team approach for sharing in the work, with intensive care being provided by board certified intensivists (instead of by surgeons), and daily rounds being performed by cardiologists, hospitalists or care extenders (such as nurse practitioners or physician assistants). Despite the attempt to relieve the residents in training of this "extra" work, many residents feel that their training experience is reduced and negatively affected by the duty hour limitations. In national surveys of both medical and surgical residents, the vast majority report either no change or a decreased quality of education after the most recent work hour restrictions (centered on reducing duty hours for interns) were released [52]. Although designed to improve patient safety and decrease burnout, this outcome has not been a clearly demonstrated result from duty-hour limitation [44]. This in part may be related to the multiple factors, besides fatigue, that contribute to burnout such as emotional well-being, job satisfaction and a sense that the work is worthwhile, and a sense of being needed—all of which might be negatively influenced by duty hour limitations [44, 53–55].

All of this has resulted in a dilemma where some residents feel compelled to "under report" their actual hours (which results in a sacrifice of personal integrity). Alternatively, the trainee can attempt to strictly adhere to the rigid duty-hour limitations; thereby missing what might be perceived as potentially valuable experiences and occasionally upsetting faculty who they believe expect them to ignore the rules (thus creating the message that "the rules don't apply to us"—which is a dangerous message). Faculty are not entirely without accountability and there are instances where the faculty has explicitly sent this message to the trainee, giving them little choice but to comply.

Concern over the consequences of duty hour restriction was expressed in the open-ended responses by some of our experts, such as this very pointed statement:

> While it goes against current residencies, I think the "maximum exposure" by ridiculous overwork for 2 or 3 years gave me the ability, experience, and knowledge to have less bad patient outcomes in my first 5 to 7 years of practice. To become an expert, exposure is the most important thing, the less exposure the more "on the job learning" which translates to poorer patient outcomes.

Striking the ideal balance between enhancing resident education and improving patient safety will require continued efforts and creative monitoring of outcomes. Perhaps the balance will be different among various sub-specialties that require diverse skills and training. Regardless, there is extensive literature on work hours and their relationship to human performance in health care and other safety-sensitive industries and further discussion is necessary on how exactly to best apply this information to physician training programs [56–63]. Ignoring the evidence about the potentially deleterious effects of sleep deprivation, fatigue and stress on patient safety and individual well-being is not prudent, and it may simply be that we need to modify our training programs in order to pack them with more of the relevant work (which is being done in some cases through the use of physician extenders), or even to extend the duration of the programs, if necessary, so that the trainee can complete their training with a minimal level of competence (which is discussed more completely later in this chapter).

Another major element introduced by the ACGME as a part of the *Outcomes* project was the introduction of six *Core Competencies* (medical knowledge, patient care, systems-based practice, practice based learning and improvement, professionalism, and interpersonal and communication skills). These were introduced on the basis of the reports of the Institute of Medicine [64–67] which emphasized the need to create quality in six domains which included healthcare that is: *patient-centered, efficient, effective, safe, timely and equitable* [65]. In order to achieve this, the core competencies enveloped a variety of skills that training programs became accountable for teaching and evaluating. The implementation of competency awareness has been perceived, in general to have improved care and to have elevated training programs from "apprenticeships" to more formal and structured educational programs designed to teach life skills.

The introduction of formal quality improvement education into residency and fellowship training (as a result of emphasizing systems-based practice, professionalism, and practice-based learning) has the potential to improve outcomes for patients. Improving quality and outcomes requires excellent technical results from a surgery, accurate diagnosis, meticulous pre and post-operative care to avoid iatrogenic injury (such as central line infections or ventilator-associated pneumonias), and careful outpatient follow-up, particularly for the most vulnerable

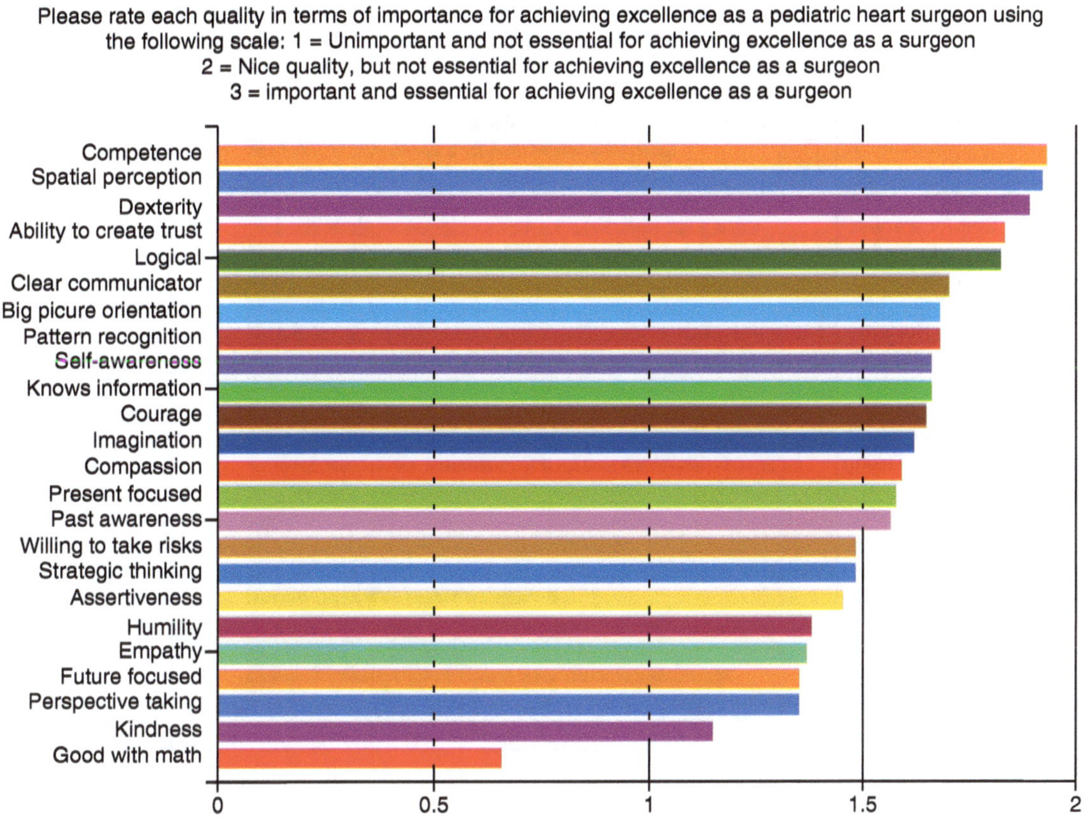

Fig. 2.8 Factors considered important in achieving excellence as a congenital heart surgeon, ranked by members of the CHSS or EACHS. The longer the bar, the more important the trait

patient populations such as the interstage single ventricle cohort. In other words, our outcomes are the result of our entire system, not just a single component. Training the next generation of surgeons, anesthesiologists, intensivists and cardiologists to examine care delivery systems and processes and to participate in rapid cycle improvement activities (related to systems-based, not just individual case-based examples) will be essential to improving the quality and outcomes for patients with congenital heart disease.

The changes to duty hours and the incorporation of more broad-based training (through the competencies) were created in an effort to not only improve quality and outcomes for our patients, but to also reduce stress, create more balance and reduce burnout for healthcare providers. Burnout is becoming recognized as an increasingly important factor in medicine that can contribute to errors [68–71]. Most disturbingly, from our own research (unpublished), burnout seems to be prevalent in medical students before they begin medical school, and increases throughout the educational journey. Awareness and recognition of burnout, and attempts to ameliorate it with programs designed to promote wellness, may have an important place in our future training programs.

In order to understand better how these changes in our educational structure fit against the backdrop of what our respondents felt was most valuable in their training, we asked pediatric cardiac surgeons about a number of qualities and had them evaluate whether or not they felt that these qualities were important to their achieving success. We believe that these data reflect the prevalent mindsets across our profession. The results are shown in Fig. 2.8 ranked in descending levels of importance.

We also inquired about whether or not they received formal education in the qualities they highlighted as important during their training.

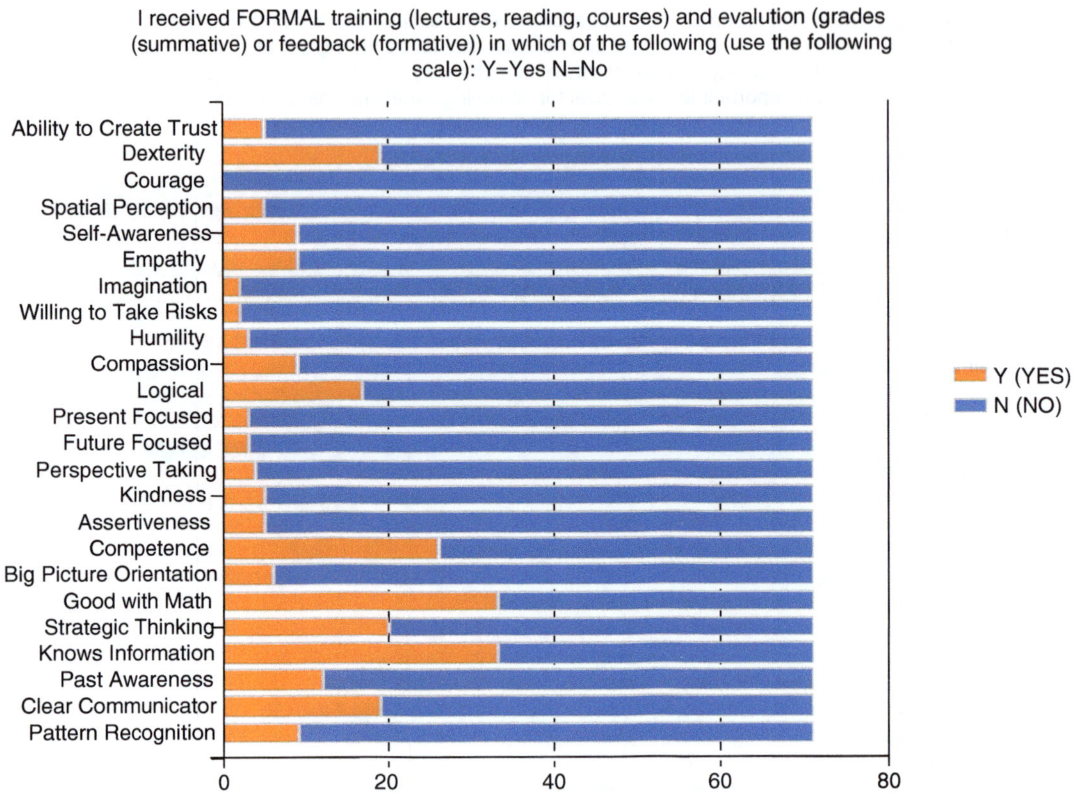

Fig. 2.9 Colored bars indicate whether or not members of the CHSS or EACHS received formal training in various areas. The longer the blue bar, the fewer number of surgeons who felt they were trained in the respective area. The data suggest that most formal training was provided with math and knowledge-based information. There was little training in courage, imagination, risk-taking, humility and kindness

The results are shown in Fig. 2.9, as stacked bars, indicating the number who felt they had received (orange) versus those who felt they did not receive (blue) formal training in these qualities.

Qualities that were deemed essential by over 75 % of the responders included: competence (meaning ability to perform a procedure without supervision) (93.0 %); spatial perception (91.5 %); dexterity (88.7 %); ability to create trust (83.1 %); and ability to be logical (81.7 %).

Other qualities that were also deemed important by over half the respondents were: clear communication (70.4 %); big picture orientation (67.6 %); pattern recognition (67.6 %); courage (66.2 %); self-awareness (66.2 %); knowledge (66.2 %); imagination (63.4 %); present focus (63.4 %); compassion (59.2 %); willingness to take risks (57.7 %); and past awareness (meaning ability to recall past events in order to incorporate them into making decisions for current events) (57.7 %).

Qualities that were felt to be "nice" but unnecessary to be successful as a pediatric cardiac surgeon (receiving votes from less than half the respondents) included: strategic thinking (47.9 %); assertiveness (46.5 %); future focus (42.3 %); humility (40.8 %); perspective taking (39.4 %); empathy (36.6 %); kindness (21.1 %); and being good with math (5.6 %).

Even though considered important to success, most surgeons did not receive formal training in ability to create trust, spatial perception, or ability to be logical. None received training in courage and very few in self-awareness, empathy, imagination, risk taking, humility, compassion, or other areas which we know to be related to developing emotional intelligence [30, 38, 72].

Most acknowledged some training (as would be expected) in math (although this was felt for the most part to be unimportant and not essential to their success), competence (ability to be self sufficient) and knowledge of medical information, as well as some training in communication and strategic thinking.

The information from this survey indicates a lack of alignment and connectedness between our training programs and the skills/attributes that will be most needed for ultimate success in our field. Self-awareness and ability to create trust are essential components for leadership and felt by many [30, 31, 38, 40, 73–79] to be the most critical foundations for successful leaders to develop. Our current training programs seem to emphasize technical skills (dexterity, medical information and "competence"—meaning the ability to do a task without help). Although not part of a "classic" surgical training curriculum, each of the other qualities listed have been associated with leadership and success, and each can be taught (and learned) [30, 33, 35, 36, 38–40, 75, 76, 79–86].

It is also notable that current training programs have no formal training or education in courage [87], imagination [83, 88–90], risk-taking [76, 78, 91], compassion [79, 84, 92, 93], perspective-taking [1, 41, 86, 94–96], pattern recognition, and many other qualities that can be taught, learned and that are associated with leadership and success [38, 40, 78, 82, 97, 98]. In fact, when choosing what they believed was most important for them to share with their colleagues, the past presidents of our national cardiac surgery organizations (American Association of Thoracic Surgery, Society of Thoracic Surgeons, Southern Thoracic Surgical Association, Western Thoracic Surgical Association) have consistently selected topics related to leadership, personal development, courage, compassion and education [1, 87, 99–101]. At this sentinel moment in their careers, these successful surgical leaders have determined that emphasizing "non-technical skills" is the message they wish to share with others.

Current training in pediatric cardiac surgery has changed in the U.S. in the past several years. As general surgery training programs have created fewer opportunities for surgical residents to work on cardiac services, and as the technical components of general surgery have transitioned more to video-assisted, robotic and other non-invasive techniques versus open, hands-on procedures that emphasize cutting and sewing, the residents entering cardiothoracic fellowship programs are less prepared for the technical challenges of cardiac and especially, pediatric cardiac surgery. Yet, these technical skills can certainly be learned and mastered in time—as long as our training programs change and adapt to the current challenges.

The aspiring pediatric cardiac surgeon must now complete an additional year of training following successful completion of cardiothoracic surgery training. This additional year of training must be completed at an ACGME accredited program for pediatric cardiac surgery training and these programs are subject to the same duty-hour restrictions that govern all ACGME accredited programs. In addition, the aspiring trainee is required to perform a specific number and diversity of procedures, show evidence of having received both summative and formative education that is structured and specific to learning congenital heart surgery, and eventually (in order to become board certified) pass a written and then an oral exam.

Many aspiring pediatric cardiologists are also encouraged to complete additional training in the current era. Advanced fellowships with specific national recommendations for the training experiences are available in a variety of subspecialties within pediatric cardiology, such as interventional cardiac catheterization, electrophysiology, echocardiography and MRI, cardiac critical care, and adult congenital heart disease. Unlike surgery, however, at this time, there is no formal exam or board certification (beyond general board certification in cardiology) for any of these subspecialties, although that may be looming on the horizon. Likewise, there is additional training available to those interested in pediatric cardiac anesthesiology. Sub-specialty certification in pediatric anesthesiology is beginning in 2013 and requires 1 year training in an ACGME accredited fellowship and then passing the subspecialty board exam. The training in pediatric anesthesiology does include training in management of

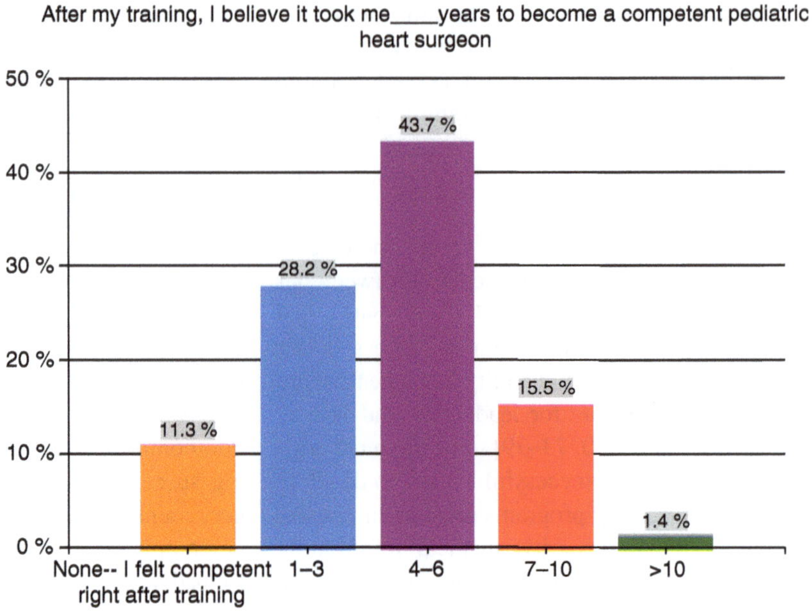

Fig. 2.10 Length of time after formal training that it took for members of the CHSS and EACHS to feel "competent"

children with complex heart disease for cardiac and non-cardiac procedures. However, at the present there is no sub-specialty certification in cardiac anesthesiology although fellowship training is recognized. Further training in pediatric cardiac anesthesiology is available, although no certification or accreditation process is in place.

Most pediatric cardiac surgeons consider themselves to either be visual learners (39.4 %–meaning they learn best by seeing or watching someone do something) or experiential learners (43.7 %–meaning they learn best by doing or having an experience of what they are trying to master). An important minority consider themselves to be perceptual learners (16.9 %–meaning they learn best by reading, reflecting and then using those processed thoughts to guide their actions). There were no surgeons surveyed who felt that they were auditory learners (learning best by listening to a talk or hearing someone describe how they do something). (A personal survey of other specialties has revealed a higher percentage of auditory learners, particularly in more medically related fields). While a minority of respondents felt that they were competent pediatric heart surgeons immediately after their training (11.3 %), the largest number felt that the journey to competence after training takes an additional 4–6 years (43.7 %) and some felt that it can take up to 10 years (15.5 %) (Fig. 2.10). For the most part, congenital heart surgeons felt that they continued to learn and develop after their formal fellowship training was completed (and many of these individuals trained in the era before duty hour limitations). The same is true for other congenital cardiac specialists such as anesthesiology, and is likely also the case for interventional cardiology, critical care, or imaging disciplines.

While competence (ability to perform routine tasks without supervision) is a likely end product of formal training, extended time to achieve expertise is more consistent with the information on development of expertise requiring focused or "deep" practice for a considerable number (10,000 or more) of hours [37, 94, 102, 103]. It may be that our experts, when responding to this question, had differing perspectives on how they valued their abilities and what, for each of them, constituted competence; with competence for some equating with expertise. Regardless, it is clear that the length of time spent in training is not sufficient to enable attainment of expertise—that takes sustained practice.

Defining stages or levels of competency may be helpful. Competency is the ability to perform a certain task for a work situation without supervision, and to know when to ask for help. It is the intent of most training programs that this is achieved by the end of training. In anesthesia training five stages of adult skill acquisition have been applied: novice, entering training; advanced beginner, at the end of first year of training; competent, at the conclusion of training; proficient, after being in practice 5 years; and expert, after practice for 10–15 years [104]. Regardless, this makes it clear that education and learning continue beyond training and are critically important to attaining the highest degree of proficiency and expertise in all possible scenarios regardless of the discipline.

Lifelong learning itself is a topic that merits discussion, since it is at the foundation of training. The environments that we create for training will ultimately shape those who will become our future educators and mentors.

It is ironic that most health care professionals learned at *Teaching Hospitals*. Teaching evolves from knowing and a desire to share with others what you know. In 1998, Parker Palmer published "*The Courage to Teach*" [105] and each year, the ACGME (Accreditation Council for Graduate Medical Education) bestows a *Courage to Teach* award on some of the nation's great teachers. All of us recall our most influential and inspiring teachers with fondness, admiration and gratitude. We can also recall some of those teachers who made our ignorance feel painful, shameful and frightening. A "teacher" who contemptuously reprimands a student for "not knowing" or worse, for being "stupid, lazy and insulting their time" does more damage than they likely can imagine. In her work on learning, Carol Dweck [76] describes the kind of attitudes that best correlate with performance excellence, and not surprisingly, they are not related to knowing the answers, but rather to asking the questions, even when the answers seem most elusive. This is why we believe it takes more courage to learn than it does to teach [1]. Learning requires that we accept the vulnerability [80, 106] that accompanies "not knowing" and then embrace a willingness to struggle—and possibly fail—while we try to challenge ourselves (and others who work with us, or who we train) to think differently or to do things we (they) have never done. We all walk because our parents likely created for us an environment that *invited learning.* You likely don't remember for yourself, but think of how babies learn to walk. When they fall, we don't criticize them for being a failure, or tell them that they will never be successful at walking. It is not likely that we compare them to a sibling who was walking sooner and admonish them that they should try to be more like that person. No. We applaud, and smile and encourage them to try again. Until they learn. And we share their joy in accomplishment. What happens that we forget how to do that in our teaching institutions? We have created a culture that rewards "knowing" (expertise) and we worry about what would happen to our patients if we weren't experts. An inviting reframe of that last statement is "What 'could' happen for our patients if we could let go of knowing and instead, keep wondering?"

It is unfortunate that we have created a culture that demands perfection, because, in the words of noted historian, Arthur Toynbee, "nothing fails like success." It is regrettable that we have been taught that "if you want a job done right, do it yourself" (ascribed to by 54.9 % of our surveyed surgeons, in lieu of "if you want a job done right, listen to ideas from others"), because this form of contempt for how other's might complete a task is a powerful way to diminish innovation and progress. (The statement instead should be "if you want a job done your way, do it yourself"). One of the babies learning how to walk today will likely set the future record for the 100-yard dash. One of our struggling young students of today may be a future leader in his or her field. But, only if we find a way to invite them to learn. Which means we have to find a way to be tolerant of their struggles, encourage them to continue to think differently, and carefully craft an environment that is safe and free from premature judgment.

In our recent survey of pediatric cardiac surgeons, 90 % of responders stated that they viewed mistakes as inevitable and therefore accepted them as opportunities to learn. (The small minority stated that mistakes are simply not acceptable in cardiac surgery and therefore cannot be tolerated). What was particularly striking, however, was their response to the next question, which was how they dealt with mistakes. Even though most responders recognized mistakes as inevitable, almost 2/3 (63.4 %) acknowledged that they were "hard on themselves" because mistakes are not tolerable. Only 36.6 % were able to view themselves with compassion as learners. And if the majority of our experts are hard on themselves when they make a mistake, how do we imagine they would treat a trainee?

What makes this even more remarkable is that when asked which teachers (mentors) left them with the most valuable lessons, the majority (76.1 %) remembered them as the ones who were supportive and nurturing—not critical and hard (see comments in section on mentoring). These numbers are compelling, and not surprising. We know we might make mistakes, and we appreciate it when someone supports and nurtures us as we learn, but we have created a cultural belief that we have to be hard on ourselves. This response from our group of professionals is not unusual and, in fact, has been recently validated as a common norm in many professions by research published from the Harvard Business School [107]. It seems that professional cultural norms in our society are to be hard on (critical of) one's-self, while simultaneously appreciating and desiring to be surrounded by those who are tolerant and nurturing of us when we err [108].

Why would we treat ourselves differently than how we wish to be treated by others? Our role as teachers (and potential mentors—addressed in the next section) makes it imperative that we recognize the incongruence behind how we want to have compassion for (and from) others, but not from within and for ourselves.

Our demand for perfection stems from the high stakes of what we do—taking care of patients with life threatening illnesses—and from our hope that all patients will survive to have a normal life [72]. Unfortunately, this demand for perfection—at all costs—is perpetuated by our cultural belief that errors are not tolerable—that they make us imperfect and unacceptable. Although it would seem nice to be perfect, perfection is an unachievable goal (since perfection is a moving target in complex adaptive systems) and it is unlikely to be achieved in our profession—particularly for those who cannot admit to, much less forgive themselves for error (as the work of Carol Dweck, cited below, emphasizes). For some, this intent to be "perfect" gets entangled with their own sense of worth and esteem—more important than the patient doing well is how they are thought of by their peers and therefore they can only be valued if all their patients survive and their peers (many of whom barely know them and have likely never worked with them) believe they are exceptional. This phenomenon in the marketing world is termed "perception management" and it revolves around creating an illusion that becomes the accepted reality. The belief that there is a "solution set" that will always create a successful outcome is not realistic in complex biological systems, in which no two patients or defects are exactly alike. Although mechanical systems are expected to perform in a consistently reliable and predictable fashion [65, 72], biologic systems do not behave this way. That is why there is an occasional mortality after ASD closure or why some patients develop early pulmonary hypertension from lesions that should be safe to follow. Unfortunately, when perfection is not possible, the delusion that it is achievable can lead to dashed expectations, disappointment and a "culture of blame." [74, 109] As trainers (and potential mentors), we have the power to transform our culture to one of curiosity (rather than blame), by modeling how we can explore (with compassion, openness and non-judgment) the creative potential that errors and failure (even when not associated with an error) have for helping us learn; and in the process of learning, truly enjoy our lifelong growth as students, as healers and as professionals.

Another unintended consequence of the striving for perfection is the lack of forgiveness for oneself and for others when the results aren't perfect. The research on self-compassion [84, 85, 92, 93] has been impressive. The ability to have compassion for oneself is directly and positively linked to the ability to learn and to the ability to be resilient and cope with difficulties [42]. (No wonder many of our surgical experts indicated resilience as the quality that was most important to their success). When contrasting high self-esteem with or without self-compassion, there is a distinct difference. Self esteem without self-awareness and self-compassion (recognition and acceptance that we all have experiences of disappointment and failure–that the self is imperfect and still deserves kindness) is often associated with grandiosity and failure to acknowledge what is "real"—a potentially dangerous trait in a cardiac surgeon, cardiologist or anesthesiologist. [84] When self-esteem is tempered by awareness of limitations, and associated with the ability to be compassionate towards oneself, this can lead to more genuine (less grandiose) self esteem that is more appropriate because it is related to the ability to hear feedback (without defensiveness), while still maintaining kindness towards oneself as a *learner* [84]. This is the challenge for us as lifelong learners—to accept that we are learners, meaning there will be times we "don't know" and have to "struggle" as we try to do new things or think in new ways [1]. A system that insists on perfection makes it very dangerous to be a learner, and ultimately, limits our ability to provide best practice.

Carol Dweck a psychologist from Stanford who has spent decades studying the learning process, has arrived at the conclusion that one of the crucial ingredients of success is the ability to learn from mistakes. Her work is thoughtfully cited by Jonah Lehrer in his book "*How we Decide*" [110] in explaining the neurobiology of learning.

Lehrer writes about Dweck's most famous, and for many, most poignant study. It was conducted in twelve different New York City schools and involved more than four hundred fifth graders. One at a time, the kids were removed from class and given a relatively easy test consisting of non-verbal puzzles. After the child finished the test, Dr. Dweck and her researchers told the student his or her score and provided a single sentence of praise. Half the kids were praised for their *intelligence*. "You must be smart at this." The other students were praised for their *effort*: "you must have worked really hard."

The students were then allowed to choose between two different subsequent tests. The first choice was described as a more difficult set of puzzles, but the kids were told that they'd learn a lot from attempting it. The other option was an easy test; similar to the test they'd just taken.

When Dweck was designing this experiment, she'd expected the different forms of praise to have a rather modest effect. After all, it was just one sentence. The results of her intervention are described below. Imagine, if a single sentence has the power to create these outcomes, what might result from a pervasive attitude in a system where the sentence is expressed as a cultural value?

Of the group of kids that had been praised for their efforts, 90 % chose the harder set of puzzles. However, of the kids that were praised for their intelligence, most went for the easier test. If we do what works because we think it makes us look good—if we aren't willing to risk failure or struggle as the condition of learning, then we are doomed to stop learning, growing and improving. We get stuck. There are surgeons who tout themselves as experts, yet they are reluctant to offer new procedures to their patients and simply state: "I don't do that operation."

> I myself (RMU) used to criticize the Ross procedure in the 1980's. I rationalized that it was a bad operation ("risk for two valve disease, etc.") and encouraged patients to avoid it. What I really meant was that "I didn't know how to do the operation and it scared me to try it", so I had to find a way to rationalize why I didn't offer it. Fortunately, at the time I was also learning about fixed vs. growth mindsets [76] and beginning to understand how to find the courage to try and master new things, even when that contributed to some outcomes that were initially "less than perfect."

This is similar to the transition that occurred in pediatric cardiac surgery when transitioning from the atrial switch to the arterial switch procedures. Surgeons had to be courageous enough to learn a new technique, even though the previous one seemed to work well, because there was likelihood that the new technique might be better. Learners recognize that they need to continue to invite the "discomfort" of not knowing and of having to adopt something new if they are to keep current. The arterial switch is now a standard procedure for infants with transposition of the great arteries and the Ross operation seems to have considerable benefits compared to other valve replacement procedures for children [111–113]. Without “inviting learning” we won’t have progress, whether it is new technology or new solutions (such as new operations or strategies). We are unlikely to develop the skills and experience necessary to deal with challenging new problems if we continually choose the “solutions” that are comfortable in order to feel better about ourselves.

When we are taught to fear failure, we suppress learning. The question for our training programs—each of them—is how do they handle failure? What happens to people who fail? Are they applauded for their efforts and encouraged to learn what they need to succeed, or are they admonished, punished, dismissed or ridiculed? Which kind of training program do you think would bring out the best in you?

Dweck went on to study this further. She gave the same fifth graders yet another test. This test was designed to be extremely difficult—it was originally written for eighth graders—but Dweck wanted to see how the kids would respond to the challenge. The students who had been praised for their efforts in the initial test worked hard at figuring out the puzzles. “They got very involved,” Dweck says. “Many of them remarked, unprovoked, ‘this is my favorite test.’” Kids that had initially been praised for their smarts, on the other hand, were easily discouraged. They viewed their inevitable mistakes as signs of failure: perhaps they really weren’t smart after all. After taking this difficult test, the two groups of students were asked to choose between looking at the exams of kids who did worse than them or looking at the exams of those who did better. Students praised for their intelligence almost invariably chose to bolster their self-esteem by comparing themselves with students who had performed worse on the test. In contrast, kids praised for their hard work were more interested in the higher-scoring exams. They wanted to understand their mistakes, to learn from their errors, to figure out how to do better.

The final round of tests was the same difficulty level as the initial test. Nevertheless, students who had been praised for their efforts exhibited significant improvement, raising their average score by 30 %. Because these kids were willing to challenge themselves, even if it meant failing at first, they ended up performing at a much higher level. This result was even more impressive when compared with students who’d been randomly assigned to the “smart” group; they saw their scores drop by an average of nearly 20 %. The experience of failure had been so discouraging for the “smart” kids that they actually regressed.

The problem with emphasizing “smart” (or natural, gifted talent) is that it misrepresents the neural reality of education, learning and development of expert skills [37, 102, 103, 110]. When neurons in a circuit become repeatedly activated, the oligodendrocytes and astrocytes (the supportive glial cells) sense that firing and wrap myelin around the interconnected neuronal circuit [41]. Myelin can increase conduction speed by 100 times. And while all neurons need to rest after firing, myelin can reduce that refractory period (resting time) by 30 times. The end result is that if we train well (and repeatedly) our learned (myelinated) circuits will function 3,000 times faster than untrained (unmyelinated) circuits [41]. “Skill is myelin insulation that wraps neural circuits and that grows according to certain signals” [37]. “Things that appear to be obstacles turn out to be desirable in the long haul.”

Spending hours training and learning is not sufficient. Research is clear that the training needs to be specific, focused and “deep.” “Deep practice feels a bit like exploring a dark and unfamiliar room. You start slowly, you bump into furniture, stop, think, and start again. Slowly, and a little painfully, you explore the space over and over, attending to errors, extending your reach into the room a bit farther each time, building a mental map until you can move through it quickly and intuitively” [37]. The essence of deep practice is to immerse yourself in an experience. In skill development, “by trying hard to do things you can barely do, in deep practice—then your skill circuits will respond by getting faster and more accurate” [37]. This process can be enhanced by a guide (mentor), but can only be learned by actual, repeated “doing.”

Struggle is not optional—it is biologically required. In order to get your skill circuit to fire optimally, you must by definition fire the circuit suboptimally; you must make mistakes and pay attention to those mistakes; you must teach your circuit. You must also keep firing that circuit—practicing, in order to keep myelin functioning properly. After all, myelin is living tissue. "Deep practice is built on a paradox: struggling in certain targeted ways—allowing yourself to make mistakes, (and having compassion for yourself—and others—as learners) to seem stupid—makes you smarter.

Emphasizing smart over continual training and learning encourages avoidance of the most useful learning activities, which is learning from mistakes. In medicine, this may be avoidance of doing the procedure we are uncertain of—staying safe doing what we know—even when the more risky procedure may be better for the long term benefit of the patient. It may manifest, as it did in the group of "smart" kids by choosing to compare our programs to those that are worse, perhaps using a non-valid criteria that favors us, in order to make us feel better. Perhaps this is accomplished by avoiding difficult cases (complex puzzles) or by doing less risky, although possibly less optimal procedures. Anything to convince ourselves and those who might judge us that we are "smart."

Leaders for creating the training programs for the future MUST create environments where it is safe for learners to struggle as they try new things, even if there is the price of occasional failure. This invites the use of more simulation, but also more tolerance, patience and presence [41, 114] by the trainers during actual cases in order to help keep the learner (and the patient) safe. In systems where leaders respond like the fifth graders who wanted to be validated, failure is feared and the eventual outcome is regression. There is no shortcut for this painstaking process.

Our data suggest four important recommendations for training.

The first is that surgical (and possibly interventional or anesthesia) training programs will do better by emphasizing time in the Operating Room for both visual and experiential learning, and that time for reading should be valued and supported. Lectures and didactic sessions, while a mainstay in our current training programs, may have less value, unless they are integrated into some form of other learning style (for example, case-based or systems-based learning through presentation by a trainee based on their reading—for perceptual learning; or based on their experience watching or doing a procedure—for visual or experiential learners). The act of the trainee personally presenting information may help them to myelinate learning circuits more effectively than simply listening to information presented by another.

Secondly, our surgical experts valued experiences where they felt nurtured and supported, despite a cultural tendency for self-criticism and intolerance of errors. Data on learning and ultimate success validates the importance of creating a model for self-compassion, acceptance of struggle and willingness to try and conquer new things (even when these new things might be difficult and challenging). In order to provide this type of training environment, faculty need permission to spend time in the OR helping guide the young learner, and it is incumbent on all of us to design ways to do this in our current organizational climates that emphasize operational efficiency, maximizing RVUs and intolerance of struggle (when struggling creates delays and potential for error). Additionally, use of simulation through case-based scenarios may play a role in accelerating experiential learning and proficiency by permitting discussion, evaluation, and debriefing in a trusting, non-threatening environment with no patient at risk.

In light of this altered concept of learning (as a process that requires courage and willingness to struggle), it would be helpful to create formal training in many of the qualities that our surgical experts felt were important or essential (qualities which are also supported as such by extensive literature) and which are currently not taught in our training programs. These qualities, can be taught and learned and might be best done through a series of reflective exercises, through carefully assigned reading related to personal development and through formative coaching that emphasizes the development of these attributes as a part of experiential learning.

Finally, our data demonstrate that "training to competence" extends beyond the formal residency-training period, and therefore, the period following formal fellowship training is critical for success. This also implies that certification of competence in pediatric cardiac specialties might be best "postponed" for a variable period of time following formal training until certain criteria are met that are more indicative that competence has been achieved, with competence including development of the attributes and qualities noted by our experts as important—qualities like resilience, self-awareness, integrity (self honesty), humility, courage and self compassion, recognizing that at this time there are no metrics to measure achievement of these qualities. The duration of the "time until competent" might actually increase in the era of duty hour restrictions, simply because of the reduced experience that our trainees will acquire before taking their first faculty/attending position. Therefore, mentoring (as discussed in the next section of this chapter) may play an even larger and more critical role in the future as training extends beyond the accredited training period.

Mentoring

The increasing complexity of congenital heart disease, the high stakes involved with decisions and performance, combined with the external demands on us as professionals (financial, social, relational) can lead to higher levels of stress—which can be experienced as both job and life related stress. All forms of stress, including the stress that is "job-related," have been linked to failing individual health and illness [115], decreased individual performance [116, 117], There is a growing body of evidence that when a young learner develops a relationship with a mentor, they experience decreased stress, improved performance and ultimately better personal and professional relationships.

Mentor was an Ithacan noble in Homer's *Odyssey*. He was a wise counselor for his friend Ulysses and was entrusted with the care, education and protection of Ulysses' son, Telemachus. Today, the term mentor generally indicates teacher, adviser, sponsor, counselor and role model. It likely is much more than that, with the whole becoming more than the sum of the parts. Mentoring creates a "powerful emotional interaction between (generally) an older and a younger person, in a relationship in which the older mentor is trusted, loving, and experienced in the guidance of the younger" [118]. Performed in accordance with this ideal, mentoring can create a resonant bond between the mentor and the mentee that reflects extraordinary and *primal* leadership [97]. Although there are certainly important similarities between leadership and mentoring (and some individuals in our field perform dual functions in this regard), there is an important distinction between leadership and mentorship. Whereas leaders are "creators and manipulators of culture," [119] mentors are "transfer agents of culture" [120]. Leadership involves a performance-oriented influence process, whereas mentoring involves a long-term role-model relationship that is primarily career and development-oriented [121, 122]. Leadership is typically a single leader influencing one or more followers, whereas mentoring usually involves one mentor and one protégé[1] (or mentee). Leadership may utilize a more formal, overt, and direct influence process, while mentoring may create a more informal, subtle, and indirect process of influence [123]. Not all effective and experienced leaders become effective mentors [122]. Some leader behaviors are primarily task-oriented (such as planning and organizing, problem solving, clarifying roles and objectives, monitoring), whereas others are more relationship oriented (such as supporting, developing, networking and recognizing). Some leaders perform task functions better than they do relationship functions, but *good mentors must perform relationship functions*. Only those leaders who

[1] The term protégé appears in the literature on mentoring, but seems to indicate an apprenticeship model where succession is handed to those who follow. We prefer the term mentee, since it more accurately implies the extended connection between an academic medical mentor and the younger students whose careers they influence, regardless of where those career paths lead.

excel at both task and relationship functions turn out to become great mentors.

Mentors perform both career and psychosocial functions. Career functions include sponsorship, exposure and visibility, coaching, protection, provision of challenging assignments (cases), and transmission of applied professional ethics. Psychosocial functions serve to enhance the mentee's sense of competence, identity and work-role effectiveness—essentially self-esteem or self-efficacy. In order to provide these psychosocial benefits, successful mentors provide role modeling, acceptance and confirmation, counseling and friendship (mutuality). Skillful mentors seamlessly blend these functions in their work with their protégés [124, 125].

Informal mentorships (those that develop spontaneously, without formal assignment by a third party) are considered by both mentors and mentees as being more effective and meaningful than formal (assigned) mentorships [126]. Most agree that mentorships in professional training should be facilitated rather than assigned.

Ideal mentors seem to exhibit specific personality characteristics and interpersonal traits that enhance their effectiveness. In terms of personality, desirable mentors are intelligent, caring, and appropriately humorous. The are flexible, empathic and patient. In addition, they are interpersonally supportive, encouraging and poised. They appear to exude "emotional intelligence." This is not at all surprising considering the fragile nature of learning (described in the previous section) and how it can be best nurtured and supported. Highly rated mentors also seem to be ethical, psychologically well-adjusted, and well-known as scholars and professionals. In essence, excellent mentors are kind, healthy and competent [118].

In a training environment, the "benefits to the mentee can be so valuable that identification with a mentor should be considered a major developmental task of the early career" [127]. These benefits include development of professional skills, enhancement of confidence and professional identity, scholarly productivity, enhanced networking, successful accomplishment of training goals, and overall satisfaction of the training program. Harder to measure, but perhaps most significant for the mentee who has had an effective mentor is their perceived "support, encouragement and blessing for their journey that leads to the 'realization of their dream" [128]. Mentors also benefit from the relationship with enhanced career satisfaction, rejuvenation of creative energy, and a sense of generativity [128].

As we look towards the future of our profession, the role of mentoring is critical. This is well recognized by our experts. Along with getting a good education and having natural ability for their profession, almost half of today's successful pediatric cardiac surgeons (42.3 %) felt that most contributory to their success was the involvement of a good mentor.

This is not surprising and is a theme that dates back to a time when stories were passed down as narratives. Each of us is on our own "hero's journey" [1, 78, 114, 129–132] which traces our path through the chapters of our lives. For each of us, the journey requires a period of searching and training (which includes connecting to our own best pieces), followed by a period of accomplishing and succeeding (as we become comfortable and confident with the competent best parts of who we are and what we can offer) and finally ends with enlightenment, transformation and satisfaction that we have achieved our goals (although these goals may be different than the ones we often set out to attain!) [1]. Along this journey, we find many who choose to help us on our quest, and we accept their help because they have something important to share with us. Some of those who choose to help us become valued guides whose wisdom and advice we gladly seek and whose influence on us becomes indelible. These mentors can take on many forms. When asked about the importance of various people as mentors in their lives, our experts told us that they included parents, family, spouses and colleagues as well as those assigned to formally train us (Fig. 2.11). Others included non-surgical colleagues (such as cardiologists) and even friends and roommates from college. There are so many opportunities to find influence in our lives when we are open to accepting it.

Ultimately, the bond between a mentor and a mentee is mutual and profound. It most often

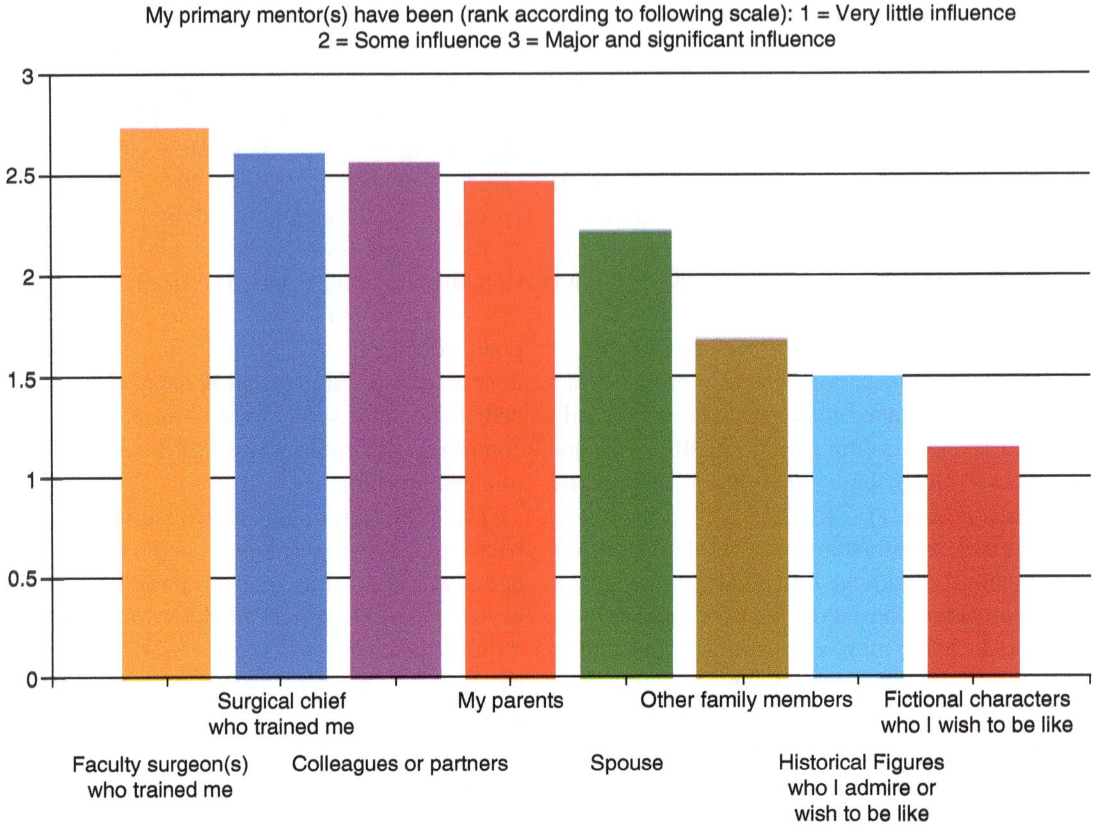

Fig. 2.11 Figure demonstrates that mentoring can come from many sources. Height of bars shows frequency that members of the CHSS or EACHS found mentors from the listed sources

develops over time and is based on shared investment in what each has to offer to the other. For the mentor, it usually includes genuine caring and concern for the mentee, but it requires much more than that to be significant. In the best circumstances, the mentor is attuned to and resonates with the mentee—and the mentee can sense this. They feel "gotten." Most importantly, the mentor accepts the learner where they are, without judgment or contempt, and the mentee can sense this [133]. As stated by one of our experts, when describing how a successful mentor should engage a learner:

> I do believe that the student should be encouraged to surpass the teacher.

Mentors attune, genuinely care, join the learner where they are and teach them how to be better. They do this by setting an example, and also by nurturing, praising and constantly allowing the learner to "work very hard at this" [76]. Mentors are patient with the process of myelination.

The importance of the mentor in creating (and transferring) a culture that nurtures a learner was expressed by one respondent to the survey (crucial identifying information deleted with editing to create anonymity):

> The attitudes of *surgeon X* as a teacher and *surgeon Y* respectively created an entirely different experience for me: 1) If, during an operation, *surgeon X* was irritated by an assistant doctor he did not like or esteem, he would not react as many of us and shout at him but rather very kindly address the person saying "why don't you go to the other side of the table, you will see much better"… 2) If, when *surgeon X* was on call, I needed to phone him at home at three o'clock in the morning, he (regardless of his age of 65) would come into the hospital to give advice or help. If an operation had to be done, *surgeon X* would assist the resident irrespective of him missing sleep. 3) *Surgeon Y* was much

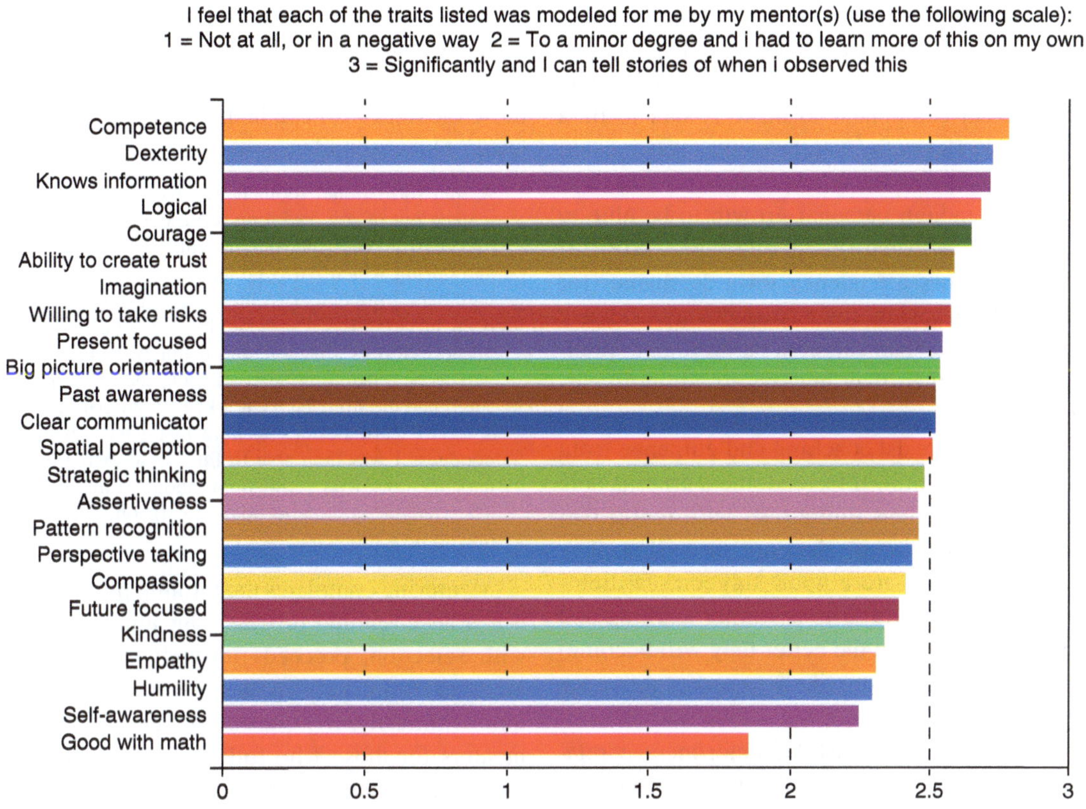

Fig. 2.12 Bar graph shows the likelihood of receiving training in a variety of areas from mentors, as perceived by members of the CHSS or EACHS. The length of the bar correlates with the likelihood that mentors provided this training. As opposed to formal training, it is more likely to receive training in courage, imagination and risk-taking from mentors. Humility and kindness still rank low on this scale

> less valuable in my training: He was known for his "let me have it!!!"... "suck!!!"... "don't!!!"... "gently, gently!!!"..."careful!!!" uttered in a rather unpleasant manner to the poor guy who had the pleasure to assist him.

In order to mentor well, a mentor needs to have achieved growth in many of the areas described as important to success as a pediatric heart surgeon, but which are ironically currently not formally taught in training programs [133]. This was indicated by our experts who responded to our survey (Fig. 2.12).

When these responses are compared to the information in Fig. 2.9, it is reassuring that qualities deemed essential for success in pediatric cardiac surgery and related specialties, but for which there is no formal educational process, are modeled by mentors; particularly qualities such as courage, ability to create trust, imagination and willingness to take risks (willingness to learn). In this sense, our education to competence (and beyond) requires mentoring to fill in the gaps that left by our current educational programs [133].

This was particularly emphasized by one respondent, who replied, in ALL CAPS:

> HAVING A MENTOR OR MENTORS IS ESSENTIAL TO BE A SUCCESSFUL PEDS HEART SURGEON. I DON'T THINK YOU CAN DO IT WELL WITHOUT ONE.

For a mentee to become receptive to a mentor, the most critical underlying condition is trust [77]. The mentee needs to feel safe—that they can expose themselves authentically and openly in the presence of their mentor, without fear for ridicule, dismissal or criticism—including all their inadequacies and imperfections [80]. It is no surprise that mentors generally scored high (Fig. 2.12) in demonstrating the quality of trust. Trust in a training environment is a very fragile and critical component to make it safe to be a learner [134]. For the mentor/mentee relationship to thrive necessitates that the mentee has achieved enough personal growth to be able to distinguish between shame and regret [106]. If the learner has a tendency towards shame (for example, they view their struggles as evidence that they are a "bad surgeon, cardiologist, intensivist," etc.) then they may try to withhold evidence of these inabilities, or feel embarrassed by them, and resist coaching and guidance from a would be mentor. If instead, the learner is able to understand their limitations with regret (for example, even though they are struggling, they accept that they are a good surgeon, cardiologist, intensivist, etc. who is simply learning and the more they learn the better they will become) then they will be more likely to accept influence from a mentor.

In the most successful mentor/mentee relationships, the mentee ultimately becomes a teacher and the mentor a grateful recipient of what can be learned from their new colleague. The relationship is never unequal—it is always shared. There are times that the learner and teacher roles reverse, but there are never times of diminished mutual caring, concern and love.

One of our experts noted that there are also negative mentors:

> I had both positive and negative mentors. A particularly bothersome realization that I have had is that I have developed some of the traits that were negatively modeled for me, even though I recognized at the time that I was observing them that they were negative behaviors.

We are not sure we would call these negative role models "mentors", since they likely lacked genuine caring or the ability to create a safe environment for learning, but they are teachers and as such, we do learn from them. It is important to recognize that we can learn a lot about what is important to us from negative experiences, just as we can from positive experiences, and when we can internalize the difference in our own behaviors or how we wish to be from how we are in the moment—when we can begin to get in touch with our own internal gyroscope or "true North", then we may be on the threshold of identifying those mentors who can help take us to "the next level." One respondent stated:

> A transformational moment for me was when I walked out of my operating room one day after a "successful" case, but one in which I felt scared, and during which I was pretty tough on my team members. I remember feeling "icky." I might have been successful as a surgeon, but I was becoming unsuccessful as a person, and if this was the only way to be a pediatric heart surgeon, then I wasn't sure I had the stomach for it. I knew then that I had a lot to learn besides technical surgery. Thank goodness I was then able to find some extraordinary mentors who I still think about to this day. They taught me how to be *as* a surgeon, not just how to be a surgeon.

Mentoring completes the training process, and it is a never-ending process. Our journey begins with selection, proceeds through training, and includes (fortunately), some very important mentors. Ultimately, if we are fortunate, we become mentors for those who follow. It is appropriate, natural and transformative.

Conclusions

We are like the boys in the parable at the beginning of this chapter. We cradle our fragile profession in our hands and in this textbook, we present it as a vibrant, living entity that is ready to take flight. Our outcomes are the best they have ever been, thanks to multidisciplinary team collaboration, incredible advances in technology, and the extraordinary people who comprise our teams—each bringing expertise, commitment and passion for excellence.

Poised and ready to join us, is our future.

Can we create and nurture the passion and commitment of those who will follow? Can we teach them how to have the courage and the compassion to learn? And can we model for them the traits that ultimately characterize what we now know are important in order for them to lead and succeed?

Will our field continue to thrive, or will it languish? It is, after all, in our hands.

References

1. Ungerleider RM. Whom does the grail serve? Ann Thorac Surg. 2007;83:1927–33.
2. Bennekom FC. Customer surveying. Bolton: Customer Service Press; 2002.
3. Curtin R, Presser S, Singer E. The effects of response rate changes on the index of consumer sentiment. Public Opin Q. 2000;64(4):413–28.
4. Keeter S, Kennedy C, Dimock M, Best J, Craighill P. Gauging the impact of growing nonresponse on estimates from a national RDD telephone survey. Public Opin Q. 2006;70:759–79.
5. Visser PS, Krosnick JA, Marquette J, Curtin M. Mail surveys for election forecasting? And evaluation of the Colombia dispatch poll. Public Opin Q. 1996;60: 181–227.
6. Lillehei CW, Varco RL, Cohen M, Warden HE, Patton C, Moller JH. The first open-heart repairs of ventricular septal defect, atrioventricular communis, and tetralogy of fallot using extracorporeal circulation by cross-circulation: a 30-year follow-up. Ann Thorac Surg. 1986;41:4–21.
7. Bell JG, Kanellitsas I, Schaffer L. Selection of obstetrics and gynecology residents on the basis of medical school performance. Am J Obstet Gynecol. 2002;186(5):1091–4.
8. Callahan CA, Mohammadreza H, Veloski J, Erdmann JB, Gonnella JS. The predictive validity of three vesions of the MCAT in relation to performance in medical school, residency, and licensing examinations: a longitudinal study of 36 classes of Jefferson Medical College. Acad Med. 2010;85:980–7.
9. Guffey RC, Rusin K, Chidiac EJ, Marsh HM. The utility of pre-residency standardized tests for anesthesiology resident selection: the place of United States Medical Licensing Examination scores. Anesth Analg. 2011;112(1):201–6.
10. Kim PY, Wallace DA, Allbritton DW, Altose MD. Predictors of success on the written anesthesiology board certification examination. Int J Med Educ. 2012;3:225–35.
11. Thundiyil JG, Modica RF, Silvestri S, Papa L. Do United States Medical Licensing Examination (USMLE) scores predict in-training test performance for emergency medicine residents? J Emerg Med. 2010;38:65–9.
12. McGaghie WC, Cohen ER, Wayne DB. Are United States Medical Licensing Exam Step 1 and 2 scores valid measures for postgraduate medical residency selection decisions? Acad Med. 2011;86:48–52.
13. Spurlock Jr DR, Holden C, Hartranft T. Using United States Medical Licensing Examination (USMLE) examination results to predict later in-training examination performance among general surgery residents. J Surg Educ. 2010;67(6):452–6.
14. Wadowski S, Mody R. Relationships between USMLE scores, clinical performance scores and in-training examination results in pediatric residents with and without Prior Clinical Training. Pediatr Res. 1998;43:329.
15. Ogunyemi D, De Taylor-Harris S. NBME Obstetrics and Gynecology clerkship final examination scores: predictive value of standardized tests and demographic factors. J Reprod Med. 2004;49:978–82.
16. Dillon GF, Clauser BE, Melnick DE. The role of USMLE scores in selecting residents. Acad Med. 2011;86(7):793.
17. Maschuw K, Schlosser K, Kupietz E, Slater EP, Weyers P, Hassan I. Do soft skills predict surgical performance?: a single-center randomized controlled trial evaluating predictors of skill acquisition in virtual reality laparoscopy. World J Surg. 2011; 35(3):480–6.
18. Goldberg AE, Neifeld JP, Wolfe LG, Goldberg SR. Correlation of manual dexterity with USMLE scores and medical student class rank. J Surg Res. 2008;147(2):212–5.
19. Rifkin WD, Rifkin A. Correlation between housestaff performance on the United States Medical Licensing Examination and standardized patient encounters. Mt Sinai J Med. 2005;72:47–9.
20. Stohl HE, Hueppchen NA, Bienstock JL. Can medical school performance predict residency performance? Resident selection and predictors of successful performance in obstetrics and gynecology. J Grad Med Educ. 2010;2(3):322–6.
21. Dirschl DR, Dahners LE, Adams GL, Crouch JH, Wilson FC. Correlating selection criteria with subsequent performance as residents. Clin Orthop Relat Res. 2002;(399):265–71.
22. Fening K, Vander Horst A, Zirwas M. Correlation of USMLE step 1 scores with performance on dermatology in-training examinations. J Am Acad Dermatol. 2011;64:102–6.
23. Dunnington GH, Pelletier MP. The future of cardiac surgery training programs (letter to the editor). Ann Thorac Surg. 2006;81:1179–80.
24. Ward ST, Smith D, Andrei AC, et al. Comparison of cardiothoracic training curricula: integrated six-year versus traditional programs. Ann Thorac Surg. 2013; 95(6):2051–6.
25. Gasparri MG, Tisol WB, Masroor S. Impact of a six-year integrated thoracic surgery training program at the Medical College of Wisconsin. Ann Thorac Surg. 2012;93:592–7.
26. Sainathan S. Integrated thoracic residency: the only pathway of thoracic surgery training in the future? Ann Thorac Surg. 2012;94:1374.
27. Chikwe J, Brewer Z, Goldstone AB, Adams DH. Integrated thoracic residency program applicants: the best and the brightest? Ann Thorac Surg. 2011; 92:1586–92.
28. Sanford EL. Pediatric anesthesia combined residency training: an applicant's perspective. Anesthesiology. 2013;116(6):1387–8.
29. Moodie D. Pediatric cardiology fellowship–the future. Congenit Heart Dis. 2013;8:181.

30. Goleman D. Emotional intelligence. New York: Bantam Books; 1994.
31. Goleman D. Working with emotional intelligence. New York: Bantam Books; 1998.
32. Goleman D. Social intelligence. New York: Bantam Books; 2006.
33. Arbinger I. Leadership and self deception. San Francisco: Berrett-Koehler; 2000.
34. Cherniss C, Goleman D. Bringing emotional intelligence to the workplace. 1998. http://www.eiconsortium.org.
35. Coulehan J. On humility. Ann Intern Med. 2010;153: 200–1.
36. Covey SR. The 8th habit. New York: Free Press; 2004.
37. Coyle D. The talent code: greatness isn't born. It's grown. Here's how. New York: Bantam; 2009.
38. Drucker PF. Managing oneself. In: Harvard Business Review: Boston, MA, the HMU guide to managing people, vol 2. 2004.
39. Feldman MD. Becoming an emotionally intelligent physician. West J Med. 2001;175:98.
40. George B, Sims P, McLean AN, Mayer D. Discovering your authentic leadership. Harv Bus Rev. 2007;85:129–37.
41. Siegel DJ. The mindful therapist. New York: W.W. Norton; 2010.
42. Sotile W, Sotile M. The resilient physician. Chicago: American Medical Association; 2002.
43. de Oliveira GSJ, Akikwala T, Kendall MC, et al. Factors affecting admission to anesthesiology residency in the United States: choosing the future of our specialty. Anesthesiology. 2012;117(2):243–51.
44. Antiel RM, Reed DA, Van Arendonk KJ, et al. Effects of duty hour restrictions on core competencies, education, quality of life, and burnout among general surgery interns. JAMA Surg. 2013;148(5):448–55.
45. Barden CB, Specht MC, McCarter MD, Daly JM, Fahey III TJ. Effects of limited work hours on surgical training. J Am Coll Surg. 2002;195(4):531–8.
46. Damadi A, Davis AT, Saxe A, Apelgren K. ACGME duty-hour restrictions decrease resident operative volume: a 5-year comparison at an ACGME-accredited university general surgery residency. J Surg Educ. 2007;64(5):256–9.
47. Fairfax LM, Christmas AB, Green JM, Miles WS, Sing RF. Operative experience in the era of duty hour restrictions: is broad-based general surgery training coming to an end? Am Surg. 2010;76(6): 578–82.
48. Simien D, Holt KD, Richter TH. The impact of ACGME work-hour reforms on the operative experience of fellows in surgical subspecialty programs. J Grad Med Educ. 2011;3(1):111–7.
49. Spencer AU, Teitelbaum DH. Impact of work-hour restrictions on residents' operative volume on a subspecialty surgical service. J Am Coll Surg. 2005;200(5): 670–6.
50. Lee DY, Myers EA, Rehmani SS, et al. Surgical residents' perception of the 16-hour work day restriction: concern for negative impact on resident education and patient care. J Am Coll Surg. 2012; 215(6):868–77.
51. Typpo KV, Tcharmtchi MH, Thomas EJ, Kelly PA, Castillo LD, Singh H. Impact of resident duty hour limits on safety in the intensive care unit: a national survey of pediatric and neonatal intensivists. Pediatr Crit Care Med. 2012;13(5):578–82.
52. Drolet BC, Christopher DA, Fischer SA. Residents response to duty-hour regulations–a follow-up national survey. N Engl J Med. 2012;366(24):e35.
53. Gopal R, Glasheen JJ, Miyoshi TJ, Prochazka AV. Burnout and internal medicine resident work-hour restrictions. Arch Intern Med. 2005;165(22): 2595–600.
54. Weatherby BA, Rudd JN, Ervin TB, Stafford PR, Norris BL. The effect of resident work hour regulations on orthopaedic surgical education. J Surg Orthop Adv. 2007;16(1):19–22.
55. West CP, Tan AD, Haermann TM, Sloan JA, Shanafelt TD. Association of resident fatigue and distress with perceived medical errors. JAMA. 2009;302(12):1294–300.
56. Blum AB, Shea S, Czeisler CA, Landrigan CP, Leape L. Implementing the 2009 Institute of Medicine Recommendations on resident physician work hours, supervision safety. Nat Sci Sleep. 2011; 3:47–85.
57. Institute of Medicine. Resident duty hours: enhancing sleep, supervision and safety. Washington, DC: National Academy Press; 2009.
58. Landrigan CP, Rothschild JM, Cronin JW, et al. Effect of reducing interns work hours on serious medical errors in intensive care units. N Engl J Med. 2004;351(18):1838–48.
59. Landrigan CP, Lockley SW, Czeisler CA. Effect of intern's consecutive work hours on safety, medical education and professionalism. Crit Care. 2005;9(5): 528–30.
60. Levine AC, Adusumilli J, Landrigan CP. Effects of reducing or eliminating resident work shifts over 16 hours: a systematic review. Sleep. 2010;33(8): 1043–53.
61. Lockley SW, Cronin JW, Evans EE, et al. Effect of reducing interns' weekly work hours on sleep and attentional failures. N Engl J Med. 2004;351(18):1829–37.
62. Lockley SW, Barger LK, Ayas NT, Rothschild JM, Czeisler CA, Landrigan CP. Effects of health care provider work hours and sleep deprivation on safety and performance. Jt Comm J Qual Patient Saf. 2007; 33(11 Suppl):7–18.
63. McCormick F, Kadzielski J, Landrigan CP, Evans B, Herndon JH, Rubash HE. Surgeon fatigue: a prospective analysis of the incidence, risk, and intervals of predicted fatigue-related impairment in residents. Arch Surg. 2012;147(5):430–5.
64. Institute of Medicine. To err is human. Washington, DC: National Academy Press; 1999.
65. Institute of Medicine. Crossing the quality chasm: a new health system for the 21st century. Washington, DC: National Academy Press; 2001.

66. Institute of Medicine. Health professionals education; the bridge to quality. Washington, DC: National Academy Press; 2003.
67. Institute of Medicine. Patient safety. Washington, DC: National Academy Press; 2004.
68. Balch CM, Freischlag JA, Shanafelt TD. Stress and burnout among surgeons. Arch Surg. 2009;144:371–6.
69. Gundersen L. Physician burnout. Ann Intern Med. 2001;135:145–8.
70. Shanafelt TD, Balch CM, Bechamps GJ, et al. Burnout and career satisfaction among American surgeons. Ann Surg. 2009;250:463–71.
71. Shanafelt TD, Balch CM, Bechamps GJ, et al. Burnout and medical errors among American surgeons. Ann Surg. 2010;251:995–1000.
72. Ungerleider JD, Ungerleider RM. Improved quality and outcomes through congruent leadership. Teamwork and life choices. Prog Pediatr Cardiol. 2011;32:75–83.
73. Boyatizis R, McKee A. Resonant leadership. Boston: Harvard Business School Press; 2005.
74. Dickey J, Damiano R, Ungerleider RM. Our surgical culture of blame: a time for change. J Thorac Cardiovasc Surg. 2003;126:1259–60.
75. Dickey J, Ungerleider RM. Teamwork: a systems-based practice. In: Gravlee GP, Davis RF, Stammers AH, Ungerleider RM, editors. Cardiopulmonary bypass: principles and practice. Philadelphia: Lippincott, Williams and Wilkins; 2007. p. 572–88.
76. Dweck CS. Mindset: the new psychology of success. New York: Bantam Books; 2008.
77. Gottman JM. The science of trust. New York: W. W. Norton; 2011.
78. Quinn RE. Deep change: discovering the leader within. San Francisco: Jossey-Bass; 1996.
79. Siegel DJ. Mindsight. New York: Random House Bantam Books; 2010.
80. Brown B. The gifts of imperfection. Center City: Hazelden; 2010.
81. Dickey J, Ungerleider RM. Professionalism and balance for thoracic surgeons. Ann Thorac Surg. 2004;77:1145–8.
82. Dickey J, Ungerleider RM. Managing the demands of professional life. Cardiol Young. 2007;17:138–44.
83. Kegan R, Lahey LL. How the way we talk can change the way we work. San Francisco: Jossey-Bass; 2001.
84. Leary MR, Tate EB, Adams CE, Hancock J. Self-compassion and reactions to unpleasant self-relevant events: the implications of treating oneself kindly. J Pers Soc Psychol. 2007;92:887–904.
85. Neff K. Self-compassion: an alternative conceptualization of a healthy attitude toward oneself. Self Identity. 2003;2:85–102.
86. Rosenberg MB. Nonviolent communication: a language of life. Encinitas: PuddleDancer Press; 2003.
87. Mavroudis C. A partnership in courage. Ann Thorac Surg. 2003;75(5):1366–71.
88. Buckingham M, Coffman C. First, break all the rules. New York: Simon and Schuster; 1999.
89. Pink DH. A whole new mind: why right-brainers will rule the future. New York: Riverhead Books; 2005.
90. Senge PM. The fifth discipline. New York: Doubleday; 1990.
91. Satir V, Banmen J, Gerber J, Gomori M. The satir model. Palo Alto: Science and Behavior Books, Inc.; 1991.
92. Neff K. The development and validation of a scale to measure self-compassion. Self Identity. 2003;2: 223–50.
93. Neff KD, Vonk R. Self-compassion versus global self-esteem: two different ways of relating to oneself. J Pers. 2009;77:23–50.
94. Coleman PT. The five percent. New York: Public Affairs Press; 2011.
95. Rifkin J. The empathic civilization. New York: Penguin; 2009.
96. Tavris C, Aronson E. Mistakes were made. Orlando: Harcourt Books; 2007.
97. Goleman D, Boyatizis R, McKee A. Primal leadership. Boston: Harvard Business Press; 2002.
98. Weinberg GM. Becoming a technical leader. New York: Dorsett House; 1986.
99. Merrill WH. Who do you say you are? Ann Thorac Surg. 2013;96(1):1–6.
100. Patterson GA. Non solus–a leadership challenge. J Thorac Cardiovasc Surg. 2010;140:495–502.
101. Verrier ED. Who moved my heart? Adaptive responses to disruptive challenges. J Thorac Cardiovasc Surg. 2004;127(5):1235–44.
102. Colvin G. Talent is overrated: what really separates world-class performers from everybody else. New York: Penguin; 2008.
103. Gladwell M. Outliers. New York: Little, Brown and Co.; 2008.
104. Matveevskii A, Moore DL, Samuels PJ. Competency and professionalism in medicine. Clin Teach. 2012; 9(2):75–9.
105. Palmer PJ. The courage to teach. San Francisco: Jossey Bass; 1998.
106. Brown B. Daring greatly. New York: Gotham Books; 2012.
107. Cuddy AJC, Kohut M, Neffinger J. Connect, then lead. Harvard Bus Rev. 2013:55–61.
108. Bosk CL. Forgive and remember: managing medical failure. Chicago: University of Chicago Press; 1979.
109. McLendon J, Weinberg GM. Beyond blaming: congruence in large systems development projects. IEEE Software. 1996:20–80 thru 20–89.
110. Lehrer J. How we decide. New York: Houghlin Mifflin Harcourt; 2009.
111. Alsoufi B, Al-Halees Z, Manlhiot C, et al. Mechanical valves versus the ross procedure for aortic valve replacement in children: propensity-adjusted comparison of long-term outcomes. J Thorac Cardiovasc Surg. 2009;137:362–70.
112. Karamlou T, Jang K, Williams WG, et al. Outcomes and associated risk factors for aortic valve replacement in 160 children: a competing-risks analysis. Circulation. 2005;112:3462–9.

113. Nötzold A, Hüppe M, Schmidtke C, Blömer P, Uhlig T, Sievers H. Quality of life in aortic valve replacement: pulmonary autografts versus mechanical prostheses. J Am Coll Cardiol. 2001; 37:1963–6.
114. Senge PM, Scharmer CO, Jaworski J, Flowers BS. Presence: human purpose and the field of the future. New York: Crown Business; 2004.
115. Kram KE, Hall DT. Mentoring as an antidote to stress during corporate trauma. Hum Resour Manage. 1989;24:493–510.
116. Jamal M. Relationship of job stress and Type-A behavior to employees' job satisfaction, organizational commitment, psychosomatic health problems, and turnover motivation. Hum Relat. 1990;43:727–38.
117. Motowidlo SJ, Packard JS, Manning MR. Occupational stress: its causes and consequences for job performance. J Appl Psychol. 1986;71: 618–29.
118. Johnson WB. The intentional mentor: strategies and guidelines for the practice of mentoring. Prof Psychol Res Pract. 2002;33:88–96.
119. Schein EH. Career dynamics: matching individual and organizational needs. Reading: Addison-Wesley; 1978.
120. Wilson JA, Elman NS. Organizational benefits of mentoring. Acad Manage Exec. 1990;4:88–93.
121. Burke RJ, McKenna CS, McKeen CA. How do mentorships differ from typical supervisory relationships? Psychol Rep. 1991;68:459–66.
122. Sosik JJ, Godshalk VM. Leadership styles, mentoring functions received, and job-related stress: a conceptual model and preliminary study. J Organ Behav. 2000;21:365–90.
123. Appelbaum SH, Ritchie S, Shapiro BT. Mentoring revisited: an organizational behaviour construct. Int J Career Manage. 1994;6:3–10.
124. Clark RA, Harden SL, Johnson WB. Mentor relationships in clinical psychology doctoral training: results of a national survey. Teach Psychol. 2000;27: 262–8.
125. Kram KE. Mentoring at work: developmental relationships in organizational life. Glenview: Scott Foresman; 1985.
126. Ragins BR, Cotton JL. Mentor functions and outcomes: a comparison of men and women in formal and informal mentoring relationships. J Appl Psychol. 1999;84:529–50.
127. Russell JEA, Adams DM. The changing nature of mentoring in organizations: an introduction to the special issues on mentoring in organizations. J Vocat Behav. 1997;51:1–14.
128. Levinson DJ, Darrow CN, Klein EB, Levinson MH, McKee B. The seasons of a man's life. New York: Ballentine; 1978.
129. Durrell S. Healing the fisher king: spiritual lessons with Parzival, Gump, the Grail, Tao and Star Wars. Miami: Art Tao Press; 2002.
130. Jaworski J. Synchronicity. San Francisco: Berrett-Koehler; 1996.
131. Johnson RA. He. New York: Harper and Row; 1989.
132. Whyte D. The heart aroused. New York: Doubleday; 2002.
133. Cohen MS, Jacobs JP, Quintessenza JA, et al. Mentorship, learning curves, and balance. Cardiol Young. 2007;17 Suppl 2:164–74.
134. Edmondson AC. Psychological safety and learning behavior in work teams. Adm Sci Q. 1999;44:350–83.

Improving Pediatric Cardiac Care with Continuous Quality Improvement Methods and Tools

3

Julie K. Johnson and Paul R. Barach

Abstract

The healthcare delivery system is overly complex, impersonal and inefficient. Stakeholders are searching for effective remedies to ensure and enable that high quality care is readily available to all no matter their socioeconomic standing and their location. High-performing healthcare organizations differentiate themselves by focusing relentlessly and continuously on process-improvement initiatives to advance patient care. Continuous quality improvement offers a powerful way of thinking about how to transform clinical operations and healthcare teams to this end. Quality improvement methods are ideally suited for applications in complex cardiac care. In particular, we find five quality improvement tools—checklists, process maps, Ishikawa diagrams, run charts, and control charts—most relevant to improving the process and outcomes of pediatric cardiac care. The tools help visualize, analyze, and track process and outcome data for both individual and groups of patients. These tools should be taught to healthcare providers and managers and should routinely be deployed by clinicians and healthcare systems to evaluate and improve care.

Keywords

Continuous quality improvement • Patient safety • Pediatric cardiac surgery • Process mapping • Control chart • Check list • Run charts • Fishbone diagrams

A History of Quality Improvement

Continuous quality improvement (CQI) is both a management philosophy and a management method. It offers an approach, a set of tools, and a way of thinking about how to more effectively assess and study clinical flow and operations to achieve better results for patients, providers and healthcare delivery systems [1].

J.K. Johnson (✉)
Department of Surgery, Center for Healthcare Studies, Institute for Public Health and Medicine, Feinberg School of Medicine, Northwestern University, 633 N. St. Clair, Chicago, IL 60611, USA
e-mail: julie.k.johnson@northwestern.edu

P.R. Barach, BSc, MD, MPH
Department of Health Management and Health Economics, University of Oslo, Oslo 1074, Norway
e-mail: pbarach@gmail.com

P.R. Barach, J.P. Jacobs, S.E. Lipshultz, P.C. Laussen (eds.),
Pediatric and Congenital Cardiac Care: Volume 2: Quality Improvement and Patient Safety,
DOI 10.1007/978-1-4471-6566-8_3,

The evolution of CQI in heath care may be traced to the pioneering work of Florence Nightingale in 1850s. Nightingale used empiric observations and robust statistical methods to link unsanitary conditions with the high number of preventable deaths during the Crimean War [2].

In the 1960s, an approach known as *Kaizen* (literally "change good" or "improvement") was introduced in Japan [3]. Grounded in Japanese local village knowledge and practices, the key features of *Kaizen* include:

- The ideas come from the workers themselves; thus they are less likely to be radically different and, and therefore, easier to implement and less prone to induce resistance
- Small improvements are less likely to require major capital investment than major process changes
- Employees will continually seek ways to improve themselves by improving their own performance while encouraging workers to take ownership for their work, thereby improving worker motivation and engagement.
- Encouraging workers to take ownership for their work, thereby improving worker motivation and engagement.

From *Kaizen* came "quality function deployment," which combined quality assurance and quality control with function deployment in value engineering [4]. Quality function deployment helped to focus improvement efforts on the customer's needs by attending to and respecting the voice of the customer (VOC) above all. Translating these needs into design and engineering characteristics could help dramatically improve a product or service [5]. The same concepts and activities are now often referred to as "quality improvement" or "quality management" or even sometimes simply as "improvement" [6]. These concepts have now spread throughout the world and across multiple economic sectors, including healthcare. What was originally called *total quality management* (TQM) in the manufacturing industry evolved into *continuous quality improvement* (CQI) as it was applied to healthcare administrative and clinical processes.

Cross-disciplinary learnings and influence between manufacturing and healthcare were spurred during the 1990s by the increasing awareness that healthcare was lagging behind other industries in providing poor and uneven value. This highlighted the need to focus on reducing waste, inefficiencies, and harms. This awareness of the limitations of traditional methods to improve patient outcomes and contain costs forced healthcare to look to other domains for solutions [7]. However, from the perspective of healthcare providers, the industrial perspective of quality is limited in that it (1) ignores the complexities and dynamic nature and nuances of the patient–practitioner relationship; (2) downplays the knowledge, skills, and intrinsic motivation, as well as the ethical obligations of practitioners; and (3) provides less emphasis on influencing professional performance through "education, retraining, supervision, encouragement, and censure" [1].

Donabedian suggested that much can be learned from industrial quality and the industrial model of quality that calls attention to several important considerations [7]:

1. The need for even greater attention to consumer requirements, values, and expectations
2. The need for greater attention to the design of systems and processes as a means of quality assurance
3. The need to extend the self-monitoring, self-governing tradition of physicians to others in the organization
4. The need for a greater role by management in assuring the quality of clinical care
5. The need to develop appropriate applications of statistical control methods to healthcare monitoring
6. The need for greater education and training in quality monitoring and assurance for all concerned.

CQI is distinguished in healthcare by the recognition that service excellence and high-value outcomes are predicated on meeting the patients' needs. Meeting these needs is the key to sustaining quality. However, these needs may change over time with changes in expectations associated with education, economics, technology, and culture. Such changes, in turn, require continuous improvements in the administrative and clinical methods vision and leadership that affect the quality of patient care.

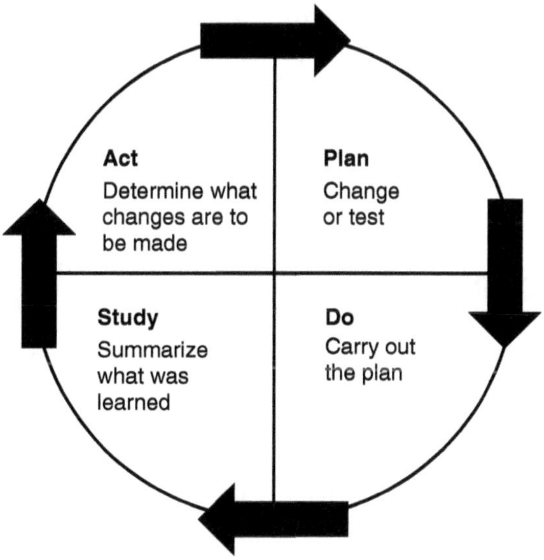

Fig. 3.1 The plan-do-study-act cycle (Adapted from Langley et al. [6])

Approaches to Quality Improvement

Several successful, multi-level, broad-based approaches have evolved across a range of healthcare disciplines, including pediatric cardiology and cardiac surgery. These approaches can be thought of as an umbrella that encompasses specific change methods. The most notable of these approaches are the plan-do-study-act (PDSA) cycle, the Model for Improvement, quality improvement collaboratives, lean manufacturing, and Six Sigma—each will be described below.

Walter Shewhart, at Bell Laboratories, introduced the iterative approach called **Plan-Do-Study-Act** (PDSA; Fig. 3.1) [8]. (Although the PDSA cycle is often attributed to Deming, he called it the Shewhart cycle.) [9] The **Model for Improvement** (Fig. 3.2), which was introduced in 1992, integrates the PDSA cycle as its core method [6]. Central to its application are three key and recurring questions:

1. What are we trying to accomplish?
2. How will we know that a change is an improvement?
3. What change can we make that will result in an improvement?

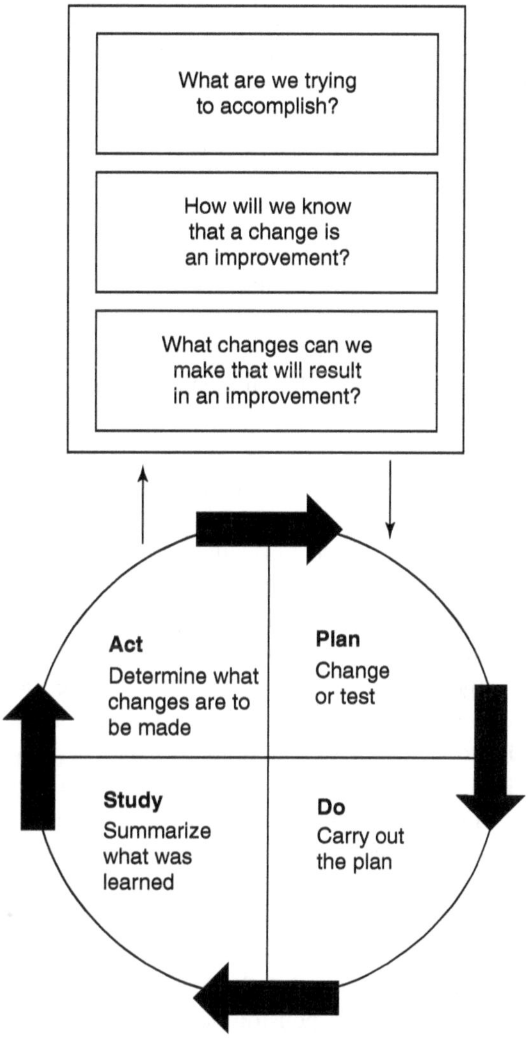

Fig. 3.2 The Model for Improvement, which incorporates the plan-do-study-act cycle (Adapted from Langley et al. [6])

The wide use of the PDSA cycle and the Model for Improvement in healthcare is the direct result of their elegance and simplicity, as well as to the transferability and application of these approaches across multiple care and non health settings.

Improvement collaboratives are another approach to quality improvement. A **quality improvement collaborative** consists of "multidisciplinary teams from various healthcare departments or organizations that join forces for several months to work in a structured way to improve their provision of care" [10].

One of the first uses of collaboratives was the Northern New England Cardiovascular Disease

Study Group in 1986 [11]. Their continuing and effective use in cardiovascular care is described in a systematic review of the management of heart failure, published in 2006, 20 years after this management process was begun. This review concluded that collaboratives "[have] significant potential to improve the outcomes of patients, particularly those with [heart failure] and chronic cardiovascular disease. The success and widespread adoption of collaboratives are directly related to the growing trust, respect, and data sharing among like-minded clinicians. This trust leads to meaningful exchanges and insights among experts and peers who then apply best practices to improve their care. Learning collaboratives can also use the PDSA approach [11] and are arguably the most effective way for systems to rapidly learn from each other about improving their process and patient outcomes.

Improvement collaboratives are successful and popular ways of improving health service delivery in disciplines ranging from cystic fibrosis, to heart failure, to trauma care [12, 13]. However, collaboratives are expensive and their results are difficult to measure with traditional epidemiological methods [14].

In the 1980s the Motorola Corporation developed the **Six Sigma Methodology** [15]. Six Sigma starts with a process mapping activity that involves elements of defining what a business does, assigning responsibilities, identifying performance standards, and deciding how success will be determined (see below). After these critical elements have been defined, Six Sigma analyzes each through the DMAIC methodology (Define, Measure, Analyze, Improve, and Control) [16].

"**Lean**," also known as "lean manufacturing," "lean enterprise," or "lean production," is a CQI approach that considers as wasteful any resources that are allocated to any goal other than creating value for the customer and that are thus targets for elimination [17]. Value is defined from the customer's perspective and includes any action or process for which a customer would be willing to pay.

For many, Lean is an approach to improvement that helps to identify and steadily eliminate waste in processes (or *muda*, in Japanese). As waste is eliminated, quality improves and production time and costs are reduced. Essentially, lean is centered on *preserving value with less work*. Lean optimizes the trade-off between productivity and quality and highlights the axiom that improved quality translates to improved profitability, or good quality is good business.

Quality Improvement Tools

Several CQI tools can help improve pediatric cardiac care and surgery [18]. The most relevant tools for pediatric cardiac surgery are listed in detail below and include checklists, process maps, Ishikawa diagrams, run charts, and control charts.

Checklists

The checklist has received the most attention (and press) for improving patient safety. Evidence supports greater adoption of checklists in surgery [19] and in other medical specialties [20–22]. In June 2008, the Safe Surgery Saves Lives Initiative of the World Health Organization (WHO) released the WHO Surgical Safety Checklist. In a little more than 2 years, more than 3,900 hospitals in more than 122 countries were registered in the Initiative. Of these 3,900 hospitals, more than 1,800 have reported using a checklist in at least one operating room [23].

The Dutch SURPASS study, conducted from October 2007 to March 2009, found that hospitals using checklists had surgical complication rates that were more than one-third lower, and death rates that were almost one-half lower (from 1.5 to 0.8 %), than they were in hospitals not using checklists [24].

Researchers at Stanford found that the observed-to-expected mortality ratio declined from 0.88 in quarter one, to 0.80 in quarter two, with the use of a modified version of the WHO Surgical Safety Checklist [25]. The use of checklists also improved communication among the surgical team, and thus the quality of care. Quality was measured by the frequency with which staff reported "Patient Safety Never Events" (i.e., the kind of events that should "never happen"). The number of Patient Safety

Never Events related to errors or complications decreased from 35.2 to 24.3 %.

The website Safesurg.org provides resources for implementing the WHO checklist or for modifying an existing checklist. Modified checklists created by other institutions can also be downloaded (http://www.who.int/patientsafety/safesurgery/checklist/en/). [26] Modifying checklists to fit local practices and needs is encouraged to enhance acceptance.

Although checklists have been widely adopted, their effectiveness has been highly variable if they are casually applied only as tick-box forms and in a top down approach [27]. Ineffective top-down engagement and inauthentic partnering with clinicians inhibits positive behavior change and encourages normalized deviance [28]. Introducing a checklist in an environment characterized by a lack of trust causes clinicians to feel jeopardized professionally and personally, encourages gaming and lead to marginal to no improvement of care or outcomes [29]. Effective adoption requires local championship, sustained clinician engagement, and a commitment to interprofessional teamwork [30, 31].

Process Maps

A process map or flowchart is a visual representation of the care process that is created with information provided by team members. The process mapping exercise can help clinicians clarify through visualization the complex and many step process of their environment and determine what they want to do to improve it. The exercise helps clinicians make assumptions and expectations explicit and can provide insight into how to improve the process of care or to overcome barriers to its improvement [32].

A high degree of process awareness often drives the design changes needed to sustain improvement. Process mapping describes precisely what an individual provider is required to do and when, in terms of cognitive processes, actions, or both, to achieve the system's goal. Data are collected from observations or interviews that carefully break down complex clinical processes into discrete, measurable, and clear tasks [32]. Team members can gain insights into how they and their colleagues perceive the same tasks and hopefully come to a shared understanding of the process.

Ultimately, improving patient outcomes requires appreciating the inherent links between structure, process and outcomes [33]. Process maps help focus improvement efforts, not solely for the individual provider, but for the entire clinical microsystem. Visualizing the process can also help identify inefficiencies (e.g., parallel or redundant processes that have emerged for whatever reason), clarify roles, and reduce ambiguity among team members, all of which can help coordinate patient care. This process is particularly useful in improving transitions of care and avoiding readmissions and patient bounce back to intensive care and high-dependency units [34, 35].

Process maps can be created at different levels of detail to illustrate the major phases or detailed activities in that process. It is important to map the current process, not the *desired process*, to identify opportunities for improvement. We have used process mapping in pediatric cardiac surgery to better understand the current process of care (Fig. 3.3) and to summarize the data on near misses and adverse events (Fig. 3.4) [32, 36].

Ishikawa Diagrams

Ishikawa diagrams, also known as "cause-and-effect diagrams," "fishbone diagrams," and "root-cause analyses," are visual representations of the sources of variation in a process [37]. The diagram is often created by brainstorming with key stakeholders to identify the causes and their effects on a process. The causes are generally allocated to five general categories: place (environment), equipment, procedures (processes), people (patients and providers), and policies (Fig. 3.5). Routine root cause analysis with Ishikawa diagrams can be very powerful in analyzing surgical adverse events. A detailed analysis in one major hospital over 4 years (Table 3.1) established the fact that excellent surgical outcomes depend on appreciating and integrating individual, team, technical, and organizational factors [38].

Reviewing the root cause categories helps the team estimate the resources needed to address the

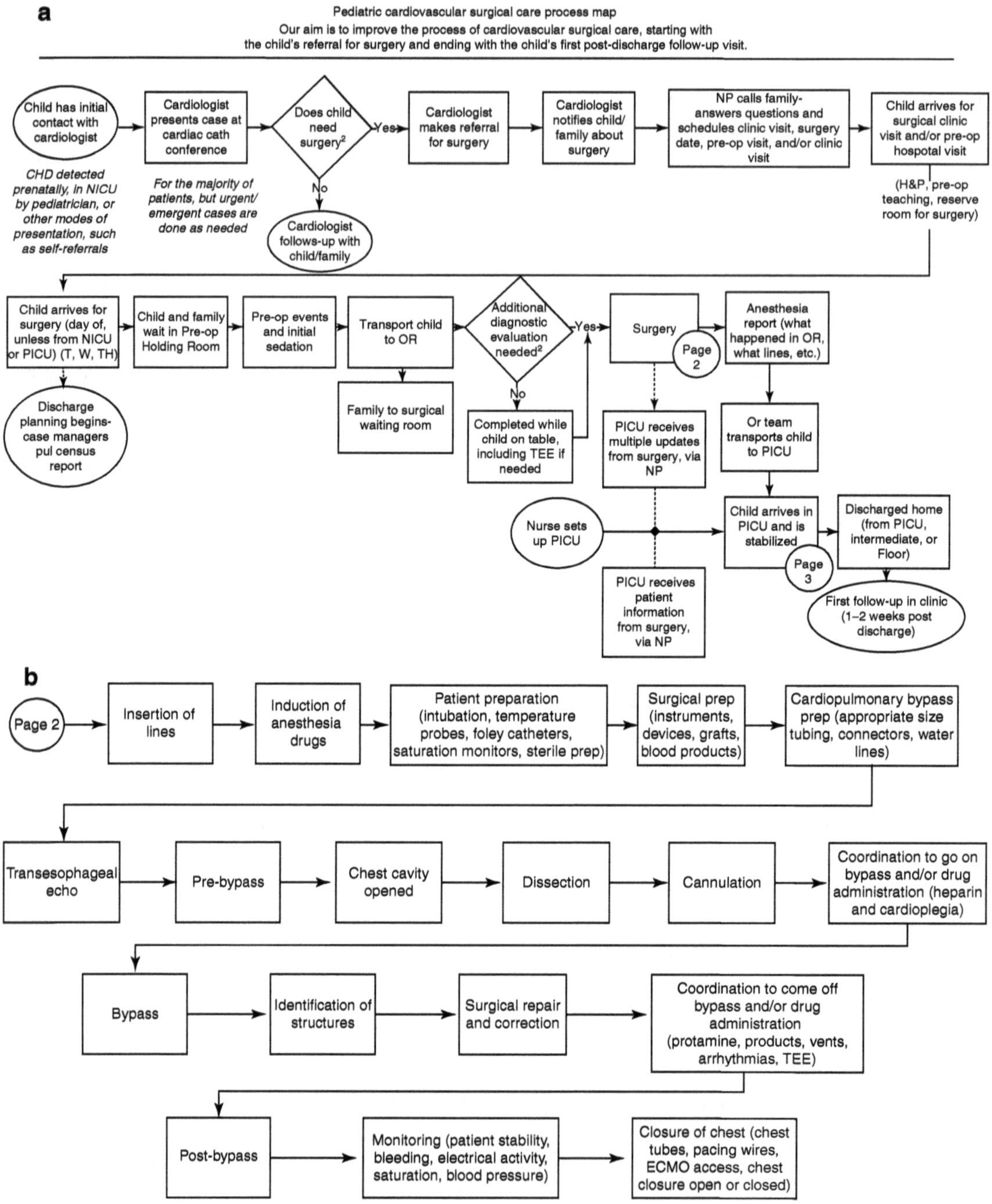

Fig. 3.3 A process map of pediatric cardiac and cardiac surgical care. (**a**) Preoperative processes. (**b**) Operative processes. (**c**) Postoperative processed (Source: Barach and Johnso [32]6). page i13. Used with permission)

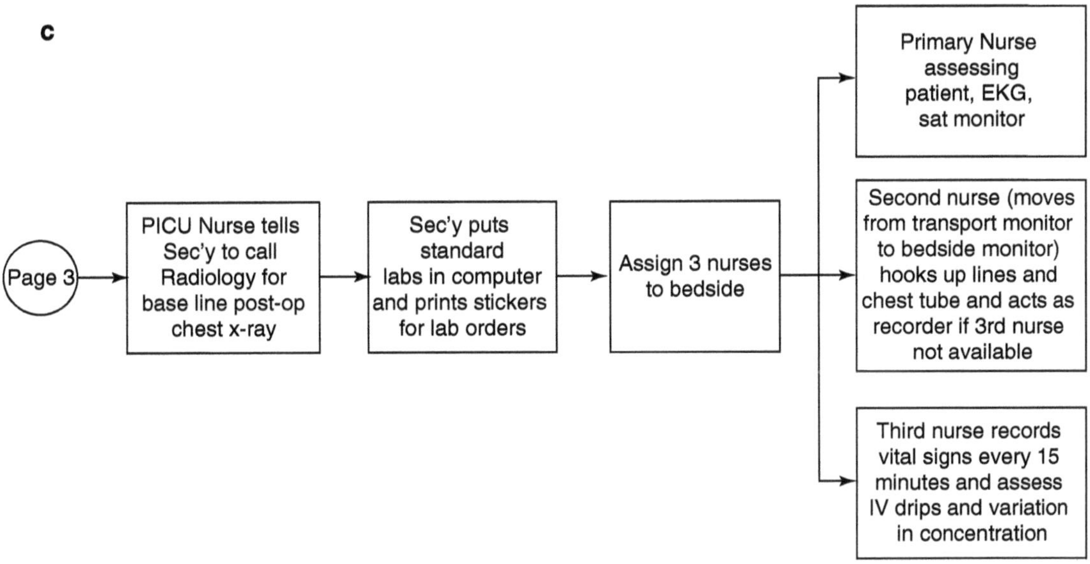

Fig. 3.3 (continued)

causes of process variation. These diagrams help identify potential improvements and which improvements might be transferable to another setting.

Run Charts and Control Charts

Two of the most powerful CQI tools are run charts and control charts [8, 39]. These tools are valuable for analyzing variability in clinical processes [40], in part because the data usually does not go beyond what is generally collected to meet reporting requirements. The run chart is a simple plot of a measurement over time with a line drawn at the median value. The data can be related to patients, organizations, or clinical units. Run charts are particularly useful because they can reveal subtle changes over time that would otherwise go unnoticed.

Important uses of the run chart for clinical improvement are to:

- Display data to make process performance visible
- Determine whether tested changes improve the process or endpoints
- Determine whether the changes are lasting
- Allow for a temporal view of data versus a static view [41].

For example, a team wanting to improve patient outcomes on mechanical ventilation might measure time-to-extubation for patients undergoing closure of atrial septal defect or ventricle septal defect. Team members start by plotting the data over time in a run chart for 30 consecutive patients (Fig. 3.6), where the time to extubation ranged from 2 to 48 h after the procedure, with a median of 14 h. As the team changes the process, they can continue plotting data to determine whether the changes decreased time-to-extubation and thus improved overall care or made no different on outcomes.

The control chart was developed by Shewhart in the 1920s to improve industrial manufacturing [8]. Like run charts, control charts display data over time, but control charts provide upper and lower control limits of variation that help determine whether a process is stable or unstable (Fig. 3.7). Control limits are calculated using median values and the moving ranges of the data. The factors leading to instability must be addressed before the process can be improved.

Shewhart and Deming define two types of variation in a process. Briefly, "common cause variation"

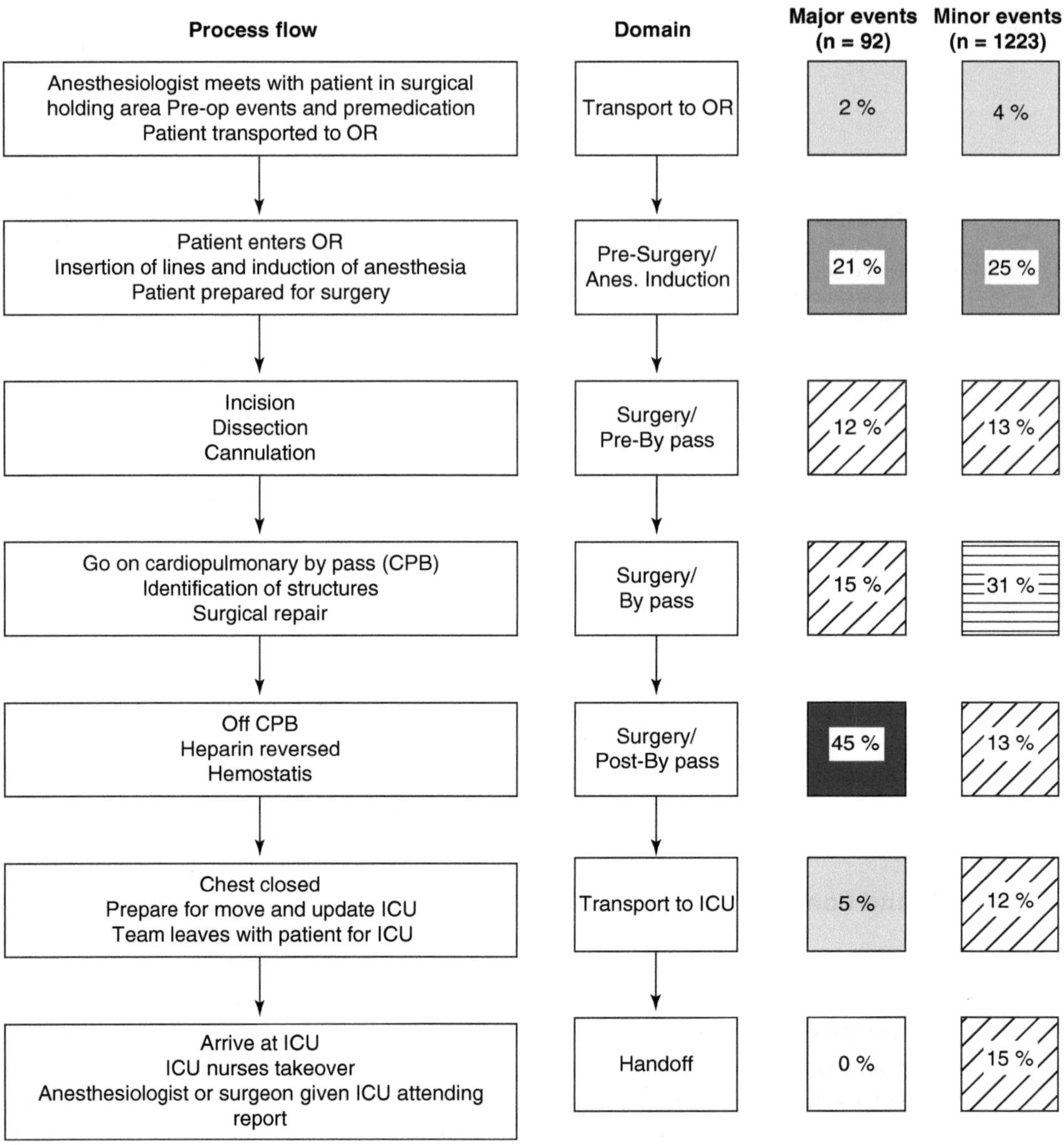

Fig. 3.4 A process map showing minor and major adverse event data in pediatric cardiac surgery (Source: Barach et al. [36]. Used with permission)

is the usual, historical, quantifiable variation in a system, whereas "special cause variation" is unusual, not previously observed, non-quantifiable variation [42]. In surgical procedures, common cause variation might include fluctuations in the severity of a patient's risk factors, the skills of operating team members, or changes in equipment settings [43]. Common cause variation suggests that improving outcomes will require changing the processes that produced the results. Special cause variation is the result of factors extraneous to the process; for example, variation introduced by a new manager, drive for more productivity or by equipment breaking during a procedure. It is not possible to predict (or control) variation caused by special causes.

If the control chart indicates that the process is currently under control (i.e., it is stable, with

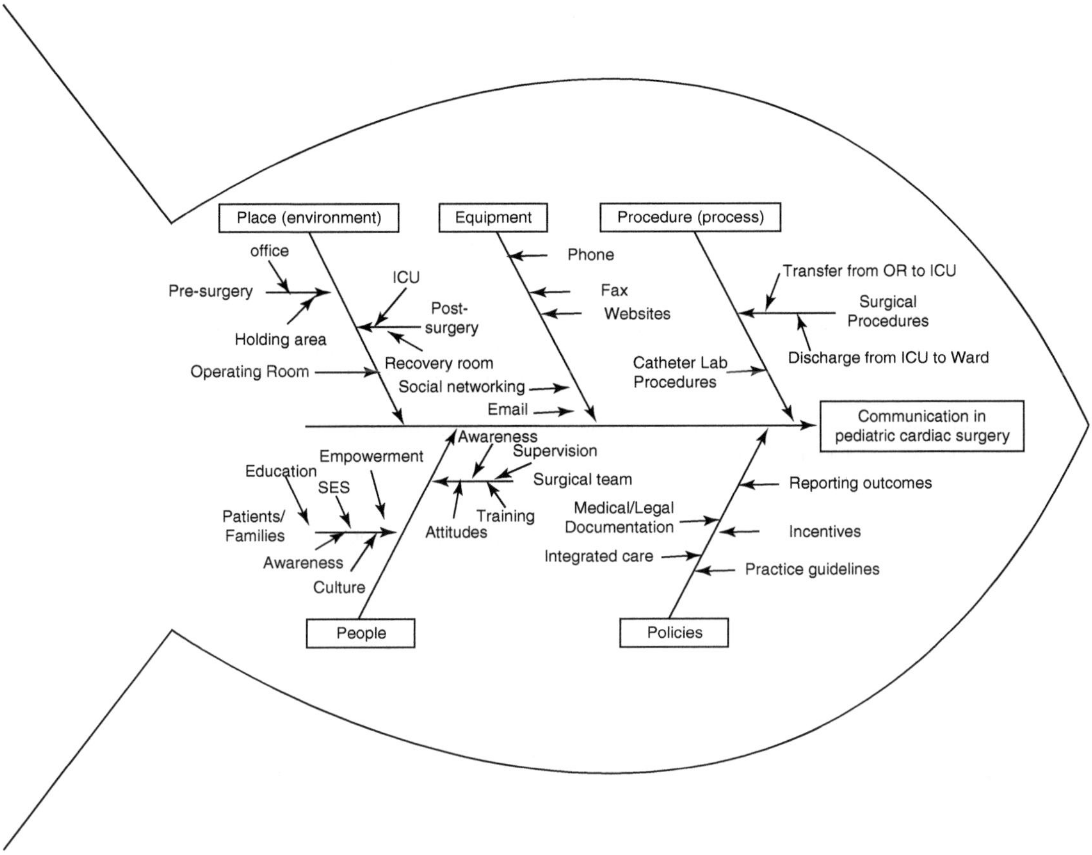

Fig. 3.5 An Ishikawa diagram for pediatric cardiac surgery

Table 3.1 Results of a root cause analysis of process variation of cardiac surgery

Theme	Issues identified
Failure to recognize or respond appropriately to the deteriorating patient within the required timeframe	Post CABG complications Postoperative sepsis Postoperative hyponatremia
Workforce availability and skills	Orientation, training, and supervising new or junior members of the surgical team, especially outside normal working hours
Transfer of patients for surgery	Difficulty in organizing an OR for surgery Failure to handover information about patient acuity
Trauma management	Coordination and response of trauma teams Clinical decision making process for trauma patients Coordination of care between multiple clinicians
Access to emergency operating room	Antepartum hemorrhage and emergency cesarean Urgent orthopedic procedure Urological complications requiring urgent OR
Missed diagnosis	Thoraco-lumbar fracture in a trauma patient Brain abscess mistaken for cerebral metastasis Sub arachnoid hemorrhage thought to be drug overdose
Unexpected procedural complications	Airway obstruction after thyroidectomy Failed intubation
Sentinel events	Wrong site procedure—spinal fusion at wrong level Retained surgical products requiring surgical removal

Adapted from Cassin amd Barach [38]

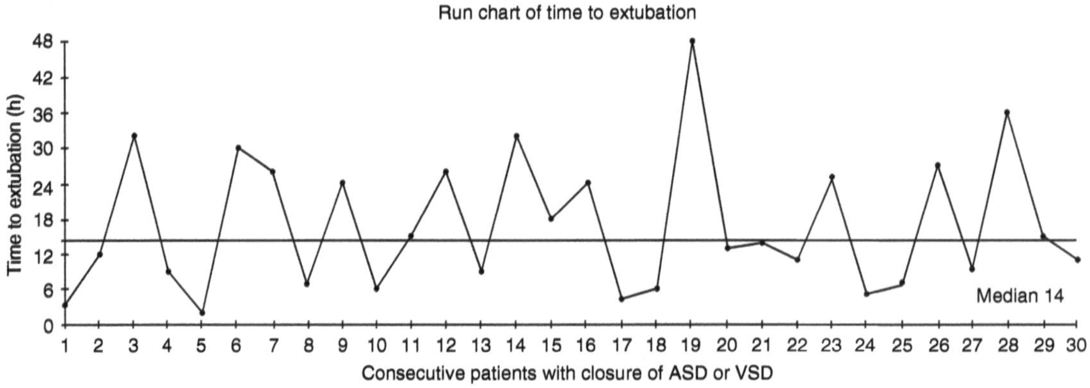

Fig. 3.6 A run chart of time to extubation for patients undergoing closure of atrial septal defect and ventricle septal defect in the intensive care unit (ICU)

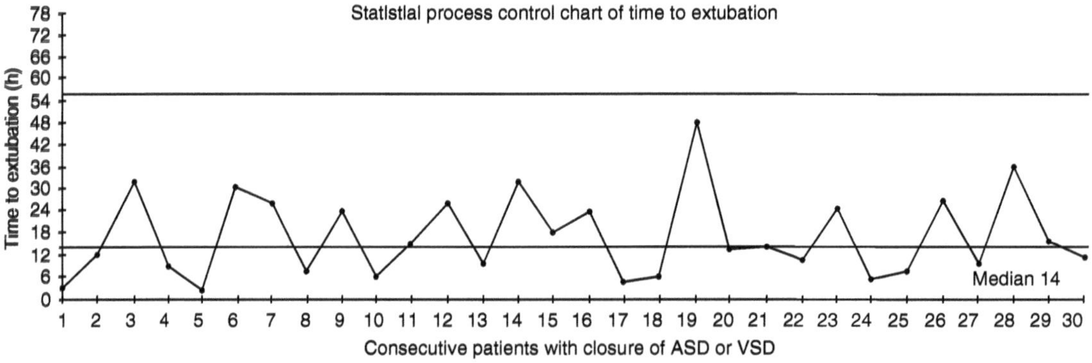

Fig. 3.7 A control chart of time to extubation for patients undergoing closure of atrial septal defect and ventricle septal defect in the ICU. The chart shows that the variation is the result of common cause variation and not special cause variation. That is, *without any changes* to the process, the time to extubation will continue to fall within a range that will not exceed the upper control limit of 55 h

variation only coming from sources common to the process), then data from the process can be used to predict the future performance of the process. If the chart indicates that the process is not under control, the chart can help determine the sources of variation, which can then be eliminated to bring the process back under control (Fig. 3.7). These data can inform the team about when to act, but also, especially in healthcare systems that are constantly tweaking their systems, when to hold and not to act, depending on the cause of the variation.

The control chart illustrates the variation that is due to a common cause and not to a special cause variation. The implications in our example about when to extubate the patient is that *without any changes* to the process it will be difficult to predict the time to extubation.

Control charts are appropriate for analyzing data from procedures that are performed frequently, consistently, and with relatively standard methods [43]. In addition, patients should be separable into more homogeneous subsets for analysis, for example, by stratifying them by procedure, and the procedures should have a documented range of favorable and unfavorable outcomes.

Conclusions

This chapter described several CQI tools that should be part of improving the processes and outcomes of pediatric cardiac care. Detailed descriptions of how to apply the tools are beyond the scope of this chapter. Improving teamwork is an important factor in improving patient outcomes. In fact, it is a requirement for using these CQI tools effectively. Indeed, ongoing quality improvement efforts are not about which tools are used but about how these tools can produce insight, provide feedback, engage the team members and track progress. Their purpose is to help people function as a team, as well as to improve patient outcomes.

References

1. Sollecito W, Johnson J, editors. Continuous quality improvement in health care. Sudbury, MA. Burlington: Jones and Bartlett Learning; 2013.
2. Neuhauser D. Florence nightingale gets no respect: as a statistician that is. Qual Saf Health Care. 2003; 12(4):317.
3. Imai M. Kaizen: the key to Japan's competitive success. New York: Random House; 1986.
4. Akao Y. Development history of quality function deployment, The customer driven approach to quality planning and deployment. Minato, Tokyo 107 Japan. Tokyo: Asian Productivity Organization; 1994.
5. Omachonu V, Barach P. Quality function development (QFD) in a managed care organization. Qual Prog: 5;36–41.
6. Langley G, Nolan K, et al. The improvement guide. San Francisco: Jossey-Bass; 1996.
7. Baker R. Avedis donabedian: an interview. Qual Health Care. 1993;2:40–6.
8. Shewhart WA. Statistical method from the viewpoint of quality control. Washington, DC: Graduate School of the Department of Agriculture; 1939.
9. Deming WE. Out of the crisis. Cambridge: Massachusetts Institute of Technology Center for Advanced Engineering Study; 1986.
10. Schouten LM, Hulscher ME, et al. Evidence for the impact of quality improvement collaboratives: systematic review. BMJ. 2008;336(7659):1491–4.
11. Newton PJ, Davidson PM, et al. An introduction to the collaborative methodology and its potential use for the management of heart failure. J Cardiovasc Nurs. 2006;21(3):161–8.
12. Brush Jr JE, Rensing E, et al. A statewide collaborative initiative to improve the quality of care for patients with acute myocardial infarction and heart failure. Circulation. 2009;119(12):1609–15.
13. Schouten LM, Hulscher ME, et al. Short- and long-term effects of a quality improvement collaborative on diabetes management. Implement Sci. 2010;5:94.
14. Overtveit J, Bate P, et al. Quality collaboratives: lessons from research. Qual Saf Health Care. 2002; 11(4):345–51.
15. Brue G. Six Sigma for managers. New York: McGraw Hill; 2002.
16. Duffy GL, Farmer E, et al. Applying lean Six Sigma in public health. In: Bialek R, Duffy GL, Moran JW, editors. The public health quality improvement handbook. Milwaukee: ASQ Quality Press; 2009.
17. Holweg M. The genealogy of lean production. J Oper Manage. 2007;25(2):420–37.
18. Johnson J, Barach P. Quality improvement methods to study and improve the process and outcomes of pediatric cardiac surgery. Prog Pediatr Cardiol. 2011; 32(2):147–53.
19. Haynes AB, Weiser TG, et al. A surgical safety checklist to reduce morbidity and mortality in a global population. N Engl J Med. 2009;360(5):491–9.
20. Pronovost P, Needham D, et al. An intervention to decrease catheter-related bloodstream infections in the ICU. N Engl J Med. 2006;355(26):2725–32.
21. Gawande A. The checklist manifesto. New York: Metropolitan Books; 2009.
22. Pronovost P, Vohr E. Safe patients, smart hospitals: how one doctor's checklist can help us change health care from the inside out. New York: Penguin Group; 2010.
23. World Health Organization. New scientific evidence supports WHO findings: a surgical safety checklist could save hundreds of thousands of lives. 2011. Retrieved 5 Aug 2011. From http://www.who.int/patientsafety/safesurgery/checklist_saves_lives/en/index.html.
24. de Vries EN, Prins HA, et al. Effect of a comprehensive surgical safety system on patient outcomes. N Engl J Med. 2010;363(20):1928–37.
25. World Health Organization. New scientific evidence supports WHO findings: a surgical safety checklist could save hundreds of thousands of lives. 2011. Retrieved 20 June 2011. From http://www.who.int/patientsafety/safesurgery/checklist_saves_lives/en/index.html.
26. Safesurg.org. A website for information on how to reduce deaths in surgical care globally. 2011. Retrieved 20 June 2011. From http://www.safesurg.org/index.html.
27. Urbach DR, Govindarajan A, et al. Introduction of surgical safety checklists in Ontario, Canada. N Engl J Med. 2014;370(11):1029–38.
28. Vaughan D. The dark side of organizations: mistake, misconduct and disaster. Ann Rev Sociol. 1999;25:271–305.

29. Barach P, Phelps G. Clinical sensemaking: a systematic approach to reduce the impact of normalised deviance in the medical profession. J R Soc Med. 2013; 106(10):387–90.
30. Bosk C, Dixon-Woods M, et al. The art of medicine: reality check for checklists. Lancet. 2009;374:444–5.
31. Aveling EL, McCulloch P, et al. A qualitative study comparing experiences of the surgical safety checklist in hospitals in high-income and low-income countries. BMJ Open. 2013;3(8):e003039.
32. Barach P, Johnson JK. Understanding the complexity of redesigning care around the clinical microsystem. Qual Saf Health Care. 2006;15 Suppl 1:i10–6.
33. Lilford R, Chilton PJ, et al. Evaluating policy and service interventions: framework to guide selection and interpretation of study end points. BMJ. 2010; 341:c4413.
34. Toccafondi G, Albolino S, et al. The collaborative communication model for patient handover at the interface between high-acuity and low-acuity care. BMJ Qual Saf. 2012;21 Suppl 1:i58–66.
35. Johnson JK, Farnan JM, et al. Searching for the missing pieces between the hospital and primary care: mapping the patient process during care transitions. BMJ Qual Saf. 2012;21 Suppl 1:i97–105.
36. Barach P, Johnson J, et al. A prospective observational study of human factors, adverse events, and patient outcomes in surgery for pediatric cardiac disease. J Thorac Cardiovasc Surg. 2008;136(6):1422–8.
37. Ishikawa K. Guide to quality control. White Plains: Kraus International Publications; 1987.
38. Cassin BR, Barach PR. Making sense of root cause analysis investigations of surgery-related adverse events. Surg Clin North Am. 2012;92(1):101–15.
39. Deming WE. The new economics for industry, government, education. Cambridge: Massachusetts Institute of Technology Center for Advanced Engineering Study; 1993.
40. Thor J, Lundberg J, et al. Application of statistical process control in healthcare improvement: systematic review. Qual Saf Health Care. 2007;16(5): 387–99.
41. Perla RJ, Provost LP, et al. The run chart: a simple analytical tool for learning from variation in healthcare processes. BMJ Qual Saf. 2011;20(1):46–51.
42. Wheeler D. Understanding variation: the key to managing chaos. Knoxville: SPC Press, Inc.; 1999.
43. Shahian DM, Williamson WA, et al. Applications of statistical quality control to cardiac surgery. Ann Thorac Surg. 1996;62(5):1351–8; discussion 1358–9.

Quality Improvement in Pediatric Cardiology: The National Pediatric Cardiology Quality Improvement Collaborative

4

Jeffrey B. Anderson, Robert H. Beekman III, Gerard R. Martin, and Carole Lannon

Abstract

Infants with congenital heart disease (CHD) manifest broad anatomical and physiological heterogeneity, often making medical decision-making complex and variable. Clinical assessments regarding medical and surgical management in an individual patient are frequently made based on individual or group heuristics and past experience rather than solely on scientific evidence [1]. The relative paucity of patients with complex CHD and the variation in their anatomy and physiology has made it difficult to perform rigorous studies defining best practices that are associated with improved outcomes in these children. The Joint Council on Congenital Heart Disease (JCCHD) developed the National Pediatric Cardiology Quality Improvement Collaborative (NPC-QIC) is the first quality improvement collaborative in pediatric cardiology. This collaborative used a multi-site network, practice-based registry data and improvement science methodology to identify variation in management and to improve outcomes in patients with complex congenital heart disease.

Keywords

Congenital heart disease • Learning networks • Quality improvement • Model for change

J.B. Anderson, MD, MPH (✉)
R.H. Beekman III, MD
Cincinnati Children's Hospital Medical Center, The Heart Institute, 3333 Burnet Avenue, ML 2003, Cincinnati, OH 45229, USA
e-mail: jeffrey.anderson@cchmc.org; rbeekman@cchmc.org

G.R. Martin, MD
Division of Cardiology, Center for Heart, Lung and Kidney Disease, Children's National Medical Center, 111 Michigan Avenue NW, Washington, DC 20010, USA
e-mail: gmartin@childrensnational.org

C. Lannon
Cincinnati Children's Hospital Medical Center, The James M. Anderson Center for Health Systems Excellence, Cincinnati, OH, USA
e-mail: carole.lannon@cchmc.org

P.R. Barach, J.P. Jacobs, S.E. Lipshultz, P.C. Laussen (eds.),
Pediatric and Congenital Cardiac Care: Volume 2: Quality Improvement and Patient Safety,
DOI 10.1007/978-1-4471-6566-8_4, © Springer-Verlag London 2015

Background

The past several decades have seen marked improvement in mortality in the most complex of congenital heart defects due to surgical and medical advancements [2]. However, despite this progress, there continues to be major adverse events, variation in management practices and outcomes among individuals and institutions caring for children with CHD [3–5]. The reasons for this variation include a continued lack of evidence-based practices in patients with rare conditions as well as limited sharing of lessons and best practices among providers. In non-health industries standardization and reduction in variation has lead to safer practices, reduced waste, cost savings and improved outcomes [6–10]. Standardization of healthcare practices can reduce process variation and provides a foundation upon which new approaches can be tested more effectively.

Role of Clinical Networks and Registries

Clinical networks and registries are useful vehicles in understanding variation in clinical care, and to test changes in clinical practice that can standardize care and improve clinical outcomes. Large networks and registries provide the infrastructure to gather information on patients between and across treatment centers and to understand differences in care processes and clinical outcomes. Regional and national networks and databases have been established to better understand care of pediatric cancer, neonatal management, and cystic fibrosis [11–14]. Implementing a registry has been demonstrated in multiple trials to reduce variation and improve care for patients with chronic illness [11]. In pediatric cardiology and cardiac surgery, registries (e.g., Pediatric Heart Network, Society for Thoracic Surgery Registry, Mid-Atlantic Group of Interventional Cardiology (MAGIC) Registry, Pediatric Cardiology Care Consortium, Pediatric Electrophysiology Society Ablation Registry, IMPACT Registry) have generated comparative data between centers and identified clinical outcomes that are related to variation in care [15–18].

A learning network is a multi-site clinical network that agrees to a set of engagement rules that relate to definitions and data collection and then uses data for ***both*** research and improvement [19, 20]. Successful models include the Northern New England Cardiovascular Disease Study Group, Vermont Oxford Network (VON), and the Children's Oncology Group (COG) [21–25].

Research and improvement networks can offer epidemiologic, statistical and translational advantages that allow for creating "laboratories" for conducting comparative effectiveness and translational research [26–28]. Creation of total population registries within and across network sites provides large, diverse, and representative study samples. These virtual laboratories facilitate spread of changes that standardize practice, reduce variations in outcomes due to variations in care delivery and offer larger statistical power. These networks linking research to care delivery and clinicians directly, can conduct research about how to effectively implement changes that improve care and outcomes. They are particularly useful to accelerate the translation of new evidence into practice. Clinician end-users are in a unique position to identify critical healthcare knowledge gaps and design interventions to bridge those gaps in effectiveness research. Finally, the care providers, along with their patients, are the final benefactors of implementing and seeing the results of the changes at the point-of-care.

Learning networks allow not only for data collection but also for structured implementation of changes in practice through quality improvement (QI) science methodology. QI methods include measurement of process and outcome metrics, applying statistical process control to those metrics and then testing interventions that may improve these processes or outcomes. Testing of interventions is carried out initially on a small scale utilizing Plan-Do-Study-Act (PDSA) cycles to determine whether the interventions work. By testing multiple interventions on a small scale more learning can take place over a shorter period of time. QI activities in the pediatric subspecialties, including pediatric cardiology, have been catalyzed in part by the adoption of new Maintenance of Certification (MOC) requirements by the American Board of Pediatrics (ABP) [20, 29, 30]. The MOC program emphasizes ongoing assessment and documentation of performance, and participation in QI activities, as a requirement for ongoing certification.

Establishment of the NPC-QIC Learning Network

The Joint Council on Congenital Heart Disease (JCCHD) was formed in 2003 as a leadership alliance to enhance communications and improve coordination among the societies representing pediatric cardiologists, congenital heart surgeons and adult congenital heart disease specialists. The leadership alliance included physician-leaders from the American Academy of Pediatrics, the American Board of Pediatrics, the American College of Cardiology, the American Heart Association, the Congenital Heart Surgery Society and International Society for Adult Congenital Cardiac Disease. The JCCHD held their initial meetings in 2005 and were funded by the American Academy of Pediatrics, the American Board of Pediatrics, the American College of Cardiology, the American Heart Association, the Congenital Heart Surgery Society and International Society for Adult Congenital Cardiac Disease. This group determined to dramatically improve the outcomes for children with CHD through a national QI collaborative network of providers working together to collect longitudinal data and conduct QI research intended to accelerate the development and transition of new knowledge into practice. In addition, participation in the collaborative was designed to meet Board requirements for maintenance of certification standards [29, 31]. The guiding principles of the Institute of Medicine (IOM) and Institute for Healthcare Improvement (IHI) were followed to provide a structure to the process. As an initial step, an Expert Conference held in January 2006 comprised of QI leadership experts, pediatric cardiologists and representatives from pediatric critical care and cardiac surgery was held in Dallas. The Expert Group developed concepts for an improvement collaborative and a shared database for QI in pediatric cardiology; defined sufficient detail for the QI initiative to pursue funding; and generated buy-in, excitement, and ownership of the QI initiative within the JCCHD. This QI initiative became the National Pediatric Cardiology Quality Improvement Collaborative.

The Children's Heart Association of Cincinnati, a parent-led organization that has a close working relationship with the Heart Institute of Cincinnati Children's Hospital Medical Center (CCHMC), provided the initial seed funding. The vision, support and guidance of key leaders in pediatric cardiology contributed to the development of a strong foundation for the collaborative. Three organizational representatives serving on the JCCHD agreed to lead the NPC-QIC; this trio invited an additional four members to constitute a seven-member Task Force. The organization brought together key leaders with expertise in content, quality measurement, and family-centered care. Parents and families were also integral partners in design of interventions and understanding clinical changes the collaborative had implemented.

Design and Management of the NPC-QIC

The NPC-QIC Task Force discussed several clinical problems to focus on in the initial phase of the collaborative and decided to focus on infants with hypoplastic left heart syndrome, a population of children with high mortality and a six-fold variation in outcomes, and whose clinical outcomes were clearly in need of improvement [32]. The risk of mortality and morbidity for infants born with hypoplastic left heart syndrome (HLHS) is amongst the highest for pediatric cardiology and cardiac surgery patients, with mortality rates over 25 % [33]. Children who survive Norwood palliation, and are discharged home while awaiting their next surgery (interstage) of the bidirectional Glenn shunt, are at risk for poor outcomes with mortality rates estimated at 10 to15% [34]. Surviving infants

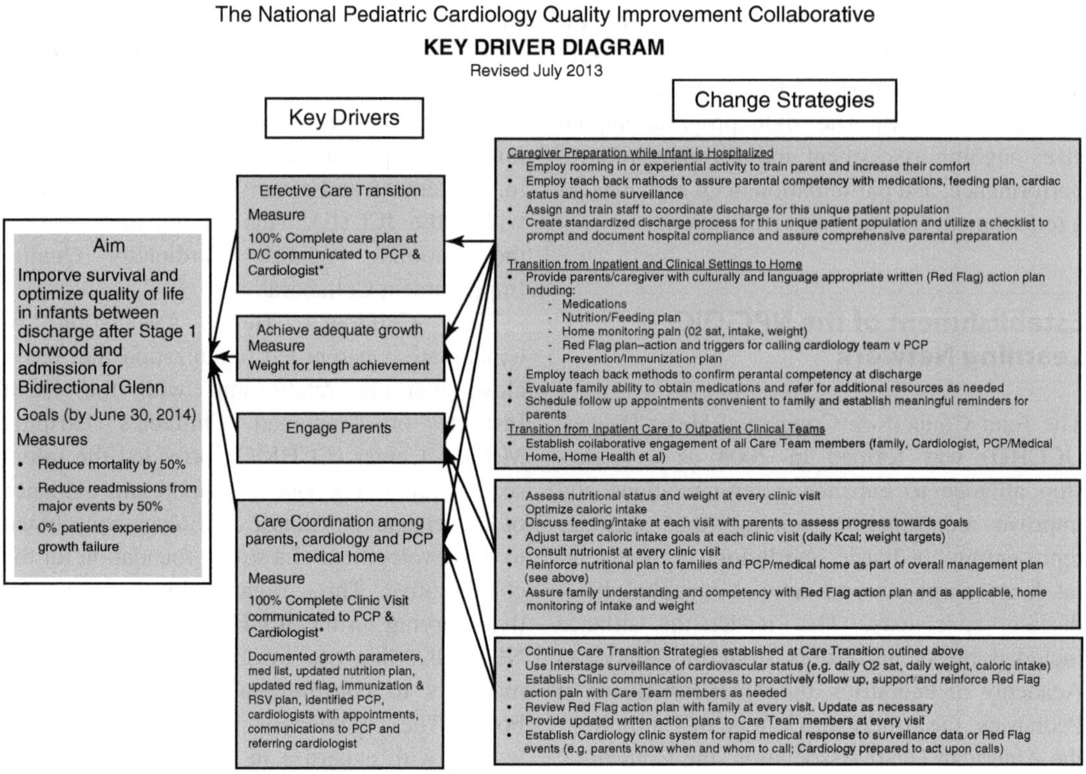

Fig. 4.1 NPC-QIC key driver diagram

experience significant morbidities, including poor feeding, chronic cyanosis, recurrent laryngeal or phrenic nerve injury, delayed growth and development and long-term mental deficiencies. This group often requires numerous unscheduled clinic visits and hospital readmissions to address these and other problems. [35] Thus, the interstage period for infants with HLHS presents children and families with major health care challenges and an opportunity for caregivers to improve clinical processes and outcomes. Because this interstage is limited to approximately 4–6 months, the committee felt that it would be an ideal interval target for improvement efforts. Finally, the taskforce felt that improved care processes identified through the study of children with HLHS would be generalizable to infants with other types of congenital heart disease.

We defined the aim of the initial project as: "Reducing the mortality and improving the quality of life of infants with hypoplastic left heart syndrome (HLHS) during the interstage period between discharge from the Norwood and admission for the bidirectional Glenn procedure" [31]. The taskforce determined that the key outcome measures important in this population were (1) reduction of mortality of infants during the interstage period; (2) reduction of readmissions during the interstage due to adverse clinical events; and (3) elimination/attenuation of growth failure commonly seen in this population. We created a Key Driver diagram, outlining the desired outcomes and the drivers, the areas we would focus on, that were deemed necessary to achieve these outcomes and a guide for the activities of the collaborative (Fig. 4.1). The drivers felt to be essential to achieve better outcomes fell into three areas: engaging parents, improving care transitions at discharge following stage 1 surgical palliation, ensuring adequate growth by optimizing nutrition, and, improving care coordination among the hospital team, the primary care team, and families. The Task Force developed metrics for using the key driver diagram as a guide to address both the outcomes and processes important to achieve the project goals. Statistical process control charts demonstrating the tracking of these key outcome measures as well as the process measures felt to be important in achieving these outcomes can be seen in Fig. 4.2. Statistical process control provides statistical boundaries, typically defined as ±3 standard deviations around the median, to a system of data points. By placing statistical boundaries around data, referred to as upper and lower control limits, changes to a system can more easily be identified helping to address and correct the variation in care processes.

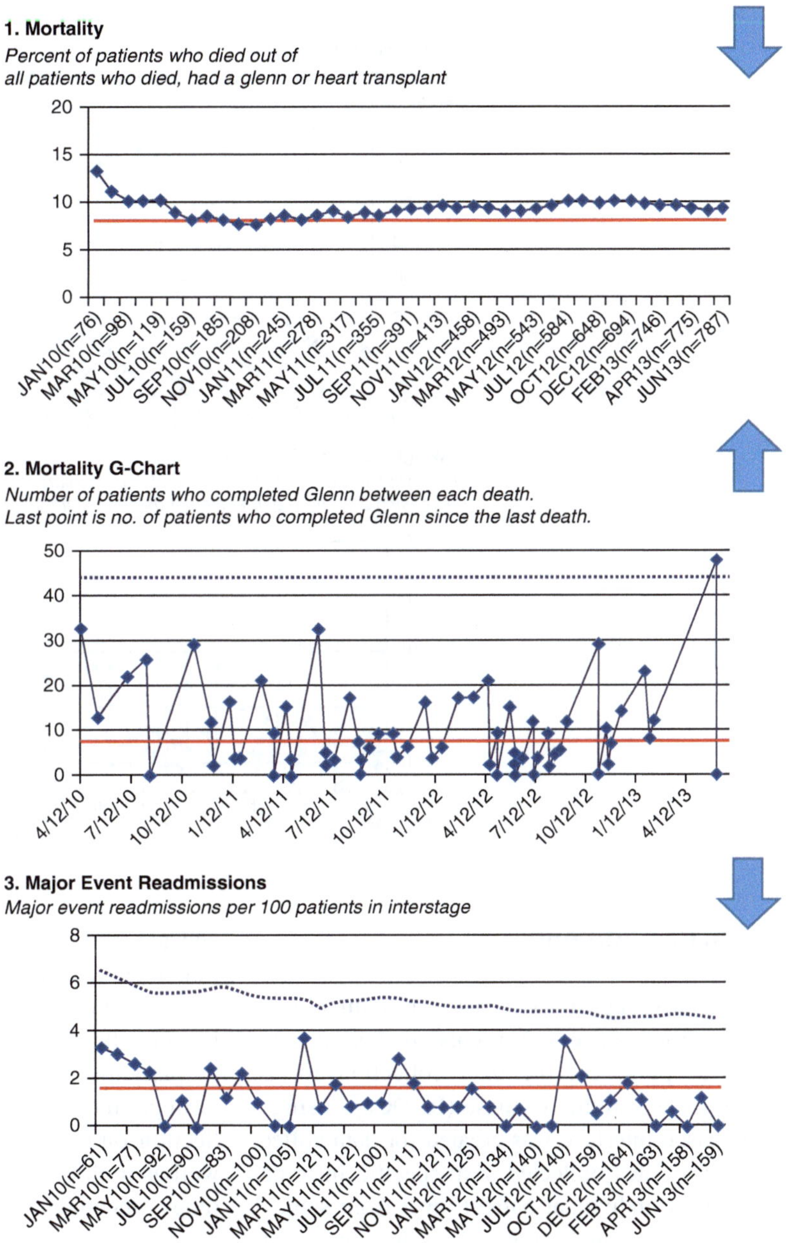

Fig. 4.2 NPC-QIC outcome measures

Fig. 4.2 (continued)

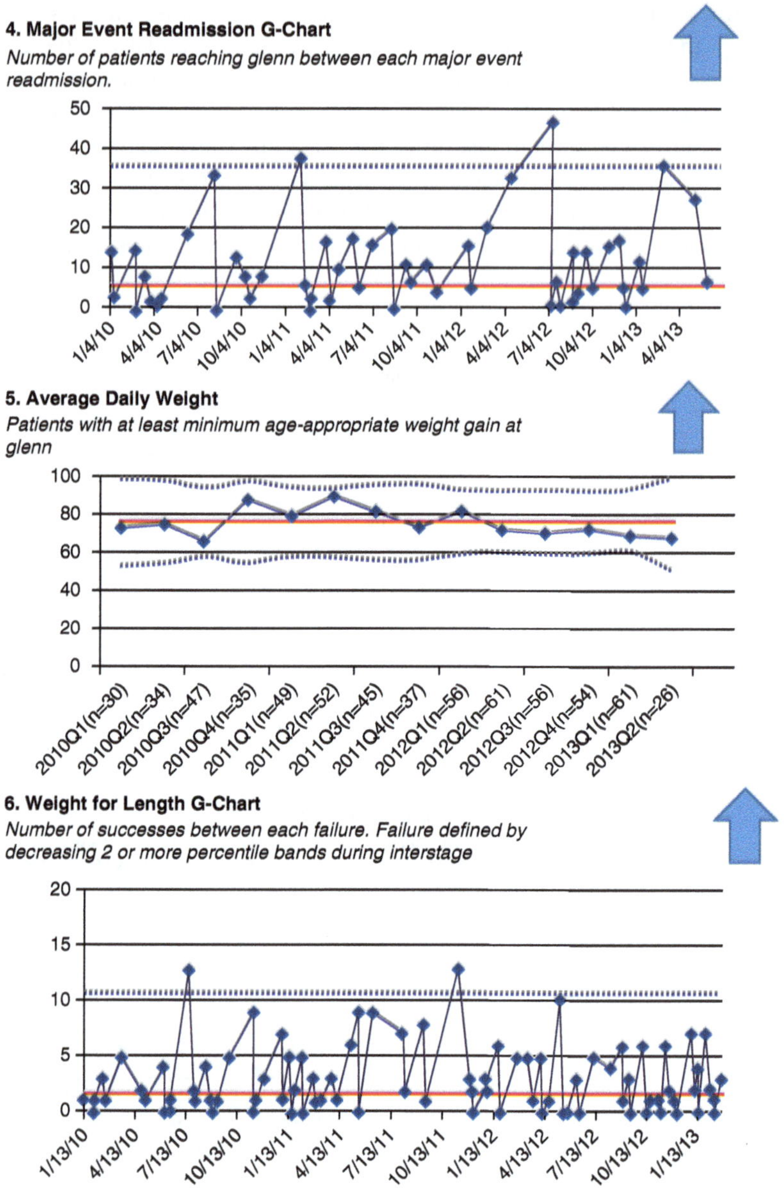

Team Recruitment

An initial group of six teams from clinical sites that perform stage 1 Norwood palliation were used to pilot test the data collection forms. A secure electronic database (REDCap) using a web-based interface was created for data collection. The sites collected visit-specific information at the individual patient level from stage 1 and stage 2 hospitalizations, interstage clinic visits and any interstage readmissions. This information included data regarding care processes as well as clinical outcome data. After the pilot testing with the initial six teams, all sites were invited to participate through an invitation circulated through the American Academy of Pediatrics Section on Cardiology and Cardiac Surgery, as well as multiple presentations at pediatric cardiology meetings. The data forms have been reviewed, updated, and revised at regular intervals

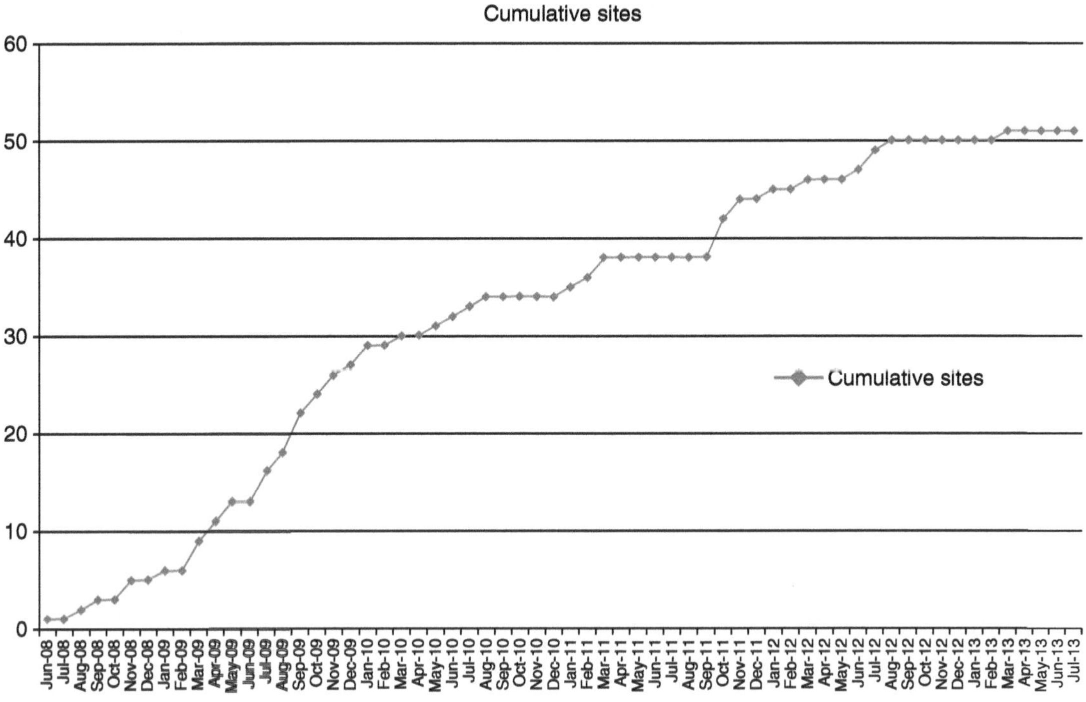

Fig. 4.3 Growth of number of NPC-QIC sites over time

to ensure accuracy and usability. In the first 3 years NPC-QIC has grown to over 40 sites in the United States (Fig. 4.3).

Collaborative structure

The collaborative is a longitudinal learning community that used the Institute for Healthcare Improvement's Breakthrough Series (BTS) Model [36–40]. The BTS model is a change management platform that utilizes effective dissemination and behavior change tools to support practice changes [41]. The BTS methods are based on educational, statistical, and systems theory. These include: (1) a focus on shared goals that are clear and explicit so that teams are aligned along a common purpose; (2) the use of data and feedback to allow teams to identify opportunities for individual improvement; and (3) the use of aggregate data, face-to-face meetings, and individual coaching to engage teams in working together to improve the systems of care for patients. The components of the BTS can be seen in Fig. 4.4 [42].

Pediatric cardiology centers participate as teams comprised of a physician champion, nursing and administrative representatives, and a nutritionist. Teams are also encouraged to include a parent or family representative. Each month, the teams collect data on patient status and care processes; post reports of their progress; participate in webinars and a listserv; and, test changes to improve their systems. Semi-annual "learning sessions" which are 1–2 day workshops bring teams together to share lessons learned. Pediatric cardiologists provide content expertise and project staff support teams as needed, particularly with implementation of changes in practice. Parents were involved in the design and implementation of the network, and work actively with clinical team member--in research work groups, at the semi-annual meetings and monthly webinars, and where aggregate data are reviewed and barriers to improvement are discussed. The NPC-QIC has encouraged and facilitated the development of parent groups at each clinical site. Clinical teams and parents have together developed practical tools (e.g. feeding algorithms,

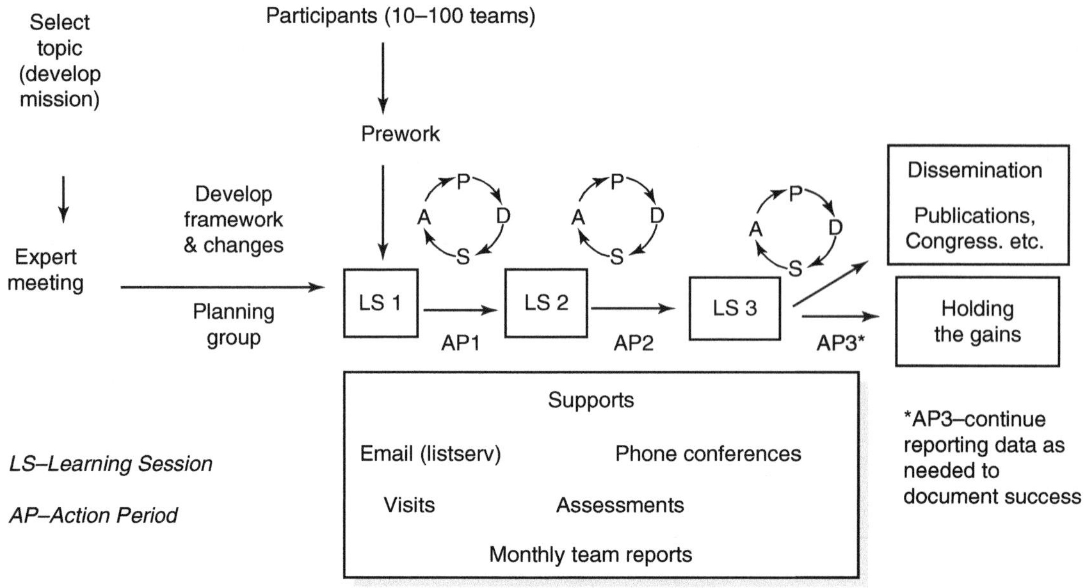

Fig. 4.4 IHI Breakthrough Series Model [36, 42] Adapted from the IHI Breakthrough Series Model [36]. *Learning session (LS)*: face-to-face team meetings, *Action Period (AP)*: period of time between learning sessions

video about discharge planning, 'red flag' checklists).In addition, along with education and support of quality improvement activities, parent-led presentations and parent panels are key components of the learning sessions. Primary care clinicians have also participated in the learning sessions and provide insight into the challenges in child handovers and coordination of care between sub-specialists and primary medical homes for these complex patients. The Anderson Center for Health Systems Excellence at Cincinnati Children's Hospital Medical Center provided the improvement, project management and data infrastructure for the NPC-QIC project. The Center has supported over 45 collaborative multi-site improvement projects involving more than 1,500 organizations [43–45].

Outcomes

One of the key findings from the NPC-QIC was the considerable variation in management and outcomes of infants with hypoplastic left heart syndrome [46–48]. This management variation was seen at several points along the process of care including pre- and post-operatively, after the Norwood procedure, as well as during the outpatient interstage. NPC-QIC has facilitated the sharing of best practices among participating centers using face-to-face meetings called Learning Sessions and monthly webinars called Action Period Calls. There has been significant improvement in and standardization of the NPC-QIC process measures as these practices have been implemented, including at additional centers. These measures capture important clinical processes at the time of discharge following the Norwood procedure and during the interstage clinic visits. Examples of improvement in process measures can be found in Fig. 4.5.

The elimination and attenuation of growth failure in this population is one of the primary outcomes of the collaborative. Analysis of growth outcomes identified significant variation in outcomes among the NPC-QIC centers [49]. This analysis determined that there were specific nutritional practices that are being used by centers that had better patient growth. These practices, when combined as a Nutritional Bundle resulted in significantly better interstage infant growth. This growth bundle included: (1)

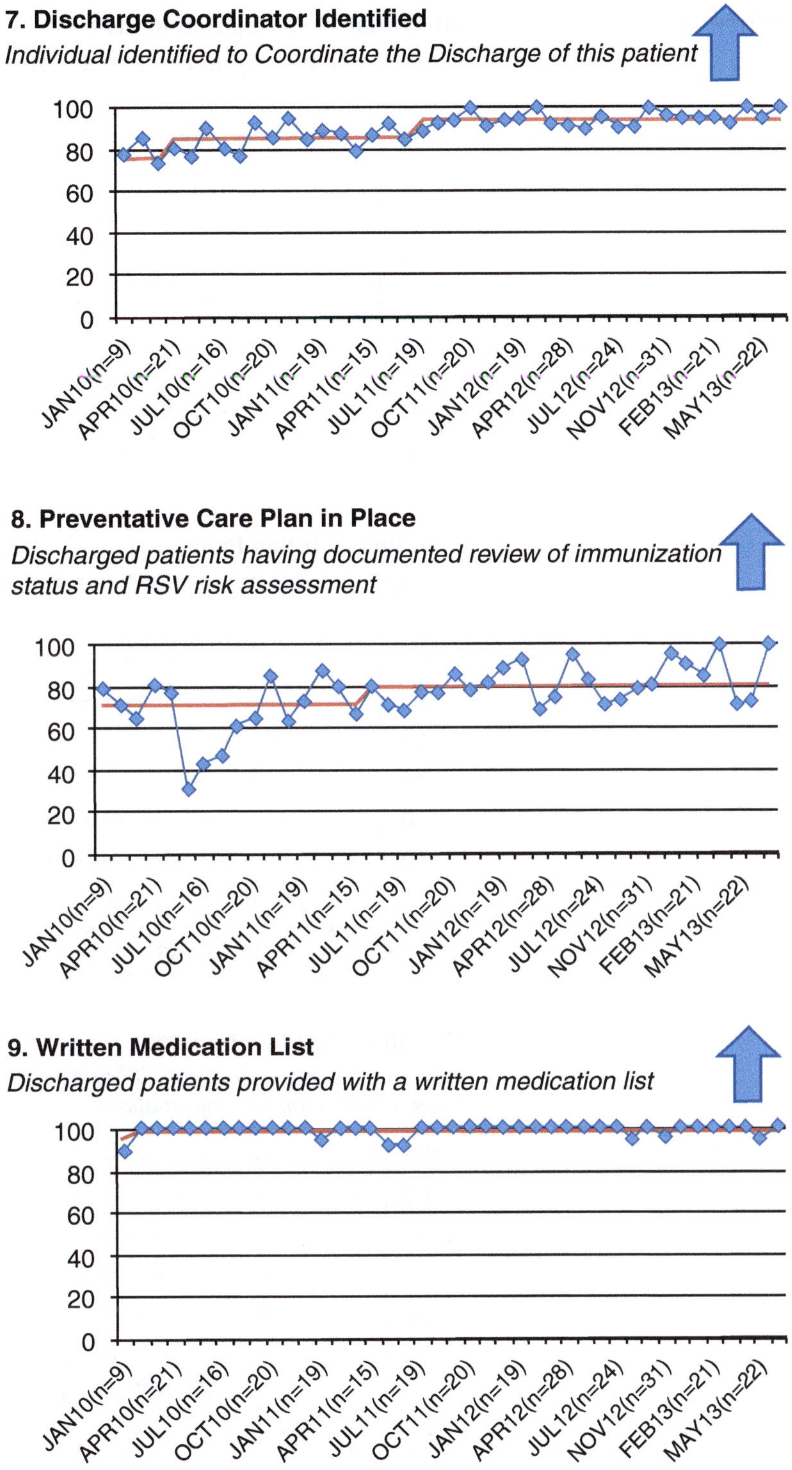

Fig. 4.5 NPC-QIC discharge and clinic visit process measures

Fig. 4.5 (continued)

10. Written Red-Flag Action Plan

Discharged patients provided with a written red-flag action plan

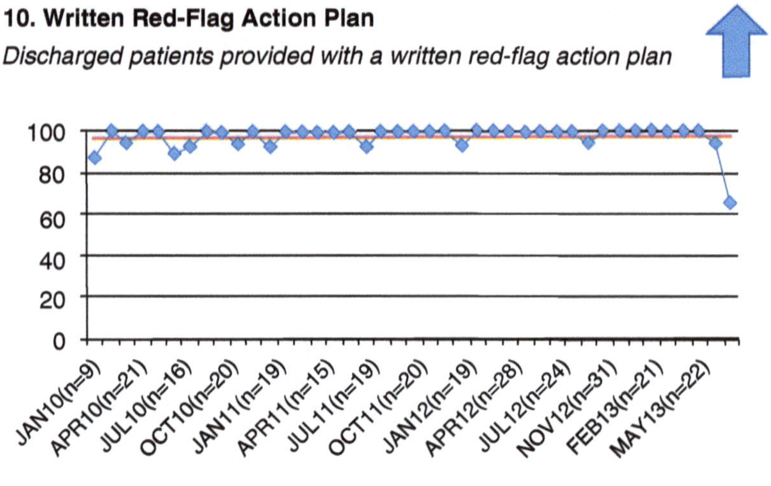

11. Written Nutrition Plan

Discharged patients provided with a written nutrition plan

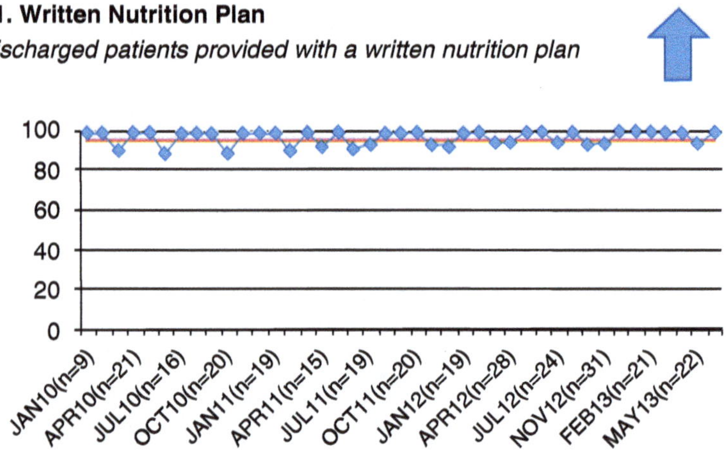

12. Follow-Up Plan Prepared

Discharged patients having PCP and cardiologist identified with follow-up appointment information

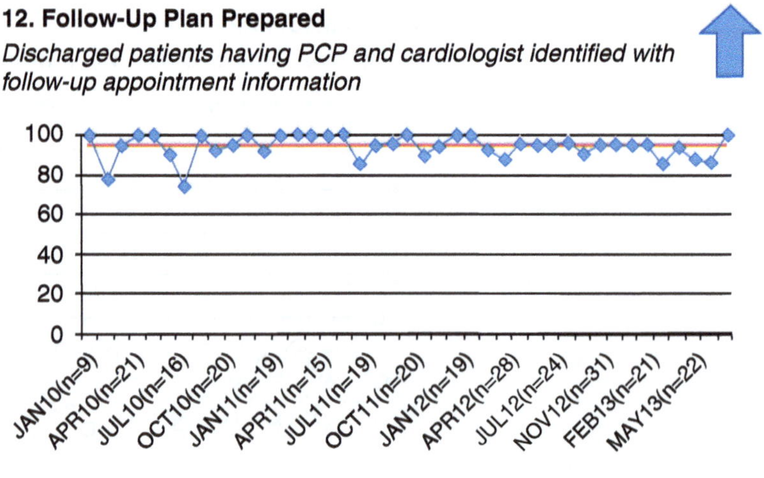

Fig. 4.5 (continued)

13. Complete Care Plan

Discharged patients with all of measures 7-12 complete

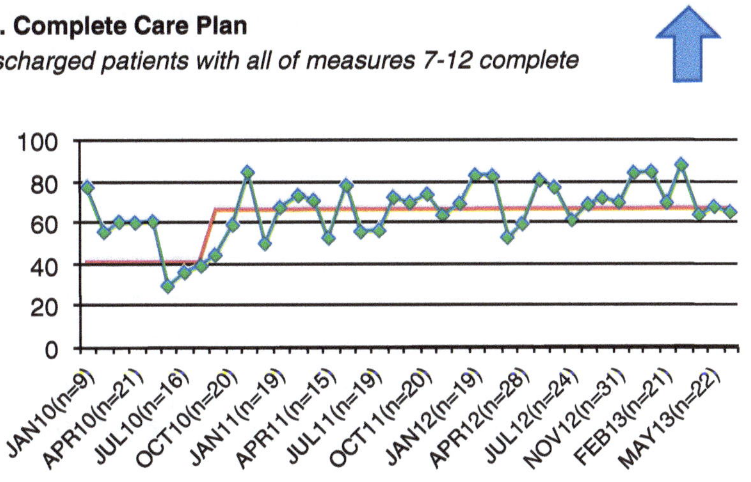

14. Complete Care Plan Communicated to PCP

Discharged patients with communication to PCP regarding measures 7-12 documented

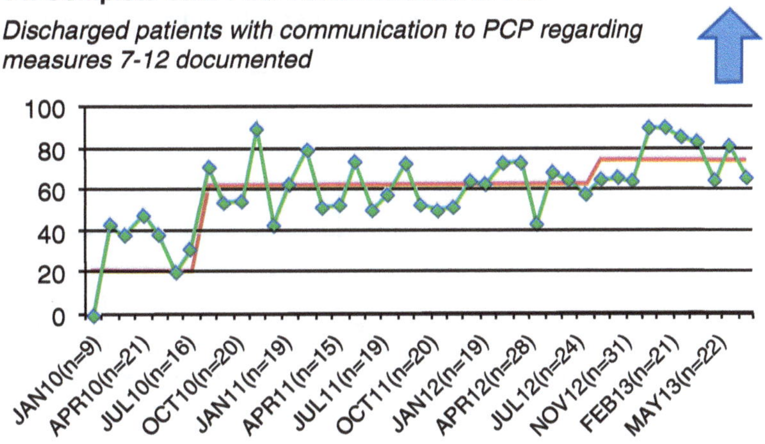

Fig. 4.5 (continued)

15. Post-Care Coordinator Identified

Individual or group identified to coordinate outpatient management of this patient

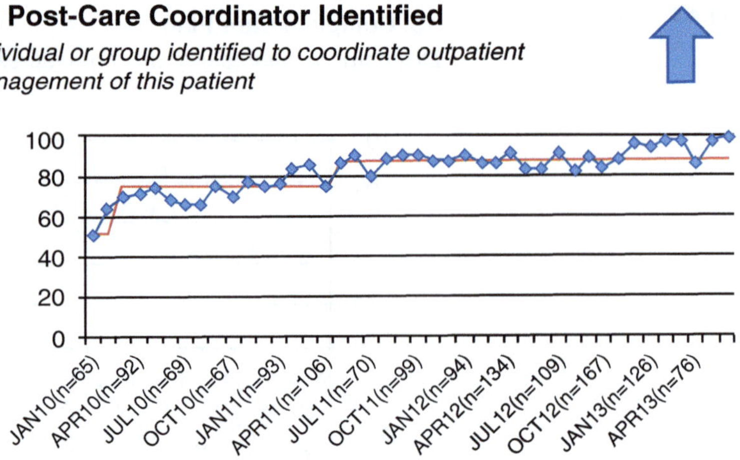

16. Preventive-Care Plan Updated

Clinic visits having documented review of immunization status and RSV risk assessment with follow-up plans

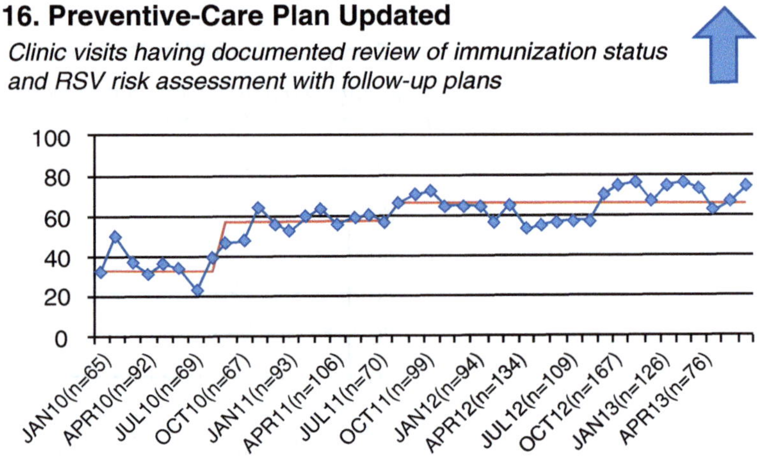

17. Written Medication List Updated

Written medication list reviewed, discussed, or updated with parents/caregivers as needed upon clinic discharge

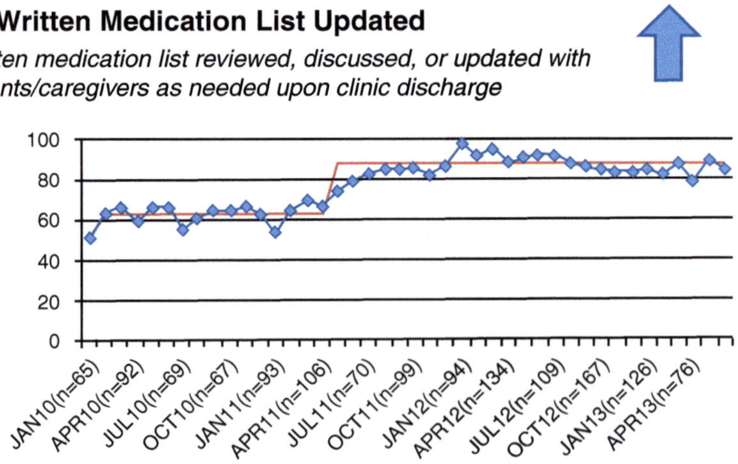

Fig. 4.5 (continued)

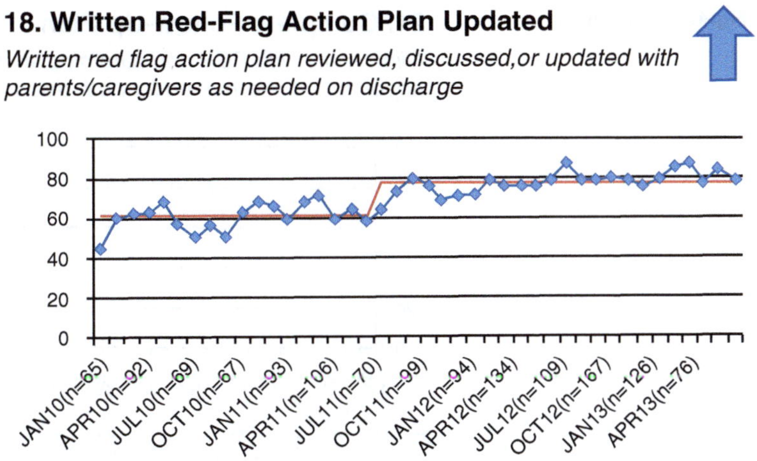

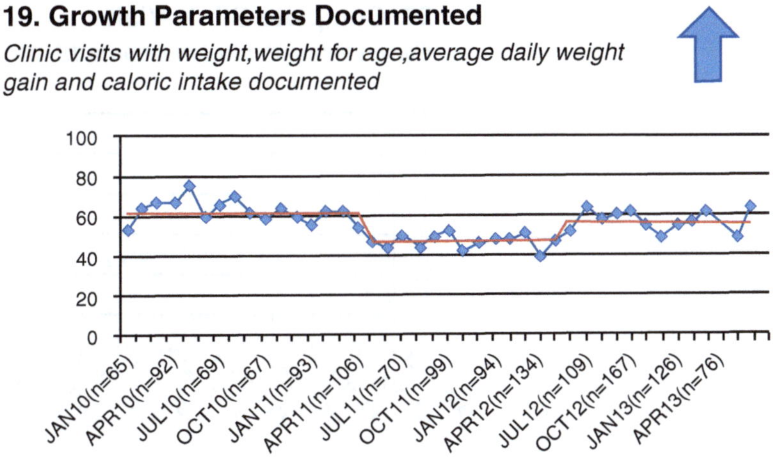

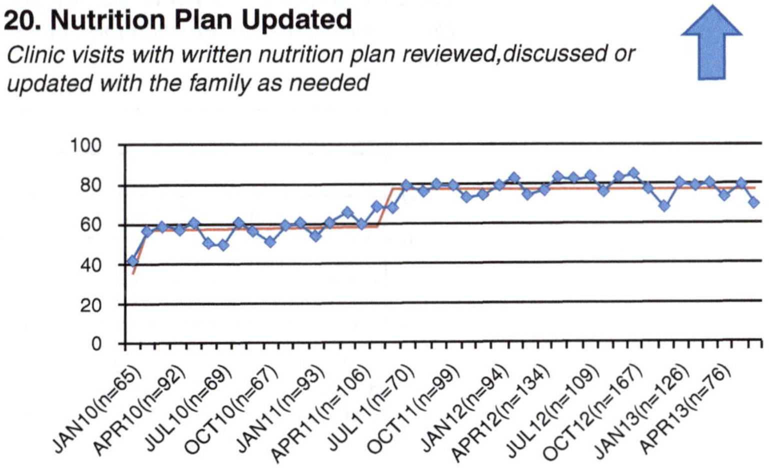

Fig. 4.5 (continued)

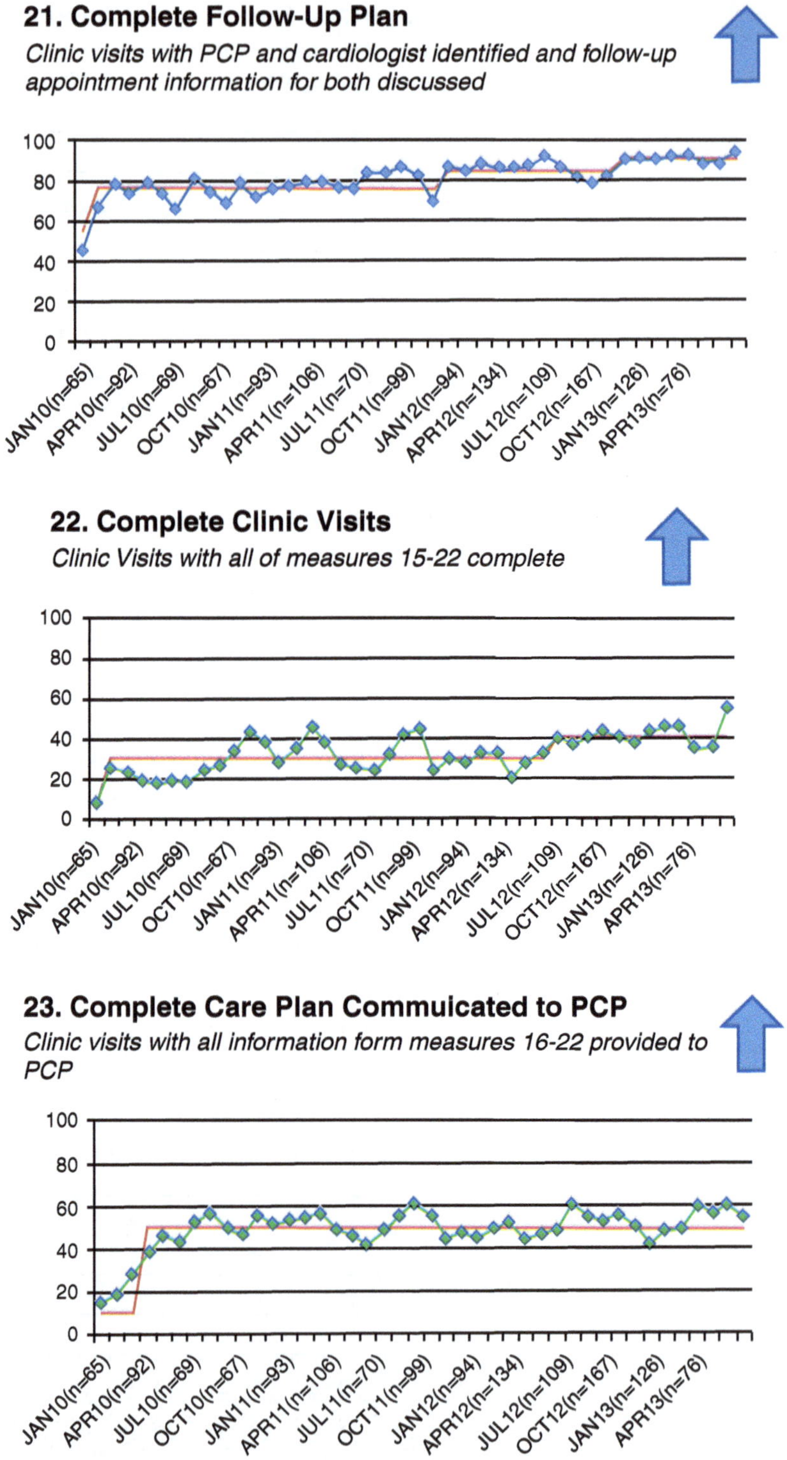

Standard evaluation of each infant prior to discharge after the Norwood procedure for any feeding dysfunction; (2) Providing families with home scales to monitor daily weight gain in the interstage phase; (3) Weekly contact with families to review interstage growth by phone/email; (4) Specific weight change "red flags" to catch growth faltering early and allow for nutritional intervention; and (5) A Dietician available for consultation, either in person or by phone, at all interstage outpatient visits. This Nutritional Bundle was provided to the NPC-QIC teams and has demonstrated great improvement in the weight and well being of these children.

The NPC-QIC brought together a Nutrition Working Group. This group comprised dieticians, nurses, speech therapists and physicians from twelve NPC-QIC sites. The Nutrition Working Group performed an extensive literature review and created algorithms for the feeding of single ventricle infants prior to Norwood, post-operatively after Norwood and in the outpatient interstage [50]. The purpose of these algorithms was to move towards reducing practice site variation by standardization of nutrition management.

Future Directions

The NPCQIC currently comprises 46 sites and includes the largest children's hospitals in the US, and *almost all programs that perform complex congenital heart surgeries*. The NPCQIC is achieving its objectives to (1) build a sustainable collaborative network of multidisciplinary pediatric cardiology teams, engaged parent partners, and scientists; and (2) use a registry to support improvement in care delivery and research projects resulting in improved survival and outcomes of infants with HLHS in the high-risk interstage. As of July 2013, the NPCQIC has amassed data from 1,000 infants in the registry, with data accrued from over 4,000 clinic visits, 1,300 readmissions and from 83 deaths.

The NPCQIC collaborative infrastructure has recently evolved to include a research subcommittee as well as a formal governance structure, consisting of seven cardiologists, five parents, a QI liaison, and three members with business expertise. Current financial support includes a 5-year grant from the Children's Heart Association of Cincinnati, participation fees from participating sites, and in-kind support for meetings from the Heart Institute of CCHMC. Previous support has included targeted project support from state and national. Grants.

The NPC-QIC has documented significant improvement in care process measures and has begun to see improvement in primary outcome measures as well. There have been single sites that have begun to show significant improvement in growth of their infants and the collaborative has seen periodic improved process measures by reducing the average time between child readmissions for major events. However, we recognize that there has been less than expected improvement in outcome measures, given the significant improvement in process measures. The collaborative has formed three multi-institution working groups in order to move to the next steps of understanding the primary outcomes including a Mortality Working Group, Readmission Working Group, and is reconvening the Nutrition Working Group. The aim of these working groups will be to determine additional information that needs to be gathered, including directly from families, define more precise metrics, and identify strategies that result in improved outcomes.

Conclusions

The National Pediatric Cardiology Quality Improvement Collaborative (NPC-QIC) is the first U.S. quality improvement collaborative in pediatric cardiology. The NPC-QIC is evolving towards the Learning Health System model described by the Institute of Medicine, in which patients, clinicians, researchers, and other stakeholders collaborate in a meaningful partnership to improve outcomes and generate new knowledge, and in which health care, health care improvement, and research are purposefully integrated [51, 52]. The NPC-QIC has successfully used a multi-site network, practice-based registry data and improvement science methodology to identify variation in management and to improve outcomes in patients with complex congenital heart disease. The NPC-QIC has seen significant improvement in process measures across participating centers and is beginning to see improvement in outcome measures. The Learning Health System model, exemplified by NPCQIC's collaborative effort, is vital to the field of pediatric cardiology, and for other clinical fields which care for patients with rare disorders [53].

References

1. Darst JR, Newburger JW, Resch S, Rathod RH, Lock JE. Deciding without data. Congenit Heart Dis. 2010;5(4):339–42.
2. Mahle WT, Spray TL, Wernovsky G, Gaynor JW, Clark 3rd BJ. Survival after reconstructive surgery for hypoplastic left heart syndrome: a 15-year experience from a single institution. Circulation. 2000;102 (19 Suppl 3):III136–41.
3. Jenkins K, Newburger J, Lock J, Davis R, Coffman G, Iezzoni L. In-hospital mortality for surgical repair of congenital heart defects: preliminary observations of variation by hospital caseload. Pediatrics. 1995;95: 323–30.
4. Stark J. Glenn lecture. How to choose a cardiac surgeon. Circulation. 1996;94(9 Suppl):II1–4.
5. Johnson B, Mussatto K, Uhing M, Zimmerman H, Tweddell J, Ghanayem N. Variability in the preoperative management of infants with hypoplastic left heart syndrome. Pediatr Cardiol. 2008;29:515–20.
6. Deming W. Out of crisis. Cambridge, MA: Massachusetts Institute of Technology, Center for Advanced Engineering Study; 1986.
7. Deming W. The new economics for industry, government, education. Cambridge, MA: Massachusetts Institute of Technology, Center for Advanced Engineering Study; 1993.
8. Institute of Medicine, Committee on Quality Health Care in America. Crossing the quality chasm – a new health system for the 21st century. Washington, DC: National Academy Press; 2001.
9. O'Connor G, Plume S, Olmstead E, et al. A regional intervention to improve the hospital mortality associated with coronary artery bypass grant surgery. The Northern New England Cardiovascular Disease Study Group. JAMA. 1996;275:841–6.
10. Simone J, Lyons J. Superior cancer survival in children compared to adults: a superior system of cancer care? Institute of Medicine: Washington, DC; 2003.
11. Bodenheimer T. Interventions to improve chronic illness care: evaluating their effectiveness. Dis Manag. 2003;6:63–71.
12. Board NCP. Childhood cancer survivorship: improving care and quality of life. Washington, DC: National Academies Press; 2003.
13. Pui C, Evans W. Acute lymphoblastic leukemia. N Engl J Med. 1998;339:605–15.
14. Hobar J, Rogowskiu J, Plsek P, et al. Collaborative quality improvement for neonatal intensive care. NIC/Q Project Investigators of the Vermont Oxford Network. Pediatrics. 2001;107:14–22.
15. Hsu DT, Zak V, Mahony L, et al. Enalapril in infants with single ventricle: results of a multicenter randomized trial. Circulation. 2010;122(4):333–40.
16. Kaltman JR, Andropoulos DB, Checchia PA, et al. Report of the pediatric heart network and national heart, lung, and blood institute working group on the perioperative management of congenital heart disease. Circulation. 2010;121(25):2766–72.
17. Ohye RG, Sleeper LA, Mahony L, et al. Comparison of shunt types in the Norwood procedure for single-ventricle lesions. N Engl J Med. 2010;362(21):1980–92.
18. Martin GR, Beekman RH, Ing FF, et al. The IMPACT registry: IMproving pediatric and adult congenital treatments. Semin Thorac Cardiovasc Surg Pediatr Card Surg Annu. 2010;13(1):20–5.
19. Billett AL, Colletti RB, Mandel KE, et al. Exemplar pediatric collaborative improvement networks: achieving results. Pediatrics. 2013;131 Suppl 4:S196–203.
20. Lannon CM, Miles PV. Pediatric collaborative improvement networks: bridging quality gaps to improve health outcomes. Pediatrics. 2013;131 Suppl 4:S187–8.
21. Malenka DJ, O'Connor GT. A regional collaborative effort for CQI in cardiovascular disease. Northern New England Cardiovascular Study Group. Jt Comm J Qual Improv. 1995;21(11):627–33.
22. Horbar JD. The Vermont Oxford Network: evidence-based quality improvement for neonatology. Pediatrics. 1999;103(1 Suppl E):350–9.
23. National Cancer Policy Board. Childhood cancer survivorship: improving care and quality of life. Washington, D.C.: National Academies Press; 2003.
24. Pui C, Evans W. Acute lymphoblastic leukemia. New Engl J Med. 1998;339:605–15.
25. Simone J, Lyons J. Superior cancer survival in children compared to adults: a superior system of cancer care? Institute of Medicine: Washington, D.C; 2003.
26. Conway P, Clancy C. Charting a path from comparative effectiveness funding to improved patient-centered health care. JAMA. 2010;303:985–6.
27. Margolis P, Provost L, Schoettker P, Britto M. Quality improvement, clinical research and quality improvement research: opportunities for integration. Pediatr Clin North Am. 2009;56(4):831–41.
28. Simpson LA, Peterson L, Lannon CM, Murphy SB, Goodman C, Ren Z, Zaijicek A. Special challenges in comparative effectiveness research on children's and adolescents' health. Health Affairs. 2010; 29(10); 1849-56.
29. American Board of Pediatrics. Maintenance of Certification (MOC) – Pediatrics. http://www.abp.org/ABPWebSite/. Accessed 15 June 2008.

30. Lannon CM, Peterson LE. Pediatric collaborative improvement networks: background and overview. Pediatrics. 2013;131 Suppl 4:S189–95.
31. Kugler JD, Beekman Iii RH, Rosenthal GL, et al. Development of a pediatric cardiology quality improvement collaborative: from inception to implementation. From the Joint Council on Congenital Heart Disease Quality Improvement Task Force. Congenit Heart Dis. 2009;4(5):318–28.
32. Pasquali SK, Jacobs JP, He X, et al. The complex relationship between center volume and outcome in patients undergoing the Norwood operation. Ann Thorac Surg. 2012;93(5):1556–62.
33. Go AS, Mozaffarian D, Roger VL, et al. Heart disease and stroke statistics–2013 update: a report from the American Heart Association. Circulation. 2013;127(1):e6–245.
34. Kogon B, Plattner C, Leong T, Simsic J, Kirshbom P, Kanter K. The bidirectional Glenn operation: a risk factor analysis for morbidity and mortality. J Thorac Cardiovasc Surg. 2008;136:1237–42.
35. Dooley K, Bishop L. Medical management of the cardiac infant and child after surgical discharge. Crit Care Nurs. 2002;25(3):98–104.
36. The breakthrough series: IHI's collaborative model for achieving breakthrough improvement. 2003; http://www.ihi.org/NR/rdonlyres/BCA88D8F-35EE-4251-BB93-E2252619A06D/0/BreakthroughSeriesWhitePaper2003.pdf. Accessed 18 May 2010.
37. Davis D, O'Brien M, Freemantle N, Wolf F, Mazmanian P, Taylor-Vaisey A. Impact of formal continuing medical education: do conferences, workshops, rounds, and other traditional continuing education activities change physician behavior ir health care outcomes? JAMA. 1999;282:867–74.
38. Davis D, Thompson M, Oxman A, Haynes R. Changing physician performance. A systematic review of the effect of continuing medical education strategies. JAMA. 1995;274:700–5.
39. Deming W. Out of crisis. Cambridge, MA: Center for Advanced Engineering Study, Massachusetts Institute of Technology; 1986.
40. Deming W. The new economics for industry, government, education. Cambridge, MA: Center for Advanced Engineering Study/Massachussets Institute of Technology; 1993.
41. Greenhalgh T, Robert G, Macfarlane F, Bate P, Kyriakidou O. Diffusion of innovations in service organizations: systematic review and recommendations. Milbank Q. 2004;82(4):581–629.
42. Kilo CM. A framework for collaborative improvement: lessons from the Institute for Healthcare Improvement's Breakthrough Series. Qual Manag Health Care. 1998;6(4):1–13.
43. Lannon C, Flower K, Duncan P, Moore K, Stuart J, Bassewitz J. The Bright Futures Training Intervention Project: implementing systems to support preventive and developmental services in practice. Pediatrics. 2008;122:e163–71.
44. Miller MR, Griswold M, Harris 2nd JM, et al. Decreasing PICU catheter-associated bloodstream infections: NACHRI's quality transformation efforts. Pediatrics. 2010;125(2):206–13.
45. Donovan EF, Lannon C, Bailit J, Rose B, Iams JD, Byczkowski T. A statewide initiative to reduce inappropriate scheduled births at 36(0/7)-38(6/7) weeks' gestation. Am J Obstet Gynecol. 2010;202(3):243 e241–248.
46. Schidlow DN, Anderson JB, Klitzner TS, et al. Variation in interstage outpatient care after the Norwood procedure: a report from the Joint Council on Congenital Heart Disease National Quality Improvement Collaborative. Congenit Heart Dis. 2011;6(2):98–107.
47. Baker-Smith CM, Neish SR, Klitzner TS, et al. Variation in postoperative care following stage I palliation for single-ventricle patients: a report from the Joint Council on Congenital Heart Disease National Quality Improvement Collaborative. Congenit Heart Dis. 2011;6(2):116–27.
48. Brown DW, Connor JA, Pigula FA, et al. Variation in preoperative and intraoperative care for first-stage palliation of single-ventricle heart disease: a report from the Joint Council on Congenital Heart Disease National Quality Improvement Collaborative. Congenit Heart Dis. 2011;6(2):108–15.
49. Anderson JB, Iyer SB, Schidlow DN, et al. Variation in growth of infants with a single ventricle. J Pediatr. 2012;161(1):16–21 e11; quiz 21 e12-13.
50. Slicker J, Hehir DA, Horsley M, et al. Nutrition algorithms for infants with hypoplastic left heart syndrome; birth through the first interstage period. Congenit Heart Dis. 2013;8(2):89–102.
51. Olsen L, Aisner D, McGinnis J. The learning healthcare system: workshop summary. Washington DC: The National Academies Press; 2007.
52. Smith M, Baigian J, Bryk A, et al. Best care at lower cost: the path to continuously learning health care in America. Washington DC: The National Academies Press; 2012.
53. Lannon CM, Miles PV, Stockman 3rd JA. The path forward: collaborative networks and the future for children's health care. Pediatrics. 2013;131 Suppl 4: S226–7.

Teams, Team Training, and the Role of Simulation

5

Paul R. Barach and Peter H. Cosman

Abstract

Many areas of acute care medicine have a low error tolerance and demand high levels of cognitive and technical performance. Growing evidence suggests that further improvements in patient outcomes depends on appreciating, measuring and improving system factors, in particular, effective team skills. In recent years, the relationship between surgical team behaviour and patient outcome has been studied by a number of researchers. Teamwork concerns the communication and coordination processes that are required to bring together the individual knowledge, skills and attitudes in the service of a common and valued team goal. Individual surgical team members are highly specialized and have their own functional taskwork (e.g., anaesthesia, nursing, surgery and perfusion), yet come together as a team towards the common goal of treating the patient. Interventions focusing on teamwork have shown a relationship with improved teamwork and safety climate. The 'working together' of a clinical microsystem is accomplished by a complex suite of 'nontechnical skills'. Teams that score low on independently observed non-technical skills make more technical errors and in cases where teams infrequently display team behaviours, patients are more likely to experience death or major complications. There is a significant correlation between subjective assessment of teamwork by team members themselves and postoperative morbidity. Good teamwork (in terms of both quality and quantity) is associated with shorter duration of operations, fewer adverse events and lower postoperative morbidity.

P.R. Barach, BSc, MD, MPH (✉)
Department of Health Management and Health Economics, University of Oslo,
Oslo 1074, Norway
e-mail: pbarach@gmail.com

P.H. Cosman, BA, MB, BS, PhD, MAICD, FRACS
Department of Surgery, St. George Private Hospital,
South St., Suite 7 L, Lvl 5, Kogarah,
NSW 2217, Australia
e-mail: peter@cosman.org

P.R. Barach, J.P. Jacobs, S.E. Lipshultz, P.C. Laussen (eds.),
Pediatric and Congenital Cardiac Care: Volume 2: Quality Improvement and Patient Safety,
DOI 10.1007/978-1-4471-6566-8_5,

Finally, this chapter addresses the importance of nurturing and sustaining team leaders. Able leaders anticipate events, prepare for them, and nurtured and grow by the effective team support and improved outcomes.

Keywords
Teams • Team training • Microsystems • Rehearsal • Debriefing • Simulation • Expert performance model • Patient safety

Introduction

The role of effective teamwork in accomplishing complex tasks is well accepted in many domains. Similarly, there is good evidence that improved outcomes in cardiac care depends on effective team performance. Teamwork during acute clinical care can be deficient in a number of different ways (Table 5.1), and multiple deficiencies may interact to impair team success and patient outcomes. This chapter focuses on understanding, assessing, and improving team performance. The need to train and evaluate the performance of clinical teams has emerged as an important topic during the past decade [1]. Deficiencies in communication and teamwork have long been cited as a frequent contributor to adverse events [2]. Conversely, team training and debriefing have been shown to reduce mortality by 18 % [3]. Precise estimates of the extent of the problem are difficult to make, given definitional issues as well as reporting and measurement problems. However, a variety of studies support the notion that teamwork and communication are critical components of safe health care systems. Previous reviews have reported linkages between various aspects of teamwork (e.g., situational monitoring, communication, leadership, trust, shared mental models) and clinical performance [4].

Teamwork requires an iterative evaluation that must include the review of the secondary management including careful delineation of team structure, thorough and ongoing team training, effective support structures, and continuous quality improvement. Valuable tools for team training and performance improvement, discussed in this chapter, include reflective learning, authentic communication, rehearsal, debriefing, simulation and videotape-based analysis.

Table 5.1 Problems and pitfalls in surgical teams

Difficulties coordinating conflicting actions
Poor communication among team members
Failure of members to function as part of a team
Reluctance to question the leader or more senior team members
Failure to prioritize task demands
Conflicting occupational cultures
Failure to establish and maintain clear roles and goals
Absence of experienced team members
Inadequate number of dedicated trauma team members
Failure to establish and maintain consistent supportive organizational infrastructure
Leaders without the "right stuff"

Modified from Schull et al. [17] and others

Role of Higher Education

Higher education methods have shifted from *providing* instruction to *facilitating* successful learning opportunities and engagement of the learner. Interactive simulation environments support learner-focused, constructivist approaches that would be unethical, inefficient, and unfeasible in actual perioperative care situations. Team training has a long history in aviation and the military, and, more recently, these experiences have been translated to health care. Studies of aviation teams reveal failures of coordination, communication, workload management, loss of group situation awareness, and inability to use available resources [5–7]. In thoroughly investigated adverse events, whether patient-or aviation-related, causes of failure were similarly multifactorial, team based, and complex [8–11].

Most of health care is performed and delivered by interdisciplinary teams – individuals with diverse specialized skills focused on a common task in a defined period of time and space, who must respond flexibly together to contingencies and share responsibility for patient outcomes. This is particularly true of cardiac surgery. Traditional specialty-centric clinical education and training are remiss because they assume that individuals acquire adequate competencies in teamwork passively without any formal training. Reviews of malpractice claims indicate that communication problems among the treating team members are major contributing factors in 24 % of cases that result in such claims [12]. Substantial evidence suggests that teams routinely outperform individuals and are required to succeed in today's complex work arenas; in these settings information, wisdom, and resources are widely distributed, technology is becoming more complicated, and workload is increasing [13]. Other studies using root cause analysis to examine contributing factors have found teamwork and communication issues cited as root causes in 2/3 of adverse events [14]. Our understanding of how medical teams coordinate in real-life situations, especially during time-constrained and crises situations, remains incomplete.

Teams and Teamwork

What Is a Team?

One must distinguish between a group of individuals sharing a common task (e.g., a jury) and a team (e.g., a marching band or a football team). A team is "a small number of people with complementary skills who are committed to a common purpose, performance goals, and approach for which they hold themselves mutually accountable" [13]. Weick and Roberts [15] defined medical teams as "a loosely coupled system of mutually interacting interdependent members and technology with a shared goal of patient care." Katzenbach and Smith [13] argued that any performance situation that warrants a team effort must meet three criteria: (1) collective work products must be delivered in real time by two or more people; (2) leadership roles must shift among the members; and (3) both mutual and individual accountability is necessary. They go on to assert that teams must have a specific team purpose (distinct from that of its individual members), shared performance goals, a commonly agreed to working approach, and, in general, make use of the team's collective work products to evaluate the team's performance. Others have suggested that smaller teams (5 to 10 members) are generally more effective than larger ones, partially because of familiarity, more cross-checking, and high interdependence of team member's roles.

There are five themes associated with effective teams (the 5 Cs [18]): Commitment, Common Goals, Competence, Consistency (of performance), and Communication. The effective team is committed to the achievement of specified goals. Team competence is measured across multiple dimensions and includes technical, decision, and interpersonal skills. The diversity of team members with complementary skills is a hallmark of many effective teams, particularly when the team is required to adapt to complex and changing circumstances. Acute-care medical teams, including trauma teams, typically excel at the first two Cs (i.e., commitment and common goal) and explicitly strive for competence, but may be much less successful in their consistency of performance (i.e., ability to sustain best practice reliably at all times), and effectiveness of communication between team members [16]. The very best trauma teams maintain an intuitive understanding and situational awareness of the evolving processes of events (see discussion below of distributed team situation awareness), appreciate and expect the unknown, and exhibit a high level of trust and respect between members [19].

Importance of Conflict

Conflicts among members are inevitable in every team, and many experts believe that conflict *and its successful resolution*, is essential to attaining maximal team performance [17, 20]. Without resolving these conflicts, trust cannot grow and thus accountability for improvement will be lacking [21]. The natural tendency of teams, especially among health care professionals, is to avoid or gloss over conflicts. However, doing so may sew the seeds of impaired team performance when the next challenge arises. There are four primary conflicts inherent in teamwork [22]. First, there are tensions between individuals and the team as a whole in terms of goals, agenda, and the need to establish an identity. Second, to attain optimal team performance, one needs to foster both support and confrontation among team members. If team members are unwilling or unable to challenge each other's decisions respectfully, then there is a real risk of poor team outcomes – a team devoid of conflict leads to "group think" [23] and the acceptance of suboptimal team decisions. Third, daily team activities must balance moment-to-moment performance against the need to continually enhance team learning and individual member development. Finally, the team leader must strike a balance between managerial authority, on the one hand, and individual team member autonomy and independence, on the other.

Teamwork Training in the Medical Domain

Surgical team performance is one of the most complex in health care and is centred around ill patients, a large and diverse range of health care providers, sophisticated equipment, and severe time constraints [24]. The cardiac team, which assembles rapidly at unpredictable times, must attempt to manage a sudden unique and chaotic situation such as acute bleeding, ruptured graft, etc. involving one or more patients presenting with complex underlying physiology.

The successful management of complex congenital malformations requires effectively coordinated prehospital care and information management followed by transfer to a well-organized and well-prepared dedicated healthcare facility. During the resuscitation, the team typically adheres to hospital protocols based on Advanced Cardiac Life Support (ACLS) principles. In most modern surgical teams, multiple team members have dedicated roles and simultaneously perform individual patient care tasks [25, 26]. While more efficient, and leading to more rapid resuscitation, this kind of horizontal structure requires team coordination, leadership, and organizational structure [27]. Studies in advanced trauma units have highlighted the difficulties of attaining effective teamwork, noting team breakdowns under dynamic and distracting conditions. Cardiac surgical teams typically consist of five to ten individuals from several clinical disciplines [28].

Medical teams, often consisting of a multidisciplinary group of members, might come together for a single clinical event (e.g., a specific surgical procedure) or be together for a short defined period (typically a month or so). Not infrequently, some team members are consistent and well defined (e.g., the intensive care unit team) while others join on an ad hoc or an as needed basis (e.g., respiratory therapists, nurses, pharmacists, anesthesiologists). Thus, a specific group of individuals do not have the opportunity to work together and develop trust and shared mental models, as a fixed team for long periods of time. Further, cardiac surgical care is often provided in academic medical centers where the trainees who make up much of the surgical team rotate on and off the team on a regular basis, which can lead to inconsistent care and awkward and ambiguous communication. Research in aviation shows that non-"rostered teams" are less effective than more stable "fixed" teams [29]. Additionally, Simon, et al. [30] have shown that rostered teams are less likely than *ad hoc* formed teams to call each other out when safety infractions occur, but, are more resilient and have better outcomes than non-rostered team when challenged.

The Team Leader

The team leader's functions may include the performance of specific tasks such as the conduct of the primary and secondary surveys (Table 5.2).

However, given sufficient personnel, the team leader must assume, as quickly as possible, a supervisory role, prioritizing and delegating tasks, and reviewing and overseeing the team's (and patient's) progress throughout the resuscitation [31]. Studies suggest that teams are less effective when the team leader spends significant time performing procedures than when delegating them to other team members and not maintaining feed forward abilities. However, the team leader should have recognized expertise in treating patients and be willing and able to intercede when other team members are not performing up to acceptable standards or the patient deteriorates.

The cardiac surgery team leader is also responsible for formulating (or at least approving) the definitive treatment plan. Thus, the team leader must quickly assimilate a large amount of disparate information from other team members with his/her own observations. This leads to an overall assessment, which includes decisions about therapeutic and diagnostic interventions, communicating with other team members, coordinating consultations, making triage decisions, and ensuring that all team members are aware of the evolving situation [32].

Although skill and experience are valuable for every member of the team, it is particularly critical for the team leader. Additionally, the personality of the team leader has a large impact on team performance. Work by Chidester and colleagues [33] led to a broad classification of three personality types of team leaders: "right stuff," "wrong stuff," and "no stuff" (Table 5.3). Teams led by individuals with the "right stuff" performed better than others. Team-oriented behaviors do not come naturally in a culture that rewards individualism above teamwork, but they can be learned and practiced with regular feedback and coaching.

Table 5.2 The team leader's responsibilities

Know the job (e.g., know guidelines expertly).
Communicate clearly and effectively, and enhance the team's communication.
Foster teamwork attitudes through tangible behaviors.
Keep the goals and approach relevant and focused.
Enhance the team's knowledge and shared expectations.
Build commitment, confidence, and trust.
Remain positive and supportive, especially under adverse conditions.
Acknowledge and manage your own limitations, and those of the team.
Strengthen the skills of each team member, and of the team as a whole across all performance dimensions: technical, functional, problem solving, decision making, interpersonal, and teamwork.
Manage relationships with outsiders and remove obstacles.
Create opportunities for others to grow into leadership roles.
Lead by example.
Reward team performance and discourage individualism that detracts from team performance.
Provide constructive feedback and opportunities for reflection.

Modified from Cooper and Wakelam [27] and others

Acquiring Expertise in the Cardiac Surgery Setting

Data from over 100 surgical root cause analysis (RCA) investigations demonstrated a number of themes that are relevant in understanding why and how surgical care can go wrong [14]. These themes (Table 5.4) represent a mixture of the outcomes of clinical care (e.g., procedural complications), and explanations relating to problems in the clinical environment (e.g., skill mix of the surgical team, and missed diagnoses).

Expert Performance Approach

The expert performance approach offers a systematic framework for examining issues related to improving patient safety [34]. It is based on an

Table 5.3 Team leader personality types

"Right Stuff"	"Wrong Stuff"	"No Stuff"
Active	Authoritarian	Unassertive
Self-confident	Arrogant	Low self-confidence
Interpersonal warmth/empathy	Limited warmth/empathy	Moderate warmth/empathy
Competitive	Impatient and irritable	Noncompetitive
Prefers challenging tasks	Prefers challenging tasks	Low desire for challenge
Strives for excellence	Strives for excellence	Doesn't strive for excellence

Modified from the work of Foushee and Helmreich [5]

Table 5.4 Themes and issues identified from surgical adverse outcomes and their related Root Cause Analysis (RCA) investigations

Theme	Issues identified
Failure to recognize or respond appropriately to the deteriorating patient within the required timeframe	Post procedure complications Infections Hypothermia
Workforce availability and skills	Orientation, training and supervision of new or junior members of the surgical team, especially outside of normal working hours
Transfer of patients for surgery	Difficulty in organizing an OR for surgery Failure to handover information about patient acuity
The management of trauma	Coordination and response of trauma teams Clinical decision making process for trauma patients Coordination of care between multiple clinicians
Access to emergency operating room	Hemorrhage and emergency bleeding Urgent orthopedic procedure Urological complications requiring urgent OR
Missed diagnosis	Thoraco-lumbar fracture in a trauma patient Sub arachnoid hemorrhage thought to be drug overdose
Unexpected procedural complications	Airway obstruction Failed intubation
Sentinel events	Wrong level procedure – chest tube thoracostomy at wrong level Retained surgical products requiring surgical removal

Source: The analysis is derived from a metropolitan health service, Sydney, NSW, Australia. Personal communication, Deputy Director for Clinical Governance, January 2007

analysis of health provider superior performance and traces the acquired processes responsible for the development of high level skills. The focus on measurable performance avoids documented shortcomings of traditional methods of identifying and studying experts, such as those based on the accumulation of knowledge, experience and/or peer nomination. The expert-performance approach proposes that learning, and improvement in performance, are not merely a passive accumulation of professional experience. Such gains are mediated by user engagement in goal-directed, self-regulated learning in a way that is quantitatively and qualitatively different from the mere accumulation of experiences [35].

Research shows that experienced and knowledgeable individuals do not always outperform naïve individuals [36]. Highly experienced financial, medical, and psychology professionals often fail to make superior forecasts or implement interventions that lead to enhanced treatment outcomes when compared with less-qualified and less-experienced professionals. Experts are typically identified on the basis of peer nomination, the degree of knowledge each seemingly possess, or their length of experience within the domain. In medicine, researchers have reported that the length of professional experience is often unrelated, and sometimes negatively related, to the quality of performance and treatment outcomes [37]. Ericsson and Smith [38] suggest that researchers interested in studying expertise should focus on trying to empirically capture performance with reliable and objective measures. They recommend a three-step approach known as the *expert performance approach.*

First, researchers must recreate the task(s) in the laboratory with sufficient fidelity to elicit the requisite expertise. Second, the antecedents of, and processes responsible for, superior performance should be identified using experimental manipulations and process tracing measures. Third, activities that lead to a performance improvement need to be identified so that the path to excellence is clearly delineated and is targeted for training and improvement [39]. Statistical process control (SPC) may be a useful tool in identifying individual clinicians and teams displaying higher levels of performance using longitudinal outcome measures.

In the 1980s, researchers began to study the way experienced people make decisions in their natural environments or in simulations that preserve key aspects of their environments called the (naturalistic decision theory) [40]. These studies showed that, in contrast to "normative decision theory," experts make real-world decisions through a serial evaluation and application ("trying on") of options that seem appropriate to the apparent situation in an iterative and rapid cycle. Naturalistic decision making (NDM) theory argues that, especially under time pressure in complex task domains (e.g., flight landing, surgical OR care), experts recognize patterns of events in situations, or their integral components, as typical or familiar, and then respond to each specific situation with appropriate pre-programmed, patterned responses. Choosing the first acceptable response that comes to them is called "recognition-primed decision making" [40, 41]. Thus, competent decision makers in complex domains are very concerned about quickly assessing and maintaining awareness of the current clinical situation.

Expertise is more than simply having extensive factual knowledge – it also includes the complementary skills, attitudes and the ability to deploy these skills in timely, measured and precise manner. Experts have specific psychologic traits (e.g., self-confidence, excellent communication skills, adaptability, risk tolerance) and cognitive skills (e.g., highly developed attention, sense of what is relevant, ability to identify exceptions to the rules, flexibility to changing situations, effective performance under stress, and ability to make decisions and initiate actions quickly based on incomplete data). Clinical experts use highly refined decision strategies such as dynamic feedback, decomposing and analyzing complex problems, and pre-thinking solutions to tough situations [42].

A key attribute of expertise in cardiac care is the ability to anticipate or to predict what might happen to a patient given his underlying pathology and the resources available. Mental simulation including rehearsal, whereby individuals *or teams* envision (simulate) a possible future clinical event or clinical action before it happens, is essential to gaining the expertise to make diagnoses and to perform or function during an evolving or future real event [43]. When expert clinicians simulate situations and actions mentally before they undertake them in real life, the evidence in this review suggests that they save time and improve performance in crucial situations (see simulation section below).

Human Factors and the Environment of Care

Human factors research on team decision-making in complex task environments is of relevance to cardiac team performance. One must carefully consider the impact of the many "performance shaping factors" that can shape and degrade cardiac surgical outcomes (Table 5.5).

Situation Awareness

One of the most important skills in cardiac surgical care is to decide what to devote attention to and what can wait. Where data overload is the rule and the patient's status changes continually, the ability to recognize clinical cues quickly and completely, detect patterns, and set aside distracting or unimportant data can be life saving. Situation awareness (or situation assessment) is a comprehensive and coherent representation of the (patient's) current state that is continuously updated based on repetitive assessment [44].

Situation awareness appears to be an essential prerequisite for safe operation of any complex dynamic system. In the case of cardiac surgical care, establishing and maintaining a "mental model" of the patient's overall situation and the associated OR/intensive care unit (ICU) facilities, equipment, and personnel are essential for developing effective situational awareness. Successful team situation awareness requiring constant communication enables members to converge around a shared mental model of the situation and course of action [45]. Effective teams adapt to changes in task requirements, anticipate each other's actions and needs, monitor the team's ongoing performance, and offer constructive feedback to other team members [46]. When team members share a common mental model of the team's ongoing activities, each may "instinctively"

Table 5.5 Performance shaping factors affecting surgical care

Performance shaping factor	Example
Individual factors	Clinical knowledge, skills, and abilities
	Cognitive biases
	Risk preference
	State of health
	Fatigue (including sleep deprivation, circadian)
Task factors	Task distribution
	Task demands
	Workload
	Job burnout
	Shiftwork
Team/communication	Teamwork/team dynamics
	Interpersonal communication (clinician–clinician and clinician – patient)
	Interpersonal influence
	Groupthink
Environment of care	Noise
	Lighting
	Temperature and humidity
	Motion and vibration
	Physical constraints (e.g., crowding)
	Distractions
Equipment/tools	Device usability
	Alarms and warnings
	Automation
	Maintenance and obsolescence
	Protective gear
Organizational/cultural	Production pressure
	Culture of safety (vs. efficiency)
	Policies Procedures Documentation requirements
	Staffing Cross coverage
	Hierarchical structure
	Reimbursement policies
	Training programs

know what each of their teammates will do next (and why), and often communicate their intentions and needs non-verbally (sometimes called implicit communication).

A Systematic Approach to the Evaluation of Teamwork Training

Assessing team performance is key to understanding methods to improve the team performance and increase the safety of patient outcomes (Table 5.6).

There is an ongoing argument in the literature that team *process* and *outcomes* must be distinguished [47]. Processes are defined by the activities, strategies, responses, and behaviors employed by the team during task accomplishment, while outcomes, are the clinical outcomes of the patients cared for by the team. Process measures are important for training when the purpose of performance measurement is to diagnose performance problems and to provide feedback to trainees. Until recently, the medical community has focused more on outcomes than on process measures. Medical educators have begun to appreciate the competencies that define

Table 5.6 Questions to ask when assessing surgical team performance

Is the team the right size and composition?
Are there adequate levels of complementary skills?
Is there a shared goal for the team?
Does everyone understand the team goals?
Has a set of performance goals been agreed upon?
Do the team members hold one another accountable for the group's results?
Are there shared protocols and performance ground rules?
Is there mutual respect and trust between team members?
Does the team leader instill trust and mutual respect by the team members?
Do team members communicate effectively?
Do team members know and appreciate each other's roles and responsibilities?
When one team member is absent or not able to perform their assigned tasks, are other team members able to pitch in or help appropriately?

effective team processes [48]. The key is to identify and measure processes that are directly related to patient outcomes (e.g., successful resuscitation). Perhaps most importantly, the results of the assessment must be translatable into specific feedback about technical or non-technical issues that can enhance the team's performance in achieving a safe outcome [49].

There are a variety of methods to support the team's reflection and evaluation of their team performance including debriefing with or without the use of videotaping, simulation with or without standardized patients, and the use of trained observers. Although metrics are available in non-medical domains, there are few well-defined validated metrics to assess competency in complex clinical team activities such as resuscitation. No rigorous evaluation studies have been undertaken that relate the training experience with actual clinical outcomes thereby validating metrics for assessing team performance.

Simulations that use pre-scripted learner-focused scenarios not only ensure that relevant competencies are being assessed, but also ease the assessment process because instructors know when key events will occur [50]. Evaluation, both formative and summative, must provide a basis for diagnosing skill deficiencies. In other words, it is not enough that a simulation captures performance outcomes; it must also evaluate the process of moment-to-moment actions and reactions to help better design effective care.

Video-Analysis of Surgical Care

Videotaping of surgical team performance can be a tremendously valuable training tool because it addresses factual challenges, helps trainees clearly visualize the event, and can be used as a permanent record or as an archive for future educational activities. Beginning with the experience of Hoyt et al. in the late 1980s [51], videotaping and review of resuscitations has become a standard quality assurance method for many trauma centers. Subsequent work has confirmed benefits from improved team education and training, more efficient and accurate quality assurance (QA) processes, interventions to improve care processes, and better patient survival [33, 52]. In a study of simulated anesthetic crises, trainees' review of their performance on videotapes of the events led to a decrease in "time to treat" and workload in subsequent simulations [53]. Scherer et al. [54] found that video-based feedback of trauma resuscitations reduced patient disposition time by 50 %.

However, videotaping of patient care requires overcoming substantial obstacles including medicolegal, confidentiality, logistical and resource issues, and analytical limitations [55, 56]. Nevertheless, the ability of multiple instructors to score performance from videotape allows the evaluation of the inter-rater reliability of performance assessment metrics. In a simulation-based study, investigators used videotape to develop and assess a systematic rating system of behavioral and clinical markers with the objective of creating effective team-training and assessment programs with high correlation among different observers [57].

Simulation for Team Training and Assessment

There are substantial ethical and educational limitations to the use of patients for the clinical training of individuals and teams. The opportunities to learn and practice desired responses to uncommon events or types of injuries can be quite limited, even in a busy medical center. In fact, actual surgical resuscitations such as massive bleeding, air embolism and acute tamponade are not optimal training opportunities because patient care takes precedence over teaching. Meaningful learning occurs after events when there is time to reflect and review events of the care, and examine what worked well and what could have been improved. Moreover, many cardiac surgical emergencies occur in an uncontrolled environment under time pressure constraints. Societal and regulatory pressures will increasingly limit the use of real patients, especially critically ill ones, for hands-on clinical training. High-fidelity patient simulators allow educators to provide repeatable, controlled clinical scenarios, affording individuals and teams the freedom to fail without jeopardising patient health [58]. The simulation environment allows concurrent assessment of response processes while increasing competency training. Simulation training enables trainees to become proficient before treating patients [59]. The fidelity offered by simulators provides the best approximation of the novelty that may be encountered when performing other complicated clinical procedures *in situ*. Although access to simulation tools and approaches is rapidly expanding, there is no general agreement about what is optimal process, device specifications, metrics to evaluate curricula or their effectiveness, standardized performance measures, or validated protocols for training.

Inroads have recently been made in this area with the development of frameworks such as Non-Technical Skills for Surgeons (NoTSS) [60], Anaesthetic Non-Technical Skills (ANTS) [61], and Scrub Practitioners List of Intra-Operative Non-Technical Skills (SPLINTS), which allow a common taxonomy and framework with which to develop process measures in the teamwork domain within the operating suite environment, and which may carry over to other settings [62]. It is important to note that these are observational frameworks, designed to be used to measure observed behaviours in the operating room. They do not establish standards of performance, and are not specifically intended for use in a training environment, although may provide useful measures in some simulation scenarios.

Table 5.7 Essential skills in surgical crew resource management courses

Adaptability
Prioritization of tasks
Shared situation awareness and distribution of the workload
Team communication before and after patient arrival
Mobilization and use of all resources in the trauma care that extends to the operating room, intensive care unit, and diagnostic facilities
Performance monitoring and cross-checking of data and team functions
Command, communication, and coordination of feedback
Leadership and management of the team members ability to accept leadership
Willingness to challenge each other and resolve conflict

Adapted from [62, 65]

Simulation has been widely touted as a tool to improve clinical care through enhanced training and evaluation. Simulations can include patient actors (e.g., standardized patients [63]), PC-based partial task trainers [59], or full-scale realistic patient simulation [58] (discussed below). Simulation is an essential training tool in almost every other high-risk domain including aviation, space flight, military operations, nuclear and hydroelectric power generation, ground and sea transportation, and chemical process control [64].

There are many benefits to be obtained from medical simulation and crew resource management (Table 5.7).

Simulations can permit clinicians to learn new or improve old techniques safely and economically without posing harm to patients or to trainees [58, 65]. Simulations can be controlled and modulated according to a team's needs [66]. Decision-making skills can be embedded into the scenario to train for reasoning, meta-cognition, risk assessment skills, and responsiveness to adverse events [67]. Guided practice with video-based feedback that incorporates measures of performance can be considered managed experience [68]. Lessons taught in a realistic simulation environment may be *retained better*, due to ability to review events again and again, active learning and focused concentration, and direct association with real-world clinical events. Thus, surgical teams using simulation can train, evaluate, and credential providers before letting them join clinical activities.

The literature has begun to provide evidence for the value of realistic patient simulation (RPS) to train and evaluate trauma teams [69]. A study by Holcomb et al. [70] evaluated ten teams of three-trainees before and after a 1-month trauma center rotation using RPS scenarios. The teams showed significant improvement on multiple measures of technical and non-technical skills, supporting the face validity of RPS-based technical performance assessment. Lee et al. [71] conducted a prospective randomized, controlled trial of surgical interns' trauma assessment and management skills after using either RPS or moulage practice training sessions. RPS-trained interns scored higher on trauma assessment skills and on the management of an acute neurologic event.

Procedural Rehearsal and Warm Up

Rehearsal and warm-up aim to improve both the operator and team performance by improving the manual dexterity, mental agility, confidence, communication and workflow. Rehearsal is considered the practice of technical and non-technical skills specific to a procedure, while warm-up is defined as 'the act or process of warming up for a contest, by light exercise or practice' [72]. In healthcare, warm-up may be considered the practice of motor or mental exercises not specific to a procedure, when undertaken immediately prior to the task being performed. For example, the use of a high-fidelity simulator by the operator, prior to performing a coronary artery angiogram, to place virtual stents is considered rehearsal; while, practicing manual dexterity skills using a low-fidelity simulator prior to arterial cannulation is considered a warm-up. Rehearsal and warm-up are gaining increasing recognition, as important processes in enhancing team performance and improving patient safety, whether for acquiring competencies or maintaining procedural and technical proficiency [73–75].

Realistic Patient Simulation

Realistic patient simulators are fully interactive physical simulations in which the device's responses to clinical interventions are scripted to be realistic. In the highest-fidelity simulators, the mannequin's response is based on detailed physiologic and pharmacologic computer models. The goal is for the simulator to respond to clinical interventions similar to how a patient would respond. Thus, the participant interacts with a realistic cognitive and physical representation of the full acute-care environment and thereby experiences emotional and physiologic responses similar to those experienced in real patient-care situations [76]. Realistic patient simulators consist of a computer-controlled system and a plastic patient mannequin that generates physiologic signals such as electrocardiogram, invasive and noninvasive blood pressure, lung sounds, and palpable pulses, which allows for realistic airway management [58, 76]. The mannequin's head contains a speaker so that the participant can converse with the patient when contextually appropriate. Participants can query the operator as needed concerning physical signs not reproduced by the mannequin, such as skin color and diaphoresis. There are multiple technical, financial, and methodologic issues that affect the design and implementation of realistic patient simulation-based training programs [64, 77]. Nonetheless, patient simulators have facilitated study of the response to critical incidents, the occurrence of medical error, the role of teamwork, and the effects of other factors on clinical performance.

Scenario Design

Oser and colleagues [78] have outlined specific steps for developing simulated scenarios for eliciting team behaviors. First, skill inventories and historical performance data are reviewed to identify *what* needs to be measured (cognitive task analysis). Identifying the core measurement objectives builds content validity into the scenario. Second, scenario events are created that provide specific reproducible opportunities to observe performance related to the objectives chosen. Third, performance measures are developed that accurately and reliably assess performance of the objectives. Measures should have the ability to describe what happened (i.e., outcome measures) in addition to describing *why* certain outcomes were or were not attained (i.e., process measures).

Setting Up the Training Program

A typical simulation-based training course will include a pretest, preparatory didactics (lecture, web, or hands-on demonstrations), the performance of one or more standardized scripted scenario(s) that are videotaped, postsimulation videotape-based debriefing, and a post training evaluation of both the trainee and the training experience. The debriefing is the most important experience, especially when doing multidisciplinary team training [79]. Debriefing should occur immediately after each simulation scenario and not uncommonly can last longer than the scenario itself [80].

Organizational Environment – The Role of Clinical Microsystems

Teams exist within the context of a system. A system is a set of interacting, interrelated, or independent elements that work together in a particular environment to perform the functions that are required to achieve a specific aim [81]. A clinical microsystem is a group of clinicians and staff working together with a shared clinical purpose to provide care for a population of patients [82]. The clinical purpose and its setting define the essential components of the microsystem, which include clinicians, patients, and support staff; information and technology; and specific care processes and behaviors that are required to provide care. The best microsystems evolve over time, as they respond to the needs of their patients and providers, as well as to the external pressures such as regulatory requirements. They often coexist with other microsystems within a larger (macro) organization, such as a hospital [83].

The conceptual theory of the clinical microsystem is based on ideas developed by Deming [84] and others. Deming applied systems thinking to organizational development, leadership, and improvement. The seminal idea for the clinical microsystem stems from the work of James Quinn [85]. Quinn's work is based on analyzing the world's best-of-best service organizations, such as FedEx, Mary Kay Cosmetics, McDonald's, and Nordstrom. Quinn focused on determining what these extraordinary organizations were doing to achieve consistent, high quality, explosive growth, high margins, and robust consumer loyalty. He found that these leading service organizations organized around, and continually engineered, the front-line relationships that connected the needs of customers with the organization's core competency. Quinn called this front-line activity that embedded the service delivery process the *smallest replicable unit* or the *minimum replicable unit*. This smallest replicable unit, or the microsystem, is the key to implementing effective strategy, information technology, and safe practices.

Nelson and his colleagues [86] have described the essential elements of a microsystem as (1) a core team of health care professionals; (2) a defined population they care for; (3) an information environment to support the work of caregivers and patients; and (4) support staff, equipment, and work environment. Linking performance and outcome data to the microsystem model provides a helpful way to identify potential areas for improvement that does not focus on the individual, but instead on the system that is producing the processes and outcomes of care [83, 87].

In the late 1990s, Donaldson and Mohr investigated high-performing clinical microsystems [88]. The research was based on a national search for the highest-quality clinical microsystems. Forty-three clinical units were identified using a sampling methodology. Semi-structured interviews were conducted with leaders from each of the microsystems. Additional research built on the Donaldson and Mohr study in which 20 case studies of high-performing microsystems were collected and included on-site interviews with every member of the microsystem and analysis of individual microsystem performance data [89]. The analysis of the interviews suggested that ten dimensions, shown in Table 5.8, were associated with effective and successful microsystems.

Table 5.8 Ten dimensions of clinical microsystems

1. Leadership
2. Organizational support of clinicians
3. Staff focus
4. Education and training
5. Interdependence of team members
6. Patient focus
7. Community and market focus
8. Performance results
9. Process improvement
10. Information and information technology

Teamwork Protocols and Patient Transitions

The most common factor cited as causing failures in teamwork is lack of effective and meaningful communication. One issue that deserves investigation is the extent to which standardized communication protocols, similar to those used in military and aviation environments, can enhance teamwork and improve patient safety. In observations focused on handoffs from the intraoperative to postoperative team [90], as well as intensive care unit (ICU) handoffs from operating room team members [91], there was no constancy in the information that was transferred nor in the order in which it was transferred. The result was that important information was sometimes omitted [92]. Recipients did not detect the missing information because they did not have the scaffolding that a standard briefing protocol with an expected set of parameters would provide. Recent papers on the power of the surgical checklists to reduce several intraoperative adverse events reinforce this point [93]. Issues raised by these studies include the need for organizing research into the types of errors that providers are susceptible to during the sign-out process, roles of personality, experience, and cultural factors, particularly as they may affect the incoming provider's inquisitiveness, and the potential impact on patient care of various methods of signing out. A standardized handoff protocol could decrease the cognitive burden on the recipients of the information [94, 95].

However, what has become clear, is that the manner a checklist is implemented and overseen can contribute to the tool's uptake and compliance by clinicians. [96]. Genuine engagement by physicians is critical to the adoption of new care models. Ineffective top-down engagement and inauthentic partnering with clinicians inhibits positive behavior change and encourages normalized deviance [97, 98].

Introducing a checklist in an environment characterized by a lack of trust may cause clinicians to feel jeopardized professionally and personally, and encourages gaming. This may explain the inordinate checklist compliance numbers in the study. Surgical checklist implementation is likely to be optimized when used as a tool in a multifaceted cultural program to strengthen patient safety and drive improvement [99]. It cannot be assumed that the introduction of a checklist will automatically lead to improved communication and clinical processes. We are reminded of Drucker's apt aphorism "culture eats strategy for breakfast" [100].

Organizational Environment

In complex organizations and environments, teams do not exist in isolation. The performance of individual teams, as well as the team's attitudes toward patient safety, is a function of the milieu, or the culture, in which the team works. Thus, the effectiveness of any particular team cannot be properly assessed without considering the larger system within which the team functions. In a hospital environment, small teams, such as operating teams, coordinate with other teams within the perioperative microsystem environment that are involved in patient care, and these teams are embedded within larger teams that are directly and indirectly involved in patient care. When looking at the effectiveness of teamwork training for patient safety, it is critical to appreciate how training is supported and reinforced by the organization in which it occurs.

Factors that need to be addressed include [90]:

- Organizational climate: Does the organizational culture support striving for patient safety? Does it allow for nonpunitive reporting of problems and near misses?
- Organizational support: Is time for training provided whereby trainees are temporarily

relieved of their regular duties? Is training viewed as more than just a necessary checkmark? Is teamwork training widespread and rewarded across the organization?
- Extent of training. Does the organization only train isolated teams? Does the training of perioperative teams incorporate the "wider" perioperative team (e.g., including for example, blood bank, radiology)?

Training Approach and Quality

There are a number of factors that impact on the effectiveness of team training, including:
- Training protocol: How is training achieved? What methods are used to impart knowledge? How are practice and feedback incorporated into training?
- Trainer skill: Is the individual who is in charge of leading the training and providing feedback adequately trained?
- Practice medium and method: How is practice carried out? What simulation environment is used (i.e., mannequin, virtual, video)? How much practice is given? It is possible that a teamwork training program that does not yield improvements in teamwork may be pedagogically sound, but may require more opportunities for practice and feedback in order to show quantitatively detectable improvements?
- Training intensity: Is it more effective to conduct training over a short time period (e.g., 1–2 days) or to conduct training over a longer time period (e.g., 2–3 h per week for several weeks)? Which is less disruptive for the trainees and for the system in which they work?

TeamSTEPPS Team Training Program[1]

Team Strategies and Tools to Enhance Performance and Patient Safety (TeamSTEPPS™) is a systematic approach developed by the Department of Defense (DoD) and the Agency for Healthcare Research and Quality (AHRQ) to integrate teamwork into practice. It is designed to improve the quality, safety, and the efficiency of health care. TeamSTEPPS is based on 25 years of research related to teamwork, team training, and culture change. As a direct outcome of the 1999 Institute of Medicine (IOM) report, *To Err is Human*, TeamSTEPPS introduced tools and strategies to improve team performance in health care.

The teamwork competencies presented and their research basis served as the foundation for TeamSTEPPS. With that information as a starting point, the goal of AHRQ and DoD was to take this academically oriented information and convert it to a framework that was meaningful from an instructional standpoint. Yet, it is difficult to directly train the skill of adaptability/flexibility, which is required when responding to unpredictable situations teams may encounter. Therefore, TeamSTEPPS instructs team members to monitor the performance of others and provide assistance, plan and organize team roles, and communicate with one another efficiently and effectively [48]. Combined, these skills can yield a highly adaptable and flexible team.

To develop the TeamSTEPPS instructional model, teamwork competencies from the literature were classified as trainable or as competencies that are the result of employing these trainable skills (i.e., outcomes). For example, shared mental models were viewed as an outcome of using monitoring and back-up behaviors [102]. The resulting TeamSTEPPS instructional framework is presented in Fig. 9, where the core competencies include the trainable skills of leadership, situation monitoring (mutual performance monitoring), mutual support (backup behavior), and communication. Performance, knowledge, and attitudinal outcomes are then depicted in the corners, resulting from proficiency on the central skills or core competencies [103].

Course Description

The TeamSTEPPS curriculum (Fig. 5.1) contains an introductory module relating to the history of team training. Four didactic-based modules discuss the core competencies/skills:

[1] This section is based on references [4, 32, 48, 101–105].

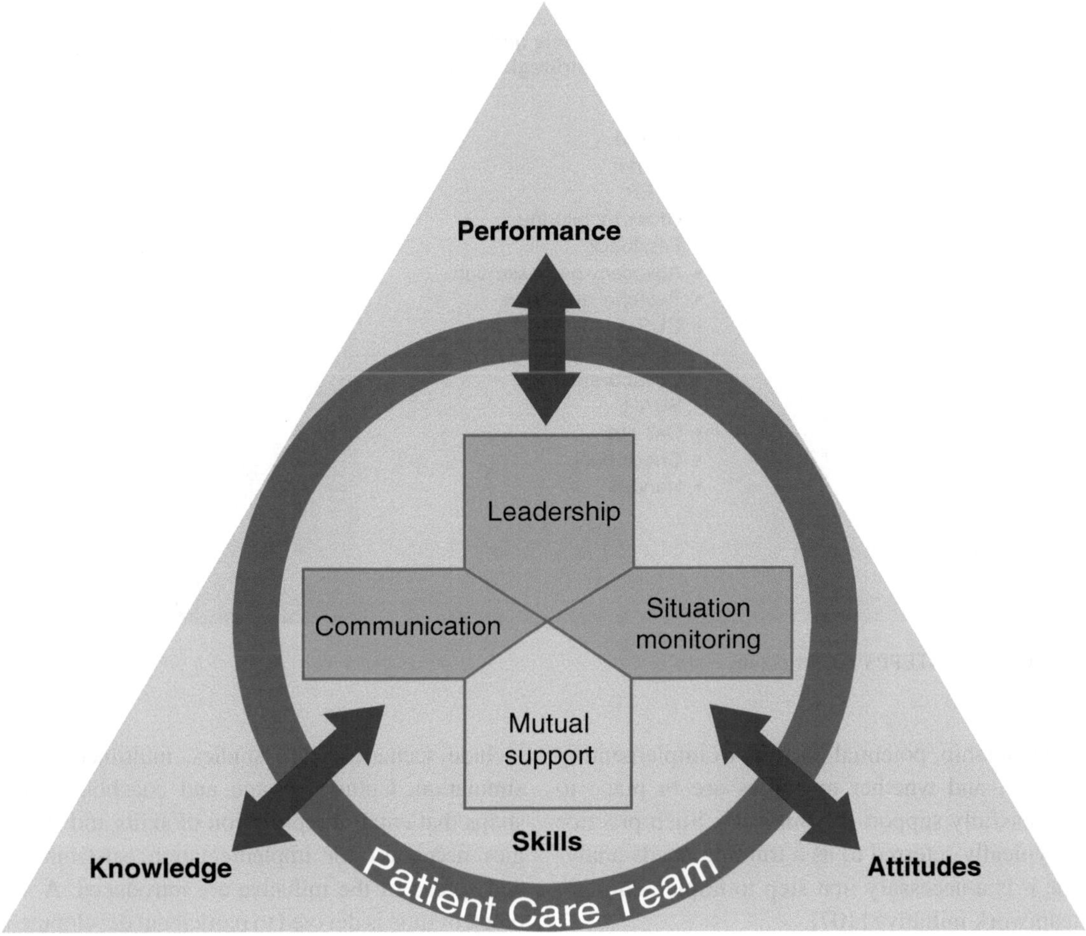

Fig. 5.1 TeamSTEPPS model

The curriculum includes modules on Leadership, Situation monitoring, Mutual support, and most importantly, Communication [103]. Emphasis is placed on defining team skills, demonstrating the tools and strategies team members can use to gain proficiency in the competencies/skills, and identification of tools and strategies that can be used to overcome common barriers to achieve desired outcomes [104]. Specialty case scenarios and video vignettes are used to further reinforce the learning [105].

The Delivery System

The TeamSTEPPS initiative also includes several sessions devoted to Implementation, a multiphase process based on John Kotter's model of organizational change [106]. A successful TeamSTEPPS Initiative requires a carefully developed implementation and sustainment plan that is captured in Figure 5.2.

Phase I: Assessment – Set the Stage

The goal of Phase I is to determine organizational readiness for undertaking a TeamSTEPPS initiative. During the pre-training assessment of Phase I, the organization or work unit identifies leaders and key champions that will make up the organization-level change team. The role of this organization-level change team is to identify specific opportunities for improvement that can be realized by employing a teamwork initiative. A site assessment is conducted to determine the readiness of the institution to include vital support

Barriers	Tools and Strategies	Outcomes
• Inconsistency in team membership	• Brief	• Shared mental model
• Lack of time	• Huddle	• Adaptability
• Lack of information sharing	• Debrief	• Team orientation
• Hierarchy	• STEP	• Mutual trust
• Defensiveness	• Cross monitoring	• Team performance
• Conventional thinking	• Feedback	• *Patient safety!!*
• Complacency	• Advocacy and assertion	
• Varying communication Styles	• Two-challenge rule	
• Conflict	• CUS	
• Lack of coordination and follow-up with co-workers	• DESC Script	
• Distractions	• Collaboration	
• Fatigue	• SBAR	
• Workload	• Call-out	
• Misinterpretation of cues	• Check-back	
• Lack of role clairty	• Handoff	

Fig. 5.2 TeamSTEPPS™ Curriculum

of leadership, potential barriers to implementing change, and whether resources are in place to successfully support the initiative. Such practice is typically referred to as a training needs analysis; it is a necessary first step to implementing a teamwork initiative [107].

A final determination is based on whether improved team performance—to include employing a TeamSTEPPS initiative—is the appropriate intervention necessary to impact change. A thorough needs analysis may uncover many underlying issues within the institution (e.g., systems problems, equipment problems, staffing shortages). The role of leadership is to assess the overall needs of the organization based on the analysis and determine the appropriate interventions.

Phase II: Planning, Training, and Implementation – Decide What To Do and Make It Happen

Phase II is the planning and execution segment of the TeamSTEPPS Initiative. Typically, the change team (or specific designees) complete a 2½-day intensive TeamSTEPPS train-the-trainer session (as described later, AHRQ is developing an infrastructure to support such training). Provided in this session is the core TeamSTEPPS curriculum to include scenarios, case studies, multimedia, and simulation. Culture change and coaching workshops that entail the provision of skills and strategies necessary for implementation, sustainment, and spread of the initiative are introduced. A 4-h block of time is devoted to participant development of a customized TeamSTEPPS Implementation and Action Plan. Each unit or department produces a tangible report detailing exactly how the initiative will be executed to best meet their unique circumstances. At the end of the session, participants are provided an opportunity to practice teach a module of the core curriculum using specialty-specific scenarios appropriate to their units or departments. Peer and instructor feedback serves to reinforce understanding of the content, along with refinement of presentation skills.

TeamSTEPPS is tailored to the organizational culture in which it is being implemented. Options include implementation of all tools and strategies throughout the entire organization, a phased-in approach that targets specific units or departments, or selection of individual tools introduced at specific intervals (a dosing strategy). As long as the primary learning objectives are maintained, the TeamSTEPPS materials are extremely adaptable.

Phase III: Sustainment—Make It Stick

The goal of Phase III is to sustain and spread improvements in teamwork performance, clinical processes, and outcomes resulting from the TeamSTEPPS Initiative. During this phase, users will:

- Integrate teamwork skills and tools into daily practice.
- Monitor and measure the on-going effectiveness of the TeamSTEPPS intervention.
- Develop an approach for continuous improvement and spread of the intervention throughout the organization or work unit.

Sustainment is managed by the designated change team through coaching and active observation of team performance. It involves continuing training of the core curriculum through refresher courses and newcomers' orientation, conducting continual evaluations of teams throughout the organization, and providing meaningful, ongoing feedback to staff members in the workplace, where day-to-day health care is provided.

Team Training Research Recommendations

Cardiac team performance measures must be grounded in team pedagogical theory, account for individual and team-level performance, capture team process and outcomes, adhere to standards for reliability and validity, and address real or perceived barriers to measurement [4]. A number of guidelines and recommendations for research on teamwork training effectiveness can be made. The recommendations are organized into those that can be achieved in nearer-term and those that can be considered after the initial research phase is well under way.

Nearer-Term Recommendations

- Clearly specify the training objectives. What knowledge, skills, and attitudes (KSAs) are being trained based on local practice?
- Design scenarios that link scenario events to training objectives. These scenarios could be developed from reported team errors or near misses in which specified teamwork skills were lacking. Ensure that the scenario includes events that trigger trainees to perform the specific competencies targeted for training in that scenario.
- Describe a set of scenarios that can be used to evaluate the effectiveness of varying training programs. Specify the training objectives that each scenario is suitable for evaluating.
- Develop, validate and apply observer-based measures of teamwork process to medical teams (Box 5.1). This will allow researchers to assess whether and, if so, which teamwork KSAs improve with training.
- Support multiple research studies in which training is evaluated using a common set of scenarios and common measurement instruments.
- Support training oriented to multidisciplinary teams so that medical team members train in the teamwork context in which they work.
- Train intact teams. In later phases, study whether training carries over to participation in newly formed teams.

Box 5.1. Recommendations for Observing Teamwork in the Operating Room

Use a detailed process map to write down observations.

Rate both moment-to-moment processes and outcomes.

Try various teamwork classification tools and adjust them to fit the observers' requirements and the context in which observations take place.

Use rating scales to judge the quality of teamwork processes; scales should be based on a single dimension (eg, impact on teamwork).

Train observers on video recordings of real operations (not scripted performance), preferably 1 to 2 hr in duration.

Discuss discrepancies in coding and settle on an accepted definition and 'gold standard,' so raters will adopt a common frame of reference.

Use video recordings repeatedly to test for inter-rater reliability.

Rate teamwork in real time and not afterwards.
Verify observations immediately after the operation with personnel involved in the operation (i.e, interviews, questionnaire).
Solicit opinions of all team members involved by distributing questionnaires before and after the operation.
Observers should remain a 'fly on the wall' during the operation and not become involved in the clinical team's work.

Longer-Term Considerations

- Introduce declarative and procedural knowledge related to the critical components of teamwork early, and reinforce this knowledge throughout the healthcare professional's school curriculum.
- Study the effect of incorporating into training communication protocols (such as readback and a standardized communication form for handoffs) for enhancing communication and team situation awareness.
- Carry out similar training in multiple environments to assess the effects of environmental (i.e., noise, distractions), organizational factors on training effectiveness.
- Research training factors (such as amount of practice and quality of feedback) that impact the degree to which teamwork training is effective in promoting high-quality patient care and patient safety.
- Develop licensure and certification process should assess and regulate health care providers teamwork-related competence.
- Assess the role of simulation in advancing team training and patient safety.

Conclusions

Teams make fewer mistakes than do individuals, especially when each team member knows his/her responsibilities, as well as those of the other team members. However, simply bringing individuals together to perform a specified task does not automatically ensure that they will function as a team. The role of the clinical microsystem as the unit of training and measurement is key [108]. Cardiac teamwork depends on a willingness of clinicians from diverse backgrounds to cooperate in varied clinical settings (i.e., clinic, operating theatre, intensive care unit, catherization laboratory, etc) toward a shared goal, communicate, work together effectively, and improve.

To achieve high reliability and consistent performance, each team member must be able to: (i) anticipate the needs of the others; (ii) adjust to each other's actions and to the changing environment; iii) monitor each other's activities and distribute workload dynamically; and (iv) have a shared understanding of accepted processes, and how events and actions should proceed (shared mental model).

Teams outperform individuals especially when performance requires multiple diverse skills, time constraints, judgment, and experience. Nevertheless, most people in health care overlook team-based opportunities for improvement because training and infrastructure are designed around individuals and incentives are all individual based. Teams with clear goals and effective communication strategies can adjust to new information with speed and effectiveness to enhance real-time problem solving. Individual behaviors change on a team more readily because team identity is less threatened by change than are individuals.

Future work should continue to evaluate the timing, duration and impact of sustainability of team training. This includes evaluating the impact of team-training on patient safety outcomes, evaluating team-training in other settings (e.g., emergency department, outpatient surgical care settings), examining the comparative effectiveness of different methods for delivering team-training, and examining implementation methods to support sustaining behavior changes achieved through training. For example, there is little evidence available to date that provides insight into the frequency of retraining or dedicated practice needed to develop and maintain effective teamwork skills. Additionally, there is a need to examine how dynamic team composition (i.e., changes in team membership, absence of key members) moderate team processes and the effects of team-training.

Turning cardiac care experts into expert teams requires substantial planning and practice. There is a natural resistance to move beyond individual roles and accountability to a team mindset. One can facilitate this commitment by: (1) fostering a shared awareness of each member's tasks and role on the team through cross-training and other team training modalities; (2) training members in specific teamwork skills such as communication, situation awareness, leadership, "followership," resource allocation, and adaptability; (3) conducting team training in simulated scenarios with a focus on both team behaviors and technical skills; (4) training team leaders in the necessary leadership competencies to build and maintain effective teams; and (5) establishing reliable methods of team performance evaluation and rapid feedback.

The roadmap for future research must include how teamwork training should be structured, delivered, and evaluated to optimize patient safety in the perioperative setting. For teamwork skills to be assessed and have credibility, team performance measures must be grounded in team theory, account for individual and team-level performance, capture team process and outcomes, adhere to standards for reliability and validity, and address real or perceived barriers to measurement. The interdisciplinary nature of work in the perioperative environment and the necessity of cooperation among the team members play an important role in enabling patient safety and avoiding errors. Training team leaders and surgical teams in this manner will lead to better satisfaction, joy at work and reduced burnout of surgical team members.

Acknowledgments This chapter is partially based or adapted from Barach P, Weinger M. Trauma team performance. In Wilson WC, Grande CM, Hoyt DB, ed. Trauma: Resuscitation, Anesthesia, & Critical Care. New York: Marcel Dekker, Inc, 2006; on, Entin E, Lei F, Barach P. Teamwork Skills Training for Patient Safety in the Perioperative Environment: A Research Agenda. Surg Innovat 2006;3:3–13; and, on the DoD funded TeamSTEPPS program for which the author (PB) was an active member of the development team.

References

1. Khetarpal S, Steinbrunn BS, McGonigal M, et al. Trauma faculty and trauma team activation: impact on trauma system function and patient outcome. J Trauma. 1999;47:576–81.
2. Weaver SJ, Rosen MA, DiazGranados D, et al. Does teamwork improve performance in the operating room? A multilevel evaluation. Jt Comm J Qual Patient Saf. 2010;36(3):133–42.
3. Neily J, Mills PD, Young-Xu Y, Carney BT, West P, Berger DH, Mazzia LM, Paull DE, Bagian JP. Association between implementation of a medical team training program and surgical mortality. JAMA. 2010;304(15):1693700.doi:10.1001/jama.2010.1506.
4. Baker D, Battles J, King H, Salas E, Barach P. The role of teamwork in the professional education of physicians: current status and assessment recommendations. Jt Comm J Qual Patient Saf. 2005;31(4): 185–202.
5. Foushee HC, Helmreich RL. Group interaction and flight crew performance. In: Wiener EL, Nagel DC, editors. Human factors in aviation. San Diego: Academic Press; 1988. p. 189–227.
6. Jones DG, Endsley MR. Sources of situation awareness errors in aviation. Aviat Space Environ Med. 1996;67:507–12.
7. Kanki BG, Lozito S, Foushee HC. Communication indices of crew coordination. Aviat Space Environ Med. 1989;60:56–60.
8. Reason J. Human error. Cambridge/London: Cambridge University Press; 1990.
9. Reason J. Understanding adverse events: human factors. Qual Health Care. 1995;4:80–9.
10. Perrow C. Normal accidents: living with high-risk technologies. New York: Basic Books; 1984.
11. Kletz T. Learning from accidents. 2nd ed. Oxford: Butterworth-Heinemann; 1994.
12. Rogers Jr SO, Gawande AA, Kwaan M, et al. Analysis of surgical errors in closed malpractice claims at 4 liability insurers. Surgery. 2006;140(1):25–33.
13. Katzenbach JR, Smith DK. The wisdom of teams: creating the high performance organization. Cambridge: Harvard Business School Press; 1993.
14. Cassin B, Barach P. Making sense of root cause analysis investigations of surgery-related adverse events. Surg Clin North Am. 2012;92:1–15. doi:10.1016/j.suc.2011.12.008.
15. Weick KE, Roberts KH. Collective mind in organizations: heedful interrelating on flight decks. Admin Sci Q. 1993;38:357–81.
16. Donchin Y, Gopher D, Olin M, et al. A look into the nature and causes of human errors in the intensive care unit. Crit Care Med. 1995;23:294–300.

17. Schull MJ, Ferris LE, Tu JV, et al. Problems for clinical judgement: thinking clearly in an emergency. CMAJ. 2001;164:1170–5.
18. Billington J. The three essentials of an effective team. Harvard Business Publishing Newsletters. 1997;2:1–4. Modified by Barach and Weinger.
19. Weick K. Prepare your organization to fight fires. Harv Bus Rev. 1996;143–148.
20. Aram JD. Individual and group. In: Dilemmas of administrative behavior. Englewood: Prentice-Hall; 1976. p. 75–95.
21. Lencioni P. The Five Dysfunctions of a Teams, Jossey-Bass; 2002. ISBN 0-7879-6075-6.
22. Hill LA. Managing your team. Harvard Business School Teaching Note. 9–494-081. 1995.
23. Janis IL. Groupthink. Psychology today. New York: Ziff-Davis Publishing Co.; 1971.
24. Barach P, Weinger M. Trauma team performance. In: Wilson WC, Grande CM, Hoyt DB, editors. Trauma: resuscitation, anesthesia, & critical care. New York: Marcel Dekker, Inc; 2006.
25. Driscoll PA, Vincent CA. Organizing an efficient trauma team. Injury. 1992;23:107–10.
26. Alexander R, Proctor H. Advanced trauma life support course. Chicago: American College of Surgeons; 2001.
27. Cooper S, Wakelam A. Leadership of resuscitation teams: "light-house leadership.". Resuscitation. 1999;42: 27–45.
28. Hoff WS, Reilly PM, Rotondo MF, et al. The importance of the command-physician in trauma resuscitation. J Trauma. 1997;43:772–7.
29. Woody JR, McKinney EH, Barker JM, Clothier CC. Comparison of fixed versus formed aircrews in military transport. Aviat Space Environ Med. 1994;65:153–6.
30. Simon R, Morey JC, Rice MM, et al. Reducing errors in emergency medicine through team performance: the MedTeams project. In: Scheffler AL, Zipperer L, editors. Enhancing patient safety and reducing errors in health care. Chicago: National Patient Safety Foundation; 1998. p. 142–6.
31. Sugre M, Seger M, Kerridge R, et al. A prospective study of the performance of the trauma team leader. J Trauma. 1995;38:79–82.
32. Barach P. Team based risk modification program to make health care safer. Theor Issues Ergon Sci. 2007;8:481–94.
33. Chidester TR, Helmrieich RL, Gregorich SE, Geis CE. Pilot personality and crew coordination: implications for training and selection. Int J Aviat Psychol. 1991;1:25–44.
34. Ericsson KA, Starkes J. Expert performance in sport. Champaign: Human Kinetics; 2003.
35. Ericsson KA, Krampe RT, Tesch-Römer C. The role of deliberate practice in the acquisition of expert performance. Psychol Rev. 1993;100:363–406.
36. Ericsson KA, Lehmann AC. Expert and exceptional performance: evidence on maximal adaptations on task constraints. Annu Rev Psychol. 1996;47:273–305.
37. Choudhrey NK, Fletcher RH, Soumerai SB. Systematic review: the relationship between clinical experience and quality of health care. Ann Intern Med. 2005;142:260–73.
38. Ericsson KA, Smith J. Toward a general theory of expertise: prospects & limits. New York: Cambridge University Press; 1991.
39. Causer J, Barach P, Williams M. Expertise in medicine: using the expert performance approach to improve simulation training. Med Educ. 2014;48: 115–23. doi:10.1111/medu.12306.
40. Klein G. Sources of power: how people make decisions. Cambridge: The MIT Press; 1998.
41. Klein GA. Recognition-primed decisions. Adv Man Machine Sys Res. 1989;5:47–92.
42. Shanteau J. Competence in experts: the role of task characteristics. Organ Behav Hum Decis Process. 1992;53:252–66.
43. O'leary J, Barach P, Shorten G. Improving clinical performance using rehearsal and warm up. A systematic review of randomized trial and observational studies. Acad Med. 2014, -D-13-00330R3.
44. Sarter NB, Woods DD. Situation awareness: a critical but ill-defined phenomenon. Int J Aviat Psychol. 1991;1:45–7.
45. Endsley MR. Measurement of situation awareness in dynamic systems. Hum Factors. 1995;37:65–84.
46. Cannon-Bowers JA, Salas E, Converse S. Shared mental models in expert team decision making. In: Castellan NJ, editor. Individual and group decision making: current issues. Hillsdale: Lawrence Erlbaum Associates; 1993. p. 221–46.
47. Cannon-Bowers JA, Salas E. A framework for developing team performance measures in training. In: Brannick MT, Salas E, Prince C, editors. Team performance assessment and measurement. Mahwah: Lawrence Erlbaum; 1997. p. 45–62.
48. Baker DP, Gustafson S, Beaubien JM, Salas E, Barach P. Medical team training programs in health care. Advances in patient safety: from research to implementation, Programs, tools, and products. AHRQ Publication No. 05-0021-4, vol. 4. Rockville: Agency for Healthcare Research and Quality; 2005.
49. Performance measurement in teams. Team training series, Book 2. Orlando: Naval Air Warfare Center Training Systems Division.
50. Uj C, Hefferman D, Barach P. Microsimulators in medical education: an overview. Simul Gaming. 2001;32:250–62.
51. Hoyt DB, Shackford SR, Fridland PH, et al. Video recording trauma resuscitations: an effective teaching technique. J Trauma. 1988;28:435–40.
52. Michaelson M, Levi L. Videotaping in the admitting area: a most useful tool for quality improvement of the trauma care. Eur J Emerg Med. 1997;4:94–6.
53. Byrne AJ, Sellen AJ, Jones JG, et al. Effect of videotape feedback on anaesthetists' performance while managing simulated anaesthetic crises: a multicentre study. Anaesthesia. 2002;57:169–82.

54. Scherer L, Chang M, Meredith J, Battistella F. Videotape review leads to rapid and sustained learning. Am J Surg. 2003;185:516–20.
55. Ellis DG, Lerner EB, Jehle DV, et al. A multi-state survey of videotaping practices for major trauma resuscitations. J Emerg Med. 1999;17:597–604.
56. Weinger MB, Gonzales DC, Slagle J, Syeed M. Video capture of clinical care to enhance patient safety: the nuts and bolts. Qual Safe Health Care. 2004;13:136–44.
57. Gaba DM, Howard SK, Flanagan B, et al. Assessment of clinical performance during simulated crises using both technical and behavioral ratings. Anesthesiology. 1998;89:8.
58. Gaba DM. Human work environment and anesthesia simulators. In: Miller RD, editor. Anesthesia. 5th ed. New York: Churchill-Livingstone; 2000. p. 2613–68.
59. Schwid HA, Rooke GA, Ross BK, Sivarajan M. Use of a computerized advanced cardiac life support simulator improves retention of advanced cardiac life support guidelines better than a textbook review. Crit Care Med. 1999;27:821–4.
60. Flin R, Yule S, Paterson-Brown S, Maran N, Rowley D, Youngson G. Teaching surgeons about non-technical skills. Surgeon. 2007;5(2):86–9.
61. Fletcher G, Flin R, McGeorge P, Glavin R, Maran N, PATEY R. Anaesthetists' Non-Technical Skills (ANTS): evaluation of a behavioural marker system. Br J Anaesth. 2003;90(5):580–8.
62. Mitchell L, Flin R, Yule S, Mitchell J, Coutts K, Youngson G. Thinking ahead of the surgeon: developing a behavioural rating system for scrub practitioners' non-technical skills (SPLINTS). Br J Anes. 2010;54(12):862–6.
63. Swanson DB, Stillman P. The use of standardized patients for teaching and assessing clinical skills. Eval Health Prof. 1990;13:79–80.
64. Tekian A, McGuire C, McGaghie W. Innovative simulations for assessing professional competence. Chicago: University of Illinois; 1999.
65. The role of the team leader. Team training series, Book 3. Orlando: Naval Air Warfare Center Training Systems Division.
66. Barach P, Fromson J, Kamar R. Ethical and professional concerns of simulation in professional assessment and education. Am J Anesth. 2000; 12:228–31.
67. Barach P, Satish U, Streufert S. Healthcare assessment and performance. Simul Gaming. 2001;32:147–55.
68. Holzman RS, Cooper JB, Gaba DM, et al. Anesthesia crisis resource management: real-life simulation training in operating room crises. J Clin Anesthesiol. 1995;7:675–87.
69. Hammond J, Bermann M, Chen B, Kushins L. Incorporation of a computerized human patient simulator in critical care training: a preliminary report. J Trauma. 2002;53:1064–7.
70. Holcomb JB, Dumire RD, Crommett JW, et al. Evaluation of trauma team performance using an advanced human patient simulator for resuscitation training. J Trauma. 2002;52:1078–86.
71. Lee SK, Pardo M, Gaba DM, et al. Trauma assessment training with a patient simulator: a prospective, randomized study. J Trauma. 2003;55:651–7.
72. Harnett MJ, Shorten GD. Address rehearsal. Eur J Anaesthesiol. 2011;28:675–7.
73. Satava RM, Hunter AM. The surgical ensemble: choreography as a simulation and training tool. Surg Endosc. 2011;25:30–5.
74. O'leary J, Barach P, Shorten G. Improving clinical performance using rehearsal and warm up: a systematic review of randomized and observations studies, Canadian Society of Anesthesia, annual meeting, 21–24 June 2013. Abstract#1635450.
75. Kahol K, Satava RM, Ferrara J, Smith ML. Effect of short-term pretrial practice on surgical proficiency in simulated environments: a randomized trial of the "preoperative warm-up" effect. J Am Coll Surg. 2009;208(2):255–68. doi:10.1016/j.jamcollsurg.2008.09.029.
76. DeAnda A, Gaba DM. Unplanned incidents during comprehensive anesthesia simulation. Anesth Analg. 1990;71:77–82.
77. Devitt JH, Kurrek MM, Cohen MM, et al. Testing internal consistency and construct validity during evaluation of performance in a patient simulator. Anesth Analg. 1998;86:1160–4.
78. Oser RL, Salas E, Merket DC, Bowers CA. Applying resource management training in naval aviation: a methodology and lessons learned. In: Salas E, Bowers CA, Edens E, editors. Improving teamwork in organizations: applications of resource management training. Mahwah: Lawrence Erlbaum; 2001. p. 283–301.
79. Christansen U, Barach P. Simulation in anesthesia. In: Romano E, editor. Anesthesia generale speciale: principles procedures and techniques. 2nd ed. Turin: Pergamon Press; 2004.
80. Christansen, U., Heffener L, Barach P. Simulation in Anesthesia. In: Anesthesia General Special, Principles Procedures and Techniques, Romano (ed.), 2nd edition, 2005, pp. 687–698.
81. Bertalanffy LV. General system theory: foundations, development, applications. New York: George Braziller, Inc.; 1968.
82. Batalden PB, Nelson EC, Mohr JJ, Godfrey MM, Huber TP, Kosnik L. Microsystems in health care: part 5. How leaders are leading. Jt Comm J Qual Saf. 2003;29(6):297–308.
83. Mohr J, Barach P, et al. Microsystems in health care: part 6. Designing patient safety into the microsystem. Jt Comm J Qual Saf. 2003;29:401–8.
84. Deming WE. Out of the crisis. Cambridge: Massachusetts Institute of Technology Center for Advanced Engineering Study; 1986.
85. Quinn JB. The intelligent enterprise. New York: Free Press; 1992.
86. Nelson EC, Batalden PB, Mohr JJ, Plume SK. Building a quality future. Front Health Serv Manage. 2000;15:3–32.

87. Wasson JH, Godfrey MM, Nelson EC, Mohr JJ, Batalden PB. Microsystems in health care. Jt Comm J Qual Saf. 2003;29:5–15.
88. Donaldson MS, Mohr JJ. Improvement and innovation in health care microsystems. A technical report for the institute of medicine committee on the quality of health care in america. Princeton: Robert Wood Johnson Foundation; 2000.
89. Batalden PB, Mohr JJ, Nelson EC, Plume SK, Baker GR, Wasson JH, Stoltz PK, Splaine ME, Wisniewski JJ. Continually improving the health and value of health care for a population of patients: the panel management process. Qual Manage Health Care. 1997;5(3):41–51.
90. Entin EB, Lai F, Dierks M, Roth E. Peri-operative readiness information management system. Technical report. Woburn: Aptima, Inc.; 2004.
91. Sharit J, Barach P. The role of patient hand-offs in health care. Proceedings of the Society of the Human Factors. 2005. p. 754–62.
92. Toccafondi G, Albolino S, Tartaglia R, Guidi S, Molisso A, Venneri F, Peris A, Pieralli F, Magnelli E, Librenti M, Morelli M, Barach P. The collaborative communication model for patient handover at the interface between high-acuity and low-acuity care. BMJ Qual Saf. 2012;21 Suppl 1:i58–66. doi:10.1136/bmjqs-2012-001178.
93. Haynes AB, Weiser TG, Berry WR, et al. A surgical safety checklist to reduce morbidity and mortality in a global population. N Engl J Med. 2009; 360:491–9.
94. Arora V, Mohr J, et al. Communication failures in patient sign-out and suggestions for improvement: a critical incident analysis. Qual Saf Health Care. 2005;14:401–7.
95. Philibert I, Barach P. Balancing scientific rigor, context and trust in a multi -nation program to improve patient handovers. BMJ Qual Saf. 2012;21 Suppl 1:i1–6.
96. Urbach DR, et al. Introduction of surgical safety checklists in Ontario, Canada. N Engl J Med. 2014;370:1029–38. doi:10.1056/NEJMsa1308261.
97. Vaughan D. The dark side of organizations: mistake, misconduct and disaster. Annu Rev Sociol. 1999;25:271–305.
98. Barach P, Phelps G. Clinical sensemaking: a systematic approach to reduce the impact of normalised deviance in the medical profession. J R Soc Med. 2013;106(10): 387–90. doi:10.1177/0141076813505045.
99. Aveling E-L, McCulloch P, Dixon- Woods M. A qualitative study comparing experiences of the surgical safety checklist in hospitals in high-income and low-income countries. BMJ Open. 2013;3:e003039. doi:10.1136/bmjopen-2013-003039.
100. Quote attributed to Peter Drucker. United Kingdom: Sage Publications.
101. Baker D, Salas E, Barach P, Battles J, King H. The relation between teamwork and patient safety. In: Carayon P, editor. Handbook of human factors and ergonomics in health care and patient safety. Mahwah: Lawrence Erlbaum Associates, Inc; 2006. p. 259–71.
102. Baker D, Gustafson S, Beaubien J, Salas E, Barach P. Medical teamwork and patient safety: the evidence-based relation. AHRQ Publication No. 05-0053. 2005. http://www.ahrq.gov/qual/medteam/.
103. Barach P, Mayer D. The role of simulation-based team training to support a safety culture. Accredit Counc Grad Med Educ Bull. 2005;29–31.
104. Sorbero M, Farley D, Mattke S, Lovejoy S, editors. Outcome measures for effective teamwork in inpatient care. Santa Monica: RAND Health; 2008. ISBN 978-0-8330-4315-3.
105. King HB, Battles J, Baker DP, et al. TeamSTEPPS™: team strategies and tools to enhance performance and patient safety. In: Henriksen K, Battles JB, Keyes MA, et al., editors. Advances in patient safety: new directions and alternative approaches, Performance and tools, vol. 3. Rockville: Agency for Healthcare Research and Quality (US); 2008. Available from: http://www.ncbi.nlm.nih.gov/books/NBK43686/.
106. Kotter J, Rathgeber H. Our iceberg is melting: changing and succeeding under any conditions. New York: St. Martin's Press; 2006. p. 39.
107. Salas E, Cannon-Bowers JA. The science of training: a decade of progress. Ann Rev Psychol. 2000;52:471–91.
108. Mohr JJ, Batalden PB, Barach P. Inquiring into the quality and safety of care in the academic clinical microsystem. In: McLaughlin K, Kaluzny A, editors. Continuous quality improvement in health care. 3rd ed. Frederick: Aspen Publishers; 2005. p. 407–23.

6 The Cardiac Intensive Care Unit and Operating Room Continuum: Quality and Safety in the Cardiac Intensive Care Unit

David S. Cooper, Darren Klugman, Angela J. Kinstler, David P. Nelson, and Stephen Muething

Abstract

In the past decade, there has been an increased focus on quality and safety in health care. Decreasing variation, increasing adherence to evidence based guidelines, monitoring processes, and measuring outcomes are critical for improving quality of care. This focus is further enhanced because of the high cost of health care and potential for harm. Patient safety is a discipline that applies safety science methods toward the goal of achieving reliable patient outcomes. The cardiac intensive care unit, in particular, brings cardiovascular surgery, anesthesia, cardiology, critical care physicians and nurses together in a critical microsystem to deliver care at the "sharp end". This group must coalesce to form a team and culture of collaboration in order to provide high quality and safe care. This team must be vested in using quality improvement and safety science to advance the care of patients with critical cardiac disease.

Keywords

High reliability teams • Situational awareness • Competency • Safety • Improvement • Culture • Microsystem

D.S. Cooper, MD, MPH (✉)
The Heart Institute, Cincinnati Children's Hospital Medical Center, University of Cincinnati College of Medicine, 3333 Burnet Avenue, MLC 2003, Cincinnati, OH 45229, USA
e-mail: david.cooper@cchmc.org

D. Klugman
Divisions of Critical Care Medicine and Cardiology, Children's National Health System, The George Washington University Medical Center, Washington, DC, USA
e-mail: dklugman@childrensnational.org

A.J. Kinstler
Department of Patient Services, Cincinnati Children's Hospital Medical Center, Cincinnati, OH, USA
e-mail: angela.kinstler@cchmc.org

D.P. Nelson
The Heart Institute, Cincinnati Children's Hospital Medical Center, University of Cincinnati School of Medicine, Cincinnati, OH, USA
e-mail: david.nelson@cchmc.org

S. Muething
The James M. Anderson Center for Health Systems Excellence, Cincinnati Children's Hospital Medical Center, Cincinnati, OH, USA
e-mail: stephen.muething@cchmc.org

P.R. Barach, J.P. Jacobs, S.E. Lipshultz, P.C. Laussen (eds.),
Pediatric and Congenital Cardiac Care: Volume 2: Quality Improvement and Patient Safety,
DOI 10.1007/978-1-4471-6566-8_6, © Springer-Verlag London 2015

Introduction

In the past decade, there has been an increased focus on quality and safety in health care. Decreasing variation, increasing adherence to evidence based guidelines, monitoring processes, and measuring outcomes are critical for improving quality of care. This focus is further enhanced because of the high cost of health care and potential for harm.

Quality Improvement (QI) initiatives in the intensive care unit, a common location for harm to occur due to the acuity of care provided, have focused on reducing preventable harm such as nosocomial infections and medication errors. These efforts have been shown to improve outcomes as well as decrease costs [1, 2].

Patient safety is a discipline that applies safety science methods toward the goal of achieving a reliable system of health care delivery. Patient safety is also an attribute of health care systems; it minimizes the incidence and impact of, and maximizes recovery from, adverse events. Patient safety is both a way of doing things and an emerging discipline.

The cardiac intensive care unit, in particular, brings cardiovascular surgery, anesthesia, cardiology, critical care physicians and nurses together in a coherent clinical microsystem to deliver care at the "sharp end". This group of driven individuals must coalesce to form a team in order to provide high quality and safe care. This team is vested in using quality improvement and safety science to advance the care of patients with critical cardiac disease. This review discusses the general principles of high reliability teams, situational awareness as a tool to enhance safety, team performance and competency.

High Reliability Teams

The term *high-reliability teams* has been used to describe teams that consistently and effectively work interdependently toward a shared goal in a complex environment [3]. Such teams are able to make good decisions in complex and changing environments and under high levels of stress consistently and effectively over time [4]. These teams are skilled in closed-loop communication, which is, the exchange of clear information, acknowledgment of receipt of that information, and confirmation of its correct understanding. A safe, honest, and transparent environment, also called psychological safety, is created where concerns can be expressed safely without defensiveness, the perception of attack or the perception of endless debate [5]. A high-reliability team is a concept that has evolved from high-reliability theory [3]. High-reliability theory focuses on organizations with complex environments, such as air traffic control systems and nuclear power plants, where ample opportunities are available for errors to lead to catastrophic consequences. What separates these organizations from other complex industries is that their errors are prevented or managed, despite incredible complex interdependencies, such that the consequences are minimized. High-reliability theory proposes that such organizations promote a culture that prioritizes safety and vigilance and responsiveness to potential accidents over blind compliance and rote rules [6]. The health care industry, as a whole, has a fairly disappointing record of reliably delivering evidence-based practice while simultaneously avoiding harm. Although pediatric intensive care unit (PICU) specific data are limited, several studies provide support that the intensive care unit is no exception. Two prospective studies in the 1990s estimated that iatrogenic adverse complications occurred in 5–8% of PICU admissions [7, 8].

High-reliability organizations (HROs) create collective mindfulness through five principles/processes aimed at the anticipation and containment of the unexpected (i.e.: errors and harm). Containment differs from anticipation in that it aims to prevent unwanted outcomes after an unexpected event has occurred rather than to prevent the unexpected event itself. The three principles of anticipation are preoccupation with failure, reluctance to simplify and sensitivity to operations. The two principles of containment are deference to expertise and commitment to resilience [9]. A pediatric cardiac intensive care unit (CICU) would serve as a microcosm of an organization with environmental complexity in which high risk is the norm and the need for high reliability is essential to its operations. Application of these principles should promote the formation of a high-reliability cardiac team.

The principle of *Preoccupation with Failure* necessitates that small, inconsequential errors be regarded as a symptom that something is wrong in the system. There is a commitment by the team to fully investigate "near-misses" and treat all failures as learning opportunities. With a consistent and constant concern over failure there is an investment in the prospective prediction of care breakdown and how it can occur. The detection of failure can be challenging in the CICU where high acuity care is delivered and cardiac arrest and death is "expected" to occur. In fact, "near-misses" may be interpreted as a success by the team in preventing more serious harm. How good are we at examining occurrences like a delay in vasoactive infusion administration or lapse in hand hygiene? Likewise, while detection of failure is important, it is of little value if it is not reported and follow-up action is taken for future process improvement. The principle of *Reluctance to Simplify* requires encouraging and supporting diversity in experience, perspective, and opinion. It emboldens the team to express differing opinions; question plans of care and share events that are suboptimal. Oversimplification can reduce sensitivity to threats and unintended consequences, which will undermine situational awareness and mask "weak signals" as mere noise not early warnings of impending harm. Teams composed of individuals with different expertise (i.e.: multidisciplinary rounds) are better able to identify variations in their environment and to see specific changes that need to be made [9]. The principle of *Sensitivity to Operations* implies attending to what is happening on the front-line. It is specifically about seeing what is actually occurring, that is the ability to process on the fly. It's the ability to pull together disparate bits of information. This is irrespective of what was supposed to be happening based on intentions, designs and plans (i.e.: How good are we at carrying out elements of infection prevention bundles?). One of the goals of care is consistency, which becomes manifest as "routine". A threat to sustained operational sensitivity is for routines to become mindless, resulting in the loss of intentionality and situation awareness. Likewise, the high-reliability team must avoid overestimating the dependability of their operation. As mentioned earlier, the "near-miss" is not a reflection of good team performance but a process warning that the system needs careful reflection and sharpening. Team situation awareness, helps all team members keep their attention focused on their key tasks within their role, but also to cross monitor the whole CICU or colleagues' activities [9].

The principle of *Commitment to Resilience* requires developing capabilities to detect, contain, and bounce-back from events that do occur. The high-reliability team is expected to adapt swiftly, communicate quickly, accurately and deploy innovative problem solving. High-reliability teams engage in simulation training to hone these skills in a safe, controlled environment. Resilience involves the ability to absorb strain and preserve functioning despite the presence of adversity, an ability to recover from untoward events and the ability to learn and develop from previous episodes of recovery [9]. There is an emerging body of literature that, in fact, complication rates tend to be similar across institutions with high performing centers (low mortality rates) not necessarily having lower rates of complications but a lower rate of harm and death in those who suffer a complication given their resilience. This concept has been described as "failure to rescue" where lower performing centers are unable to contain the consequences of an error or complication [10]. The principle of *Deference to Expertise* necessitates pushing decision-making down and around to the people at the sharp end, those with the most related knowledge and expertise, even if junior in hierarchy. The high-reliability team looks to the front-line staff to find credible and practical expertise and knowledge about the problem at hand. It is key to have flattening of the authority gradient to allow for informed, dynamic and flexible decision-making. Authority flows from trust, respect, experience, and a shared mental model of what is happening, what needs to happen and who best can make the difficult decision [9].

Situational Awareness

Intensive care units (ICU) provide complex care for patients at risk for harm and mortality. The complexity and demanding urgency of treatment interventions coupled with advances in healthcare technology and medical procedures create numerous opportunities for serious harm in the ICU. Over-stimulation can obscure human cognitive function and impede precision, attention span, knowledge retrieval, concentration, and skill performance [11]. The Institute of Medicine report "To Err is Human: Building a Safer Health System", launched the patient safety movement to reduce preventable medical harm. The Agency for Healthcare Research and Quality (AHRQ) recommends healthcare institutions adopt human factors strategies for situation awareness (SA) to optimize patient safety, teamwork and decision support.

Human factors engineer, Mica Endsley, is renowned for her innovative work in designing and evaluating systems to support human situation awareness and decision-making. Endsley defines situation awareness as, "the perception of elements in the environment within a volume of time and space, the comprehension of their meaning, and the projection of their status in the near future" [12]. Endsley's model for situation awareness illustrates three levels of SA formation: perception, comprehension, and projection. An individual can perceive the status, attributes, and dynamics of relevant elements in their environment, comprehend the elements through the processes of pattern recognition, interpretation, and evaluation and then project the ability to predict how these elements will affect future states of the operational environment [12].

Healthcare systems provide multidisciplinary care and without proper integration, these multiple care providers can compromise the healthcare team. Endsley describes situation awareness as instrumental to the success of a team and defines team SA as "the degree to which every team member possesses the SA required for his or her responsibilities" [12]. Endsley and Jones later created the model of team situation awareness to conceptualize how individuals share SA within a team. They define "shared SA" as the degree to which team members possess the same SA on shared SA requirements. There are four factors that build shared SA in a team [13]:

1. *Team SA Requirements*: The information the team members know to share, including higher-level assessments, projections, task status and current capabilities.
2. *Team SA Devices*: Devices available in an environment to directly communication information.
3. *Team SA Mechanisms*: Systems which facilitate creating a shared mental model in order to support the team's ability to interpret information in the same way and make accurate projections regarding each other's actions. A shared mental model can significantly facilitate communication and coordination within a team.
4. *Team SA Processes*: Team members employ effective system processes to share SA information. These systems may develop processes to question assumptions, check for conflicting information or perceptions, coordinate and prioritize tasks, and establish contingency plans.

The success or failure of a team is dependent on the success or failure of each member. The model theorizes how high-performing teams develop high level of shared SA among team members. Situation awareness strategies have been utilized to create a culture of safety for the purpose of reducing serious safety events and patient harm [1]. Brady and colleagues [14] developed a sophisticated SA system to proactively identify patients at risk for acute clinical deterioration. The system processes consisted of individual and team SA. A patient identification system was established to create a shared mental model among the care team for patients at risk for acute decompensation (Fig. 6.1). Patients were identified as "watchers" based on the following criteria: an elevated pediatric early warning score, administration of high risk therapies, the expressed concerns of a care provider or family member and/or communication concerns. To facilitate this process, the team conducted a unit-based huddle to develop mitigation plans addressing the patients' signs and symptoms. An escalation algorithm outlined the process to heighten awareness at the organizational level. Three organizational wide huddles occurred daily

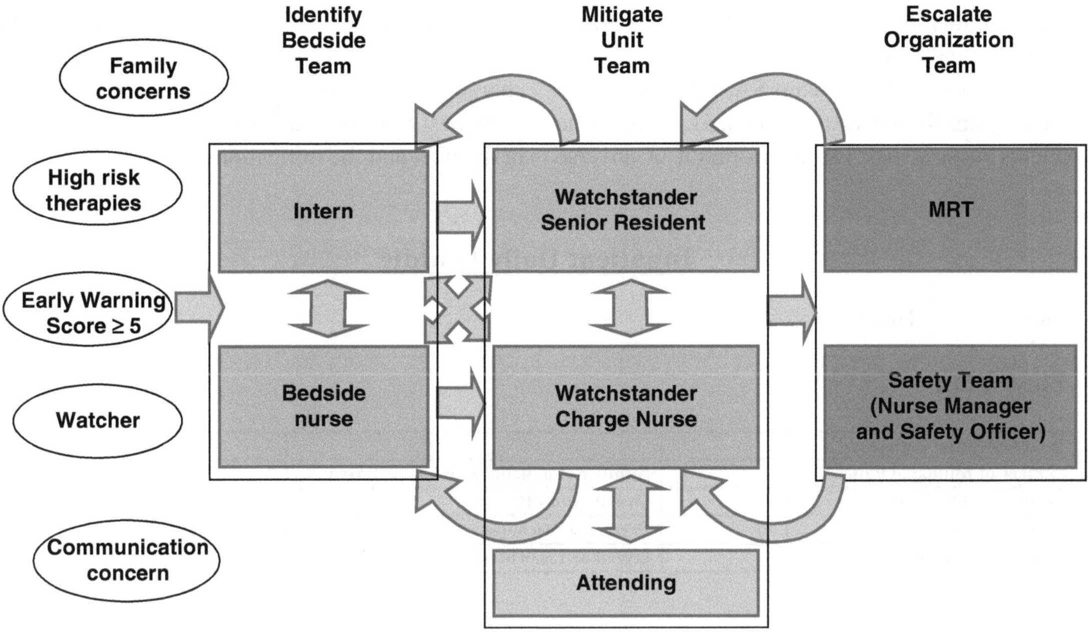

Fig. 6.1 Identify, mitigate, and escalate model illustrates which risk factors were systematically identified and how standardized communication about risk occurs throughout Cincinnati Children's Hospital Medical Center. Reproduced with permission from *Pediatrics*, Vol. 131, pages e298–e308, Copyright (c) 2013 by the AAP

to review patients at risk for acute clinical deterioration. These SA techniques prompted timely activation of the medical response team (MRT) to transfer patients to an ICU prior to acute decompensation. This helped decrease cardiac code events outside of the ICU and serious safety events [14].

Utilization of SA systems in the CICU environment has been limited. Reader and colleagues reported a system to assess the SA of an ICU team and observed that members of the team formed conflicting anticipations regarding the likelihood of patient deterioration [15]. The SA systems utilized in general care units could be generalizable to most inpatient healthcare environments, including the ICU. Although ICUs are typically considered high acuity environments with patients at risk for further clinical deterioration, failure to recognize acute decompensation in patients can lead to serious safety events. In order to recognize patients at highest risk for clinical deterioration or mortality, SA techniques could be utilized to proactively identify patients at highest risk for deterioration and mitigate potential acute events. As noted by Reader and colleagues a key goal of the ICU team is to create a shared mental model of the patients' status. Similar to Brady and colleagues identification system, criteria to identify those ICU patients at highest risk for deterioration would foster better SA among members of the ICU team [15].

Instituting principles of high-reliability over a 24 hour span assures more consistent communication of SA within a CICU care team. Conducting a quick 10 min unit huddle prior to morning rounds offers an opportunity for the clinical care team to generate an emerging shared mental model for the identified-at-risk patients they are caring for over the next shift. The lead physician and charge nurse facilitate the huddle to foster a partnership between physicians and nursing. Creating consistent, scripted processes when facilitating huddles and rounds can lead to more timely discussion and clear communication of plans reducing unnecessary delay when emergent treatment is necessary [16]. During the huddle the team reviews the previous 24 hours discussing predicted events, mitigation plans utilized and unexpected patient and/or operational outcomes (complications, medication errors, equipment issues, inadequate staffing)

(Fig. 6.2). Identifying and reviewing safety events provides timely awareness and appreciation of system issues. To foster team SA, the team would discuss plans for the next 24 hours, focusing on the patients most at risk for deterioration or adverse events. Potential topics for the huddle might include: census review, admissions, transfers, discharges, surgical and medical procedures, patients at highest risk for acute events, infection patterns in the ICU and the mitigation plans.

Inpatient Daily Huddle

Date: **Time:**

Flow Plan

Total number of patients			
Number of Intubated Patients		**Number of patients with Critical Airway**	
Current Available Beds		**Overflow in PICU**	
Expected Transfers		**Predicted Discharges**	
Expected Admissions		**Overflow Elsewhere**	

Anticipated Admissions

Patient Name	**Room #**	**Expected Arrival Time**	**Procedure/Direct Admissions** - If critical safety risk identified, add to CSR section	**Procedure/ eqpmnt that pose critical safety risk?** (Yes/No, name of procedure/ equipment)

Transfers/Discharge – LISTED IN PRIORITY ORDER

Patient Name	**Unit to Transfer**	**Room #**	**Expected Transfer Time or D/C**	**What needs to be done before Transfer or D/C**

Looking Back

Predicted Events

All CSRs predicted in the past 24 hours. **Only POIs with a predicted event** and or a significant change in the past 24 hours.

Patient Name	**Remains CSR or POI**	**Did a Predicted Event occur? (Yes/No) If yes, brief description**	**Was there a mitigation plan in place? (Yes/No)**	**Mitigation Plan Utilized (Yes/No)**	**Follow Up/ Comments –** What worked well? Opportunities for improvement?

Fig. 6.2 Cincinnati Children's Hospital Medical Center Heart Institute Inpatient Huddle Model

Unexpected Patient Outcomes *UPO* (Critical Events not Predicted with a Mitigation Plan)
Any unexpected changes in pt condition during prior day not predicted and discussed: Cardiac Instability - increasing support, monitoring, adding gtts, Respiratory Instability - increasing support, possible reintubation; **Unexpected complication** - bleeding, infection, return to OR; **Medical Treatment Errors.**

Patient/ Description of Event – (was the patient predicted as a CSR or POI?)	**Could this event be predicted? (Yes/No)**	**Could this event have been prevented? (Yes/No/TBD)**	**Follow Up/ Comments** –Opportunities for improvement?

Unexpected Operational Outcomes (Critical Events)
Medical Treatment Delays; Unplanned Admissions- without staffing to absorb safely; **Overflow; MRTs; Late transfers**
Suboptimal Staffing- #RN assignments> #RNs, RTs not at Core.

Patient/ Description of Event	**Could this event be predicted? (Yes/No)**	**Could this event have been prevented? (Yes/No)**	**Follow Up/ Comments** –Opportunities for improvement?

Looking Forward

PATIENTS of INTEREST (*POI*)
Predicted Safety Risks/Concerns: Risk for acute decompensation, Extubations for the day & post 24 hours, Radiology Procedures w/o Cardiac Anesthesia, Road trips, New procedure/ equipment/ standard of care.

Room	**Patient Name & description of activity/ event**	**Comments:** Specific Mitigation Plan when necessary

CRITICAL SAFETY RISK PATIENTS (*CSR*)
Predicted Critical Safety Risks/Concerns: Risk for Mortality - Cardiac Instability - increasing support, monitoring, adding gtts, **Respiratory Instability** - increasing support, possible reintubation, **Complex post op management**, **Unclear condition, Pts potential to code in the next 24 hours.**

Room	**Patient Name & Diagnosis**	**Concerns:** What is pt at risk for:	**Mitigation plan:** Specific & Measurable Mitigation Plan developed & updated on Morning rounds & SA Rounds with Care Team

Fig. 6.2 (continued)

Morning care rounds are an existing system that could be utilized to foster SA of the CICU team. Implementing new processes in existing systems leads to higher reliability. During morning care rounds, the entire care team gathers to plan the care for each individual patient. Embedding SA into rounds discussion could stimulate a shared mental model for the patient's plan of care. For example, the provider could initiate a time-out for safety, explaining the specific mitigation plan for the identified risks when concluding the patient's plan of care. Clear communication of a specific plan of care may enable timely interventions to reduce the possibility of severe

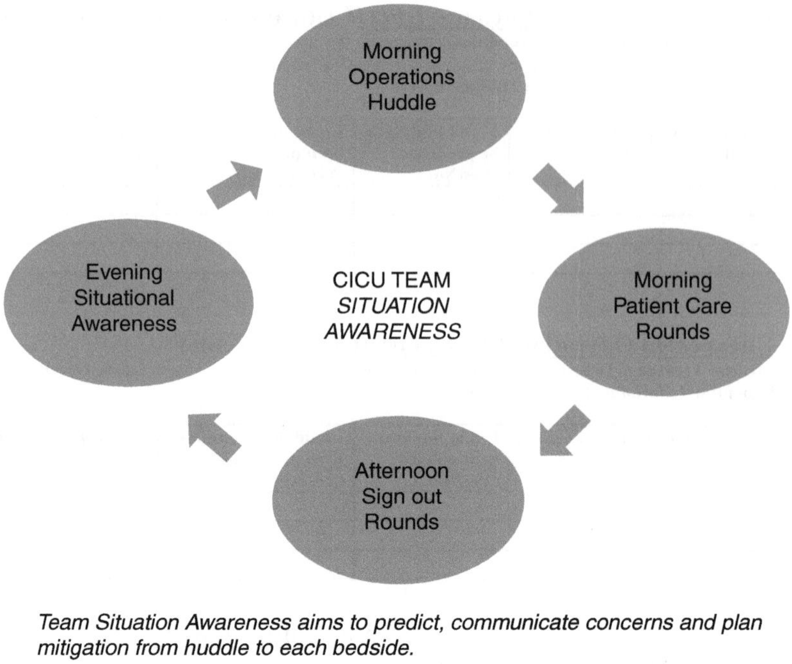

Fig. 6.3 Model of team situational awareness over a 24-hour period

cardiopulmonary decompensation. Creating additional SA opportunities is essential to assure utilization of mitigation plans and the sustainability of a shared mental model across the 24 hour span. A huddle at the time of nighttime handover presents another opportunity to briefly review the identified high-risk patients and their mitigation plans to ensure a shared mental model. Acute events such as cardiopulmonary resuscitation are equally common during night shift hours in an intensive care unit. During the night shift, availability of clinicians to respond to acute events is reduced. Instituting SA efforts during the night shift hours has tremendous potential to prevent serious patient safety events. By establishing evening SA rounds, the shared mental model for high-risk patients and their mitigation plans can be communicated, allowing for an ongoing shared mental model of patient care. The model illustrated in Fig. 6.3 demonstrates the key SA touch points throughout a 24 hour time period.

Situation awareness in a CICU can generate significant clinical impact. Since episodes of clinical deterioration can exacerbate organ system injury and increase patient length of stay, early recognition can prevent increased morbidity, delay ICU discharge and eliminate unnecessary costs. Establishment of a CICU situation awareness model may improve patient safety, clinical outcomes and the overall patient experience.

Performance

Health-care providers share a common goal – providing high quality care to their patients. Measuring performance can help one understand how well your team is accomplishing this goal. It allows for an analysis of where and what changes need to be made in order to improve performance and the quality of care provided. Measuring performance also allows providers to reflect and consider what is working well; information that can be shared with other providers who can learn from their success and failure. Performance measurement is the regular collection of data to assess whether the correct processes are being performed and desired results are being achieved [17]. It analyzes the success of a team, program, or organization's efforts by comparing data on what actually happened to what was planned or intended. The focus of performance measurement is less on the individual provider and more on the team as a whole to evaluate whether an adequate structure and correct processes are in place to achieve the stated goals.

Avedis Donabedian, an influential leader in the study of health care quality, developed a widely used, three-element model of quality measurement in 1966, which included measuring health care *structures* (the characteristics associated with a health care setting), *processes* (the activities done in a health care setting), and *outcomes* (the results achieved for a patient after a given set of interventions) [18]:

1. *Structural measures* include requirements imposed by payers and regulators, such as specifications for the facilities, management systems, health IT systems, board certification, and staffing ratios. Examples of structural measures include physician staffing, computerized physician order entry, pharmacist participation during rounds, rate of unplanned CICU readmission and cancelled OR cases.
2. *Process measures* determine whether evidence-based care guidelines were followed, but do not indicate whether a patient's health actually improved. Process measures, in essence, are used on the assumption that better outcomes should result from evidence-based care processes. Examples of process measures include rates of unplanned extubation, nutrition support, multidisciplinary daily rounds, effective assessment of pain, appropriate use of blood transfusions and appropriate gastric ulcer prophylaxis.
3. *Outcome measures* seek to determine whether the desired results are achieved. This could include whether the patient/family was satisfied with the care received. Examples of clinical outcome measures are catheter-associated bloodstream infection, CICU mortality rate and patient/family satisfaction.

Additionally, the team usually identifies a *balancing measure* to ensure that changes to improve one part of the system are not causing new problems or unexpected consequences in other parts of the system. The next step is to use the information to measure performance and improve care. Performance measures provide a picture of the team's quality, but further investigation is necessary to determine the factors that influence the measure results and how you can learn from positive results and make changes where performance is not at an optimal level.

Performance management is when a team uses performance measures and standards to achieve desired results. It is a forward-looking, continuous and purposeful process. This practice involves strategic use of performance measures and standards to establish performance targets and goals. Performance management practices can also be used to prioritize and allocate resources; to inform leaders about needed adjustments or changes in policy or program direction to meet goals and to frame reports on the success in meeting performance goals. Performance management includes the following components [19]:

1. *Performance standards* – establishment of organizational or system performance standards, targets, and goals to improve public health practices.
2. *Performance measures* – development, application, and use of performance measures to assess achievement of such standards.
3. *Reporting of progress* – documentation and reporting of progress in meeting standards and targets and sharing of such information through feedback.
4. *Quality improvement* – establishment of a program or process to manage change and achieve quality improvement in programs or infrastructure based on performance standards, measurements, and reports.

Performance improvement requires substantial investments in the underlying science of measurement, transparent communication of measurement results, attention to the role of measures in quality improvement efforts, and using performance data in focused and strategic ways [17].

Competency

Pediatric cardiac critical care has undergone tremendous growth and expansion over a short period of time. The growth of this field has paralleled expansive growth in general pediatric critical care over the same time period [20]. Over the past 20 years, pediatric cardiac critical care has developed into a robust clinical, scientific and research entity and, as a result, a well-recognized subspecialty within pediatrics. As surgical techniques and management have advanced, survival in infants and children with congenital heart disease has improved [21], and greater emphasis has been placed on the reliability of care in the intensive care unit. Increasing attention is being paid to optimizing outcomes, preventing harm, and delivering safe and cost-effective care rather than simply preventing mortality.

Training

The need to ensure appropriately trained staff to care for these complex patients has been scrutinized and debated. As surgical techniques have advanced, so too has the complexity of patients cared for in the cardiac intensive care unit. Pushing the surgical envelope has demanded more from the postoperative care team; however, the best training for the physicians and other team members responsible for the care of children in the cardiac intensive care unit remains unclear.

While some have argued that patients in the pediatric cardiac intensive unit are best taken care of by critical care trained providers [22, 23], care models for children with critical cardiac disease vary greatly across the United States [24]. Guidelines for pediatric cardiovascular centers set forth by the American Academy of Pediatrics (AAP) stipulate the need for dedicated space in either a specialty cardiac intensive care unit, or a pediatric or neonatal intensive care unit prepared to offer comprehensive care to the postoperative patient. The AAP recommends that the cardiac intensive care unit patient should be cared for by surgeons, intensivists and cardiologists [25]. However, comparison of outcomes for patients cared for in a dedicated cardiac intensive care unit (closed) to those cared for in other non-dedicated and open intensive care unit care models demonstrated no difference in postoperative morbidity or mortality [26]. According to the American College of Cardiology, American Heart Association and American College of Physicians Task Force on Clinical Competence, board eligible/certified pediatric cardiologists require at least 9 months of additional advanced training to be primarily responsible for the comprehensive care of children with critical congenital or acquired heart disease [27]. Training and proficiency is needed in many aspects of critical care including mechanical ventilation, invasive procedures and management of multi-system organ failure [27]. While the skills specified are largely inclusive of the care and knowledge needed to care for critically ill children with heart disease, specific measures of competency are not documented and there is no standardization of the training elements.

There is evidence that 24-hours care by trained pediatric intensive care providers decreases the duration of mechanical ventilation and intensive care unit length of stay [28]. Data such as these support the concept that the skill set of the providers are likely more important than the training path taken to acquire those skills, and research in adult critical care has shown that the base subspecialty training does not impact outcomes [29]. Rather than focus on the training background of the physician, emphasis should be placed on the competency and quality of care delivered by the teams managing critically ill children with heart disease.

Assessment of Competency

The diverse training background of physicians delivering care in the cardiac intensive care unit makes the assessment of competency challenging, and the lack of standardization in training contributes to difficulty in defining appropriate competencies. The absence of standardized competencies has led to the development of scoring systems to assess outcomes and the performance of the intensive care unit as a whole. The Pediatric Risk of Mortality (PRISM) III scoring system assesses mortality risk based on physiologic variables within 12 and 24 hours of admission and has been validated as a discriminatory tool to assess the mortality risk [30]. However, the PRISM III scoring system is not designed specifically for children with heart disease and does not take into account provider variables. Similarly, the Pediatric Index of Mortality score (PIM) II assesses mortality risk at the time of intensive care unit admission [31], but is not dynamic and also has similar shortcomings to the PRISM III score.

Two validated surgical complexity-scoring systems include the RACHS-1 scoring system and the comprehensive Aristotle score, both developed specifically for children with congenital heart disease undergoing cardiac surgery [32, 33]. The Aristotle score was developed with the idea that perhaps performance is a function of complexity. Child survival where complexity is a constant is based on the lesion and operation to be performed. Survival then is dependent on performance which is measured as Performance = complexity × survival [32]. While the Aristotle score introduces this interesting concept, we are still without a means to assess performance. If a patient has a low-risk lesion and an uncomplicated operation with an experienced surgeon yet suffers a bad outcome, does this reflect the poor performance of the cardiac intensive care unit physician or the surgeon or the entire team? Any assessment of competency and performance must ideally be linked to patient outcomes while under the care of a specific provider or providers.

Multiple surrogate means for assessing competency have been developed. Simulation-based training develops clinical scenarios and assesses individual and team performance in management of a clinical case. Simulation in pediatric cardiac critical care has demonstrated perceived improvements in provider confidence and ability to function as a member of a resuscitation team [34, 35]. Further, simulation training for cardiac surgical trainees in cannulation skills for extracorporeal membrane oxygenation demonstrated improvement in time to cannulation following sustained simulation training [36]. While these studies suggest that competency might be assessed by simulation, in order for any measure of performance or competency assessment to be truly valid, it needs to correlate with improved process and outcomes. Thus far this has been elusive.

Studies examining outcomes of pediatric cardiac intensive care unit patients have demonstrated that care delivered in the intensive care unit does impact outcomes [37–39]. Patients who returned to the cardiac intensive care unit within 72 h of discharge with respiratory symptoms were noted to have changes on chest radiograph prior to discharge from the intensive care unit and have higher rates of death compared to similar patients [37]. In a study of 342 postoperative patients, Brown and colleagues demonstrated that preoperative mechanical ventilation and postoperative complications including necrotizing enterocolitis had statistically significant impact on length of stay [38]. Critically ill children with hospital-acquired conditions in the ICU have increased morbidity and length of stay [40, 41]. In addition, provider compliance with bundled care to prevent hospital-acquired infections has been shown to reduce morbidity [42, 43]. These data present challenges when assessing competency. Does the provider who missed the changes on chest radiograph prior to discharge from the intensive care unit or the provider responsible for care when the patient developed postoperative necrotizing enterocolitis or a hospital acquired condition lack sufficient competency to care for these complex patients? Furthermore, should these questions be focused on the individual provider or the entire clinical team?

As pediatric cardiac critical care continues to develop as a subspecialty, accurate assessment of provider competency and performance is essential. The cardiac intensive care unit is a high stress environment with complex systems and an expected low mortality for children surviving congenital heart surgery. In such an environment, providers are prone to make mistakes [44] and those physicians who are more effective leaders have been shown to deliver more efficient care [45]. Failure to rescue, otherwise described as the probability of death following a complication, is a new concept, which attempts to assess the impact of errors or complications and the resilience of the system when processes have failed. Initial data suggest that centers with a lower failure to rescue rate have higher mortality rates; however, they do not actually have fewer complications [46]. These data might reflect increased resiliency and safety infrastructure amongst centers with high failure to rescue rates. However, more research is necessary to understand what failure to rescue rates actually tell us about a specific center's care delivery system.

Pediatric cardiac intensive care currently relies on large databases such as the Society of Thoracic Surgeons database, to assess center-based performance and center variations in care. Current literature on team dynamics provide evidence that high functioning teams provide more efficient care delivery; however, have not shown improvement in patient safety, outcomes or increased provider competency [47]. Analysis of individual provider competency and performance must begin with an effort to standardize training competencies. Training pathways for cardiac critical care include (although not exclusively): dual training in cardiology and critical care; fellowship training in pediatric anesthesia, critical care or cardiology followed by a fourth year advanced fellowship in cardiac critical care which is not currently standardized between institutions. Establishment of an integrated 4 year training program for pediatric cardiac intensivists that provides key baseline clinical elements of both cardiology and critical care training programs as well as research and elective time in specialized areas such as heart failure, pulmonary hypertension and neonatology might create standardized training metrics. This could be the foundation for the development of a single accreditation across professional societies [48]. The use of methods such as simulation can then be used to incorporate and evaluate the competencies outlined in standardized training requirements. In addition, improvements must be made in our ability to capture real-time clinical data from the electronic medical record and bedside monitors to allow for early recognition of complications.

Longevity

The American Heart Association policy statement on the evolution of critical care cardiology published in 2012 addresses future challenges in the adult field of cardiac intensive care and highlights the expanding training models and intensive care unit staffing as important issues [49]. The field of pediatric cardiac intensive care faces similar issues. In order to maintain growth and support the capacity needed in the field, training additional competent staff must keep pace with the clinical demands and growth in patient volumes. Whether we are training enough pediatric cardiac intensive care personnel remains uncertain [50].

As the field of pediatric critical care moves toward wider acceptance of 24-hour intensive care trained staff presence in cardiac intensive care units, staff longevity may be compromised. While 24-hour coverage and the number of nights spent in the hospital has been associated with burn out in adult intensive care units [51], there are possible benefits including improved trainee education and patient outcomes. As clinical needs continue to grow, the importance of career fulfillment, financial constraints and job satisfaction must be addressed [52, 53]. Patient safety and clinical needs must be paramount when considering staffing; however, providers in academic hospitals must also be given opportunities and time to pursue academic endeavors. Burn out and job dissatisfaction can be offset by non-clinical pursuits in research and education. In order to be successful in research and academic pursuits, the expectation for 24-hour in-house call coverage must be balanced with the need to develop and retain staff while maintaining a high level of satisfaction.

The clinical burden can be minimized and academic productivity optimized in a number of ways: limit a single provider to care for 10–12 patients during day shifts, limit 24 hour shifts, increase 12 hour and night float-type coverage and keep total overnight calls in an academic year below 50. All efforts to improve career satisfaction and longevity must be accomplished while prioritizing patient safety and optimizing outcomes. In 2010, the Pediatric Heart Network and the National Heart Lung and Blood Institute outlined a number of goals for future research and advancements in perioperative management of congenital heart disease, including limiting practice variation and advancing quality improvement [54].

Conclusions

The Institute of Medicine reported that there is a quality chasm in healthcare. The report suggested that the delivery of healthcare should be improved, so that it is safe, effective, patient-centered, timely, efficient and equitable [55]. Both medical leadership and frontline staff need to work together to achieve such a healthcare system. Quality improvement and patient safety initiatives in the intensive care unit have been shown to improve outcomes as well as decrease costs. The pediatric cardiac intensive care unit team through the use of high-reliability behaviors, situational awareness tools and performance management methods can advance the care of patients with critical cardiac disease. Understanding how to assess competency and ensure longevity of both the individual practitioner and the team will be paramount to achieving the maximal benefit and outcomes for patients with critical cardiac disease.

References

1. Muething SE, Goudie A, Schoettker PJ, et al. Quality improvement initiative to reduce serious safety events and improve patient safety culture. Pediatrics. 2012;130:e423–31.
2. Brilli RJ, McClead Jr RE, Crandall WV, et al. A comprehensive patient safety program can significantly reduce preventable harm, associated costs, and hospital mortality. J Pediatr. 2013;163(6):1638–45.
3. Wilson KA, Burke CS, Priest HA, Salas E. Promoting health care safety through training high reliability teams. Qual Saf Health Care. 2005;14(4):303–9.
4. Powell SM, Hill RK. My copilot is a nurse: using crew resource management in the OR. AORN J. 2006; 83(1):178–206.
5. Edmondson A. Psychological safety and learning behavior in work teams. Adm Sci Q. 1999;44(2): 350–83.
6. Weick KE, Sutcliffe KM, Obstfeld D. Organizing for high reliability: processes of collective mindfulness. In: Shaw B, Sutton R, editors. Research in organizational behavior, vol. 21. Greenwich: JAI Press; 1999. p. 81–123.
7. Stambouly JJ, McLaughlin LL, Mandel FS, et al. Complications of care in a pediatric intensive care unit: a prospective study. Intensive Care Med. 1996; 22:1098–104.
8. Stambouly JJ, Pollack MM. Iatrogenic illness in pediatric critical care. Crit Care Med. 1990;18:1248–51.
9. Weick KE, Sutcliffe KM. Managing the unexpected: resilient performance in an age of uncertainty. San Francisco: Jossey-Bass; 2007.
10. Gonzalez AA, Dimick JB, Birkmeyer JD, Ghaferi AA. Understanding the volume-outcome effect in cardiovascular surgery: the role of failure to rescue. JAMA Surg. 2014;149(2):119–23. Epub ahead of print 2013 Dec 11.
11. Moray N. Error reduction as a systems problem. In: Roper MS, editor. Human error in medicine: thinking/problem solving. Mahwah: Lawrence Erlbaum Associates; 1994. p. 67–91.
12. Endsley MR. Toward a theory of situation awareness in dynamic systems. Hum Factors. 1995;37(1): 32–64.
13. Endsley MR, Jones WM. Situation awareness, information dominance, and information warfare (No. AL/CF-TR-1997-0156). Wright-Patterson AFB: United States Air Force Armstrong Laboratory; 1997.
14. Brady PW, Muething S, Kotagal U, et al. Improving situation awareness to reduce unrecognized clinical deterioration serious safety events. Pediatrics. 2013;131:e298–308.
15. Reader TW, Flin R, Mearns K, Cuthbertson BH. Team situation awareness and the anticipation of patient progress during ICU rounds. BMJ Qual Saf. 2011; 20(12):1035–42.
16. Goldenhar LM, Brady PW, Sutcliffe KM, et al. Huddling for high reliability and situation awareness. BMJ Qual Saf. 2013;22:899–906.
17. Langley GL, Nolan KM, Nolan TW, Norman CL, Provost LP. The improvement guide: a practical approach to enhancing organizational performance. 2nd ed. San Francisco: Jossey-Bass Publishers; 2009.
18. Donabedian A. Evaluating the quality of medical care. Milbank Mem Fund Q. 1996;44(3):166–206.
19. Public Health Foundation. From silos to systems: using performance management to improve the public's health. Seattle, WA: Turning Point National Program Office at the University of Washington, 2010.
20. Randolph AG, Gonzales CA, Cortellini L, Yeh TS. Growth of pediatric intensive care units in the United States from 1995 to 2001. J Pediatr. 2004;144(6): 792–8.
21. Boneva RS, Botto LD, Moore CA, Yang Q, Correa A, Erickson JD. Mortality associated with congenital heart defects in the United States: trends and racial disparities, 1979–1997. Circulation. 2001;103(19):2376–81.
22. Baden HP, Berger J, Brilli RI, et al. Pediatric cardiac critical care patients should be cared for by intensivists. J Am Coll Cardiol. 2006;48(1):221–2.
23. Baden HP, Zimmerman JJ, Brilli RJ, et al. Intensivist-led team approach to critical care of children with heart disease. Pediatrics. 2006;117(5):1854–6.
24. Burstein DS, Rossi AF, Jacobs JP, et al. Variation in models of care delivery for children undergoing congenital heart surgery in the United States. World J Pediatr Congenit Heart Surg. 2010;1(1):8–14.
25. Guidelines for pediatric cardiovascular centers. Pediatrics. 2010;109(3):544–9.

26. Burstein DS, Jacobs JP, Li JS, et al. Care models and associated outcomes in congenital heart surgery. Pediatrics. 2011;127(6):e1482–9.
27. Kulik T, Giglia TM, Kocis KC, et al. ACCF/AHA/AAP recommendations for training in pediatric cardiology. Task force 5: requirements for pediatric cardiac critical care. J Am Coll Cardiol. 2005;46(7):1396–9.
28. Nishisaki A, Pines JM, Lin R, et al. The impact of 24-hr, in-hospital pediatric critical care attending physician presence on process of care and patient outcomes. Crit Care Med. 2012;40(7):2190–5.
29. Matsushima K, Goldwasser ER, Schaefer EW, Armen SB, Indeck MC. The impact of intensivists' base specialty of training on care process and outcomes of critically ill trauma patients. J Surg Res. 2013;184(1):577–81.
30. Pollack MM, Patel KM, Ruttimann UE. PRISM III: an updated Pediatric Risk of Mortality score. Crit Care Med. 1996;24(5):743–52.
31. Slater A, Shann F, Pearson G. PIM2: a revised version of the Paediatric Index of Mortality. Intensive Care Med. 2003;29(2):278–85.
32. Lacour-Gayet F, Clarke D, Jacobs J, et al. The Aristotle score: a complexity-adjusted method to evaluate surgical results. Eur J Cardiothorac Surg. 2003;25(6):911–24.
33. Jenkins KJ, Gauvreau K, Newburger JW, et al. Consensus-based method for risk adjustment for surgery for congenital heart disease. J Thorac Cardiovasc Surg. 2003;123(1):110–8.
34. Allan CK, Thiagarajan RR, Beke D, et al. Simulation-based training delivered directly to the pediatric cardiac intensive care unit engenders preparedness, comfort, and decreased anxiety among multidisciplinary resuscitation teams. J Thorac Cardiovasc Surg. 2010;140(3):646–52.
35. Figueroa MI, Sepanski R, Goldberg SP, Shah S. Improving teamwork, confidence, and collaboration among members of a pediatric cardiovascular intensive care unit multidisciplinary team using simulation-based team training. Pediatr Cardiol. 2013;34(3):612–9.
36. Allan CK, Pigula F, Bacha EA, et al. An extracorporeal membrane oxygenation cannulation curriculum featuring a novel integrated skills trainer leads to improved performance among pediatric cardiac surgery trainees. Simul Healthc. 2013;8(4):221–8.
37. Bastero-Minon P, Russell JL, Humpl T. Frequency, characteristics, and outcomes of pediatric patients readmitted to the cardiac critical care unit. Intensive Care Med. 2012;38(8):1352–7.
38. Brown KL, Ridout DA, Goldman AP, Hoskote A, Penny DJ. Risk factors for long intensive care unit stay after cardiopulmonary bypass in children. Crit Care Med. 2003;31(1):28–33.
39. Gaies MG, Clarke NS, Donohue JE, et al. Personnel and unit factors impacting outcome after cardiac arrest in a dedicated pediatric cardiac intensive care unit. Pediatr Crit Care Med. 2012;13(5):583–8.
40. Connor JA, Gauvreau K, Jenkins KJ. Factors associated with increased resource utilization for congenital heart disease. Pediatrics. 2005;116(3):689–95.
41. Dominguez TE, Chalom R, Costarino AT. The impact of adverse patient occurrences on hospital costs in the pediatric intensive care unit. Crit Care Med. 2001; 29(1):169–74.
42. Miller MR, Niedner MF, Huskins WC, et al. Reducing PICU central line-associated bloodstream infections: 3-year results. Pediatrics. 2011;128(5):e1077–83.
43. Muszynski JA, Sartori J, Steele L, et al. Multidisciplinary quality improvement initiative to reduce ventilator-associated tracheobronchitis in the PICU. Pediatr Crit Care Med. 2013;14(5):533–8.
44. Donchin Y, Gopher D, Olin M, et al. A look into the nature and causes of human errors in the intensive care unit. Crit Care Med. 1995;23(2):294–300.
45. Stockwell DC, Slonim AD, Pollack MM. Physician team management affects goal achievement in the intensive care unit. Pediatr Crit Care Med. 2007; 8(6):540–5.
46. Pasquali SK, He X, Jacobs JP, et al. Evaluation of failure to rescue as a quality metric in pediatric heart surgery: an analysis of the STS Congenital Heart Surgery Database. Ann Thorac Surg. 2012;94(2):573–9.
47. Rehder KJ, Uhl TL, Meliones JN, et al. Targeted interventions improve shared agreement of daily goals in the pediatric intensive care unit. Pediatr Crit Care Med. 2012;13(1):6–10.
48. Penny DJ, Shekerdemian LS. The American Heart Association's recent scientific statement on cardiac critical care: implications for pediatric practice. Congenit Heart Dis. 2013;8(1):3–19.
49. Morrow DA, Fang JC, Fintel DJ, et al. Evolution of critical care cardiology: transformation of the cardiovascular intensive care unit and the emerging need for new medical staffing and training models: a scientific statement from the American Heart Association. Circulation. 2012;126(11):1408–28.
50. Stromberg D. Pediatric cardiac intensivists: are enough being trained? Pediatr Crit Care Med. 2004;5(4):391–2.
51. Embriaco N, Azoulay E, Barrau K, et al. High level of burnout in intensivists: prevalence and associated factors. Am J Respir Crit Care Med. 2007;175(7): 686–92.
52. Ward NS, Afessa B, Kleinpell R, et al. Intensivist/patient ratios in closed ICUs: a statement from the Society of Critical Care Medicine Taskforce on ICU Staffing. Crit Care Med. 2013;41(2):638–45.
53. Shugerman R, Linzer M, Nelson K, et al. Pediatric generalists and subspecialists: determinants of career satisfaction. Pediatrics. 2001;108(3):E40.
54. Kaltman JR, Andropoulos DB, Checchia PA, et al. Report of the pediatric heart network and national heart, lung, and blood institute working group on the perioperative management of congenital heart disease. Circulation. 2010;121(25):2766–72.
55. Institute of Medicine. Crossing the quality chasm: a new health system for the 21st century. Washington, DC: National Academy Press; 2001.

7 Professional Formation of Physicians Focused on Improving Care

Ingrid Philibert and Paul V. Miles

Abstract

There is evidence that many patients do not receive optimum care despite efforts to improve health care quality. Society expects physicians to improve care for their patients, and to lead and function as members of quality improvement (QI) teams. A range of educational approaches exist to prepare physicians for this important role. Education in QI across the educational continuum is supported by the requirements of educational accrediting organizations and the expectation of specialty certification board. These regulatory bodies expect that physicians develop these skills during training, and that physicians in practice maintain QI competence, and assess and improve their patients' care. At the same time, no coordinated curriculum for teaching QI across the continuum of medical education exists to date. An effective approach to QI education encompasses both didactics and immersive experiences that enable learners to apply their developing competence to real-world problems. Given the importance of team-based approaches in the care of complex patients, new multidisciplinary QI approaches, informed by research on what makes care effective, will contribute to care that improves the patient experience. These will be supported by advances in medical training and assessment, healthy populations, and will lead to improved quality and lower per capita cost of health care to benefit patients and society.

I. Philibert, PhD, MBA (✉)
Department of Field Activities,
Accreditation Council for Graduate
Medical Education, 515 North State Street,
Suite 2000, Chicago, IL 60654, USA
e-mail: iphilibert@acgme.org

P.V. Miles, MD
Quality Improvement and Assessment Programs in
Pediatric Practice, American Board of Pediatrics,
12 Wedgewood Rd, Chapel Hill, NC 27514, USA
e-mail: pvm@abpeds.org

P.R. Barach, J.P. Jacobs, S.E. Lipshultz, P.C. Laussen (eds.),
Pediatric and Congenital Cardiac Care: Volume 2: Quality Improvement and Patient Safety,
DOI 10.1007/978-1-4471-6566-8_7,

Keywords
Medical education • Professional development • Patient safety • Quality improvement • Educational continuum • Multi-specialty and team-based care • Triple aim • Practice-based learning and improvement • Systems-based practice

The Quality Imperative

Quality and safety of care are important in all healthcare settings. Assuring safe care is particularly challenging for critically ill patients, complex care, human-technology interactions, and care by multiple health professionals and teams. Donabedian provided a framework for assessing and addressing quality problems in healthcare in a groundbreaking book published in 1966 [1]. Despite innovative work and critical thinking over more than four decades to develop and implement quality improvement (QI) programs, studies still show significant variations in the quality, safety, utilization and cost of healthcare services [2]. Children, for example, receive only 46 % of recommended services [3], and a study using national data for Medicare beneficiaries found that increased use of specialists and larger healthcare expenditures did not always translate into better outcomes and at times increased pain and suffering [4].

Crossing the Quality Chasm, a 2001 report by the Institute of Medicine of Medicine (IOM) asserted that gaps in quality of care result in part from health professions education that has not kept pace with new team-based approaches to care, use of technology and informatics, and understanding patient expectations for their experience of care [5]. To address these concerns, the IOM put forth six aims for the healthcare system: care should be effective, safe, patient-centered, timely, efficient, and equitable [5]. The IOM's seminal report on patient safety, *To Err is Human*, also noted that besides problems with the design of the care system, educating health professionals about avoiding errors and adverse events is critical to safe and effective healthcare, but that these concepts are not included in the educational curricula in most health professions [6].

Research has shown that quality and safety of care are inextricably linked to the education and ongoing professional development of physicians, and that the quality of formal training has a long-term and profound effect on the quality of care a physician delivers over a lifetime of practice. A study of the effect of training on obstetrician-gynecologists' performance in practice showed that the complication rates for patients cared for by physicians who had trained in programs who ranked in the bottom quintile for risk-standardized major maternal complications was one-third higher than the rate for patients cared for by graduates of programs in the top quintile [7]. Enhancing formal education and continuing professional development related to QI and improvement science is essential to close these gaps. The aim of these programs is to develop physicians who are lifelong learners who can continuously self-assess and improve their performance and outcomes. Needed skills include a comprehensive understanding of QI, the ability to reflect on the patient and the processes of care, and the skills to apply these principles in day-to-day practice to enhance quality and avoid medical errors and preventable adverse events. The Dartmouth Health Atlas' website, citing long term influence of the training program on the quality of care physicians deliver in practice, emphasizes that residents should know the quality of care delivered by institutions and clinical departments as a key factor in selecting their residency program [8].

While the earliest professional group with involvement in quality improvement is nursing, going back to Florence Nightingale during the Crimean War [9], the history of physician involvement in efforts to improve the quality of care traces back to Ernest Codman and his efforts to improve surgical care at the Massachusetts General Hospital in the early twentieth century [10]. Codman developed a system to assess where problems with the quality of care originated, address the causes [11], and use these principles to inform a set of standards for hospitals that over time evolved into the Joint Commission for the Accreditation of Healthcare Organization (now TJC) [10]. Quality improvement in industrial production began in the 1940s, through the work of Shewhart, Deming and others [12]. These concepts did not become widely disseminated and applied in healthcare until the late 1980s [13]. Prior to the adoption of QI concepts from industry, efforts to manage quality in healthcare largely were separate from medicine and medical education, and focused on meeting regulatory and accreditation requirements, compliance and utilization review [14]. Once QI principles were introduced in the healthcare sector, another decade passed before Headrick, Batalden, Leach, Davidoff, Berwick and others introduced these concepts into medical education [15]. Out of this work emerged organizing principles for quality improvement that include: (1) understanding healthcare as processes within a system; (2) understanding variation in care and the need to measure it; (3) knowing the effect of illness and healthcare on patients; (4) understanding the process of making changes in healthcare and the roles of leading and participating in these efforts; (5) collaborating in teams and groups; (6) dealing with social context and accountability; and (7) developing and applying locally useful knowledge [16].

Following the publication of the IOM's "To Err is Human" [6] and "Crossing the Quality Chasm" [5] reports, the IOM addressed the needs for education and professional development of health professionals related to QI in a third report, entitled *Health Professions Education: A Bridge to Quality* [17]. Collectively, the three IOM reports have contributed to more widespread teaching of quality and patient safety concepts across the continuum of medical education [18], and the education of nurses [19] and other health professionals [20].

This chapter discusses the components of the professional formation of physicians related to improving the quality and safety of patient care across the continuum from undergraduate and graduate education to continuing professional development. It also describes the barriers and facilitators to QI learning, and the assessment of educational and clinical outcomes related to improvement learning. Practical examples of physicians' professional formation in quality and safety improvement are presented throughout. The chapter concludes with a research agenda to promote physicians' professional development relevant to quality and safety.

Components of Health Professional Formation Related to Improvement

The IOM's 2003 report *Health Professions Education: A Bridge to Quality* identified five core competencies to meet the needs of the twenty-first century healthcare system, which span the various professions involved in healthcare [17]. The IOM competencies have been used to define goals and objectives for professional formation and development across a range of professions. They build on earlier efforts to define common competencies across the different health professions [21–23], and a growing recognition that much of the work to improve healthcare is done in interprofessional teams.

The aim of educating physicians in quality improvement is to ensure they develop skills and competencies that enable them to improve care in their local clinical context, as well as in the larger system of care. Knowledge of QI science is relevant, yet equally important is the ability to apply these tools in a real-world, organizational context. Added competencies particularly relevant to the implementation components of QI work include communication, teamwork, analytic skills and an understanding of healthcare systems. *Crossing the Quality Chasm* also identified commitment to lifelong learning as an important competency [5]. Lifelong learning consists of formal education and ongoing professional development that is required for physicians and other licensed professionals, along with learning through self-directed studies, reflection and interaction with peers.

Recognition that the predominant focus on medical knowledge and clinical skills underemphasized other areas relevant to the delivery of high-quality care prompted the Accreditation Council for Graduate Medical Education (ACGME) and the American Board of Medical Specialties (ABMS) to develop a broader approach to defining the skills and attributes that physicians should have to deliver quality are. At its core are six competencies relevant to the work of physicians: (1) patient care, (2) medical knowledge, (3) interpersonal and communication skills, (4) professionalism, (5) practice-based learning and improvement (PBLI), and (6) system-based practice (SBP). In 1999, these competencies were formally endorsed by the ACGME for the education and assessment of physicians in training [24], and by the American Board of Medical Specialties (ABMS) for the certification and ongoing professional development of physicians in practice [25]. While all ACGME/ABMS competencies are relevant to the delivery of high-quality care, PBLI and SBP – are particularly pertinent to the role physicians need to play in ensuring quality of care. There is considerable conceptual overlap between the ABMS/ACGME core competencies aimed at individual physicians, and the IOM competencies for a safer and more effective healthcare system.

PBLI encompasses the process physicians use to assess and improve their knowledge and skills relevant to their practice, including development of learning and improvement goals, initiating professional development activities, and evaluating the outcomes in a self-guided approach [26]. Improvement often begins with the identification of a clinical area or the care of a specific group of patients, with a focus on tailoring interventions to address gaps in quality and safety identified via self-assessment or external information such as clinical outcomes or patient satisfaction. Resources for this process include new medical evidence, and there is conceptual overlap between PBLI and evidence-based medicine [27].

Embedded in SBP is an understanding of the systems of care, along with participation in efforts to improve them. Activities include advocating for high-quality patient care; working in interprofessional teams to enhance the quality and safety of services; and participating in identifying and diagnosing system errors and implementing solutions.

There have been a number of attempts to define quality and safety curricula, including, among other, an annotated bibliography on teaching quality and safety during formal medical education [28], a patient safety program for physicians in practice developed [29], and a curriculum for residents in surgical specialties [30]. Recently, the Institute of Healthcare Improvement's (IHI's) Open School has made publicly available a broad range of curricular materials relevant to healthcare quality and safety, and these resources are being used in the education of residents and medical students, and in nursing and other health professions [31, 32]. While there are differences across curricula, and no universally accepted quality and safety curriculum exists to date, there is considerable overlap across professions and different formulations.

The Educational Continuum

A model of education that encompasses all forms of learning, from formal education and instruction to the ongoing learning that continues throughout an individual's professional career is important for a concept of professional formation [33]. For physicians, this encompasses undergraduate medical education, residency and fellowship training, and ongoing professional development for physicians in practice.

Undergraduate Medical Education

A century after Codman's pioneering work to introduce outcome based medicine into healthcare and 30 years after the introduction of quality improvement, it is gratifying that more medical schools are including these concepts in their curricula and approaches for teaching and assessing students [34]. Ideally, these concepts are taught at the beginning of student clinical experiences and become an integral part of the ongoing development of physicians' clinical improvement skills

[34]. Some medical schools have implemented focused QI electives for students in the clinical years [35]. The World Health Organization (WHO) emphasizes that patient safety and QI should be taught to medical students [36]. In contrast, the standards of the Liaison Committee on Medical Education, which accredits US and Canadian medical schools, do not yet include formally mention curricular elements or require competence in healthcare quality and safety [37]. Recommendations from the National Patient Safety Foundation (NPSF) on enhancing patient safety call for medical schools to emphasize the ACGME/ABMS competencies, patient-centered care, and working in interdisciplinary teams [38]. The NPSF also has recommended that teaching about patient safety should begin on the first day of medical school and should encompass the science of error causation and mitigation, the study of human factors, safety improvement science, systems theory and analysis, and systems design [38].

Graduate Medical Education

Graduate medical education is the phase of the educational continuum during residency and fellowship training where much of physicians' education about healthcare quality and safety occurs. While many of the first QI curricula targeted medical students, a few were aimed at both students and residents. In 2002, recommendations called for a broader approach to teaching QI to physicians, including expanded curricula, a focus on creating an organizational culture conducive to improvement and assessing outcomes at the individual and program levels [39]. Early efforts focused on non-mandatory "QI electives" [40], while more recent implementation of QI in the residency curriculum entails mandatory QI rotations and experiences for all residents [41–43].

Some teaching efforts have used active engagement in projects that integrate didactics with the application of what is learned [44]. This is based on the principles of experiential learning [45, 46]. The underlying theory is that teaching should be grounded in learners' experiences and that these experiences themselves represent a valuable educational resource [46]. Learning by doing and "just in time training," are related approaches that have been found useful in teaching QI principles and practices to learners across a range of health professions [47]. Efforts have also focused on the creation of templates that guide learners through the QI process, and that allow QI efforts to be recorded like other scholarly projects [48].

Currently, five approaches are commonly used for teaching residents PBLI, SBP and related concepts: (1) didactic sessions, including lectures, case studies, journal clubs and online self-study modules; (2) incorporating QI principles and concepts into clinical events such as morbidity and mortality (M&M) and clinical case conferences, and morning report [49–51]; (3) resident-initiated quality improvement projects [52, 53]; (4) resident participation in program-level QI projects; and (5) participation in multi-disciplinary institutional QI efforts [54]. Readily implementable modules, some of which are online, are being used to facilitate improvement in outcomes for common diagnoses such as diabetes and asthma are being used particularly in ambulatory and primary care settings [55–57]. Some improvement efforts have a longer term focus, multiple PDSA cycles, and include a focus on spread and sustainability of improvement [58]. A matrix that crosslinks the Institute of Medicine (IOM) aims with the ACGME competencies has also been used to make QI concepts meaningful to residents [59]. Efforts to involve residents in larger department or institutional QI efforts are less common. Some examples include addressing waiting times in pediatric urgent care [60]; improving patient flow in a resident continuity clinic [40]; use of practice data to enhance compliance with immunization guidelines [61]; standard order sets for patients with community-acquired pneumonia [62]; and a resident-led initiative to improve communication between the inpatient medical staff and ambulatory physicians [63]. The AAMC's Teaching for Quality report offers broad recommendations for medical schools and teaching hospitals to incorporate the principles and practice of Quality Improvement and

Patient Safety (QI/PS), including learning experiences and use of these concepts in the assessment of physicians across the continuum of education and practice [64].

Continuing Professional Development for Physicians in Practice

Since the 1970s, medicine, nursing and several other health professions require continuing education to maintain a professional license [65]. To ensure the effectiveness and quality of continuing education for physicians, providers of continuing medical education must be accredited by the Accreditation Council for Continuing Medical Education (ACCME) [66]. A review of the literature on the effectiveness of continuing medical education (CME) found a positive effect on attitude and practice behaviors, and some improvement in outcomes [67]. At the same time, the value of traditional CME is being challenged, with critics noting that CME is mostly delivered in lectures, with little post-participation assessment beyond learner reactions and self-reported changes in behaviors [68, 69]. In contrast, interactive learning, and participating in multiple activities focused on the same topic are effective in producing moderate to significant change in participants' behavior [70, 71]. A 2010 IOM report on redesigning continuing education in the health professions noted flaws in existing approaches that include narrow curricula, a failure to focus education on individual and collective knowledge and capability gaps [72], and gaps related to quality and safety of care.

The responsibility for assessing ongoing professional development of physicians in practice lies with the member boards of the American Board of Medical Specialties (ABMS). Board certification grew out of concerns about the quality of physician education and preparation for practice at the turn of the twentieth century, resulting in the establishment of the Advisory Board of Medical Specialties, the precursor of the American Board of Medical Specialties in 1933 [73].

Initially, board certification was achieved by passing a secure written and for some specialties and oral examination at the end of formal training and was valid over a physicians' entire career. Starting in the 1970s, several ABMS boards, acknowledging that medical knowledge changes rapidly over the course of a physician's career initiated a process of periodic re-certification through repeat secure knowledge examinations. Over time all member boards gradually moved from life-time certificates to time-limited certificates and periodic repeat examinations [74, 75]. The American Board of Family Medicine has required periodic recertification since its inauguration in 1969 [76]. Research on the effect of board certification has found a positive and statistically significant association between specialty board certification and greater compliance with recommended treatments and improved outcomes. Certification for internists is associated with improved patient care [77], and prevention of medical errors [78]. Examples from the surgical field include lower mortality and complication rates for surgical procedures, including carotid endarterectomies and aortic aneurysm surgery [79], colon surgery [80], and surgery for peptic ulcers [81].

In 1999, prompted by documented gaps in quality and safety of care in almost all areas of medicine and a growing focus on improving care, the ABMS redesigned the certification process to ensure ongoing competence by including expectations that all diplomates engage in measuring and improving the quality of care they provide, using the framework of the six competencies first developed by the ACGME and adopted by ABMS [73]. Over the past decade, certifying boards have moved from assessing professional development primarily based repeated assessment of medical knowledge through a secure examinations and participation in CME to use of self- and peer assessments of other competencies such as communication, professionalism, actual delivery of care, the ability to function in complex systems and the ability to assess and improve quality of care in practice [74]. The resulting four part Maintenance of Certification® (MOC) framework became official ABMS policy in 2000 and by 2006 all 24 member specialty boards had established time lines for implementing MOC [74].

The MOC has four components. Part I requires physicians maintain an unrestricted medical license [74], and surgeons must document they have privileges or a staff appointment in a hospital accredited by the Joint Commission [82]. Part II requires completion of a specified amount of CME or acquisition of specialty specific medical knowledge, some of which must relate to the physician's clinical practice [83]. Part III, "Cognitive Expertise," consist of a completing a periodic secure specialty examination, and Part IV, "Performance in Practice," requires physicians to assess their practice performance, with some boards requiring improvement data for a sample of patients, such as data extracted from medical records and clinical databases, or results of patient surveys [74]. Physicians may use Web-based improvement modules, such as the Patient Safety Improvement Program developed by the ABMS [84], or the improvement modules developed by the American Board of Pediatrics, American Board of Family Medicine and the American Board of Internal Medicine. Physicians are encouraged to aggregate their performance data into a portfolio that documents how their diagnostic and clinical decisions and outcomes compare to those of peers and available national comparisons. For surgeons, the MOC Part IV offers credit for ongoing participation in a national, regional or local outcomes registry or quality assessment program, and the American Board of Surgery requires that this improvement program address areas specific to the individual physician's practice [82]. The concept of continuous professional development integrated with PBLI is considered important in helping surgeons improve the care they provide to patients [85].

Physicians are encouraged to participate in proven QI efforts that have been shown to improve care to address gaps in quality in areas in need of improvement. Part IV activities in several specialties use Practice Improvement Modules (PIMs), which facilitates collaborative, QI efforts within practices and across practices [86, 87]. An added advantage of PIMs is that they can be used in teaching settings to collect longitudinal improvement data for individual residents [86, 87]. Several of the MOC programs also award Part IV MOC credit for diplomate participation in approved ongoing QI efforts in their practice setting. Some of these efforts are multi-center prospective ongoing QI networks that have demonstrated significant improvement in outcomes of care and at times reduction in cost of care [88]. Other examples include medication reconciliation [89], prevention of childhood obesity [90], and prevention and management of cardiac disease [91], among others. Some boards have made significant gains in introducing improvement activities into the professional development of practicing physicians while for other specialties MOC is still early in its implementation. Fifteen of the ABMS boards have agreed to common standards for awarding credit for MOC Part IV to diplomates who participate in organizationally sponsored QI efforts through the Multi-Specialty Portfolio Program [92]. Data on the effectiveness of MOC in improving the safety and quality of care is growing and can be tracked on the ABMS website (http://www.ABMS.org).

Physicians' role in institutional healthcare improvement requires a new skill set for individuals who function as institutional leaders in quality and safety, with a formal description of the role and its responsibilities [93], and the requisite knowledge and training, including implementation science and policy work [94, 95]. Examples of programs for training these quality experts are found in the Department of Veterans Affairs [96], Dartmouth College [97], and George Mason University [98].

Interprofessional and Team Learning

Given the variability in how and to what degree curricula and educational approaches in health professions education emphasize improving quality and patient safety, one solution that has been proposed is interprofessional education, which has been generally found to enhance quality and reduce cost in healthcare [99]. The value of interprofessional education has been emphasized since the 1970s [100], and beginning in 2013, the LCME standards require medical schools to prepare students to function collaboratively on teams that include other health professionals in training and practice [101].

The "Retooling for Quality and Safety" initiative of the Josiah Macy Jr. Foundation and the Institute for Healthcare Improvement has developed a curriculum focused on interprofessional training, involving both medical and nursing students [102]. The initiative fostered integration of improvement and patient safety curricula in undergraduate medical and nursing education, emphasizing the value of interprofessional learning because the didactic curriculum is taught the same way actual improvement occurs, in interprofessional teams addressing quality problems in a real clinical setting. The advantage of this approach is that "learning how to do quality improvement and actually carrying out quality improvement are essentially one and the same; both are special forms of experiential learning" [103]. A few successful models exist for the prelicensure phase of education [104], and there is a need to expand this work to the continuum of health professions formation.

Curricula for interprofessional learning have included train-the-trainer exercises that facilitate hands-on training [105]. For patient safety, curricular components have included patient safety basics, developing academic leadership, improving the culture of practice, changing the response to error, and applying principles of interprofessional teaching and learning [106]. Interprofessional learning is also being proposed for continuing education in the health professions. A 2010 IOM report on the redesign of continuing education recommended that it be carried out in interprofessional teams that mirror the team composition in the healthcare setting [107]. A recommendation for advancing team-based learning and practice also has called for the development of community learning sites to serve as venues for interprofessional learning and practice [108]. This type of interprofessional learning and practice does not yet occur in many settings, although there are efforts to conduct e-learning activities that provide a matched curriculum to multiple health professions, to promote interprofessional learning [109]. In addition the IHI Open School modules are suitable for use across difference health professions [31], and many of the quality improvement efforts approved for MOC Part 4 credit involve interdisciplinary care teams [74].

Barriers and Facilitators to QI Learning

Some of the barriers that account for the slow spread of QI in health professions education include a shortage of faculty able and prepared to teach these concepts in the clinical setting, discipline-specific educational "silos" that conflict with the need to teach and practice quality and safety improvement in multi-professional and inter-professional teams, perceptions that physicians in training must first acquire "clinical skills" before engaging in quality improvement, and a shortage of time and opportunity to insert hands-on experiences in quality and safety into packed medical education curricula. A final barrier to learner involvement in QI is the availability of real time patient quality and safety data related to the populations served by residency and fellowship programs. Even in organizations with well-developed quality improvement efforts, capabilities for assessing clinical outcomes of care in training programs lag behind most other areas.

The most frequently cited barrier is the lack of clinically based faculty members with the skills to teach improvement of care and the effect this has on the "informal curriculum" at the bedside and in the clinic. For example, the Macy Foundation's effort to promote interprofessional education in quality and safety found that a common challenge was the lack of sufficient faculty across all health professions trained in the principles and processes of improvement [102]. Teaching of quality and safety thus far has relied to a large degree on a small core of regional and national experts presenting lectures and educational modules. Many frontline teachers, not familiar or comfortable with quality and safety principles fail to enforce these concepts in the clinical context in training programs. Learning is influenced by organizational culture and the "informal curriculum" that can undermine teaching and valuing quality and safety especially when the faculty physicians are not engaged in meaningful quality improvement and safety efforts in their own practices. The informal curriculum is important because it teaches the "values of the profession," [110] and deeply influences professional formation [111]. Through this, it can enhance or thwart formal efforts to introduce new concepts, including added emphasis on approaches to enhance the quality and safety of care [110, 112, 113]. Work to overcome the informal curriculum as a barrier to meaningful, effective QI exposure for residents has focused on faculty development to improve their bedside QI teaching [64, 113], and enhancing faculty understanding of the power of the informal curriculum.

Recommendations for overcoming these barriers have focused on the alignment between the formal and informal curriculum to contribute to a learning healthcare system, including appropriate role modeling of QI practice by teaching faculty [113]. The AAMC's recommendations for integrating quality improvement and patient safety into faculty competencies include a focus on faculty development in these areas [64]. Practical efforts congruent with these principles have focused on QI becoming a more integral part of the residency curriculum by coordinating teaching of PBLI and SBP with resident engagement in improvement activities. This gives residents the opportunity to apply their new learning in a local context and to contribute to improving care. Active involvement of learners was recommended as early as the mid-1990s [114]. Nearly two decades later, models to achieve this are being developed and tested, with a focus on five components of a meaningful QI experience for leaners: (1) curricula and education models that ground learners in the principles of QI; (2) faculty preparation for teaching QI and practicing it in clinical settings; (3) ensuring all learners receive QI education; and (4) overcoming time and other constraints to allow them to apply newly developed QI skills, and (5) assessing the effect of exposure to QI on learners' competence [115].

The final barriers to effective QI education for physicians are the constraints on available time posed by packed clinical curricula and the time intensive nature of a meaningful QI immersion experience. This makes it challenging to meet expectations that all learners should be exposed in a meaningful way to QI, and have the opportunity for active participation in efforts to improve care. Efforts to overcome this barrier include revisions to the scheduling of residents' QI experiences. At one institution this resulted in a change of the QI experience first from a 1-month experience at 100 % time, to a 3-month experience at 50 % of the residents' time and ultimately to 9 months at 15 % protected time for QI to allow residents to initiate or participate in longitudinal improvement projects [116]. QI immersion programs for residents in several institutions have shown that it is possible to achieve meaningful resident involvement in QI within the established duty hour limits for medical residents [42, 117].

Assessing Educational and Clinical Outcomes of QI Education

Established methods of evaluation, such as examinations that test the acquisition of knowledge are not optimally designed competence in an applied concept like QI, which both requires experiential learning and application of the concepts in practice [118]. Assessment has focused on a broader set of learning outcomes such as gains in knowledge, changes in attitude, acquisition of skills and ability to engage in QI activities, actual clinical outcomes, and whether an intervention produced other benefits for patients or the healthcare system.

The Kirkpatrick framework for assessing the outcomes of learning is the approach most commonly used, and has been the basic model for assessing educational and training interventions across a range of industries [119]. Developed more than 50 years ago, it offers a comprehensive approach that assesses adult learning, taking into consideration the needs of the learner, the instructor, the larger system and the stakeholders, such as patients and the larger healthcare system, that the adult learning program is intended to benefit [119]. Kirkpatrick emphasized that the assessment of training should go beyond obtaining information in immediate reactions of the attendees, and assessment should be carried out on four different levels [119]. The four levels consist of: (1) **Reaction** - How well did the learners like the learning process; (2) **Learning** - What did they learn? (gains in knowledge and skills); (3) **Behavior** - (What changes in job performance resulted from the learning process? (gains in capability to perform the newly learned skills while on the job); and (4) **Results** - What are the tangible results of the learning process in terms of reduced cost, improved quality or efficiency [119].

Research on the outcomes of medical education has consistently found that involvement in QI benefitted residents' PBLI competence, including skill in designing projects and conducting plan-do-study-act cycles as well as their self-ratings of knowledge and efficacy related to QI [120]. Activities such as improvement exercises, multidisciplinary rounds, chart audits, and opportunities to compare residents' patient outcomes to relevant benchmarks were found to enhance proficiency in PBLI and SBP [121, 122]. The limitations of the literature on learning outcomes of residents' exposure to QI principles include the small samples for most studies, the narrow scope and brief follow-up period for many interventions, and the fact that outcomes often are limited to Kirkpatrick Levels 1 or 2. Studies that assessed the outcomes of training in general have found that level 3 is rarely attained and Level 4 is never assessed [123]. A systematic review of patient feedback in improving physician consult behavior found four studies that assessed interventions at Level 4 [124], and another review showed that most QI curricula in the literature resulted in improvement in learner knowledge or confidence to perform QI, yet only a few studies offered evidence that QI education had an actual impact on meaningful behavior change, as well as clinical outcomes [125]. A small number of studies have assessed the effect of a safety or quality curriculum to Level 3 of the Kirkpatrick framework [126].

Some studies that have involved residents have produced meaningful outcomes in the inpatient and ambulatory setting, including efforts to reduce sternal wound infections [127], improving surgical start and end times [128], and reducing catheter-associated bloodstream infections [129]. Despite these beneficial outcomes, there are practical challenges to assessing the effectiveness of teaching QI to residents in improving care. They include residents moving through rotations, delayed feedback, and the multifactorial inputs in the inpatient settings, making it difficult to attribute the improvement to a single intervention such as resident education and involvement in QI.

One reason for the small number of QI studies in the literature prior to the most recent decade may be that in the past, QI was given less attention and academic recognition than research, including non-acceptance for publication in research-focused academic journals. This contributed to a dearth of papers in the clinical literature on approaches that were successful in other settings for adoption or adaptation, as well as descriptions of what did not work. It also contributed to QI not being considered an area worthy of academic scholarly pursuit [130, 131], Over the past decade, availability of clinical outcomes of QI education has been facilitated by the emergence of QI as an area for formal scholarly work [132, 133], aided by the pioneering work of a few high-profile institutions to implement, test and report on clinical improvement. This type of collaborative work, including efforts coordinated by the Institute for Healthcare Improvement, has produced a number of high-profile, successful cross-institutional efforts to improve care. Examples include interventions to reduce adverse drug events [134], the study of the organizational climate for quality and patient safety [135], and efforts to improve the safety of pediatric anesthesia [136].

A growing body of literature describes QI collaborations in teaching settings, including interventions to reduce bloodstream catheter infections and other elements of the IHI patient safety campaigns [137–140], as well as efforts to link clinical quality and improvement education for physicians with other health professionals [141–143]. Additional efforts have focused on sharing QI data and best practices, with positive outcomes for care for patients with cardiovascular disease [144], premature infants [145], patients with chronic disease [146], glycemic control in the ICU environment [147], reductions in adverse events [148], prevention of complications in the surgical ICU [149], and the identification of expert-evaluated patient safety approaches [150]. Multi-institution collaborations include the Academic Chronic Care Collaborative, and the Academic Rapid Response Collaborative, which have adapted QI approaches to teaching settings with an emphasis on resident involvement [151, 152], and successful national multi-site QI improvement networks in pediatrics [153]. Other areas important to high performance and quality of care such as team work and the dimensions of effective team-based care have remained more elusive from an assessment perspective. Recommendations for the assessment of teamwork skills have focused on the importance of theory, capturing team and individual performance and outcome data, ensuring reliability and validity, and overcoming real and perceived barriers to measurement [154].

Recognizing the need to disseminate successful improvement efforts and the difficulty getting quality improvement articles accepted into leading medical journal, a group of leading QI experts and health researchers developed the Standards for Quality Improvement Reporting Excellence (SQUIRE) guidelines [155]. The guidelines are designed to facilitate the reporting of quality improvement work in healthcare. The SQUIRE standards provide clear, useful guidelines on how to organize articles for publication to facilitate dissemination of QI [156, 157]. In addition to SQUIRE, standards for the protection of human subjects, including informed consent, study integrity and ensuring the scientific value of protocols also are being adapted to QI interventions [158].

Areas for Future Research

The work of improving care has benefitted from research and scholarship by dedicated experts. There is a growing field of improvement research that includes studies on how to advance quality improvement theory and its application to real-world problems. Many of the unanswered questions and areas in need for further study involve QI and patient safety education in training programs. Addressing them will improve theory and practice in physician education and professional development relevant to healthcare quality and safety. Practical areas for study include identifying curricula that "fit" the processes for teaching QI in medical school and residency, with a focus toward preparing learners for interprofessional practice. A related question is how soon QI should be introduced in the health professions curriculum, as there may be benefits making QI an established part of the core curriculum in undergraduate medical education and pre-licensure education for other health professions. Also needed is research on how to adapt QI education for residents to the system constraints posed by the organization of the residency program, largely consisting of brief clinical rotations that do not permit longer-term immersion and learning within a given clinical context. A relevant research question is whether optimal engagement of learners in QI will necessitate changes in the structure and duration of residency. Work also is needed to explore the mechanisms for spreading of knowledge about QI, and how existing social networks in teaching institutions could be leveraged to facilitate wider learner engagement in QI, to overcome the "silos" of professional learning that have been found to deter the spread of innovation [159]. Finally, research is needed to advance the assessment of the outcomes of QI, including the benefits to quality when care is delivered by individuals who have had meaningful involvement and exposure to safety, root cause analyses and QI during their education [160]. Benefits should be assessed in terms of clinical and functional outcomes, health systems outcomes, such as costs and population health, and patient, staff and learner satisfaction. Future research will address questions relevant to healthcare quality that are just now being posed, but have not yet been framed as formal research topics. Topics include whether the medical school acceptance process could be refined, to target individuals that will providing high-quality care throughout their career; efforts to identify the most effective ways for students and residents to learn about quality and safety; and optimal approaches for learners to acquire judgment, systems-thinking and sensitivity to the multiple institutional and cultural contexts in which they function in their lifetime of practice.

No chapter on education for quality and safety is complete without a discussion of "value," defined as outcomes relative to costs [161]. Value is a topic in need of added research because to date, despite a realization of the importance of "value" to a high-functioning healthcare system, value and related concepts around stewardship of resources occupy a very limited space in the medical education curriculum. Recommendations for addressing cost along with quality, such as the IHI's "Triple Aim" framework [162] for optimizing health system performance are important for quality, safety and value of healthcare, but are largely conceptual and aspirational to date. The Triple Aim calls for a design of the health system to:

1. Improve the patient experience of care (including quality and satisfaction);
2. Improve the health of populations; and
3. Reduce the per capita cost of health care.

Further study is needed to identify optimum ways of teaching these concepts, as well as assessing the impact of this on medical practice, cost and patient and health system outcomes. Other new areas, not yet fully explored, include approaches to population health that involve improving the nation's health status [163, 164], and overcoming racial and ethnic disparities in healthcare [165, 166].

Improving healthcare is a professional obligation. Physicians put patients' lives at risk if the quality of care they and their care teams deliver is suboptimal, and they owe it to their patients to know the quality of the care they and their care teams deliver, and to address gaps in quality and safety. This is a continuous process of life lone professional development for those who choose to enter medicine. It begins with medical school and continues throughout their professional career.

References

1. Donabedian A. Evaluating quality of medical care. Milbank Q. 1966;44:166–206.
2. Wennberg JE. Variation in use of medicare services among regions and selected academic medical centers: is more better? New York: New York Academy of Medicine; 2005.
3. Mangione-Smith R, DeCristofaro AH, Setodji CM, et al. The quality of ambulatory care delivered to children in the United States. N Engl J Med. 2007;357(15):1515–23.
4. Fisher ES, Wennberg DE, Stukel TA, et al. Variations in the longitudinal efficiency of academic medical centers. Health Aff (Millwood). 2004;23.
5. Committee on Quality of Health Care in America, Institute of Medicine. Crossing the quality chasm: a new health system for the 21st century. Washington, DC: National Academies Press; 2001.
6. Kohn LT, Corrigan JM, Donaldson MS, editors. To err is human: building a safer health system. Washington, DC: National Academy Press; 2000.
7. Asch DA, Nicholson S, Srinivas S, Herrin J, Epstein AJ. Evaluating obstetrical residency programs using patient outcomes. JAMA. 2009;302(12):1277–83.
8. Dartmouth Health Atlas, Dartmouth College, Hanover. http://www.dartmouthatlas.org/pages/residency. Accessed 10 Mar 2014.
9. Gallagher L. Continuing education in nursing: a concept analysis. Nurse Educ Today. 2006;27(8).
10. Mallon WJ. Ernest Amory Codman: the end result of a life in medicine. Philadelphia: Saunders; 2000.
11. Cooper M. Quality assurance and improvement. In: Wolper LF, editor. Health care administration: planning, implementing, and managing organized delivery systems. Gaithersburg: Aspen Publishers, Inc; 1999.
12. Langley GJ, Nolan KM, Norman CL, Provost LP, Nolan TW. The improvement guide: a practical approach to enhancing organizational performance. 2nd ed. San Francisco: Jossey-Bass; 2009.
13. Berwick DM, Jain SH. The basis for quality care prepaid group practice. In: Enthoven AC, Tollen LA, editors. Toward a 21st century health system: the contributions and promise of prepaid group practice. San Francisco: Jossey-Bass; 2004.
14. Luce JM, Bindman AB, Lee PR. A brief history of health care quality assessment and improvement in the United States. West J Med. 1994;160(3):263–8.
15. Kenney CC. The best practice. New York: Public Affairs Books; 2008.
16. Batalden PB, Davidoff F. What is "quality improvement" and how can it transform healthcare? Qual Saf Health Care. 2007;16:2–3.
17. Greiner AC, Knebel E, editors. Health professions education: a bridge to quality. Washington, DC: National Academies Press; 2003.
18. The Academic Medical Center Working Group of the Institute for Healthcare Improvement. The imperative for quality: a call for action to medical schools and teaching hospitals. Acad Med. 2003;78:1085–9.
19. Thompson SA, Tilden VP. Embracing quality and safety education for the 21st century: building interprofessional education. J Nurs Educ. 2009;48(12):698–701.
20. Batalden P. Developing health professionals capable of continually improving health care quality, safety and value: the health professional educator's work. http://www.ihi.org/offerings/ihiopenschool/resources/Pages/ImprovementStories/DevelopingHealthProfessionalsCapableOfContinuallyImproving-HealthCare.aspx. Accessed 10 Mar 2014.
21. Batalden P, Leach D, Swing S, Dreyfus H, Dreyfus S. General competencies and accreditation in graduate medical education. Health Aff. 2002;21(5):103–11.
22. Commission on Collegiate Nursing Education. 2002. "CCNE Accreditation." Online. Available at http://www.aacn.nche.edu/Accreditation. Accessed 10 Mar 2014.

23. Byrd G. Can the profession of pharmacy serve as a model for health informationist professionals? J Med Libr Assoc. 2002;90(1):68–75.
24. Leach DC. Competence is a habit. JAMA. 2002; 287(2):243–4.
25. Johnson JK, Miller SH, Horowitz SD. Systems-based practice: improving the safety and quality of patient care by recognizing and improving the systems in which we work. In: Henriksen K, Battles JB, Keyes MA, Grady ML, editors. Advances in patient safety: new directions and alternative approaches, Culture and redesign, vol. 2. Rockville: Agency for Healthcare Research and Quality (US); 2008.
26. Knowles MS. Self-directed learning: a guide for learners and teachers. Englewood Cliffs: Prentice Hall; 1975.
27. Chatterji M, Graham MJ, Wyer PC. Mapping cognitive overlaps between practice-based learning and improvement and evidence-based medicine: an operational definition for assessing resident physician competence. J Grad Med Educ. 2009;1(2):287–98.
28. Moskowitz EJ, Nash DB. Teaching trainees the tenets of quality and safety: an annotated bibliography. Am J Med Qual. 2009;24(4):333–43.
29. American Board of Medical Specialties. ABMS® Patient Safety Improvement Program. 2009. http://www.abms.org/Products_and_Publications/pdf/ABMS_PS_ImprovementProgram.pdf. Accessed 10 Mar 2014.
30. Sachdeva AK, Philibert I, Leach DC, Blair PG, Stewart LK, Rubinfeld IS, Britt LD. Patient safety curriculum for surgical residency programs: results of a national consensus conference. Surgery. 2007;141(4):427–41.
31. Martin L, Joyner, B. IHI Open School as a framework for resident education in safety and quality. Institute for Healthcare Improvement. 2013. http://www.ihi.org/offerings/IHIOpenSchool/resources/Pages/UniversityOfWashingtonResidentEducation.aspx. Accessed 10 Mar 2014.
32. More Medical and Nursing Schools to Require IHI Open School Basic Certificate. Institute for Healthcare Improvement. 2013. http://www.ihi.org/offerings/IHIOpenSchool/resources/Pages/MoreMedicalAndNursingSchoolsRequireBasicCertificate.aspx. Accessed 17 June 2013.
33. Houle CO. Continuing learning in the professions. San Francisco: Jossey-Bass; 1980.
34. Wong BM, Etchells EE, Kuper A, Levinson W, Shojania KG. Teaching quality improvement and patient safety to trainees: a systematic review. Acad Med. 2010;85(9):1425–39.
35. Levitt DS, Hauer KE, Poncelet A, Mookherjee S. An innovative quality improvement curriculum for third-year medical students. Med Educ Online. 2012;17. doi:10.3402/meo.v17i0.18391.
36. Walton M, Woodward H, Van Staalduinen S, Lemer C, Greaves F, Noble D, Ellis B, Donaldson L, Barraclough B. The WHO patient safety curriculum guide for medical schools. Qual Saf Health Care. 2010;19(6):542–6. doi:10.1136/qshc.2009.036970.
37. Liaison Committee on Medical Education. Functions and structure of a medical school. http://www.lcme.org/functions.pdf. Accessed 10 Mar 2014.
38. Foundation NPS, Institute LL. Unmet needs: teaching physicians to provide safe patient care. National Patient Safety Foundation; 2010. http://www.npsf.org/about-us/lucian-leape-institute-at-npsf/lli-reports-and-statements/the-patient-safety-imperative-for-health-care-reform/unmet-needs. Accessed 10 Mar 2014.
39. Aron DC, Headrick LA. Educating physicians prepared to improve care and safety is no accident: it requires a systematic approach. Qual Saf Health Care. 2002;11(2):168–73.
40. Weingart SN, Tess A, Driver J, Aronson MD, Sands K. Creating a quality improvement elective for medical house officers. J Gen Intern Med. 2004;19(8):861–7.
41. Reardon CL, Ogrinc G, Walaszek A. A didactic and experiential quality improvement curriculum for psychiatry residents. J Grad Med Educ. 2011;3(4): 562–5.
42. Akins RB, Handal GA. Utilizing quality improvement methods to improve patient care outcomes in a pediatric residency program. J Grad Med Educ. 2009;1(2):299–303.
43. Sepulveda D, Varaklis K. Implementing a multifaceted quality-improvement curriculum in an obstetrics-gynecology resident continuity-clinic setting: a 4-year experience. J Grad Med Educ. 2012;4(2): 237–41.
44. Singh R, Naughton B, Taylor JS, Koenigsberg MR, Anderson DR, McCausland LL, Wahler RG, Robinson A, Singh G. A comprehensive collaborative patient safety residency curriculum to address the ACGME core competencies. Med Educ. 2005;39(12):1195–204.
45. Stanton F, Grant J. Approaches to experiential learning, course delivery and validation in medicine. A background document. Med Educ. 1999;33(4):282–97.
46. Kolb DA. Experiential learning: experience as the source of learning and development. Englewood Cliffs: Prentice Hall; 1984.
47. Hall LW, Headrick LA, Cox KR, Deane K, Gay JW, Brandt J. Linking health professional learners and health care workers on action-based improvement teams. Qual Manag Health Care. 2009;18(3):194–201.
48. McClain EK, Babbott SF, Tsue TT, Girod DA, Clements D, Gilmer L, Persons D, Unruh G. Use of a structured template to facilitate practice-based learning and improvement projects. J Grad Med Educ. 2012;4(2):215–9.
49. Folcik MA, Kirton OC, Ivy ME. A two-tiered quality management program: Morbidity and Mortality conference data applied to resident education. Conn Med. 2007;71(8):471–8.
50. Kravet SJ, Howell E, Wright SM. Morbidity and mortality conference, grand rounds, and the ACGME's core competencies. J Gen Intern Med. 2006;21(11):1192–4.

51. Stiles BM, Reece TB, Hedrick TL, Garwood RA, Hughes MG, Dubose JJ, Adams RB, Schirmer BD, Sanfey HA, Sawyer RG. General surgery morning report: a competency-based conference that enhances patient care and resident education. Curr Surg. 2006;63(6):385–90.
52. Ogrinc G, Headrick LA, Morrison LJ, Foster T. Teaching and assessing resident competence in practice-based learning and improvement. J Gen Intern Med. 2004;19(5 Pt 2):496–500.
53. Krajewski K, Siewert B, Yam S, Kressel HY, Kruskal JB. A quality assurance elective for radiology residents. Acad Radiol. 2007;14(2):239–45.
54. Varkey P, Reller MK, Smith A, Ponto J, Osborn M. An experiential interdisciplinary quality improvement education initiative. Am J Med Qual. 2006;21(5): 317–22.
55. Hussain KA, Kelton GM. Utilization of health care quality markers in a family medicine outpatient setting. Fam Med. 2006;38(7):490–3.
56. Canal DF, Torbeck L, Djuricich AM. Practice-based learning and improvement: a curriculum in continuous quality improvement for surgery residents. Arch Surg. 2007;142(5):479–82.
57. Frey K, Edwards F, Altman K, Spahr N, Gorman RS. The 'Collaborative Care' curriculum: an educational model addressing key ACGME core competencies in primary care residency training. Med Educ. 2003; 37(9):786–9.
58. Oyler J, Vinci L, Johnson JK, Arora VM. Teaching internal medicine residents to sustain their improvement through the quality assessment and improvement curriculum. J Gen Intern Med. 2011;26(2):221–5.
59. Quinn DC, Bingham JW, Garriss GW, Dozier EA. Residents learn to improve care using the ACGME core competencies and institute of medicine aims for improvement: the health care matrix. J Grad Med Educ. 2009;1(1):119–26.
60. Singleton AF, Bazargan M, Ilagan B, Yan L, Eugenio J. Using resident focus groups to improve subspecialty consultations in a pediatric urgent care setting. J Natl Med Assoc. 2006;98(9):1478–82.
61. Mohr JJ, Randolph GD, Laughon MM, Schaff E. Integrating improvement competencies into residency education: a pilot project from a pediatric continuity clinic. Ambul Pediatr. 2003;3(3):131–6.
62. Fishbane S, Niederman MS, Daly C, Magin A, Kawabata M, de Corla-Souza A, Choudhery I, Brody G, Gaffney M, Pollack S, Parker S. The impact of standardized order sets and intensive clinical case management on outcomes in community-acquired pneumonia. Arch Intern Med. 2007;167(15):1664–9.
63. Kalanithi L, Coffey CE, Mourad M, Vidyarthi AR, Hollander H, Ranji SR. The effect of a resident-led quality improvement project on improving communication between hospital-based and outpatient physicians. Am J Med Qual. 2013;28(6):472–9.
64. Association of American Medical Colleges. Integrating quality improvement and patient safety across the continuum of medical education. Report of an Expert Panel. 2013. https://members.aamc.org/eweb/upload/Teaching%20for%20Quality%20Report.pdf. Accessed 10 Mar 2014.
65. Landers MR, McWhorter JW, Krum LL, Glovinsky D. Mandatory continuing education in physical therapy: survey of physical therapists in states with and states without a mandate. Phys Ther. 2005;85(9):861–71.
66. ANCC (American Nurses Credentialing Center). ANCC accreditation application manual. http://www.nursecredentialing.org/ContinuingEducation/Accreditation/AccreditationProcess.aspx. Accessed 10 Mar 2014.
67. Marinopoulos SS, Dorman T, Ratanawongsa N, Wilson LM, Ashar BH, Magaziner JL, Miller RG, Thomas PA, Prokopowicz PG, Qayyum R, Bass EB. Effectiveness of continuing medical education, Evidence report/technology assessment no. 149. Rockville: Agency for Healthcare Research and Quality; 2007.
68. Davis D, O'Brien MA, Freemantle N, Wolf FM, Mazmanian P, Taylor-Vaisey A. Impact of formal continuing medical education: do conferences, workshops, rounds, and other traditional continuing education activities change physician behavior or health care outcomes? JAMA. 1999;282(9):867–74.
69. Bloom BS. Review effects of continuing medical education on improving physician clinical care and patient health: a review of systematic reviews. Int J Technol Assess Health Care. 2005;21(3):380–5.
70. Mansouri M, Lockyer J. A meta-analysis of continuing medical education effectiveness. J Contin Educ Health Prof. 2007;27(1):6–15.
71. Forsetlun L, Bjørndal A, Rashidian A, Jamtvedt G, O'Brien MA, Wolf FM, Davis D, Odgaard-Jensen J, Oxman AD. Continuing education meetings and workshops: effects on professional practice and health care outcomes. Cochrane Database Syst Rev. 2009. http://onlinelibrary.wiley.com/doi/10.1002/14651858.CD003030.pub2/full. Accessed 10 Mar 2014.
72. Institute of Medicine. Redesigning continuing education in the health professions. Washington, DC: The National Academies Press; 2009.
73. Miller S. ABMS' maintenance of certification. Clin Orthop Relat Res. 2006;449:155–8.
74. American Board of Medical Specialties. ABMS maintenance of certification. http://abms.org/Maintenance_of_Certification/ABMS_MOC.aspx. Accessed 10 Mar 2014.
75. Miller SH, Thompson JN, Mazmanian PE, Aparicio A, Davis D, Spivey B, Kahn N. Continuing medical education, professional development, and requirements for medical licensure: a white paper of the conjoint committee on continuing medical education. J Contin Educ Health Prof. 2008;28(2):95–8.
76. Sumner 2nd W, Truszczynski M, Marek VW. A formal model of family medicine. J Am Board Fam Pract. 1996;9(1):41–52.
77. Holmboe E, Wang Y, Mechan T, et al. Association between maintenance of certification examination scores and quality of care for medicare beneficiaries. Arch Intern Med. 2008;168(13):1396–403.

78. Brennan TA, Horwitz RI, Duffy FD, Cassel CK, Goode LD, Lipner RS. The role of physician specialty board certification status in the quality movement. JAMA. 2004;292(9):1038–43.
79. Pearce W, Parker M, Feinglass J, Ujiki M, Manheim L. The importance of surgeon volume and training in outcomes for vascular surgical procedures. J Vasc Surg. 1999;299:768–76.
80. Prystowsky J, Bordage G, Feinglass J. Patient outcomes for segmental colon resection according to surgeon's training, certification, and experience. Surgery. 2002;132:663–70.
81. Kelly J, Hellinger F. Physician and hospital factors associated with mortality of surgical patients. Med Care. 1986;24:785–800.
82. The American Board of Surgery, MOC Part 4 – practice assessment resources. http://www.absurgery.org/default.jsp?exam-mocpa. Accessed 10 Mar 2014.
83. American Board of Pediatrics. Part IV maintenance of certification. http://www.aap.org/en-us/professional-resources/practice-support/quality-improvement/Quality-Improvement-Innovation-Networks/pages/American-Board-of-Pediatrics-Part-4-Maintenance-of-Certification.aspx?nfstatus. Accessed 10 Mar 2014.
84. ABMS® Patient Safety Improvement Program. http://www.abms.org/Products_and_Publications/pdf/ABMS_PS_ImprovementProgram.pdf. Accessed 10 Mar 2014.
85. Sachdeva AK. The new paradigm of continuing education in surgery. Arch Surg. 2005;140(3):264–9.
86. Caverzagie KJ, Bernabeo EC, Reddy SG, Holmboe ES. The role of physician engagement on the impact of the hospital-based practice improvement module (PIM). J Hosp Med. 2009;4(8):466–70.
87. Vinci LM, Oyler J, Johnson JK, Arora VM. Effect of a quality improvement curriculum on resident knowledge and skills in improvement. Qual Saf Health Care. 2010;19(4):351–4.
88. Lannon CM, Miles PV, Stockman 3rd JA. The path forward: collaborative networks and the future for children's health care. Pediatrics. 2013;131 Suppl 4:S226–7.
89. Rappaport DI, Collins B, Koster A, Mercado A, Greenspan J, Lawless S, Hossain J, Sharif I. Implementing medication reconciliation in outpatient pediatrics. Pediatrics. 2011;128(6):e1600–7.
90. Huang JS, Chun S, Sandhu A, Terrones L. Quality improvement in childhood obesity management through the maintenance of certification process. J Pediatr. 2013;26.
91. Bernabeo EC, Conforti LN, Holmboe ES. The impact of a preventive cardiology quality improvement intervention on residents and clinics: a qualitative exploration. 13. Am J Med Qual. 2009;24(2):99–107.
92. Multispecialty MOC Portfolio Approval Program. http://mocportfolioprogram.org/. Accessed 9 Mar 2014.
93. Pronovost PJ, Miller MR, Wachter RM, Meyer GS. Perspective: physician leadership in quality. Acad Med. 2009;84(12):1651–6.
94. Pronovost PJ, Goeschel CA, Marsteller JA, Sexton JB, Pham JC, Berenholtz SM. A framework for patient safety research and improvement. Circulation. 2009;119:330–7.
95. Ackerly DC, Parekh A, Stein D. Perspective: a framework for career paths in health systems improvement. Acad Med. 2013;88(1):56–60.
96. Department of Veterans Affairs National Quality Scholars Fellowship Program. http://www.va.gov/oaa/specialfellows/programs/SF_NQSF_default.asp?p=10. Accessed 10 Mar 2014.
97. Center for Leadership and Improvement, The Dartmouth Institute. http://tdi.dartmouth.edu/faculty/tina-foster-md-mph. Accessed 10 Mar 2014.
98. Quality Improvement and Outcomes Management in Health Care Systems, Graduate Certificate, George Mason University. http://chhs.gmu.edu/quality/. Accessed 10 Mar 2014.
99. Baldwin Jr DC. Some historical notes on interdisciplinary and interprofessional education and practice in health care in the USA. 1996. J Interprof Care. 2007;21 Suppl 1:23–37.
100. Institute of Medicine. Educating for the heath team. Washington, DC: National Academy of Sciences; 1972.
101. Liaison Committee on Medical Education. New Accreditation Standard ED-19-A Approved. http://www.lcme.org/. Accessed 10 Mar 2014.
102. Headrick LA, Barton AJ, Ogrinc G, Strang C, Aboumatar HJ, Aud MA, Haidet P, Lindell D, Madigosky WS, Patterson JE. Results of an effort to integrate quality and safety into medical and nursing school curricula and foster joint learning. Health Aff (Millwood). 2012;31(12):2669–80.
103. Batalden P, Davidoff F. Teaching quality improvement: the devil is in the details. JAMA. 2007;298:1059–61.
104. Westberg SM, Adams J, Thiede K, Stratton TP, Bumgardner MA. An interprofessional activity using standardized patients. Am J Pharm Educ. 2006;70(2):34.
105. Mitchell PH, Robins Lynn S, Schaad D. Creating a curriculum for training health profession faculty leaders. http://www.ahrq.gov/professionals/quality-patient-safety/patient-safety-resources/resources/advances-in-patient-safety/vol4/Mitchell.pdf. Accessed 10 Mar 2014.
106. Cleghorn GD, Baker GR. What faculty need to learn about improvement and how to teach it to others. J Interprof Care. 2000;14(2):147–59.
107. Institute of Medicine. Redesigning continuing education in the health professions. Washington, DC: The National Academies Press; 2010.
108. Team-Based Competencies: Building a Shared Foundation for Education and Clinical Practice. Macy Foundation. Conference Proceedings. Washington, DC. 2011. http://macyfoundation.org/docs/macy_pubs/Team-Based_Competencies.pdf. Accessed 10 Mar 2014.
109. Segrave S, Holt D. Contemporary learning environments: designing e-learning for education in the professions. Distance Educ. 2003;24(1):7–24.

110. Hafferty F. Beyond curriculum reform: confronting medicine's hidden curriculum. Acad Med. 1998;73: 403–7.
111. Cooke M, Irby DM, O'Brien BC. Educating physicians: a call for reform of medical school and residency. San Francisco: Jossey-Bass; 2010.
112. Stern DT. In search of the informal curriculum: when and where professional values are taught. Acad Med. 1998;73(10 Suppl):S28–30.
113. Pingleton SK, Horak BJ, Davis DA, Goldmann DA, Keroack MA, Dickler RM. Is there a relationship between high-quality performance in major teaching hospitals and residents' knowledge of quality and patient safety? Acad Med. 2009;84(11):1510–5.
114. Weingart SN. House officer education and organizational obstacles to quality improvement. Jt Comm J Qual Improv. 1996;22(9):640–6.
115. Philibert I, Johnstone MJ. Initiating and sustaining resident involvement in quality improvement: top-down and bottom-up approaches. Chicago: Accreditation Council for Graduate Medical Education; 2008.
116. Philibert I, Gonzalez del Rey JA, Lannon C, Lieh-Lai M, Weiss KB. Quality improvement skills for pediatric residents: from lecture to implementation and sustainability. Acad Pediatr. 2014;14(1):40–6.
117. Shaikh U, Natale JE, Nettiksimmons J, Li ST. Improving pediatric health care delivery by engaging residents in team-based quality improvement projects. Am J Med Qual. 2013;28(2):120–6.
118. Cooke M, Ironside PM, Ogrinc GS. Mainstreaming quality and safety: a reformulation of quality and safety education for health professions students. BMJ Qual Saf. 2011;20(Suppl_1):i79–82.
119. Kirkpatrick D. Evaluating training programs: the four levels. San Francisco: Berrett-Koehler; 1998.
120. Djuricich AM, Ciccarelli M, Swigonski NL. A continuous quality improvement curriculum for residents: addressing core competency, improving systems. Acad Med. 2004;79(10 Suppl):S65–7.
121. Ziegelstein RC, Fiebach NH. "The mirror" and "the village": a new method for teaching practice-based learning and improvement and systems-based practice. Acad Med. 2004;79(1):83–8.
122. Lyman J, Schorling J, May N, Scully K, Sarafian N, Nadkarni M, Voss J. Customizing a clinical data warehouse for housestaff education in practice-based learning and improvement. AMIA Annu Symp Proc. 2006;1017.
123. Catalanello R, Kirkpatrick D. Evaluating training programs: the state of the art. Train Dev J. 1968; 22(5):2–9.
124. Reinders ME, Ryan BL, Blankenstein AH, van der Horst HE, Stewart MA, van Marwijk HW. The effect of patient feedback on physicians' consultation skills: a systematic review. Acad Med. 2011;86(11):1426–36.
125. Boonyasai RT, Windish DM, Chakraborti C, Feldman LS, Rubin HR, Bass EB. Effectiveness of teaching quality improvement to clinicians: a systematic review. JAMA. 2007;298(9):1023–37.
126. Lee P, Allen K, Daly M. A 'Communication and Patient Safety' training programme for all healthcare staff: can it make a difference? BMJ Qual Saf. 2012; 21(1):84–8.
127. Woodward CS, Son M, Taylor R, Husain SA. Prevention of sternal wound infection in pediatric cardiac surgery: a protocolized approach. World J Pediatr Congenit Heart Surg. 2012;3(4):463–9.
128. Varughese AM, Adler E, Anneken A, Kurth CD. Improving on-time start of day and end of day for a pediatric surgical service. Pediatrics. 2013;132(1): e219–28.
129. Wheeler DS, Giaccone MJ, Hutchinson N, Haygood M, Bondurant P, Demmel K, Kotagal UR, Connelly B, Corcoran MS, Line K, Rich K, Schoettker PJ, Brilli RJ. A hospital-wide quality-improvement collaborative to reduce catheter-associated bloodstream infections. Pediatrics. 2011;128(4):e995–1004; quiz e1004–7.
130. Blumenthal D, Kilo CM. A report card on continuous quality improvement. Milbank Q. 1998;76(4): 625–48.
131. Shortell SM, Bennet CL, Byck GR. Assessing the impact of continuous quality improvement on clinical practice: what it will take to accelerate progress. Milbank Q. 1998;76(4):593–624.
132. Lynn J. When does quality improvement count as research? Human subject protection and theories of knowledge. Qual Saf Health Care. 2004;13:67–70.
133. Reinhardt AC, Ray LN. Differentiating quality improvement from research. Appl Nurs Res. 2003; 16(1):2–8.
134. Leape LL, Kabcenell AI, Gandhi TK, Carver P, Nolan TW, Berwick DM. Reducing adverse drug events: lessons from a breakthrough series collaborative. Jt Comm J Qual Improv. 2000;26(6):321–31.
135. Pronovost PJ, Weast B, Holzmueller CG, Rosenstein BJ, Kidwell RP, Haller KB, Feroli ER, Sexton JB, Rubin HR. Evaluation of the culture of safety: survey of clinicians and managers in an academic medical center. Qual Saf Health Care. 2003;12(6):405–10.
136. Kurth CD, Tyler D, Heitmiller E, Tosone SR, Martin L, Deshpande JK. National pediatric anesthesia safety quality improvement program in the United States. Anesth Analg. 2014;119(1):112–21.
137. Berenholtz SM, Pronovost PJ, Lipsett PA, Hobson D, Earsing K, Farley JE, Milanovich S, Garrett-Mayer E, Winters BD, Rubin HR, Dorman T, Perl TM. Eliminating catheter-related bloodstream infections in the intensive care unit. Crit Care Med. 2004;32(10): 2014–20.
138. Johnson T, Currie G, Keill P, Corwin SJ, Pardes H, Cooper MR. NewYork-Presbyterian Hospital: translating innovation into practice. Jt Comm J Qual Patient Saf. 2005;31(10):554–60.
139. Pronovost PJ, Berenholtz SM, Goeschel CA, et al. Creating high reliability in health care organizations. Health Serv Res. 2006;41(4 Pt 2):1599–617.
140. Pronovost PJ, King J, Holzmueller CG, Sawyer M, Bivens S, Michael M, Haig K, Paine L, Moore D, Miller M. A web-based tool for the Comprehensive

Unit-based Safety Program (CUSP). Jt Comm J Qual Patient Saf. 2006;32(3):119–29.
141. Jagsi R, Kitch BT, Weinstein DF, Campbell EG, Hutter M, Weissman JS. Residents report on adverse events and their causes. Arch Intern Med. 2005;165(22): 2607–13.
142. Lypson ML, Frohna JG, Gruppen LD, Woolliscroft JO. Assessing residents' competencies at baseline: identifying the gaps. Acad Med. 2004;79(6):564–70.
143. Afessa B, Kennedy CC, Klarich KW, Aksamit TR, Kolars JC, Hubmayr RD. Introduction of a 14-hour work shift model for housestaff in the medical ICU. Chest. 2005;128(6):3910–5.
144. Likosky DS, Nugent WC, Ross CS, Northern New England Cardiovascular Disease Study Group. Improving outcomes of cardiac surgery through cooperative efforts: the northern New England experience. Semin Cardiothorac Vasc Anesth. 2005;9(2):119–21.
145. Ohlinger J, Kantak A, Lavin Jr JP, Fofah O, Hagen E, Suresh G, Halamek LP, Schriefer JA. Evaluation and development of potentially better practices for perinatal and neonatal communication and collaboration. Pediatrics. 2006;118 Suppl 2:S147–52.
146. Wagner EH, Glasgow RE, Davis C, Bonomi AE, Provost L, McCulloch D, Carver P, Sixta C. Quality improvement in chronic illness care: a collaborative approach. Jt Comm J Qual Improv. 2001;27(2):63–80.
147. Martinez EA, Chavez-Valdez R, Holt NF, Grogan KL, Khalifeh KW, Slater T, Winner LE, Moyer J, Lehmann CU. Successful implementation of a perioperative glycemic control protocol in cardiac surgery: barrier analysis and intervention using lean six sigma. Anesthesiol Res Pract. 2011;2011:565069.
148. Resar RK, Rozich JD, Simmonds T, Haraden CR. A trigger tool to identify adverse events in the intensive care unit. Jt Comm J Qual Patient Saf. 2006;32(10): 585–90.
149. Shake JG, Pronovost PJ, Whitman GJ. Cardiac surgical ICU care: eliminating "preventable" complications. J Card Surg. 2013;30.
150. Shekelle PG, Pronovost PJ, Wachter RM, McDonald KM, Schoelles K, Dy SM, Shojania K, Reston JT, Adams AS, Angood PB, Bates DW, Bickman L, Carayon P, Donaldson L, Duan N, Farley DO, Greenhalgh T, Haughom JL, Lake E, Lilford R, Lohr KN, Meyer GS, Miller MR, Neuhauser DV, Ryan G, Saint S, Shortell SM, Stevens DP, Walshe K. The top patient safety strategies that can be encouraged for adoption now. Ann Intern Med. 2013; 158(5 Pt 2):365–8.
151. Stevens DP, Wagner EH. Transform residency training in chronic illness care – now. Acad Med. 2006;81(8):685–7.
152. Wood KA, Ranji SR, Ide B, Dracup K. Use of rapid response systems in adult academic medical centers. Jt Comm J Qual Patient Saf. 2009;35(9):475–82.
153. Lannon CM, Miles PV. Pediatric collaborative improvement networks: bridging quality gaps to improve health outcomes. Pediatrics. 2013;131 Suppl 4:S187–8. doi:10.1542/peds.2012-3786D.
154. Baker DP, Salas E, King H, Battles J, Barach P. The role of teamwork in the professional education of physicians: current status and assessment recommendations. Jt Comm J Qual Patient Saf. 2005;31(4): 185–202.
155. Davidoff F, Batalden P, Stevens D, Ogrinc G, Mooney SE, SQUIRE Development Group. Publication guidelines for quality improvement studies in health care: evolution of the SQUIRE project. BMJ. 2009;338:a3152.
156. Standards for quality improvement reporting excellence. http://squire-statement.org/. Accessed 10 Mar 2014.
157. Oermann MH. SQUIRE Guidelines for reporting improvement studies in healthcare: implications for nursing publications. J Nurs Care Qual. 2009; 24(2):91–5.
158. Harrington L. Quality improvement, research, and the institutional review board. J Healthc Qual. 2007; 29(3):4–9.
159. Ferlie E, Fitzgerald L, Wood M, et al. The nonspread of innovations: the mediating role of professionals. Acad Manage J. 2005;48(1):117–34.
160. Vohra P, Daugherty C, Mohr J, Wen M, Barach P. Housestaff and medical student attitudes towards adverse medical events. JCAHO Journal of Quality and Safety. 2007;33:467–76.
161. Porter ME. Defining and introducing value in health care. In: Evidence-based medicine and the changing nature of health care: 2007 IOM annual meeting summary. Washington, DC: Institute of Medicine; 2008. p. 161–72.
162. Institute for Healthcare Improvement. Triple aim: the best care for the whole population at the lowest cost. http://www.ihi.org/offerings/Initiatives/TripleAim/Pages/default.aspx. Accessed 10 Mar 2014.
163. Anderson GF, Squires DA. Measuring the U.S. health care system: a cross-national comparison. Issue Brief (Commonw Fund). 2010;90:1–10.
164. The National Association of County and City Health Officials. A strategic approach to community health improvement: MAPP field guide. National Association of City and County Health Officials; City of publication is Washington, DC. 2007.
165. Chin MH, Chien AT. Reducing racial and ethnic disparities in health care: an integral part of quality improvement scholarship. Qual Saf Health Care. 2006;15:79–80.
166. Weiss KB, Wagner R, Nasca TJ. Development, testing, and implementation of the ACGME Clinical Learning Environment Review (CLER) program. J Grad Med Educ. 2012;4(3):396–8.

Surgical Volume and Outcome Relationship in Pediatric Cardiac Surgery

8

David Kalfa, Danielle Gottlieb, Jonathan M. Chen, and Emile Bacha

Abstract

A significant inverse relationship between surgical institutional and surgeon volume and patient outcome has been demonstrated in many high-stakes surgical specialties. By in large, the same results were found in pediatric cardiac surgery, where a more thorough analysis has demonstrated that this relationship is mediated by case complexity and the type of surgical procedures. Lower-volume programs tend to underperform in comparison to larger programs as case complexity increases. High-volume pediatric cardiac surgeons have better results compared with low-volume surgeons, especially with complex procedures such as with the Norwood procedure. Nevertheless, this trend towards lower mortality at larger centers is not universal: all larger programs do not perform better than all smaller programs. Moreover, surgical volume seems to account for only a small proportion of the overall between-center variation in outcome. Thus the use of center-specific risk adjusted outcomes as a tool for quality assessment may be more reliable than relying upon surgical volume alone. Indeed, a patient's risk factors and their level of disease severity may play a more important

D. Kalfa, MD, PhD (✉)
Department of Pediatric Cardiac Surgery, Morgan Stanley Children's hospital – New York Presbyterian Hospital, 3959 Broadway, New York, NY 10032, USA
e-mail: dk2757@cumc.columbia.edu

D. Gottlieb, MS, MD, MPH
Department of Pediatric Cardiac Surgery, Columbia University Medical Center, Morgan Stanley Children's Hospital, 3959 Broadway CHN-276, New York, NY 10032, USA
e-mail: dgottlieb1@gmail.com

J.M. Chen, MD
Department of Pediatric Cardiac Surgery, Congenital Cardiac Surgery, University of Washington School of Medicine, Seattle, WA 98105, USA

Heart Center, Seattle Children's Hospital, 4800 Sand Point Way NE, Seattle, WA 98105, USA
e-mail: jonathan.chen@seattlechildrens.org

E. Bacha, MD
Division of Cardiothoracic and Vascular Surgery, Department of Surgery, Columbia University Medical Center, Columbia/NewYork-Presbyterian, 3959 Broadway North Room 274, New York, NY 10032, USA
e-mail: eb2709@cumc.columbia.edu

P.R. Barach, J.P. Jacobs, S.E. Lipshultz, P.C. Laussen (eds.),
Pediatric and Congenital Cardiac Care: Volume 2: Quality Improvement and Patient Safety,
DOI 10.1007/978-1-4471-6566-8_8, © Springer-Verlag London 2015

role in determining their individual outcome than the impact of the surgeon or program's volume. Nevertheless, the relationship between surgical volume and outcome in pediatric cardiac surgery is strong enough that it ought to shape and influence public policy around the decision to centralise pediatric cardiac surgery and support strategies that support higher center and surgeon volumes and their impact on patients and providers.

Keywords
Case complexity • Norwood procedure • Outcome • Pediatric cardiac surgery • Quality assessment • Surgical volume

Introduction

Pediatric cardiac surgery is a high-risk field that depends on safe practices, continuous research into improvement of outcomes and measurement of quality [1]. However, the definition and measurement of quality in pediatric cardiac surgery is in its infancy [2]. One of the most simple and easily available tools for health quality measures in all surgical specialities is the surgical volume of a hospital. Birkmeyer et al. demonstrated that Medicare patients undergoing selected cardiovascular or cancer procedures can significantly reduce their risk of operative death by simply selecting a high-volume hospital for their procedure [3]. Two extensive reviews [4, 5] systematically assessed the methodology and results of studies dealing with this volume/outcome relationship in varied surgical and medical fields. Many of these studies were found to be compromised by the use of retrospective administrative data [6], inadequate risk adjustment and problematic statistical methodology [7]. In pediatric cardiac surgery, the specific relationship between institutional and surgeon volumes and outcome (mortality, complications) is currently the subject of numerous investigations and remains controversial. The conclusions drawn from these studies might have an outstanding impact internationally on the intra institution, inter institution and national organization of pediatric cardiac services.

This chapter aims at highlighting (1) current evidence of surgical volume on patient outcome relationships in pediatric cardiac surgery; (2) the specific volume/outcome relationship depending on case complexity, type of surgical procedures and surgeon volume; and, (3) the potential consequences in terms of quality improvement initiatives and regional/national public health policies.

Overall Relationship Between Institutional Surgical Volume and Outcome in Pediatric Cardiac Surgery

Studies Based on Administrative Data or Single-state Clinical Data

In 1995, Jenkins et al. reported preliminary observations of variation of in-hospital mortality in pediatric cardiac surgery depending on hospital caseload [8]. This study, based on retrospective assessment of administrative databases included children undergoing surgery for congenital heart disease in California or Massachusetts. These patients were identified by the presence of procedure codes indicating surgical repair of a congenital heart defect in computerized aggregated hospital discharge abstract databases in the two states. It was shown that centers performing less than 300 cases per year had higher risk-adjusted odds of in-hospital mortality when compared with thoses performing more than 300 cases (OR = 7.7, <10 cases; OR = 2.9, 10 to 100 cases; OR = 3, 101 to 300 cases). This study, limited by the absence of clinical detail in discharge abstract databases, concluded that, for children with a congenital heart defect who underwent surgery in

California in 1988 or Massachusetts in 1989, the risk of dying in-hospital was much lower if the surgery was performed at an institution performing more than 300 cases annually.

These preliminary findings were then confirmed by two investigations performed in New York State. In 1999, Sollano et al. examined the relationship between hospital volume and in-hospital mortality in 3 cardiovascular procedures: coronary artery bypass grafting, elective repair of abdominal aortic aneurysms, and repair of congenital cardiac defects [9]. Using a New-York State clinical database, this study demonstrated a significant inverse relationship between volume and death in pediatric cardiac surgery (OR, 0.944 for every 100 additional cases), which was most pronounced for neonates (OR, 0.636 for every 100 additional cases). It also demonstrated the absence of such a relationship in patients who benefited from coronary artery bypass grafting. The authors hypothesized that the NY State quality improvement program for bypass operations might explain the difference.

The other New-York State-based study was specifically designed to evaluate the effects of hospital and surgeon volume on in-hospital mortality after pediatric cardiac surgery [10]. This population-based retrospective cohort study used a single-state clinical database and demonstrated that both hospital volume and surgeon volume were significantly associated with risk-adjusted in-hospital mortality (8.26 % for center <100 cases versus 5.95 % for centers >100 cases). Moreover, these differences persisted for both high-complexity and low-complexity pediatric cardiac procedures.

The topic was addressed again in the early 2000s by two studies exploring two parallel hypotheses. In 2002, Chang et al. hypothesized that reducing the numbers of centers performing pediatric cardiac surgery in a given region would improve outcome [11]: based on abstracted statewide hospital discharge data from California from 1995 to 1997, they showed that a theoretical regionalization of pediatric cardiac surgery in this State during this period was associated with a reduction in surgical mortality from 5.34 % to 4.08 % when all cases were referred to high-volume hospitals, or, mortality was decreased to 4.60 % when only high-risk cases were referred. They identified mean annual volume cut-off points of 70 and 170 cases per year. However, a group from Israel reported in 2003 that an increase in caseload in a department of pediatric cardiac surgery tended to decrease the complications-related mortality rate [12].

This evidence in favour of a significant inverse relationship between caseload and death in pediatric cardiac surgery has been consistent in five studies despite different methodologies including different databases, risk adjustments, and hospital volume cut-offs. This association was further reinforced in the late-2000s by two further studies. In 2007, Bazzani et al. reevaluated the volume-outcome relationship for pediatric cardiac surgery using a larger, more contemporary hospital discharge database (1998 –2003) from the state of California [13]. He and his team found a weaker and less consistent volume-mortality relationship than had been reported previously when he replicated the methodology of the previously mentioned studies [8–11]. A newly developed and updated model demonstrated a volume-mortality relationship but it was dependent on highly leveraged covariate patterns found in the largest-volume hospital. The attenuated relationship over time could be explained, according to the authors, by the avoidance of high-risk surgical procedures by low-volume hospitals on the one hand, and, by technological advances adopted at higher-volume centers sooner and more reliably than lower-volume centers [14]. Finally, the authors felt that the impact of quality improvement initiatives [15, 16] at larger hospitals were more pronounced and sustained.

Welke et al. demonstrated in 2008, the important need of risk-adjusted models to further understand the volume/outcome relationship in pediatric cardiac surgery [17]. They demonstrated using the national administrative data from the Nationwide Inpatient Sample (NIS), that, as a discriminator of mortality, volume alone performed significantly worse than a model with Risk Adjustment for Congenital Heart Surgery, version 1 (RACHS-1) category and age (ROC curve area, 0.60 vs 0.81). Indeed the unadjusted mortality rate at very small hospitals was not different than at large hospitals. Nevertheless, after adjustment for RACHS-1 category and age, large hospitals performed *significantly better* than all other volume groups, demonstrating that large-volume hospitals performed more complex operations and achieved superior results when compared to smaller ones.

These findings demonstrated the need for sophisticated risk-adjusted models. It also pointed to the limited reliability and predictive abilities of administrative data regarding the ability to adjust for patient-level risk factors and surgical case-mix designation. New studies exploring the volume/outcome relationship in pediatric cardiac surgery are now based on national or multicentric clinical databases.

Studies Based on Multi-state or National Clinical Data

Welke et al. first demonstrated in 2009, the inverse association between pediatric cardiac surgical volume and mortality in a national clinical database [18]. Using the Society of Thoracic Surgeons Congenital Heart Surgery Database, and after adjustment for patient-level risk factors and surgical case mix (Aristotle Basic Complexity ABC and RACHS-1 categories), they showed an inverse relationship between overall surgical volume as a continuous variable and mortality (P=.002), with an inflection point between 200 and 300 cases per year. This study also proved for the first time the modifying role played by case complexity in mediating the strength of the volume/outcome relationship. Indeed, surgical centers with less than 150 cases per year performed significantly worse those with more than 350 cases per year, especially for difficult operations (Aristotle technical difficulty component score more than 3.0), whereas all groups performed in similar manner for low-difficulty (Aristotle score less than 2.0) operations.

Pasquali et al. confirmed this volume/outcome relationship in 2012, in a national clinical database using a surgical risk category-adjusted multivariable risk analysis [19]. This study also explored the effect of the institutional volume on the occurrence of complications and the mortality rate in patients who suffered from complications. Interestingly, this study demonstrated that the higher mortality observed at centers with more than 150 cases per year compared to centers with more than 350 cases per year may be related to a higher rate of mortality in patients with postoperative complications (OR=1.59), rather than a higher rate of complications alone. This association of volume with complication-related mortality was more marked in the higher surgical risk categories, which was consistent with data from Welke et al. [18].

Volume/Outcome Relationship According to the Case Complexity and the Type of Procedure

Volume/Outcome Relationship by Case Complexity

Welke et al. first explored the impact of case complexity in 2009, by showing the volume/outcome relationship in pediatric cardiac surgery [18]. They showed that this relationship was most apparent for difficult operations (Aristotle technical difficulty component score more than 3.0), for which mortality decreased from 14.8 % at programs less than 150 cases per year to 8.4 % at programs with more than 350 cases (OR, 2.41; P<.0001). The same was true for the subgroup of patients who underwent a Norwood procedure (36.5 % vs 16.9 %). To further investigate the volume–mortality relationship, they analyzed volume as a continuous variable and used logistic regression to adjust for patient-level risk factors and surgical case mix. The inverse relationship between surgical volume as a continuous variable and mortality was not significant for low-complexity cases (P=0.06) but was consistent for high-complexity cases (P=0.007) (Fig. 8.1). This suggests that lower-volume programs significantly underperformed in comparison to larger programs as case complexity increased, whereas volume was not associated with mortality for low-complexity cases in this study.

Pasquali et al. similarly confirmed a significant association between center volume and mortality in the higher risk patients (STS-EACTS or STAT categories 4–5) but not in the lower risk patients (STAT categories 1–3) [19].

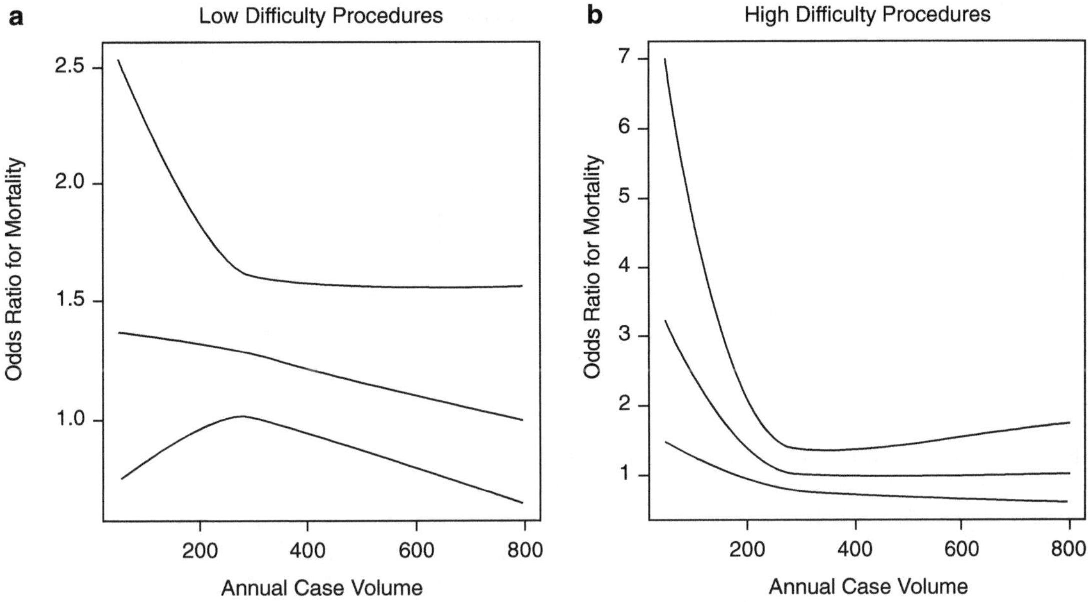

Fig. 8.1 Association between surgical volume and risk-adjusted mortality by Aristotle difficulty: (**a**) low difficulty, ≤3 (P=0.059); (**b**) high difficulty,>3 (P=0.007) (Reprinted from Welke et al. [18], copyright 2009 with permission from Elsevier)

Volume/Outcome Relationship by the Type of Procedure

Hirsch et al. used the administrative Kids' Inpatient Database (KID) in 2008 to explore the institutional volume/outcome relationship for the Norwood and arterial switch operations (ASO), that represent the most complex neonatal cardiac procedures [20]. They demonstrated that in-hospital mortality significantly decreased for both the ASO and the Norwood procedure as institutional volume increased. For ASO, mortality rates were 9.4 % for institutions performing two ASOs per year, 3.2 % for 10 ASOs/year, and 0.8 % for 20 ASOs oer year; for Norwood procedure, these rates were 34.8 % for two Norwood procedures per year, 25.7 % for 10 Norwood procedures/year, and only 16.7 % when 20 Norwood procedures were done per year.

Interestingly, Karamlou et al. showed in a Congenital Heart Surgeons Society (CHSS) study in 2010 the impact of institutional volume on the risk-adjusted mortality after ASO or repair of interrupted aortic arch, but not after a Norwood procedure or repair of a pulmonary atresia with intact ventricular septum [21]. The absence of a strong volume/outcome association in regards to the Norwood procedure in this study by Karamlou et al. was not confirmed in following studies that specifically investigated this topic. Finally, the same group investigated the volume/outcome relationship in 2013 after extracorporeal membrane oxygenation (ECMO) in patients younger than 20 years, using the Project Kids' Inpatient Database [22]. After adjustment to case complexity (RACHS-1 categories), the lower ECMO volume remained a significant determinant of in-hospital death (OR=1.75; CI:1.03–2.94).

Volume/Outcome Relationship and the Norwood Procedure

Several recent studies have investigated the volume–mortality relationship specifically for the Norwood procedure because of the high level of system knowledge and coordination that this procedure requires. Welke et al. demonstrated that programs that do over 350 cases per year outperformed all other volume groups for the Norwood procedure [18] (Fig. 8.2).

Checchia et al. showed using the Pediatric Health Information System database including

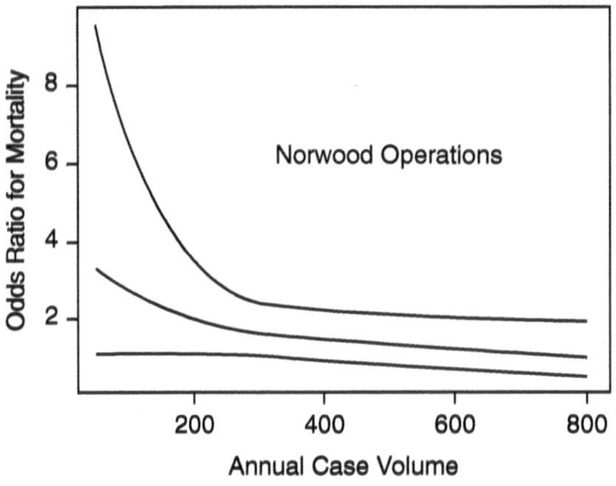

Fig. 8.2 Association between hospital volume and risk-adjusted mortality for Norwood operations (P<.001) (Reprinted from Welke et al. [18], copyright 2009 with permission from Elsevier)

801 Norwood procedures, that the survival after the Norwood procedure was associated with institutional Norwood procedure volume (p=0.02) [23]. Hirsch et al. evaluated 624 Norwood patients in the Kids' Inpatient Database and confirmed this significant inverse association between volume and mortality (35 % in low-volume centers versus 17 % in high-volume centers) [20].

A 2010 study by Karamlou et al. called the volume/outcome relationship into question [21]. The authors explained the absence of such a relationship in their study by three factors. First, the higher dependence of outcomes after Norwood procedure on preoperative and postoperative care, compared to the arterial switch operation; second, the higher anatomic heterogeneity of hypoplastic left ventricle compared to TGA; and third, the fact that this study missed the learning curve effect in the Norwood cohort compared to the arterial switch cohort. Moreover, the volume estimates in this CHSS study were based on the number of patients from each center enrolled in a cohort of patients with aortic atresia or stenosis selected for a Norwood operation, and not on the overall number of patients at each center undergoing the Norwood operation.

In 2012, Pasquali et al. demonstrated in a study using a large multicenter registry (The Society of Thoracic Surgeons Congenital Heart Surgery Database) that, after adjustment for patient

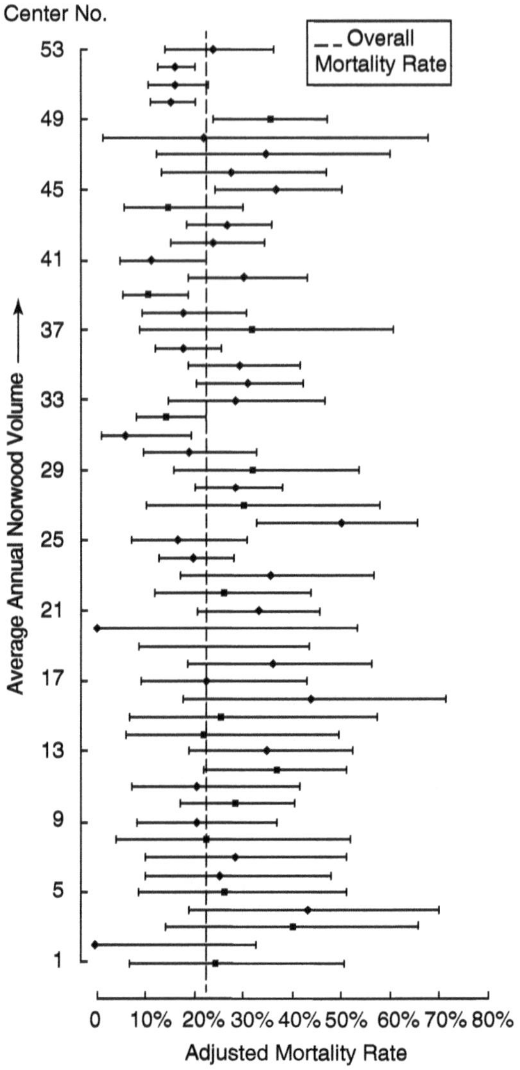

Fig. 8.3 Adjusted mortality rate displayed by increasing center volume (Reprinted from Pasquali et al. [24], copyright 2012 with permission from Elsevier)

characteristics, a lower Norwood center volume remained modestly but significantly associated with higher in-hospital mortality when evaluated as a continuous and categorical variable (OR=1.54 (1.02 to 2.32), p=0.04) [24]. Such a relationship did not vary significantly across preoperative risk tertiles but did not hold true across all centers (Fig. 8.3). Indeed, there are some middle volume centers with Norwood mortality rates comparable to those of higher volume centers, and some higher volume centers with mortality rates similar to those of lower volume groups. Finally, this study showed that the Norwood volume explained an estimated 14 % of the between-center variation in mortality observed after this procedure, and that the majority of between-center variation in mortality remained after adjusting for Norwood volume ($p<0.001$). Based on these results, the authors concluded that the use of *institutional volume alone* is not a good quality metric for the Norwood procedure, and, that we would be better off to rely on center-specific risk adjusted outcomes.

Institutional Volume, Surgeon Volume or Volume-Independent Center Effect?

Relative Impact of Surgeon and Center Volume in Pediatric Cardiac Surgery

Studies in adult cardiac surgery have concluded that the observed insitutional volume/ mortality association was largely mediated by individual surgeon volume [25]. It has even been suggested in adult vascular surgery that a means to improve one's chances of survival would be to select a surgeon who performs a specific operation frequently [26, 27]. In pediatric cardiac surgery, this issue was investigated by 4 groups. In 1998, Hannan et al. showed, using a New-York State clinical database, that surgeons with pediatric cardiac surgical cases volumes of less than 75 per year had significantly higher mortality rates (8.77 %) than surgeons with surgical volumes more than 75 cases per year (5.90 %) [10]. But this result was not confirmed by 2 subsequent studies that addressed this issue in the specific population of patients that required a Norwood procedure. Indeed, Checcia et al. found using a large administrative database that surgeon volume was not associated with patient outcomes after a Norwood procedure [23]. In 2010, the CHSS study by Karamlou et al. showed that neither center nor surgeon volume were associated alone with Norwood outcomes [21]. The results of these two studies might have been limited by the use of administrative data and the methodology used for calculating surgical volume.

More recently, Hornik et al. evaluated the relative impact of surgeon and center volume on mortality in a large Norwood cohort, using the Society of Thoracic Surgeons Congenital Heart Surgery Database [28]. They showed that, when analyzed individually, both lower center and surgeon volumes were associated with higher in-hospital mortality (odds ratio for surgeons with 0–5 cases versus surgeons with more than 10 cases per year = 1.60). This surgeon volume/mortality association after Norwood procedure was true in all center volume strata: lower volume surgeons had higher adjusted in-hospital mortality rates across low, medium, and high volume centers. A low-volume surgeon's outcomes were worse regardless of center volume, but the surgeons's results were mitigated by a large center volume. These results have been reproduced most potently in a recent analysis of the Single Ventricle Reconstruction trial, which also showed a significant survival advantage for high-volume surgeons [29]. This association can be easily understood as it has been shown that surgical technical performance improves outcomes irrespective of preoperative physiologic status or case complexity in the Stage 1 norwood procedure [30] and in other neonatal cardiac surgical procedures [31, 32]. These data could lead to the development of regional collaboration and centralization policies within and across centers through enhanced mentoring program by the highest-volume surgeons. Nevertheless, this impact of surgeon volume on Norwood mortality demonstrated by Hornik et al. was less strong when compared to the impact of surgeon volume in adult cardiac surgery [25]. This could be explained by the key role played by other providers, human factors and hospital-related factors impacting on the preoperative and postoperative management of complex single-ventricle physiology, thus decreasing the direct consequences of the impact of surgeon volume in pediatric vs adult cardiac surgery.[33]

A Volume-Independent Center Effect?

Recent studies have demonstrated that a volume-independent center-effect seems to contribute substantially to the between-center variability in outcomes. This center effect was has been demonstrated after orthotopic heart transplantation [34]: Kilic et al. demonstrated that institutional volume alone only accounted for 16.7 % of the variability in mortality between centers, and that a significant between-center variability persisted after adjusting for this factor ($P<0.001$). This finding was confirmed in pediatric cardiac surgery in 2013 by Vincour et al. [35]. Vinocur et al. aimed at characterizing the relative contribution of patient factors, center surgical volume, and a volume-independent center effect on early postoperative mortality in a retrospective cohort study of North American centers in the Pediatric Cardiac Care Consortium. Although the center volume was inversely associated with outcome in all age groups and risk categories (except the lowest one), a volume-independent center effect contributed substantially more to the risk model than did the volume.

Another group revealed the impact of prior hospital performance on the current outcomes after surgery for congenital heart disease [36]. They demonstrated using the Pediatric Health Information Systems database, that prior hospital postoperative mortality was significantly associated with mortality across all risk strata of congenital heart surgery, whereas, prior hospital surgical volume tended to be associated with improved mortality after only higher-risk operations. These intriguing recent results suggest that center-specific variation in outcomes after pediatric cardiac surgery is only partially explained by operative volume and that other factors have yet to be clearly identified.

Controversies and Perspectives

The Volume Alone as a Quality Metric?

The results of the most recent previously mentioned studies demonstrate that a relationship between case volume and mortality should be interpreted with caution. The trend for lower mortality at larger centers is not universal: all larger programs do not perform better than all smaller programs. Morevover, it has been shown that the volume accounted for only a small proportion of the overall between-center variation in outcome [24, 35, 36]. The lack of long-term follow-up (beyond 30 days) in most of these studies also limits the evaluation to the very early mortality. This serious challenge prevents the authors from addressing the long-term mortality, morbidity, functional status, and neurologic status which is quite significant in single vessel pathologies even after repair [18]. Thus, the center or surgeon volume alone may not be reliable enough to measure and compare center outcomes. The use of center-specific risk adjusted outcome as a proxy tool for quality assessment may be more reliable than relying upon volume alone [17, 37]. Such an adjustment should consider at the minimum both surgical case complexity and patient specific factors [24]. Indeed, a patient's risk factors and their level of disease severity may play a more important role in determining their individual outcome than the impact of the program's volume.

The Confounding Bias of the Volume Factor

The true mechanism of the volume/outcome association remains controversial. Higher volume centers probably have other organizational, logistical, technical and/or human characteristics that at least partially explain this relationship. These factors include the availability of highly equipped operating rooms and cath labs, better management of health resources, ergonimic design and deployment of new technologies, composition of the care team, advanced training programs, improved preoperative and intraoperative care, multidisciplinary discussions, the use of standardized management protocols, and better resilience and timely recognition and treatment of complication [18, 19, 28, 38–41]. That suggests that higher center volume may be a surrogate for other aspects of care that are more likely to be provided at larger centers. These process measures and structural characteristics of systems that lead to better outcomes are not currently captured in available databases. These aspects including the role of human factors, team training and debriefing and non technical team skills should be extensively studied to determine their respective roles in outcomes after pediatric cardiac surgery [33, 42, 43]. The increasing mobility of skillful and experienced surgical, anesthesia and ICU staff should also be taken into account when studying the volume/outcome relationship [44]. Finally, we could also wonder whether high case volumes may lead to the improvement of outcomes thanks to an increased practice or better results attract more referrals, thus leading to higher volumes [11]. The relation between high volume and better outcomes remains strong and persistent in the field of pediatric cardiac surgery. [24, 28, 29], What then should policy makers do? what should parents and healthcare mangers do? and in view of the results of the latest studies [45, 46].

What Do We Do with These Results?

The regionalization of care and the selective referral of patients to high performing centers have been proposed based on these results of the volume/outcome relationship in pediatric cardiac surgery. Chang et al., suggested that regionalization of services in California may result in decreased mortality in children undergoing cardiac surgery [11]. Such a regionalization of care has already been done in some European countries, most pronounced in Sweden, Norway, UK, the Netherlands and Poland. For example, in Sweden, care was centralized to two centers with the lowest mortality and early national mortality rates were reduced from 9.5 to 1.9 % [47]. In the US, Mainwaring et al. showed that a model based on affiliation of low volume programs with a larger academic program within the same region, including referral of high-complexity cases such as Norwood operations to the high volume program, was associated with lower overall mortality [48]. Whether regionalization of care for children undergoing heart surgery in the United States is politically and financially feasible or even desirable remains under debate. We suggest that regionalization should be conducted on a region-by-region basis, according to the characteristics of local geography, demographics, and healthcare markets [41].

Alternative strategies to regionalisation of care have been proposed to reduce the present unacceptable large variation between centers. Quality improvement initiatives, quality assurance initiatives, development of evidence-based best practice guidelines [24], (for instance standardizing the way we recognize and manage complications [19]) could lead to major improvement of outcomes in pediatric cardiac surgery. Recent quality improvement activities including widespread use of learning collaboratives in adult cardiac surgery involving the adult cardiac surgery programs in Michigan [49] or the Northern New England Cardiovascular Disease Study Group [50] proved the feasibility and impact of quality improvement initiatives and could be applied to the field of the pediatric cardiac surgery. The National Pediatric Cardiology Quality Improvement Collaborative (NPC-QIC) is a potential model for applying system improvement and learning collaboratives.[51]

Conclusions

There is a significant inverse relationship between surgical institutional and surgeon volume and outcomes in pediatric cardiac surgery. This relationship depends on case complexity and the type of surgical procedures. Lower-volume programs tend to underperform larger programs as case complexity increases. High-volume pediatric cardiac surgeons also tend to have better results compared with low-volume surgeons, especially in the Norwood procedure. Nevertheless, this trend for lower mortality at larger centers is not universal: all larger programs do not perform better than all smaller programs. Morevover surgical volume seems to account for only a small proportion of the overall between-center variation in outcome. Thus the use of a center-specific risk adjusted outcome as a tool for quality assessment may be more reliable than relying upon surgical volume alone. However, the relationship between surgical volume and outcomes in pediatric cardiac surgery is strong enough that it ought to guide regional and national healthcare policies around centralization of complex pediatric cardiac surgery.

References

1. Bacha EA. Patient safety and human factors in pediatric cardiac surgery. Pediatr Cardiol. 2007;28(2):116–21. PubMed PMID: 17487540.
2. Welke KF, Jacobs JP, Jenkins KJ. Evaluation of quality of care for congenital heart disease. Semin Thorac Cardiovasc Surg Pediatr Card Surg Annu. 2005;8(1):157–67. PubMed PMID: 15818372.
3. Birkmeyer JD, Siewers AE, Finlayson EV, Stukel TA, Lucas FL, Batista I, et al. Hospital volume and surgical mortality in the United States. N Engl J Med. 2002;346(15):1128–37. PubMed PMID: 11948273.
4. Dudley RA, Johansen KL, Brand R, Rennie DJ, Milstein A. Selective referral to high-volume hospitals: estimating potentially avoidable deaths. JAMA. 2000;283(9):1159–66. PubMed PMID: 10703778.
5. Halm EA, Lee C, Chassin MR. Is volume related to outcome in health care? A systematic review and methodologic critique of the literature. Ann Intern Med. 2002;137(6):511–20. PubMed PMID: 12230353.
6. Welke KF, Peterson ED, Vaughan-Sarrazin MS, O'Brien SM, Rosenthal GE, Shook GJ, et al. Comparison of cardiac surgery volumes and mortality rates between the Society of Thoracic Surgeons and Medicare databases from 1993 through 2001. Ann Thorac Surg. 2007;84(5):1538–46. PubMed PMID: 17954059.
7. Shahian DM, Normand SL. The volume-outcome relationship: from Luft to Leapfrog. Ann Thorac Surg. 2003;75(3):1048–58. PubMed PMID: 12645752.
8. Jenkins KJ, Newburger JW, Lock JE, Davis RB, Coffman GA, Iezzoni LI. In-hospital mortality for surgical repair of congenital heart defects: preliminary observations of variation by hospital caseload. Pediatrics. 1995;95(3):323–30. PubMed PMID: 7862467.
9. Sollano JA, Gelijns AC, Moskowitz AJ, Heitjan DF, Cullinane S, Saha T, et al. Volume-outcome relationships in cardiovascular operations: New York State, 1990–1995. J Thorac Cardiovasc Surg. 1999;117(3):419–28; discussion 28–30. PubMed PMID: 10047643.
10. Hannan EL, Racz M, Kavey RE, Quaegebeur JM, Williams R. Pediatric cardiac surgery: the effect of hospital and surgeon volume on in-hospital mortality. Pediatrics. 1998;101(6):963–9. PubMed PMID: 9606220.
11. Chang RK, Klitzner TS. Can regionalization decrease the number of deaths for children who undergo cardiac surgery? A theoretical analysis. Pediatrics. 2002;109(2):173–81. PubMed PMID: 11826192.
12. Dagan O, Birk E, Katz Y, Gelber O, Vidne B. Relationship between caseload and morbidity and mortality in pediatric cardiac surgery–a four year experience. Isr Med Assoc J. 2003;5(7):471–4. PubMed PMID: 12901239.
13. Bazzani LG, Marcin JP. Case volume and mortality in pediatric cardiac surgery patients in California, 1998–2003. Circulation. 2007;115(20):2652–9. PubMed PMID: 17485577.
14. Hannan EL, Siu AL, Kumar D, Kilburn Jr H, Chassin MR. The decline in coronary artery bypass graft surgery mortality in New York State. The role of surgeon volume. JAMA. 1995;273(3):209–13. PubMed PMID: 7807659.
15. Gauvreau K. Reevaluation of the volume-outcome relationship for pediatric cardiac surgery. Circulation. 2007;115(20):2599–601. PubMed PMID: 17515477.
16. Ho V. Evolution of the volume-outcome relation for hospitals performing coronary angioplasty. Circulation. 2000;101(15):1806–11. PubMed PMID: 10769281.
17. Welke KF, Diggs BS, Karamlou T, Ungerleider RM. The relationship between hospital surgical case volumes and mortality rates in pediatric cardiac surgery: a national sample, 1988–2005. Ann Thorac Surg. 2008;86(3):889–96; discussion –96. PubMed PMID: 18721578.
18. Welke KF, O'Brien SM, Peterson ED, Ungerleider RM, Jacobs ML, Jacobs JP. The complex relationship between pediatric cardiac surgical case volumes and mortality rates in a national clinical database. J Thorac Cardiovasc Surg. 2009;137(5):1133–40. PubMed PMID: 19379979.
19. Pasquali SK, Li JS, Burstein DS, Sheng S, O'Brien SM, Jacobs ML, et al. Association of center volume with mortality and complications in pediatric heart surgery. Pediatrics. 2012;129(2):e370–6. PubMed PMID: 22232310. Pubmed Central PMCID: 3269112.
20. Hirsch JC, Gurney JG, Donohue JE, Gebremariam A, Bove EL, Ohye RG. Hospital mortality for Norwood and arterial switch operations as a function of institutional volume. Pediatr Cardiol. 2008;29(4):713–7. PubMed PMID: 18080151.
21. Karamlou T, McCrindle BW, Blackstone EH, Cai S, Jonas RA, Bradley SM, et al. Lesion-specific outcomes in neonates undergoing congenital heart surgery are related predominantly to patient and management factors rather than institution or surgeon experience: a Congenital Heart Surgeons Society Study. J Thorac Cardiovasc Surg. 2010;139(3):569–77 e1. PubMed PMID: 19909989.
22. Karamlou T, Vafaeezadeh M, Parrish AM, Cohen GA, Welke KF, Permut L, et al. Increased extracorporeal membrane oxygenation center case volume is associated with improved extracorporeal membrane oxygenation survival among pediatric patients. J Thorac Cardiovasc Surg. 2013;145(2):470–5. PubMed PMID: 23246046.
23. Checchia PA, McCollegan J, Daher N, Kolovos N, Levy F, Markovitz B. The effect of surgical case volume on outcome after the Norwood procedure. J Thorac Cardiovasc Surg. 2005;129(4):754–9. PubMed PMID: 15821640.
24. Pasquali SK, Jacobs JP, He X, Hornik CP, Jaquiss RD, Jacobs ML, et al. The complex relationship between center volume and outcome in patients undergoing the Norwood operation. Ann Thorac Surg. 2012;93(5):1556–62. PubMed PMID: 22014746. Pubmed Central PMCID: 3334400.

25. Birkmeyer JD, Stukel TA, Siewers AE, Goodney PP, Wennberg DE, Lucas FL. Surgeon volume and operative mortality in the United States. N Engl J Med. 2003;349(22):2117–27. PubMed PMID: 14645640.
26. McPhee JT, Robinson 3rd WP, Eslami MH, Arous EJ, Messina LM, Schanzer A. Surgeon case volume, not institution case volume, is the primary determinant of in-hospital mortality after elective open abdominal aortic aneurysm repair. J Vasc Surg. 2011;53(3):591–9 e2. PubMed PMID: 21144692.
27. Wu C, Hannan EL, Ryan TJ, Bennett E, Culliford AT, Gold JP, et al. Is the impact of hospital and surgeon volumes on the in-hospital mortality rate for coronary artery bypass graft surgery limited to patients at high risk? Circulation. 2004;110(7):784–9. PubMed PMID: 15302792.
28. Hornik CP, He X, Jacobs JP, Li JS, Jaquiss RD, Jacobs ML, et al. Relative impact of surgeon and center volume on early mortality after the Norwood operation. Ann Thorac Surg. 2012;93(6):1992–7. PubMed PMID: 22516833. Pubmed Central PMCID: 3469698.
29. Tweddell JS, Sleeper LA, Ohye RG, Williams IA, Mahony L, Pizarro C, et al. Intermediate-term mortality and cardiac transplantation in infants with single-ventricle lesions: risk factors and their interaction with shunt type. J Thorac Cardiovasc Surg. 2012;144(1):152–9. PubMed PMID: 22341427. Pubmed Central PMCID: 3359406.
30. Karamichalis JM, Thiagarajan RR, Liu H, Mamic P, Gauvreau K, Bacha EA. Stage I Norwood: optimal technical performance improves outcomes irrespective of preoperative physiologic status or case complexity. J Thorac Cardiovasc Surg. 2010;139(4):962–8. PubMed PMID: 20074754.
31. Shuhaiber J, Gauvreau K, Thiagarjan R, Bacha E, Mayer J, Del Nido P, et al. Congenital heart surgeon's technical proficiency affects neonatal hospital survival. J Thorac Cardiovasc Surg. 2012;144(5):1119–24. PubMed PMID: 22421402.
32. Nathan M, Karamichalis JM, Liu H, Emani S, Baird C, Pigula F, et al. Surgical technical performance scores are predictors of late mortality and unplanned reinterventions in infants after cardiac surgery. J Thorac Cardiovasc Surg. 2012;144(5):1095–101.e7. PubMed PMID: 22939862.
33. Galvan C, Bacha B, Mohr J, Barach P. A human factors approach to understanding patient safety during pediatric cardiac surgery. Prog Pediatr Cardiol. 2005;20:13–20.
34. Kilic A, Weiss ES, Yuh DD, Shah AS, Cameron DE, Baumgartner WA, et al. Institutional factors beyond procedural volume significantly impact center variability in outcomes after orthotopic heart transplantation. Ann Surg. 2012;256(4):616–23. PubMed PMID: 22964734.
35. Vinocur JM, Menk JS, Connett J, Moller JH, Kochilas LK. Surgical volume and center effects on early mortality after pediatric cardiac surgery: 25-year North American experience from a multi-institutional registry. Pediatr Cardiol. 2013;2. PubMed PMID: 23377381.
36. Oster ME, Strickland MJ, Mahle WT. Impact of prior hospital mortality versus surgical volume on mortality following surgery for congenital heart disease. J Thorac Cardiovasc Surg. 2011;142(4):882–6. PubMed PMID: 21571324.
37. Khuri SF, Henderson WG. The case against volume as a measure of quality of surgical care. World J Surg. 2005;29(10):1222–9. PubMed PMID: 16151664.
38. Goh AY, Lum LC, Abdel-Latif ME. Impact of 24 hour critical care physician staffing on case-mix adjusted mortality in paediatric intensive care. Lancet. 2001;357(9254):445–6. PubMed PMID: 11273070.
39. Srinivasan C, Sachdeva R, Morrow WR, Gossett J, Chipman CW, Imamura M, et al. Standardized management improves outcomes after the Norwood procedure. Congenit Heart Dis. 2009;4(5):329–37. PubMed PMID: 19740187.
40. Ghaferi AA, Birkmeyer JD, Dimick JB. Complications, failure to rescue, and mortality with major inpatient surgery in medicare patients. Ann Surg. 2009;250(6): 1029–34. PubMed PMID: 19953723.
41. Smith PC, Powell KR. Can regionalization decrease the number of deaths for children who undergo cardiac surgery? A theoretical analysis. Pediatrics. 2002;110(4):849–50; dicsussion –50. PubMed PMID: 12359811.
42. Section on C, Cardiac S, American Academy of P. Guidelines for pediatric cardiovascular centers. Pediatrics. 2002;109(3):544–9. PubMed PMID: 11875158.
43. Barach P, Johnson J, Ahmed A, Galvan C, Bognar A, Duncan R, Starr J, Bacha E. Intraoperative adverse events and their impact on pediatric cardiac surgery: a prospective observational study. J Thorac Cardiovasc Surg. 2008;136(6):1422–8.
44. Mosca RS. Invited commentary. Ann Thorac Surg. 2012;93(5):1562. PubMed PMID: 22541186.
45. Bacha E. Invited commentary. Ann Thorac Surg. 2012;93(6):1998. PubMed PMID: 22632495.
46. Winlaw D, d'Udekem Y, Barach P. Where to now for paediatric surgery? ANZ J Surg. 2011;81:659–60.
47. Lundstrom NR, Berggren H, Bjorkhem G, Jogi P, Sunnegardh J. Centralization of pediatric heart surgery in Sweden. Pediatr Cardiol. 2000;21(4):353–7. PubMed PMID: 10865012.
48. Mainwaring RD, Reddy VM, Reinhartz O, Lamberti JJ, Jacobson JG, Jimenez DL, et al. Outcome analysis for a small, start-up congenital heart surgery program. J Card Surg. 2008;23(6):622–6. PubMed PMID: 19016985.
49. Prager RL, Armenti FR, Bassett JS, Bell GF, Drake D, Hanson EC, et al. Cardiac surgeons and the quality movement: the Michigan experience. Semin Thorac Cardiovasc Surg. 2009;21(1):20–7. PubMed PMID: 19632559.
50. Likosky DS, Nugent WC, Ross CS, Northern New England Cardiovascular Disease Study Group. Improving outcomes of cardiac surgery through cooperative efforts: the northern new England experience. Semin Cardiothorac Vasc Anesth. 2005;9(2):119–21. PubMed PMID: 15920635.
51. Lannon CM, Miles PV. Pediatric collaborative improvement networks: bridging quality gaps to improve health outcomes. Pediatrics. 2013;131 Suppl 4:S187–8.

9 The Pediatric Perioperative Cardiac Arrest (POCA) Registry

Nathaniel H. Greene, Sanjay M. Bhananker, Karen L. Posner, and Karen B. Domino

Abstract

The Pediatric Perioperative Cardiac Arrest (POCA) Registry was one of the first registries of its kind to generate an accurate incidence of perioperative cardiac arrest in pediatric patients undergoing surgery in the United States. This task was accomplished by collaboration with 62 medical centers including both academic institutions and community hospitals. While the POCA Registry faced some methodological challenges unique to the time it was created, it was able to answer important questions about factors associated with perioperative cardiac arrest in pediatric patients requiring anesthesia for surgery. POCA Registry data demonstrate that high American Society of Anesthesiologists physical status and emergency surgery were independent predictors of mortality from perioperative cardiac arrest, and that patients with congenital heart disease were at a significant and increased of perioperative cardiac arrest while undergoing noncardiac procedures. POCA Registry data also suggested that the use of halothane was particularly hazardous for infants. Future efforts to address perioperative cardiac arrest will benefit from utilization of electronic-based resources, although their widespread implementation is several years away.

Keywords

Cardiac arrest • Pediatric • Anesthesia • Cardiac arrest outcomes • Mortality • Perioperative cardiac arrest • Registry • Incidence • Patient safety

N.H. Greene, MD
Department of Anesthesiology and Pediatrics, Duke University School of Medicine, DUMC, 3094, Durham, NC 27710, USA
e-mail: nathaniel.greene@duke.edu

S.M. Bhananker, MD
Department of Anesthesiology, Harborview Medical Center, 325 Ninth Avenue, 359724, Seattle, WA 98104, USA
e-mail: sbhanank@uw.edu

K.L. Posner, PhD • K.B. Domino, MD, MPH (✉)
Department of Anesthesiology and Pain Medicine, University of Washington School of Medicine, 1959 NE Pacific Street, 356540, Seattle, WA 98195, USA
e-mail: posner@uw.edu; kdomino@uw.edu

P.R. Barach, J.P. Jacobs, S.E. Lipshultz, P.C. Laussen (eds.), *Pediatric and Congenital Cardiac Care: Volume 2: Quality Improvement and Patient Safety*, DOI 10.1007/978-1-4471-6566-8_9,

POCA Registry Beginnings

While it was first suggested in 1954 that children were at higher risk for anesthesia-related death [1], the mechanisms of anesthesia-related death and risk factors for anesthesia-related death had not been described. The impetus to establish the Pediatric Perioperative Cardiac Arrest (POCA) Registry arose from an analysis of closed pediatric anesthesia malpractice claims using American Society of Anesthesiologists (ASA) Closed Claims Project data [2]. The Closed Claims Project is a longitudinal study of malpractice claims filed against anesthesiologists in the United States. Closed Claims Project data includes detailed clinical information on events and outcomes allegedly causing anesthesia-related injury from 1970 to the present (excluding injury to teeth), regardless of whether the claim was dropped, settled, or adjudicated. Closed Claims Project data showed that pediatric patients had higher perioperative mortality rates and more respiratory events than adults [2]. The differences observed between adult and pediatric patients was striking, with respiratory events 43 % more common and mortality rates 43 % higher in pediatric claims. In the claims examined, the complications in pediatric patients were thought to be more commonly preventable with better monitoring, and anesthetic care was judged to be less than appropriate in a majority of the cases. The relative contributions of patient disease, anesthesia, and surgery to these complications were not well understood.

Examining each pediatric anesthetic malpractice claim closely revealed insufficiently detailed information surrounding the intraoperative event of interest, as the focus of the Closed Claims Project was not cardiac arrest and resuscitation, but rather any complication of anesthesia and resultant lawsuits which may or may not have led to payouts [3]. As such, details pertaining to resuscitation and cardiac arrest were particularly lacking [4]. Using the Closed Claims Project to examine this topic would likely lead to a biased sample as it would be more likely to capture arrests with poor outcomes. Also, as cardiac arrest in children was still a relatively rare event, even a relatively large database such as the Closed Claims Project yielded insufficient numbers of cases for robust analyses. Efficient study of this process would require multiple institutions to participate in a registry in order to be able to collect a large number of events in a timely fashion. Thus, the POCA Registry was started by the Closed Claims Study Group in the Department of Anesthesiology and Pain Medicine at the University of Washington in Seattle, where the ASA Closed Claims Project database [5] was housed. The POCA Registry was guided by its own steering committee of pediatric anesthesiologists from Children's Hospital in Seattle and Stanford University Medical Center, with guidance and oversight by the Closed Claims Project.

Startup funding for the POCA Registry was provided by the ASA Committee on Professional Liability within the Closed Claims Project. The POCA Registry was further endorsed by the American Academy of Pediatrics (AAP) Section on Anesthesiology Committee on Quality Assurance. The infrastructure for the Registry was put in place by the Closed Claims Project investigators, and case reports of pediatric perioperative cardiac arrests began to be collected in 1994, just 1 year following the initial publication of pediatric closed claims analysis. The POCA Registry did not have any independent funding or staff specifically devoted to the project.

Registry Design

The POCA Registry study group initially obtained voluntary participation from not only academic medical centers, but also community hospital groups in a hope to truly understand risk factors for pediatric cardiac arrest in all surgical operating rooms. Each participating center submitted pediatric case volume data annually to create a denominator for registry case data. Case report data collection forms were sent to participating institutions each year to gather detailed reports of cases of cardiac arrest that occurred at each institution. New

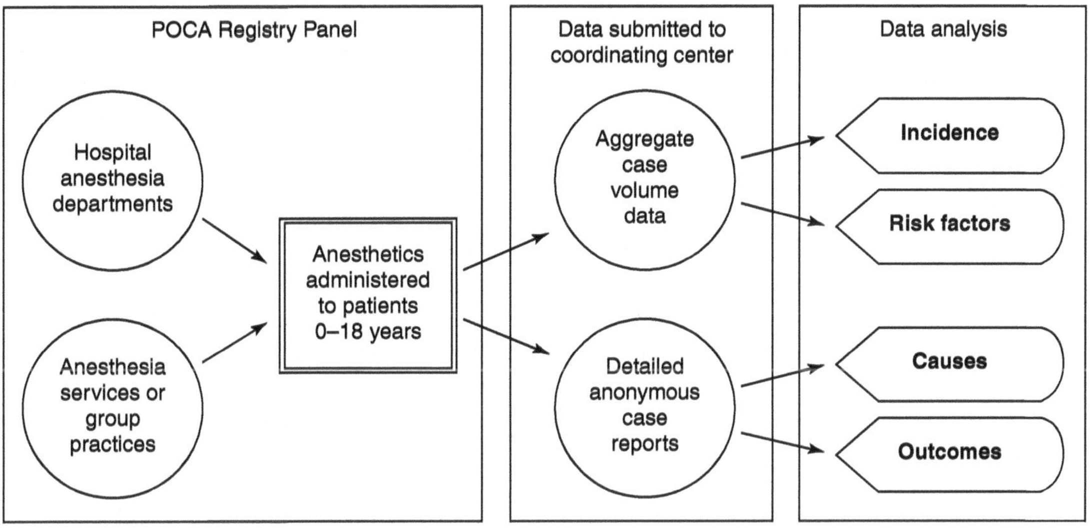

Fig. 9.1 Methodological overview of POCA registry (Reproduced from *BMJ Quality and Safety*; Posner et al. [4], copyright 2002 with permission from BMJ Publishing Group Ltd)

forms were sent to every participating institution each year, occasionally with updated questions and data entry fields. Centers were allowed to join or leave each calendar year on January 1st in an effort to have an accurate estimation of which centers were still participating and submitting cases, so that we could track the denominator. The panel of participating institutions remained fairly stable at approximately 70 each year. Each participating center designated an anesthesiologist volunteer that was the institutional representative, responsible for sending in the data to the Registry.

Cardiac arrest was defined as cardiopulmonary resuscitation (including administration of chest compressions) or death [4]. Cases were included if a cardiac arrest occurred in a child 18 years of age or younger during administration of or recovery from anesthesia. Neonatal resuscitations and resuscitations in the pediatric intensive care unit or on the ward were excluded to ensure that cardiac arrests captured were likely to be associated with anesthesia. Failure to wean from cardiac bypass was captured on a short case report form. Basic demographic data was collected on these cases to have an accurate count, but these cases were assumed to be surgical complications or related to patient disease rather than anesthesia-related arrests. The data collection process for the POCA Registry is outlined in Fig. 9.1 [4].

For each case, an 8-page case report form with 14 sections was completed by the institutional representative and submitted to the Registry. These 14 sections included patient data (demographic variables, ASA status), procedure data (surgical procedure and type, type of anesthetic, time of induction), personnel involvement (all providers involved in care at time of arrest including amount of training of attending anesthesiologist and if the attending was present at the time of arrest), sedation (details on type of sedation techniques used, if applicable), premedications, regional anesthesia use, general anesthesia use (types of medications used to induce and maintain anesthesia including details on anesthetic depth), status immediately prior to cardiac arrest (position of patient, level of airway support, monitors used, and clinical warnings prior to arrest), status during cardiac arrest (including location of arrest, and the presumed cause of arrest), resuscitation data (times of and all treatments given during resuscitation), outcome of cardiac arrest (including severity of injury after arrest), an overall assessment section, follow up criteria, and a written narrative of the events. A follow up form was submitted if certain information regarding the arrest had yet to be clarified, or if the injury sustained during the arrest had not yet fully evolved.

Findings

There were three main analyses using POCA Registry data and each contributed something different to understanding the incidence and factors associated with pediatric anesthesia cardiac arrest.

First Analysis

The first report from the POCA Registry [6] confirmed what was suspected by some pediatric anesthesiologists, that the use of halothane, even in acceptable doses, appeared to have contributed to many cases of cardiac arrest. The most common mechanisms of anesthesia-related cardiac arrest in children in POCA Registry case reports were medication (mostly halothane alone or in combination with other anesthetic agents) and cardiovascular events. Infants (less than 12 months of age) accounted for greater than half of POCA Registry case reports of cardiac arrest related to anesthesia. This finding was consistent with previous reports of higher risk of cardiac arrest in infants. Other causes of arrest included respiratory system problems (20 %, most commonly laryngospasm and airway obstruction) and equipment (7 %, mainly central venous catheters). Interestingly, the proportionate causes of arrest varied significantly between healthy (ASA physical status 1–2) and chronically ill (ASA physical status 3–5) patients (Fig. 9.2) [6]. The most common cause of anesthesia-related arrest in healthy children was medication-related while arrest in chronically ill children was more often cardiovascular in nature. The figure represents proportionate risk data within the POCA Registry sample of anesthesia-related perioperative arrests and *not* a representation of absolute risk within the general pediatric population.

Another major finding from this initial report was analysis of factors associated with mortality from perioperative cardiac arrest. ASA physical status of 3–5 (odds ratio of 13, 95 % CI 2.9–57.7) and emergency surgery (odds ratio of 4, 95 % CI 1.6–9.6) were associated with mortality following anesthesia-related cardiac arrest in the POCA Registry data. After adjusting for these factors, age group and type of surgery were not predictive of mortality. Although infants represented a higher proportion of cardiac arrest cases in the POCA Registry, and this seemed to be related to cardiovascular suppression effects of halothane, outcome (mortality) from a cardiac arrest was only related to ASA physical status and whether or not the surgery was emergent (rather than age). While anesthesia-related cardiac arrest was more common in infants, once arrest occurred, healthier patients undergoing elective surgery were more likely to be successfully resuscitated than sick infants.

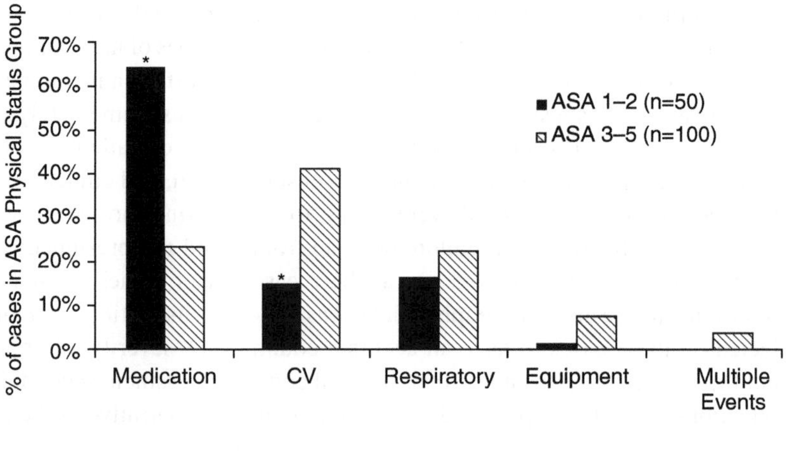

Fig. 9.2 Cause of Cardiac Arrest by Category, Stratified by ASA Physical Status. *p < 0.01 compared with ASA physical status 3–5 patients. *CV* cardiovascular (Reproduced from Morray et al. [6] with permission from Wolters Kluwer Health)

Table 9.1 Incidence estimates of perioperative cardiac arrest in pediatric patients including POCA results (*in italics*)

Source	Years represented	Sample size	No. of hospitals	Country	Perioperative CA rate[a]	Perioperative CA mortality[b]	Case fatality (%)[c]
Morray et al. [6]	***1994–1997***	***1,089,200***	***63***	***US/Canada***	***1.4***	***0.36***	***26***
Kurth et al. [7]	2010–2013	736,365	19	US	3.27[d]	1.06	32
van der Griend et al. [8]	2003–2008	101,885	1	Australia	NR	0.98	NR
Flick et al. [9]	1988–2005	92,881	1	US (Minnesota)	0.65	0.22	33
Murat et al. [10]	2000–2002	24,165	1	France	0.8	0	0
Ahmed et al. [11]	1992–2006	20,216	1	Pakistan	2.0	0.49	25
Newland et al. [12]	1989–1999	16,051	1	US (Nebraska)	1.9	0	0
Tay et al. [13]	1997–1999	10,000	1	Singapore	1[d]	0	0

CA cardiac arrest, *NR* none reported
[a]Anesthesia-related cardiac arrests/10,000 anesthetics
[b]Anesthesia-related deaths/10,000 anesthetics
[c]% of anesthesia-related cardiac arrests resulting in death
[d]Relationship to anesthesia not reported

The data from this first report was the best data to capture an accurate incidence estimate of cardiac arrest (1.4 arrests per 10,000 anesthetics delivered) given the participation and compliance was most likely highest during the first few years of the Registry. Several subsequent studies would later estimate similar rates of anesthetic-related perioperative cardiac arrest and mortality (Table 9.1) [6–13], but most had nowhere near the number of patients studied as were enrolled in the POCA Registry. This incidence estimate may not be as relevant today since halothane is rarely used in the United States, but it was relevant at the time it was published and is not far from more recent estimates. While this estimate of the rate of cardiac arrest was considered an accurate estimate based on the POCA Registry institutions, it represented only those institutions participating in the POCA Registry. As in all similar estimates, its relationship to total US incidence of cardiac arrest among pediatric anesthesia patients was impossible to assess.

Second Analysis

The second report from the POCA Registry [14] comparing anesthesia-related cardiac arrest from 1998–2004 to those from 1994–97 suggested a shift in the causes of cardiac arrest from the first report, as halothane use for pediatric anesthesia had declined substantially over time. Medication-related arrests decreased by approximately half between the first and second report (Fig. 9.3) [14], with halothane-related arrests decreasing from 25 % of all anesthesia-related arrests in the first publication to only 5 % in 1998–2004. Additionally, cardiac arrest in ASA 1 patients was less common in the second analysis compared to the earlier report (7 % vs. 15 %). The more prevalent causes of arrest being reported in 1998–2004 were cardiovascular (41 % of anesthesia-related arrests in 1998–2004, Fig. 9.3) with the most common identifiable cardiovascular mechanisms of arrest identified as hypovolemia from blood loss or complications from inappropriate fluid resuscitation and blood transfusion (usually hyperkalemia). As hypovolemia associated with blood loss was the most common cause, the cause of this hypovolemia was analyzed in detail. This analysis revealed that an underestimation of blood loss was the most common cause of hypovolemia leading to cardiovascular-related cardiac arrest in children (48 % of cases). The next most common cardiovascular causes of perioperative cardiac arrest were inadequate peripheral venous access (22 %) and not having (or not transducing) a central venous catheter, thus underestimating the patient volume status (22 %).

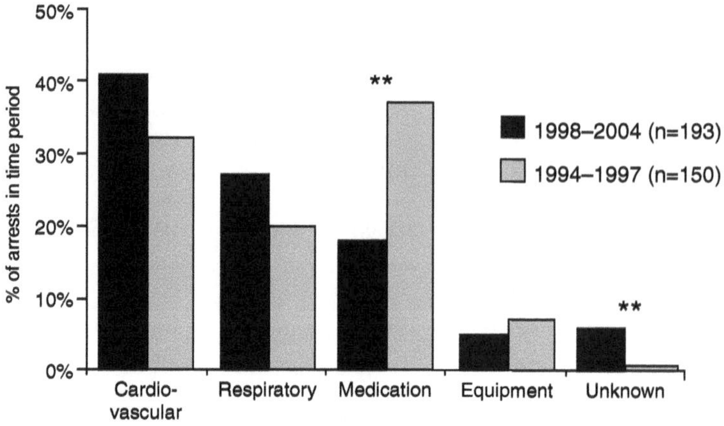

Fig. 9.3 Cause of Cardiac Arrest by Time Period. **p<0.01, 1998–2004 vs. 1994–1997 by z-test (Reproduced from Bhananker et al. [14] with permission from Wolters Kluwer Health)

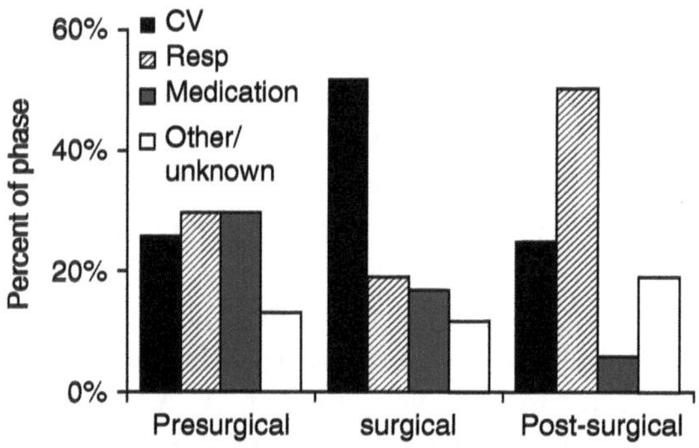

Fig. 9.4 Cause of Cardiac Arrest by Phase of Anesthetic Care. *CV* cardiovascular (Reproduced from Bhananker et al. [14] with permission from Wolters Kluwer Health)

An additional analysis presented in this second POCA Registry report examined causes of arrest by phase of patient care (Fig. 9.4) [14]. While most (58 %) arrests occurred during the surgical procedure (maintenance phase of anesthesia), 24 % occurred prior to incision (pre-induction or induction) and 19 % after completion of surgery (emergence, transport or recovery). The predominant cause of arrest during anesthesia maintenance was cardiovascular in origin (52 %), usually related to fluid resuscitation during craniotomy or spine surgery, while the predominant cause of arrest during the post-surgical phase was respiratory in origin (50 %), usually in patients with an unprotected airway during emergence or recovery. A majority of the respiratory related arrests were observed in airway/ear, nose, throat surgery highlighting this type of surgery as a potential risk factor for cardiac arrest.

The mortality from anesthesia-related cardiac arrest observed in this second report was 28 %, which was similar to the estimate from the first analysis (26 %). Similarly, the only factors predictive of mortality from cardiac arrest were ASA physical status 3–5 (odds ratio 3.6, 95 % CI 1.3–9.8) and emergency surgery (odds ratio 2.8, 95 % CI 1.3–5.9).

The incidence of cardiac arrest was not reported in this second report from the POCA Registry. It was suspected that compliance and reporting had declined over time and incidence calculations might be inaccurate. Nevertheless, analysis of proportionate causes of cardiac arrest was still very useful. Pediatric anesthesia practice today is similar to that being practiced during the time frame of this second report, so the results from this analysis are still applicable today and form the basis for our understanding of perioperative cardiac arrest risk in all children who undergo surgery.

Final Analysis

The final report from the POCA Registry [15] examined all available data in the Registry (case reports from 1994 to 2005) with the aim of comparing anesthesia-related arrests in children with heart disease to those without heart disease.

Table 9.2 Cardiac lesion surgical status and mortality

		Lesion surgical status[a]			
Cardiac lesion	No. of cases	Unrepaired	Palliated	Repaired	Mortality died
Single ventricle	24	5 (21 %)	19 (79 %)	0 (0 %)	6 (25 %)
Left to right shunts (ASD, VSD)	23	14 (61 %)	0 (0 %)	9 (39 %)	4 (17 %)
Obstructive (coarctation/AS/PS)	20	15 (75 %)	3 (15 %)	2 (10 %)	9 (45 %)
Aortic stenosis	13	10 (77 %)	2 (15 %)	1 (8 %)	8 (62 %)
Cardiomyopathy	16	15 (94 %)	1 (6 %)	0 (0 %)	8 (50 %)
Tetralogy of fallot	15	5 (36 %)	7 (50 %)	2 (14 %)	3 (20 %)
Truncus arteriosus	6	5 (83 %)	0 (0 %)	1 (17 %)	2 (33 %)

Reproduced from Ramamoorthy et al. [15] with permission from Wolters Kluwer Health.
Percentages based on number of cases with this lesion (row total)
ASD atrial septal defect, *VSD* ventricular septal defect, *coarctation* coarctation of the aorta, *AS* aortic stenosis, *PS* pulmonary stenosis
[a]Cases with unknown status excluded

Children were classified as having heart disease if they had congenital or acquired disease, with the most common conditions including single ventricle, left to right shunts (septal defects), obstructive lesions (coarctation of the aorta, aortic stenosis, pulmonary stenosis), cardiomyopathy, tetralogy of Fallot, and truncus arteriosus. It was additionally noted whether or not their disease was surgically repaired, palliated, or unrepaired. Patients with heart disease were sicker at the time of arrest (92 % ASA physical status 3–5). This analysis found that cardiac arrests in children with heart disease were more commonly reported during elective non-cardiac procedures than during cardiac surgery or cardiac catheterization procedures. The cause of cardiac arrest in these patients was usually cardiovascular in nature, but the precise cause could not be specified in more than half of the cardiovascular-related cases.

Although patients with heart disease were less likely to be successfully resuscitated after an arrest compared to those without heart disease, this was associated with their disease and underlying health status rather than simply the presence of heart disease itself. When adjusted for ASA physical status, the mortality was similar between patients with heart disease and patients without heart disease after anesthesia-related cardiac arrest. An additional analysis also showed an interesting mortality stratification by the status of the surgical lesion: 43 % for those with unrepaired lesions, 27 % for those with palliated lesions, and only 6 % for those with completely repaired lesions (Table 9.2).[15]

Although six percent of the cardiac arrests in the heart disease population were associated with halothane, the vast majority of the cases in this final report were related to other anesthetic agents or causes unrelated to anesthetic agent. The results are therefore largely still applicable to today's practice of anesthesia. Nine of the 11 equipment-related cardiac arrests in the heart disease population were related to central line placement, 7 in newborns (less than 30 days old), although it is not clear if these occurred before ultrasound was routinely used to place these lines.

The findings from this analysis were particularly striking and alerted the anesthesiology community to the risk of perioperative cardiac arrest in patients with congenital heart disease undergoing non-cardiac surgery. As a result of this work, some have advocated [16] for having pediatric cardiac anesthesiologists available to assist in the care of pediatric patients with heart disease undergoing non-cardiac procedures, although this is not a consensus opinion.

Limitations of the POCA Registry

When the POCA Registry started, there were no consistent legal protections in place for collecting quality improvement data, which led the study designers to make all submissions anonymous. The case reports had no physician, patient, or institutional identifiers, and the POCA Registry could not trace case reports back to the submitting institution. One limitation of anonymous data collection was that POCA Registry staff could not keep track of which centers were submitting cases and verify data or compliance in reporting.

It should be noted that the POCA Registry continued to collect cases for 12 years, making it one of the longest running registries in medicine at the time. Although the study staff suspected reporting compliance may have declined in the later years of POCA Registry operation, cases continued to be submitted until the time data collection was halted. While a substantial number of community hospitals collaborated and submitted cases, most participating centers came from academic groups and specialty children's hospitals, resulting in a less healthy study population than generally represented by pediatric anesthesia patients in North America.

Since determining the cause of each cardiac arrest was a difficult endeavor, a large amount of data was required from each submission to accurately capture causes and ensure quality conclusions. As such, submitting one case could take several hours of a participant's time, and this time usually came from a participant's spare time, outside of work. The POCA Registry did not provide any funding to participating centers to compensate for time or effort of participation. The submission process for POCA Registry case reports relied exclusively on postal mail. Conversion to electronic data submission was not initiated for concern that it may have excluded centers that did not use electronic medical records, thus leading to biased estimates of epidemiologic parameters. Even today, a significant number of anesthetic records are still maintained on paper. While some centers have automated data capture and have made a full transition, we are still very far from being able to streamline this type of reporting using online methods.

In the future, electronic records will help streamline electronic reporting of such events, but we are still several years away from the capability to include all types of centers in electronic data capture registries. Lack of interoperability between electronic health record systems, even with the same vendor, is currently a major limitation to pooling of health information. Some multi-institutional efforts have since started to pool electronic data. The Multicenter Perioperative Outcomes Group (MPOG) and the Anesthesia Quality Institute (AQI) began repositories of anesthetic cases which can be searched by participants to examine rare events and outcomes, but these efforts are still in their infancy and are far from providing robust, broadly generalizable incidence estimates of the type that POCA provided.

The data collected by the POCA Registry was important in that it provided answers to long-standing questions about pediatric anesthesia cardiac arrest. The findings from the POCA Registry proved very useful to the field of anesthesia and resuscitation. Twelve years after its inception, the POCA Registry stopped collecting data. The major lesson learned from the POCA Registry is that the quality and richness of the Registry results depends upon the use of standard clinical definitions, careful registry construction, and systematic database verification, irrespective of whether a paper or electronic system is used to capture registry data. As submission rates to the POCA Registry declined over time, minimization of physician effort through automated electronic data capture may lead to more sustained and improved registries. Linkage of physician payment to participation in registries (already in use with pay-for-performance programs), will encourage broader physician participation and has the potential to yield data that is generally representative of all U.S. patients.

Conclusions

The POCA Registry has had a tremendous impact on anesthesia care and contributed to change in use of anesthesia inhalational agents from almost complete reliance on halothane to nearly universal non-use of halothane in pediatric anesthesia [14]. Additional major changes that occurred since the POCA formation include the flourishing of the health information technology sector making the capture and sharing of information easier, and federal legal protections put in place for quality improvement data reporting through the Patient Safety Organization framework [17].

The POCA Registry provided important answers to challenging questions that are still relevant to anesthesiology today. Since it has ended, other registries have been created to answer similar questions about rare perioperative events. One such registry is the Society for Pediatric Anesthesia's Wake Up Safe program, a multi-institutional patient safety organization that records not only perioperative cardiac arrests, but other significant rare events, and utilizes today's information technology protected by federal law from legal discovery [7]. Several challenges remain this registry that won't be addressed until we are able to create a linked system that is representative of all anesthetic care provided in the United States. We are still years, if not decades, away from such systems becoming a practical reality.

The POCA Registry offers important lessons to future investigators to learn from the POCA Registry experience, and continue to improve upon registry design while striving to improve the safety and quality of clinical care.

References

1. Beecher HK, Todd DP. A study of the deaths associated with anesthesia and surgery: based on a study of 599, 548 anesthesias in ten institutions 1948–1952, inclusive. Ann Surg. 1954;140(1):2–35.
2. Morray JP, Geiduschek JM, Caplan RA, Posner KL, Gild WM, Cheney FW. A comparison of pediatric and adult anesthesia closed malpractice claims. Anesthesiology. 1993;78(3):461–7.
3. Cheney FW, Posner K, Caplan RA, Ward RJ. Standard of care and anesthesia liability. JAMA. 1989;261(11): 1599–603.
4. Posner KL, Geiduschek J, Haberkern CM, Ramamoorthy C, Hackel A, Morray JP. Unexpected cardiac arrest among children during surgery, a North American registry to elucidate the incidence and causes of anesthesia related cardiac arrest. Qual Saf Health Care. 2002;11(3):252–7.
5. Cheney FW. The American Society of Anesthesiologists Closed Claims Project: what have we learned, how has it affected practice, and how will it affect practice in the future? Anesthesiology. 1999;91(2):552–6.
6. Morray JP, Geiduschek JM, Ramamoorthy C, Haberkern CM, Hackel A, Caplan RA, et al. Anesthesia-related cardiac arrest in children: initial findings of the Pediatric Perioperative Cardiac Arrest (POCA) Registry. Anesthesiology. 2000;93(1): 6–14.
7. Kurth CD, Tyler D, Heitmiller E, Tosone SR, Martin L, Deshpande JK. National Pediatric Anesthesia Safety Quality Improvement Program in the United States. Anesth Analg. 2014;119:112–21.
8. van der Griend BF, Lister NA, McKenzie IM, Martin N, Ragg PG, Sheppard SJ, et al. Postoperative mortality in children after 101,885 anesthetics at a tertiary pediatric hospital. Anesth Analg. 2011;112(6):1440–7.
9. Flick RP, Sprung J, Harrison TE, Gleich SJ, Schroeder DR, Hanson AC, et al. Perioperative cardiac arrests in children between 1988 and 2005 at a tertiary referral center: a study of 92,881 patients. Anesthesiology. 2007;106(2):226–37.
10. Murat I, Constant I, Maud'huy H. Perioperative anaesthetic morbidity in children: a database of 24,165 anaesthetics over a 30-month period. Paediatr Anaesth. 2004;14(2):158–66.
11. Ahmed A, Ali M, Khan M, Khan F. Perioperative cardiac arrests in children at a university teaching hospital of a developing country over 15 years. Paediatr Anaesth. 2009;19(6):581–6.
12. Newland MC, Ellis SJ, Lydiatt CA, Peters KR, Tinker JH, Romberger DJ, et al. Anesthetic-related cardiac arrest and its mortality: a report covering 72,959 anesthetics over 10 years from a US teaching hospital. Anesthesiology. 2002;97(1):108–15.
13. Tay CL, Tan GM, Ng SB. Critical incidents in paediatric anaesthesia: an audit of 10 000 anaesthetics in Singapore. Paediatr Anaesth. 2001;11(6):711–8.
14. Bhananker SM, Ramamoorthy C, Geiduschek JM, Posner KL, Domino KB, Haberkern CM, et al. Anesthesia-related cardiac arrest in children: update from the Pediatric Perioperative Cardiac Arrest Registry. Anesth Analg. 2007;105(2):344–50.
15. Ramamoorthy C, Haberkern CM, Bhananker SM, Domino KB, Posner KL, Campos JS, et al. Anesthesia-related cardiac arrest in children with heart disease: data from the Pediatric Perioperative Cardiac Arrest (POCA) registry. Anesth Analg. 2010;110(5):1376–82.
16. Steven JM. Congenital heart disease and anesthesia-related cardiac arrest: connecting the dots. Anesth Analg. 2010;110(5):1255–6.
17. The Patient Safety and Quality Improvement Act of 2005. Overview, June 2008. Rockville: Agency for Healthcare Research and Quality. Available from: http://www.ahrq.gov/legacy/qual/psoact.htm. Accessed 28 May 2013.

Reporting in Pediatric Resuscitation: Get with the Guidelines-Resuscitation Registry

10

Heather A. Wolfe, Robert M. Sutton, Alexis Topjian, Akira Nishisaki, Dana E. Niles, Peter A. Meaney, Robert A. Berg, and Vinay M. Nadkarni

Abstract

High quality CPR and post-resuscitation care is associated with improved survival and functional outcomes following pediatric cardiac arrest. The evidence suggests that the quality of in-hospital resuscitation often does not achieve current resuscitation guideline targets and poor quality CPR contributes to poor patient outcomes. The Get With the Guidelines-Resuscitation (GWTG-R) database is a national evidence-based hospital quality improvement and patient safety program focused on improving resuscitation following cardiac arrest. Registry participation is voluntary with an annual fee that includes data support and report generation. The primary purpose of GWTG-R is to improve outcomes from in-hospital cardiac arrests through individual hospital cardiac arrest resuscitation process and outcome measurement. A secondary purpose is to generate a large, multi-institutional database of adult and pediatric cardiac arrests that facilitates comparison between the international consensus on resuscitation science and treatment recommendations with the actual implementation of guidelines and resultant outcomes. Limitations of the dataset include the

H.A. Wolfe, MD (✉) • R.M. Sutton, MD MSCE
A. Topjian, MD, MSCE • A. Nishisaki, MD, MSCE
D.E. Niles, MS
Department of Anesthesiology and Critical Care Medicine, The Children's Hospital of Philadelphia, Philadelphia, PA USA
e-mail: wolfeh@email.chop.edu; suttonr@email.chop.edu; topjian@email.chop.edu; nishisaki@email.chop.edu; niles@email.chop.edu

P.A. Meaney, MD MPH
Department of Anesthesiology and Critical Care Medicine, The Children's Hospital of Philadelphia, University of Pennsylvania, Philadelphia, PA USA
e-mail: meaney@email.chop.edu

R.A. Berg, MD • V.M. Nadkarni, MD, MS
Department of Critical Care Medicine, The Children's Hospital of Philadelphia, 3400 Civic Center Boulevard 8th Floor, 8NE8566, Philadelphia, PA 19104, USA
e-mail: bergra@email.chop.edu; nadkarni@email.chop.edu

P.R. Barach, J.P. Jacobs, S.E. Lipshultz, P.C. Laussen (eds.),
Pediatric and Congenital Cardiac Care: Volume 2: Quality Improvement and Patient Safety,
DOI 10.1007/978-1-4471-6566-8_10, © Springer-Verlag London 2015

lack of illness severity scores, risk-adjusted classification for congenital heart surgery scoring, and long-term neurologic, behavioural and functional outcome data. Exciting prospects for the future include linkage with other existing large databases such as the Extracorporeal Life Support Organization (ELSO) and Society for Thoracic Surgery (STS) databases.

Keywords
American Heart Association • Get With the Guidelines • Resuscitation • Cardiopulmonary resuscitation • Quality

Introduction

In-hospital cardiac arrest is a relatively uncommon condition among children. The estimates vary between two to six percent of hospitalized children in the intensive care units (ICUs) [1–5], and 4–6 % of cardiac ICU patients after cardiac surgery have arrested [6–8]. In the administrative Kids' Inpatient Database cardiac arrest occurred in 7 per 1,000 hospital admissions for children with cardiovascular disease, nearly ten-fold higher than that of children without cardiovascular disease. The risk for cardiac arrest was amplified in patients with myocarditis (3 % of admissions), heart failure (2 %) and coronary artery disease (2 %), with the highest mortality among patients with single ventricle physiology [9].

The data suggests that the burden of in-hospital pediatric cardiac arrest is shifting to the ICU setting, possibly due to the impact of hospital rapid response teams. Survival to discharge following in-hospital cardiac arrests has improved from 9 % in 1987 to almost 40 % over the last several years, with favorable neurologic outcome at discharge in more than 75 % of survivors [3, 6, 10–14]. Although children who undergo cardiac surgery are at greater risk for cardiac arrest, they also show excellent potential for survival and survival with favorable neurological outcomes [6–8], even when prolonged CPR is required. The American Heart Association's (AHA) national registry of cardiopulmonary resuscitation (Get With The Guidelines-Resuscitation = GWTG-R, formerly known as NRCPR or the National Registry of Cardiopulmonary Resuscitation) database has both served as a quality improvement tool for benchmarking with local and national guidelines and as a repository of data for scientific investigation.

Get with the Guidelines-Resuscitation (GWTG-R) Database

The Get With the Guidelines-Resuscitation (GWTG-R) database is a multisite, in-hospital resuscitation registry sponsored by the AHA. The registry started in 1999 as the National Registry for Cardiopulmonary Resuscitation (NRCPR) to collect resuscitation data from hospitals nationwide and create evidence based guidelines for inpatient cardiopulmonary resuscitation (CPR). The mission was to reduce disability and death from cardiac and respiratory emergencies by providing an evidence-based quality improvement program to support patient safety, medical emergency team response, effective resuscitation and post-resuscitation care [15]. In 2010 NRCPR was incorporated into GWTG to provide additional resources and benefits to members. Membership is voluntary and fee based (which includes data support and report generation). The primary purpose of the database is to improve outcomes from in-hospital CPR through individual hospital cardiac arrest resuscitation process and outcome measurement encouraging performance quality improvement. Process and outcome data are provided at each institution over time and benchmarking data are available for comparisons with national and peer standards.

Trained research coordinators at each participating institution abstract data from each cardiopulmonary arrest from hospital medical charts. Data sheets are completed for cardiopulmonary arrests, acute respiratory compromise events and medical emergency team activations. Recently the important component of post-resuscitation care has been added. The database contains precisely defined variables derived from the Utstein-style data reporting guidelines for cardiac arrest [16]. Data abstractors complete a certification examination consisting of multiple-choice questions and a mock scenario covering operational definitions and criteria for inclusion and exclusion. Case study methods are used to evaluate data abstraction, the accuracy of entries, and compliance with operational definitions before data are accepted.

The six major categories of variables are facility data, patient demographics, pre-event data, event data, outcomes, and quality improvement data. Explicit operational definitions have been generated for every data element. Each patient is assigned a unique code, and specific patient identifiers are not transmitted to the central database repository, which is in compliance with the Health Insurance Portability and Accountability Act. Patients with multiple events have each event captured separately. Table 10.1 shows a list of the updated event specific data points (August, 2013). The data are securely submitted to a central data repository (Patient Management Tool, Outcomes Sciences, Inc, Cambridge, MA). The AHA oversees the entire process of data collection, analysis, and reporting through its national center staff, scientific advisory board, and executive database steering committee.

Multiple benefits exist for using the database, including continuous process improvement opportunities and benchmarking with hospitals according to size, region, type of hospital (e.g., children's hospital), and type of patient (e.g., surgical cardiac patients, medical cardiac patients, etc.). National and local awards and recognition are possible for hospital teams that demonstrate continued compliance with pre-defined metrics. The program also offers various professional education opportunities to improve resuscitation quality of care including web-based conferences and monthly newsletters.

Table 10.1 Data points for GWTG-R October 2012

Admission/Discharge Form:
1. System Entry Time
2. Age
3. Born this Admission
4. Gender
5. Race
6. Hispanic Ethnicity
7. Weight
8. Residence Prior to System Entry
9. Admission Adult and Pediatric Cerebral Performance Category
10. Newborn/Neonate Specific Data (a) Prenatal Care Received (b) Maternal Conditions (c) Delivery Details (i) Fetal Monitoring (ii) Delivery Mode (iii) Presentation (iv) Apgar Scores (v) Cord pH (vi) Gestational Age (d) Special Circumstances Recognized at Birth
11. Discharge Data (a) Discharge Disposition (b) Date/Time of Discharge/Death (c) Do Not Attempt Resuscitation Order During this Admission (Date/Time) (d) Life Support Withdrawn (e) Organs Recovered (f) Discharge Destination (g) Adult and Pediatric Cerebral Performance Category at Discharge
Cardiopulmonary Arrest Form:
1. Date/Time Need for Chest Compression and/or Defibrillation Recognized
2. Pre-event Data (Optional data element) (a) Patient Status Prior to Event (b) Pre-event Vital Signs
3. Pre-Existing Conditions
4. Interventions Already in Place at Time of Event
5. Event data
6. Initial Condition Data
7. Defibrillation Data
8. Types of Ventilation/Airways Used
9. Epinephrine/Vasopressin Bolus Data
10. Other Drug Interventions
11. Non-drug Interventions
12. Event Outcome data
13. Post Return of Circulation Data

(continued)

Table 10.1 (continued)

(a) Induced Hypothermia (yes/no)
(b) Highest Temperature in First 24 h.
14. CPR Quality
(a) End Title CO2 Data
(b) Arterial Line Data
(c) Quality of Compression Data
15. Resuscitation Related Events and Issues
Acute Respiratory Compromise Event Form:
1. Date/Time Need for Emergency Assisted Ventilation Recognized
2. Pre-Event Data
3. Pre-Existing Conditions (Optional data element)
4. Interventions Already in Place at Time of Event
5. Event data
6. Immediate Cause Data
7. Ventilation Data
8. Other Interventions
9. Event Outcome data
10. Resuscitation Related Events and Issues
Medical Emergency Team Event Form:
1. Date/Time of Team Activation
2. Pre-Event Data
(a) Patient Status Prior to Event
(b) Pre-Event Vital Signs
3. Event data
(a) Team Arrival and Departure Date/Time
(b) Subject type and Illness Category
(c) Event Location
(d) Vital Signs at the Time of Event
4. Team Activation Triggers
5. Drug Interventions
6. Non Drug Interventions (diagnostic and therapeutic)
7. Event Outcome
(a) Reason Event Ended
(b) Transfer Location
8. Review of MET Response
(a) Response Delays
(b) Equipment or Medication Delays
(c) Communication Issues

Perhaps as important as the data generated for local quality improvement and benchmarking, is the wealth of published research from the registry. Participating hospitals are able to apply to GWTG-R for access to the de-identified dataset to answer specific research questions. Strict standards and requirements exist for data requests from the registry and all requests are reviewed by the GWTG- R Committee. Each project is reviewed for feasibility, validity and novelty and performed in an expeditious manner; publications are expected to occur within a year of attaining data. More than 50 pediatric and adult resuscitation science papers have been generated based on data gathered from the GWTG-R Registry, and a multitude of studies are currently in the review process. A list of all studies published and all current research requests are available on the American Heart Association website.

Literature Review

We will briefly review a few important pediatric and adult GWGT-R investigations. Notably, recent GWTG-R publications have established that outcomes of in-hospital cardiac arrest have improved over the last decade in GWTG-R hospitals; patients with prolonged CPR can survive with favorable neurological outcomes; and resuscitation process failures are associated with worse outcomes. In addition, a GWTG-R study has raised questions about the optimal pediatric defibrillation dose.

Girotra et al. established that outcomes following in-hospital pediatric cardiac arrest have improved in GWTG-R hospitals from 2000 to 2009. The rate of survival to discharge increased (risk adjusted rates: 14.3 % in 2000 to 43.4 % in 2009; adjusted Risk Ratio per year 1.08; 95 % CI 1.01–1.16; p for trend = 0.02). The improved outcome was primarily driven by an increase in the rate of return of spontaneous circulation from 42.9 % in 2000 to 81.2 % in 2009. In a similar adult study Girotra showed that despite an increase in cardiac arrests due to PEA or asystole, the risk-adjusted rates of survival to discharge after adult in-hospital cardiac arrest increased 13.7–22.3 % from 2000 to 2009 [17].

One of the biggest decisions clinicians face when initiating CPR is when to stop resuscitative efforts. Limited evidence is available to guide these difficult decisions. In contrast to widely held beliefs that pediatric resuscitation is futile after 30 min [14], Matos et al. established that

12 % of children survived to hospital discharge after >35 min of CPR in a GWTG-R study of 3,400 pediatric in-hospital cardiac arrests over a 10-year period [4]. Importantly, 60 % of these survivors of prolonged CPR had favorable neurological outcomes. As in previous published data from the GWTG-R, pediatric surgical cardiac patients had superior survival rates when compared to all other categories [6]. Goldberger et al. found similar trend in survival from prolonged cardiac arrest duration in adults. In another GWTG-R study of 64,339 adult cardiac arrest patients at 435 US hospitals, Goldberger et al. also demonstrated that prolonged CPR can result in successful resuscitation among adults: 12 % of all adults who attained ROSC did so after >30 min of CPR, nearly 10 % of adults with CPR >25 min survived to hospital discharge and 78 % of these patients who survived after >30 min of CPR had favorable neurological outcomes [18]. Of course, both the pediatric study and adult study showed that survival rates were lower after prolonged CPR compared with shorter duration CPR. These GWTG-R studies have been instrumental in increasing our understanding regarding the relationship of CPR duration to outcome.

CPR duration was overall inversely associated with survival to discharge with favorable neurologic outcomes [4]. This multi-center study captured over 3,400 pediatric in hospital arrests over a 10-year period, and data collected allowed for stratification of patients by illness category. This study reinforced the previously published data from the GWTG-R by Ortmann et al. that, surgical cardiac patients had improved survival outcomes when compared to all other categories [18].

The GWTG-R data has been evaluated to address best practices during CPR as well as quality and patient safety measures that correlate with outcomes. Meaney et al. analyzed the first defibrillation events during pediatric cardiac arrest in order to identify appropriate pediatric defibrillation dosage. Among 285 ventricular fibrillation or pulseless ventricular tachycardia (VF/pVT) events in 266 children, defibrillation attempts with 2 J/kg (J/kg) successfully terminated VF/pVT in only 56 % compared with 91 % in previous data from a much smaller series (57 defibrillation attempts). Disappointingly, 4 J/kg was not superior to 2 J/kg in terms of rates of successful defibrillation or rates of survival [19]. The optimal defibrillation dosage in pediatrics still remains unknown.

In another GWTG-R registry, Phelan et al. showed that tracheal intubation during CPR was documented as confirmed by capnography or an esophageal detector device in only 56.8 % of patients. Importantly, confirmation by capnography or esophageal detector device was significantly associated with both increased likelihood of ROSC (adjusted OR 1.229 [1.179,1.282]) and survival to hospital discharge (adjusted OR 1.093 [1.033,1.157]) [20]. In addition, Ornato and colleagues demonstrated that documented resuscitation process errors (i.e., delay in medication administration, defibrillation, airway management and chest compression performance) were also associated with decreased survival from in-hospital cardiac arrest. [21] We have briefly reviewed several relevant publications from the Get With the Guidelines-Resuscitation database to highlight the type of data and uses of the registry.

Limitations of Dataset

Several limitations exist for the Get With The Guidelines-Resuscitation dataset. The database does not include information regarding severity of illness. Risk adjustment is limited to age, pre-arrest characteristics and interventions in place at time of arrest, and broad disease illness categories. There is no delineation of cardiac anatomy or type and stage of congenital heart disease repair within the database, nor are risk-adjusted classification for Congenital Heart Surgery (e.g., RACHS-1) determined [22]. While there is specific event and patient level data, there is limited institutional specific data.

The data are self-reported and not independently checked. Variability in coding can be another source of bias as resuscitation record documentation can be suboptimal and ambiguous. The two potential biases are addressed by explicit training for data coordinators and abstractors using robust Utstein-style reporting guidelines. Another limitation is the dataset lacks *quantitative* measures of CPR quality, such as depth or rate of chest compression, however indirect measures such as end tidal CO2, arterial blood pressure data despite clear evidence in both animal and human studies that the quality of CPR relates to both short and long term outcomes [23–25]. Many of these limitations are not unique to the GWTG-R database and are inherent to large national surveillance databases.

Future Goals of Get with the Guidelines – Resuscitation Database

The future is exciting for resuscitation science. Limitations of the GWTG-R database are being addressed by attempted linkage with the Extracorporeal Life Support Organization (ELSO) and Society for Thoracic Surgery (STS) databases. Additional links to large administrative database such as Pediatric Health Information System (PHIS) and Kids' Inpatient Database (KIDS), and quality improvement databases such as the Virtual PICU Systems (VPS) will enhance the detail, richness and scope of analyses.

In addition, linkage of training (mock code performance and outcomes) using simulated cardiac arrest scenarios with real cardiac arrest CPR quality performance and outcomes is under development (e.g., a mock-GWTG-R registry to complement the real GWTG-R registry). Using highly standardized simulated cases, this mock registry could provide abundant data on quality of resuscitation and may further clarify current gaps [26].

Conclusions

Pediatric in-hospital cardiac arrest is rare but still poses major morbidity and mortality risk for patients. Furthermore, it is more common among patients with congenital heart disease compared to hospitalized patients without cardiac disease [9]. The Get With the Guidelines- Resuscitation database is a multisite, in-hospital resuscitation database that was developed to assess process of resuscitation care and outcomes to improve survival from in-hospital cardiac arrest. This registry links the international and national guidelines with actual implementation of process of care and the resultant impact on benchmarked patient outcomes. Exciting prospects for the future include linkage with other existing large administrative and quality improvement databases such as the Extracorporeal Life Support Organization (ELSO) and Society for Thoracic Surgery (STS) databases, and the development of a mock-GWTG-R registry to characterize and improve the linkage of resuscitation guideline training and implementation with improved patient safety, survival and neurological outcomes.

References

1. Suominen P, Olkkola KT, Voipio V, Korpela R, Palo R, Räsänen J. Utstein style reporting of in-hospital paediatric cardiopulmonary resuscitation. Resuscitation. 2000;45(1):17–25.
2. de Mos N, van Litsenburg RRL, McCrindle B, Bohn DJ, Parshuram CS. Pediatric in-intensive-care-unit cardiac arrest: incidence, survival, and predictive factors*. Crit Care Med. 2006;34(4):1209–15. doi:10.1097/01.CCM.0000208440.66756.C2.
3. Nadkarni VM, Larkin GL, Peberdy MA, Carey SM, Kaye W, Mancini ME, et al. First documented rhythm and clinical outcome from in-hospital cardiac arrest among children and adults. JAMA. 2006;295(1):50–7.
4. Matos RI, Watson RS, Nadkarni VM, Huang H-H, Berg RA, Meaney PA, Carroll CL, Berens RJ, Praestgaard A, Weissfeld L, Spinella PC, American Heart Association's Get With The Guidelines–Resuscitation (Formerly the National Registry of Cardiopulmonary Resuscitation) Investigators. Duration of cardiopulmonary resuscitation and illness category impact survival and neurologic outcomes for in-hospital pediatric cardiac arrests. Circulation. 2013;127(4):442–51. doi:10.1161/CIRCULATIONAHA.112.125625.
5. Slonim AD, Patel KM, Ruttimann UE, Pollack MM. Cardiopulmonary resuscitation in pediatric intensive care units. Crit Care Med. 1997;25(12):1951–5.
6. Ortmann L, Prodhan P, Gossett J, Schexnayder S, Berg R, Nadkarni V, Bhutta A, for the American Heart Association's Get With the Guidelines-Resuscitation (formerly National Registry of Cardiopulmonary Resuscitation) Investigators, The American Heart Association GWTG-R Investigators. Outcomes after in-hospital cardiac arrest in children with cardiac disease: a report from Get With the Guidelines-Resuscitation. Circulation. 2011;124(21):2329–37. doi: 10.1161/CIRCULATIONAHA.110.013466.

7. Parra DA, Totapally BR, Zahn E, Jacobs J, Aldousany A, Burke RP, et al. Outcome of cardiopulmonary resuscitation in a pediatric cardiac intensive care unit. Crit Care Med. 2000;28(9):3296–300.
8. Rhodes JF, Blaufox AD, Seiden HS, Asnes JD, Gross RP, Rhodes JP, Griepp RB, Rossi AF. Cardiac arrest ins infants after congenital heart surgery. Circulation. 1999;100(Supplement 2):II-194–9. doi:10.1161/01.CIR.100.suppl_2.II-194.
9. Lowry AW, Knudson JD, Cabrera AG, Graves DE, Morales DLS, Rossano JW. Cardiopulmonary resuscitation in hospitalized children with cardiovascular disease: estimated prevalence and outcomes from the kids' inpatient database. Pediatr Crit Care Med. 2013;14(3):248–55. doi:10.1097/PCC.0b013e3182713329.
10. Reis AG, Nadkarni V, Perondi MB, Grisi S, Berg RA. A prospective investigation into the epidemiology of in-hospital pediatric cardiopulmonary resuscitation using the international Utstein reporting style. Pediatrics. 2002;109(2):200–9.
11. Tibballs J, Kinney S. A prospective study of outcome of in-patient paediatric cardiopulmonary arrest. Resuscitation. 2006;71(3):310–8. doi:10.1016/j.resuscitation.2006.05.009.
12. Girotra S, Spertus JA, Li Y, Berg RA, Nadkarni VM, Chan PS, American Heart Association Get With the Guidelines–Resuscitation Investigators. Survival trends in pediatric in-hospital cardiac arrests: an analysis from Get With the Guidelines-Resuscitation. Circ Cardiovasc Qual Outcomes. 2013;6(1):42–9. doi:10.1161/CIRCOUTCOMES.112.967968.
13. Samson RA, Nadkarni VM, Meaney PA, Carey SM, Berg MD, Berg RA, American Heart Association National Registry of CPR Investigators. Outcomes of in-hospital ventricular fibrillation in children. N Engl J Med. 2006;354(22):2328–39. doi:10.1056/NEJMoa052917.
14. Zaritsky A, Nadkarni V, Getson P, Kuehl K. CPR in children. Ann Emerg Med. 1987;16(10):1107–11.
15. Hunt EA, Mancini ME, Smyth M, Truitt TL. Using the American Heart Association's National Registry of Cardiopulmonary Resuscitation for performance improvement. Jt Comm J Qual Patient Saf. 2009;35(1):13–20. Available at: http://www.ingentaconnect.com/content/jcaho/jcjqs/2009/00000035/00000001/art00003.
16. Jacobs I, Nadkarni V, Bahr J, Berg RA, Billi JE, Bossaert L, Cassan P, Coovadia A, D'Este K, Finn J, Halperin H, Handley A, Herlitz J, Hickey R, Idris A, Kloeck W, Larkin GL, Mancini ME, Mason P, Mears G, Monsieurs K, Montgomery W, Morley P, Nichol G, Nolan J, Okada K, Perlman J, Shuster M, Steen PA, Sterz F, Tibballs J, Timerman S, Truitt T, Zideman D, International Liaison Committee on Resuscitation, American Heart Association, European Resuscitation Council, Australian Resuscitation Council, New Zealand Resuscitation Council, Heart and Stroke Foundation of Canada, InterAmerican Heart Foundation, Resuscitation Councils of Southern Africa, ILCOR Task Force on Cardiac Arrest and Cardiopulmonary Resuscitation Outcomes. Cardiac arrest and cardiopulmonary resuscitation outcome reports: update and simplification of the Utstein templates for resuscitation registries: a statement for healthcare professionals from a task force of the International Liaison Committee on Resuscitation (American Heart Association, European Resuscitation Council, Australian Resuscitation Council, New Zealand Resuscitation Council, Heart and Stroke Foundation of Canada, InterAmerican Heart Foundation, Resuscitation Councils of Southern Africa). Circulation. 2004;110(21):3385–97. doi:10.1161/01.CIR.0000147236.85306.15.
17. Girotra S, Nallamothu BK, Spertus JA, Li Y, Krumholz HM, Chan PS. Trends in survival after in-hospital cardiac arrest. N Engl J Med. 2012;367(20):1912–20. doi:10.1056/NEJMoa1109148.
18. Goldberger ZD, Chan PS, Berg RA, Kronick SL, Cooke CR, Lu M, et al. Duration of resuscitation efforts and survival after in-hospital cardiac arrest: an observational study. Lancet. 2012;380(9852):1473–81.
19. Meaney PA, Nadkarni VM, Atkins DL, Berg MD, Samson RA, Hazinski MF, Berg RA, for the American Heart Association National Registry of Cardiopulmonary Resuscitation Investigators. Effect of defibrillation energy dose during in-hospital pediatric cardiac arrest. Pediatrics. 2011;127(1):e16–23. doi: 10.1542/peds.2010-1617.
20. Phelan MP, Ornato JP, Peberdy MA, Hustey FM, Investigatorsc FTAHAGWTG-R. Appropriate documentation of confirmation of endotracheal tube position and relationship to patient outcome from in-hospital cardiac arrest. Resuscitation. 2013;84(1):31–6. doi:10.1016/j.resuscitation.2012.08.329.
21. Ornato JP, Peberdy MA, Reid RD, Feeser VR, Dhindsa HS, Investigatorsc FTN. Impact of resuscitation system errors on survival from in-hospital cardiac arrest. Resuscitation. 2012;83(1):63–9. doi:10.1016/j.resuscitation.2011.09.009.
22. Jenkins KJ, Gauvreau K, Newburger JW, Spray TL, Moller JH, Iezzoni LI. Consensus-based method for risk adjustment for surgery for congenital heart disease. J Thorac Cardiovasc Surg. 2002;123(1):110–8. doi:10.1067/mtc.2002.119064.
23. Abella BS, Alvarado JP, Myklebust H, Edelson DP, Barry A, O'Hearn N, et al. Quality of cardiopulmonary resuscitation during in-hospital cardiac arrest. JAMA. 2005;293(3):305–10.
24. Wik L, Kramer-Johansen J, Myklebust H, Sørebø H, Svensson L, Fellows B, et al. Quality of cardiopulmonary resuscitation during out-of-hospital cardiac arrest. JAMA. 2005;293(3):299–304.
25. Edelson DP, Litzinger B, Arora V, Walsh D, Kim S, Lauderdale DS, et al. Improving in-hospital cardiac arrest process and outcomes with performance debriefing. Arch Intern Med. 2008;168(10):1063–9.
26. Griswold S, Ponnuru S, Nishisaki A, Szyld D, Davenport M, Deutsch ES, et al. The emerging role of simulation education to achieve patient safety: translating deliberate practice and debriefing to save lives. Pediatr Clin North Am. 2012;59(6):1329–40. doi:10.1016/j.pcl.2012.09.004.

Addressing Nutrition and Growth in Children with Congenital Heart Disease

11

Jeffrey B. Anderson and Robert H. Beekman III

Abstract

Adequate nutrition is required for infants and children to grow and develop normally. Children with congenital heart disease commonly experience growth failure early in life with major potential consequences. This is especially true for those children who require surgery during the first several weeks of life. The etiology of this growth failure poorly understood but often results in both short and long term adverse outcomes. Careful attention to growth monitoring and appropriate intervention when needed can alleviate some growth problems in children with congenital heart disease. This can be accomplished by standardization of monitoring and nutrition practices. Feeding infants with congenital heart disease also poses some risks including a higher risk of necrotizing enterocolitis and risks associated with enteral feeding via nasogastric tube. While there has been considerable improvement in our understanding of feeding problems in congenital heart disease, there is much work to be done to help understand and alleviate this problem.

Keywords

Congenital heart disease • Growth failure • Nutrition • Clinical outcomes • Neurodevelopment

Introduction

Normal growth and development for infants and children requires adequate nutrition. Nutrition affects somatic and neurodevelopmental growth as well. Nutrients required for normal growth and development include carbohydrates, fats, proteins, vitamins, minerals and water. During

J.B. Anderson, MD, MPH (✉)
R.H. Beekman III, MD
Cincinnati Children's Hospital Medical Center,
The Heart Institute,
3333 Burnet Avenue, ML 2003,
Cincinnati, OH 45229, USA
e-mail: jeffrey.anderson@cchmc.org;
rbeekman@cchmc.org

P.R. Barach, J.P. Jacobs, S.E. Lipshultz, P.C. Laussen (eds.),
Pediatric and Congenital Cardiac Care: Volume 2: Quality Improvement and Patient Safety,
DOI 10.1007/978-1-4471-6566-8_11, © Springer-Verlag London 2015

periods of rapid growth and development, infants and children require increased supplies of these nutrients, compared to adults. It is essential for central nervous system development during critical periods of neural growth

Malnutrition is defined as inadequate intake of essential nutrients and calories leading to growth failure. Growth failure is a term that describes an infant or child who has indexed weight-for-age or weight-for-length that is less than the 5th-centile or has crossed two major centile lines on a standardized growth curve [1]. Failure-to-thrive is a clinical term that describes an infant or child who is failing to meet growth goals over a period of time. The National Research Council has defined minimum energy needs for healthy infants and children [1]. A healthy infant requires from 108 to 117 kilocalories (kcal) per kilogram (kg) of body weight per day. This caloric intake is sufficient to allow for homeostasis but also provides the energy for rapid muscle and neural growth during the first several months of life [2]. As children get older the caloric intake needed to meet their energy needs drops (indexed to body weight) [1].

Adequate monitoring of growth is essential to ensure that nutritional needs are met as infants and children grow and develop. Monitoring is especially critical in infants and children with chronic medical problems that put them at risk for growth failure and in cases where growth problems need to be addressed with nutritional interventions. *Anthropometric measurements*, including weight, length or height, and weight-for-length/height, are the most important tools to follow growth in infants and children. These measurements, and their changes over time, should be age indexed using National Center for Health Statistics growth curves [3]. These measurements should be made at each clinical encounter, using the same equipment if possible. Other anthropometric measurements such as upper arm and lower leg length, skinfold thickness and body composition can also be followed in cases of concern for growth faltering.

Other tools can also be used to assess for nutritional and growth adequacy. A three-day *dietary journal* can provide much needed information about actual nutritional intake. *Laboratory measurements* of nutritional status can be used as an adjunct to anthropometric measures of growth and nutrition. These tests are typically not helpful in understanding the etiology of growth problems, but rather help understand the severity of the problem. Laboratory measurements can include albumin, which indicates nutrient intake during the past several weeks, and pre-albumin, which reflects nutrient intake during the past several days. Finally, measurement of *energy expenditure* can be performed to assess caloric needs. The World Health Organization provides comparative data for resting energy expenditure based on age, gender and weight [4].

Growth in Congenital Heart Disease

Growth failure is well recognized and common in infants with congenital heart disease (CHD) [5–7]. While anthropometric measurements are often normal at birth, even in infants with the most complex forms of congenital heart disease, because fetal growth and development is typically not affected. However, growth problems often become evident in the first several weeks and months of life and can subsequently persist through childhood in some cases [8–10]. Infants and children with congenital heart disease require higher caloric intake than their healthy counterparts, often in excess of 120 kcal/kg per day as infants, and some can require more than 160 kcal/kg per day for catch-up growth [2, 11].

Children with congenital heart disease face many challenges that impair their ability to achieve adequate growth, both peri-operatively and longer term [12–14]. The etiologies for these challenges include frequent interruption of feeds around diagnostic and therapeutic procedures (adequate nutrition can be interrupted for weeks in the peri-operative period), prolonged hospital stays, post-operative fluid restrictions, gastroesophageal reflux, and oral feeding aversion [2, 15, 16]. Physiologic problems may also adversely affect nutritional intake. Gastrointestinal malabsorption may occur in patients with high filling pressure or in conjunction with low cardiac output and impaired systemic perfusion [15].

A hypermetabolic state, which may be due to congestive heart failure and manifested by tachycardia, diaphoresis or tachypnea, has also been reported as a cause for growth failure in this population [15, 17].

Poor nutrition and growth can lead to both short and long-term adverse consequences for infants and children with congenital heart disease. Many forms of congenital heart disease require surgical repair or a series of palliative surgical procedures. Not only do these procedures and their associated hospitalizations affect concurrent nutrition and growth, but importantly it is becoming apparent that short term surgical outcomes can be adversely affected by a worse nutritional status at the time of surgery [8–10]. Nutrition and growth problems have an adverse effect on perioperative outcomes. Poor nutrition in adults, as defined by low fat-free mass, low body mass index, or low serum albumin or pre-albumin levels has been associated with longer hospital stays and increased rate of readmission following discharge [18, 19]. Increased rates of mortality and post-surgical infection have been described in children with diverse types of congenital heart disease with poor nutritional status at the time of surgery [20, 21]. Infants and children with single ventricle heart disease and growth problems also have longer post-operative hospital lengths of stay and increased infection risks following palliative surgical procedures [8, 10].

Children with growth failure early in life may also experience poor long-term neurodevelopmental outcomes, which have been widely reported among children with complex congenital heart disease [22–24]. These deficits include impairment in intelligence [25], language development [26], visual construction and perception [27], gross and fine motor skills [28], and behavioral adjustment [29]. Early growth failure in infancy is associated with later deficits in intelligence [30], fine and gross motor skills [31], and behavior adjustment [32]. This connection between early growth failure and later neurodevelopmental deficits in children with congenital heart disease is strongly suspected, but causality has not yet been established.

Nutritional Management in Congenital Heart Disease

Growth Monitoring

Close monitoring for feeding and growth problems is essential for early identification of growth faltering in infants and children with congenital heart disease. In patients with the most complex congenital heart disease there is considerable variation in practices surrounding nutrition and growth of patients among centers caring for these infants. This has been most clearly demonstrated by the work of the National Pediatric Cardiology Quality Improvement Collaborative (NPC-QIC) that followed infants with a single ventricle who had undergone stage 1 palliation through their first interstage period [33]. Figure 11.1 demonstrates the variation in growth of interstage patients among several centers involved in the NPC-QIC [34]. The etiology of growth variation among centers was in part due to variation in nutrition and monitoring methods at these surgical sites. The most significant factors associated with better patient growth among centers were related to closer monitoring of growth failure during the months comprising the interstage and involvement of a Registered Dietician in the outpatient team caring for these infants.

All infants and children with congenital heart disease who are at risk for growth failure require close monitoring of anthropometric measurements during periods of increased risk for growth failure. Early detection of growth failure is essential to assure that appropriate nutritional interventions are accomplished with sufficient time to improve growth before subsequent surgical procedures are undertaken. It is recommended that weight, length/height, head circumference as well as weight-for-age, length-for-age, head circumference-for-age and weight-for-length be obtained at each clinic visit in infants with complex heart disease. These measurements will help determine when a nutritional change or intervention needs to be made. Involvement of a Registered Dietician in the care of at-risk infants and children allows for appropriate monitoring and consultation when interventions are needed.

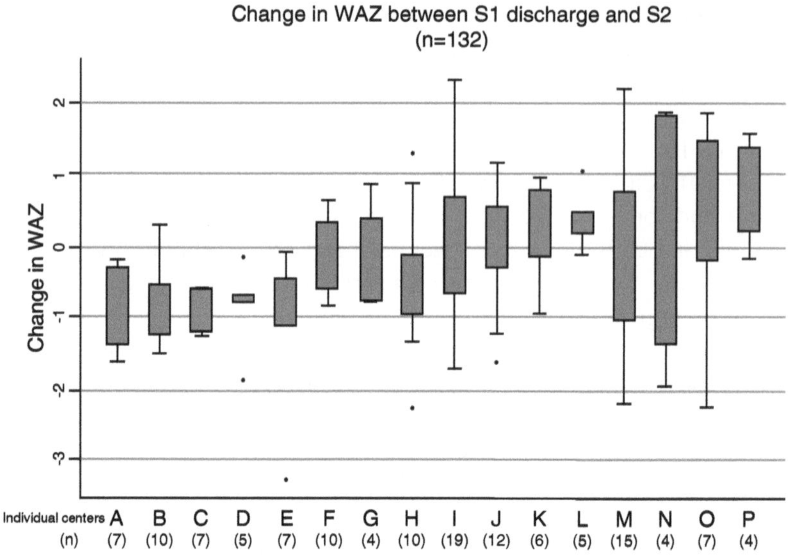

Fig. 11.1 Growth variation in infants with single ventricle. Variation in weight for age z-score changes, by surgical site caring for the patient, measured from stage 1 discharge to presentation for stage 2 palliation (Reprinted from Anderson et al. [34], copyright 2012, with permission from Elsevier)

Standardization of Feeding Practices

Standardization of feeding practices can improve growth and long term outcomes. The NPC-QIC has published recommended feeding algorithms for infants with a single ventricle, with the intent to help centers standardize their nutritional approach to these challenging patients (Figs. 11.2, 11.3, 11.4, and 11.5). Using standardized feeding algorithms have been shown to increase nutrient delivery, decrease length of stay, and minimize morbidities [12, 35–37]. In addition to improving nutritional intake, feeding protocols both before and after cardiac surgery have been shown to reduce the incidence of necrotizing enterocolitis (NEC), minimize interruptions in feeding, improve oral intake, decrease cost and hospital length of stay as well as improve overall outcomes [38, 39]. The use of an interdisciplinary team also has been shown to improve oral intake and overall nutritional management in high-risk neonates and infants [40]. The use of a standardized approach has been successful in infants with hypoplastic left heart syndrome following stage 1 palliation. Braudis et al. demonstrated significantly reduced post-operatively times to reach the recommended daily allowance of calories from 13 days to 9 days in this group of patients [36]. Suboptimal growth in cardiac patients is multifactorial leading to a complex process of feeding and dysfunctional feeding postoperatively. Implementation of care bundles driven by multidisciplinary teams is a strategy that can address not only the medical and physical needs of the infant but also the behavioral and environmental factors that may affect nutrition and growth [38].

Preoperative Feeding

In infants undergoing surgical repair or palliation of congenital heart disease there are practices that can be instituted that may help the patients meet nutritional needs and goals. During the preoperative period feeding is helpful to promote normal development of feeding patterns in neonates, prevent translocation of bacteria and to promote immunologic and gut mucosal health. Current evidence suggests that enteral feeding can be attempted with close monitoring and vigilance in patients with hemodynamic stability. In most cases, sick neonates will need supplemental parenteral nutrition to provide adequate nutrition. Postoperatively there should be a goal for early introduction of enteral feeding. Intermittent oral and nasogastric feeding preoperatively has been successful and safe in many studies of infants with congenital heart disease although it has been shown that continuous feeding requires more time to reach the caloric goals [41, 42]. Initiation of enteral nutrition should be started at 20–25 mL/kg/day. Human or Donor milk is the preferred fluid but if not available a standard infant formula is an acceptable alternative. Advancement of feeds should be increased by 20 mL/kg/day to a goal of 120–150 ml/kg/day. Feeding intolerance is an important clinical sign that can suggest poor systemic perfusion in conjunction with poor cardiac output. If an infant cannot feed preoperatively or for a prolonged period of time post-operatively, non-nutritive measures should be provided to continue to develop oral motor skills.

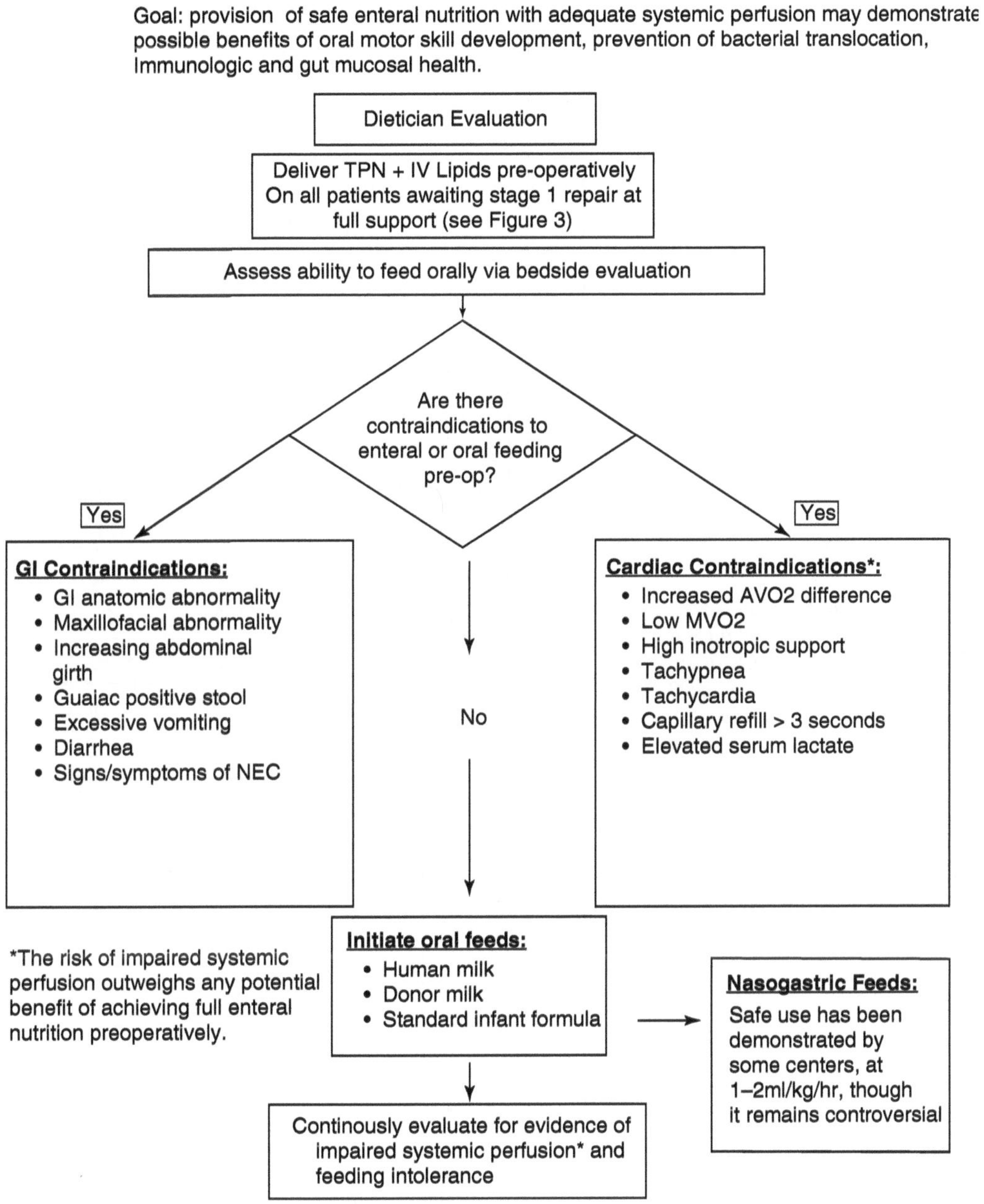

Fig. 11.2 Pre-operative enteral feeding protocol

Goal: All infants that will not receive full EN in </=3–5 days post-operatively should receive PN to achieve electrolyte balance and full nutrition support as soon as fluid regulation allows for cost effective adequate nutrition.

Initiate TPN

Fluids:
Start @ 100mL/kg total fluids or volume allowed by fluid restriction

Dextrose:
Start with a Glucose Infusion Rate (GIR) of 6-9 mg/kg/min or 10-12.5% Dextrose

Amino Acids:
Start with 1.5-3 gm/kg/day and increase daily by 1 gm/kg to a goal of 3-4 gm/kg/day. Restrict protein if needed for renal dysfunction

Lipids:
Start with 1-2 gm/kg/day and advance by 0.5-1 gm/kg/day to a goal of 3 gm/kg/day

Micronutrients/Trace Elements:
- Sodium 2-5 mEq/kg/day
- Potassium 2-4 mEq/kg/day
- Calcium 0.5-4 mEq/kg/day
- Phosphorus 0.5-2 mMol/kg/day
- Magnesium 0.3-0.5 mEq/kg/day
- Zinc 50-250 mcg/kg/d
- Copper 20 mcg/kg
- Manganese 1 mcg/kg/day
- Selenium 2 mcg/kg
- Chromium

Additional considerations:
- Increase Zinc to 250-400 mcg/kg/day
- Levocarnitine: 8-10 mg/kg/day
- Cysteine (essential amino acid) is sometimes added to PN to help decrease the pH of the solution which increases the solubility of calcium and phosphorus. Recommend 40 mg/gm of amino acid.
- Albumin/PreAlbumin are commonly monitored, though they are not relevant to nutritional status in the critically ill population

Central Access is most desirable →

Advance TPN to goal

Goal Calories:
- 90-100 kcal/kg/day (may be decreased if paralyzed)

Fluids:
- Maintain 100-120 mL/kg or liberalize per team

Dextrose:
- Increase GIR daily by 1-2 mg/kg/min to a goal of 12-14 mg/kg/min

Amino Acids:
- Increase daily by 1-1.5 gm/kg to a goal of 3-4 gm/kg/day. Restrict protein if needed for renal dysfunction

Lipids:
- Goal of 3 gm/kg/day

Criteria for Cautious use of PN:

Hyperglycemia	Glucose >300 mg/dL
Azotemia	BUN >100 mg/dL
Hyperosmolality	Serum >350 mOsm/kg
Hypernatremia	Na >150 mEq/L
Hypokalemia	K <3 mEq/L
Hyperchloremic	Cl >115 mEq/L
Hypochloremic	Cl <85 mEq/L
Hypophosphatemia	Phos <2 mg/dL
Acidosis/ alkalosis	

Monitoring TPN

Daily:
- Na, K, Chloride, CO2, BUN, Creatinine, Glucose
- Calcium
- Magnesium
- Phosphorus

1-2 x Weekly:
- Triglycerides, bile acids, Bilirubin, Alk phos, ALT/AST, GGT

Fig. 11.3 Post operative Total Parental Nutrition Protocol (TPN)

Potential Post-operative Feeding and Nutrition Difficulties

Vocal cord injury is a common post-operative complication following congenital heart repairs involving aortic arch reconstruction, particularly after the Norwood operation in infants with hypoplastic left heart syndrome and due to prolonged intubation [43, 44]. Infants with vocal cord injury often have difficulty feeding

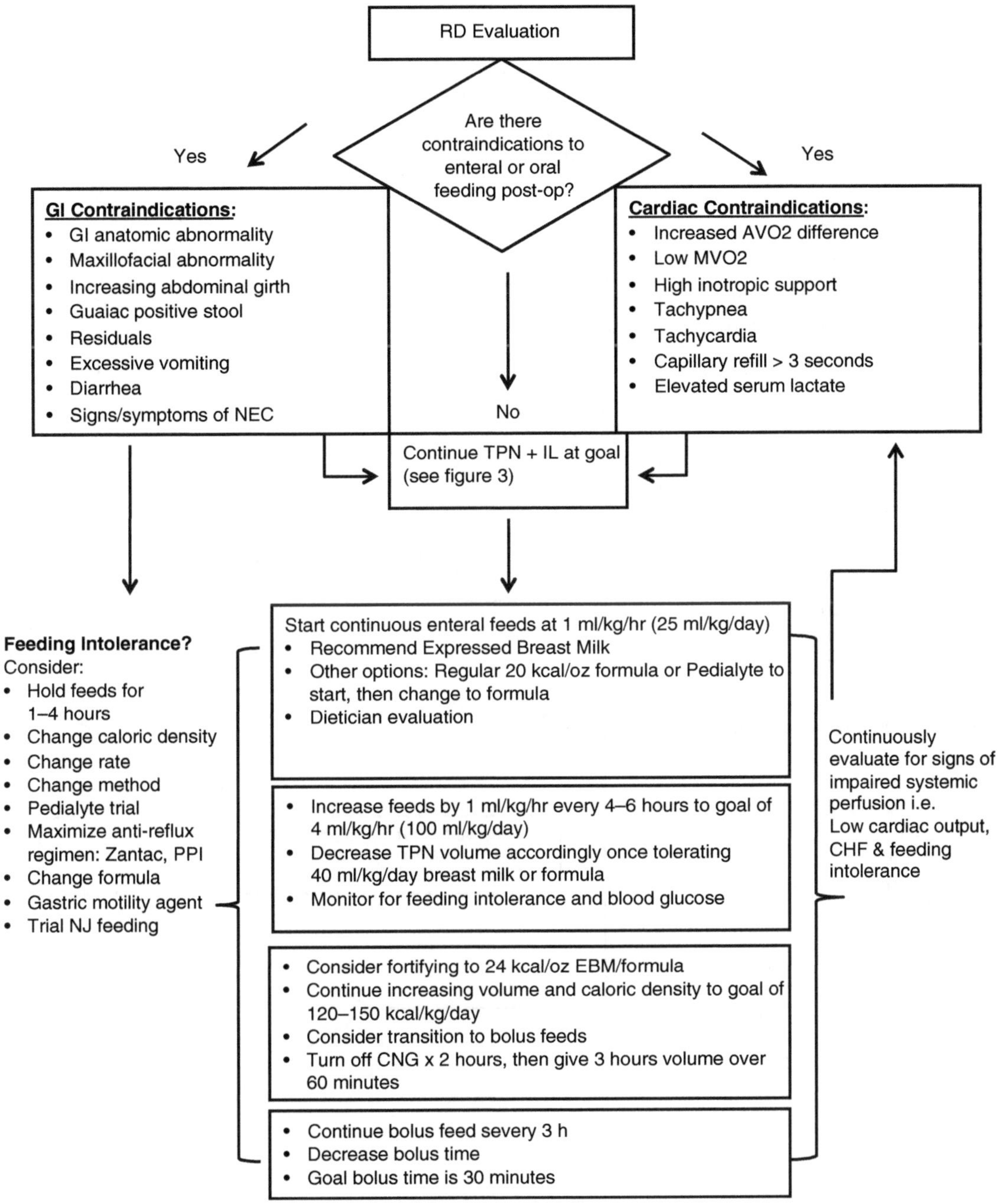

Fig. 11.4 Post operative Enteral Feeding (EN)

and require speech therapy during its resolution [12]. Because of this common finding it is recommended that thorough speech and feeding evaluations be performed following infant aortic arch reconstruction surgery. This highlights the importance of multidisciplinary teams in the care of these complex infants. Speech and language pathologists offer critical assessment skills in the area of feeding and swallowing dysfunction diagnosis and management.

Chylous effusion can be a serious complication following cardiovascular surgery and can significantly impair efforts at feeding in the post-operative period. The incidence of chylous effusion is reported to be from 0.05 to 9 % of infants

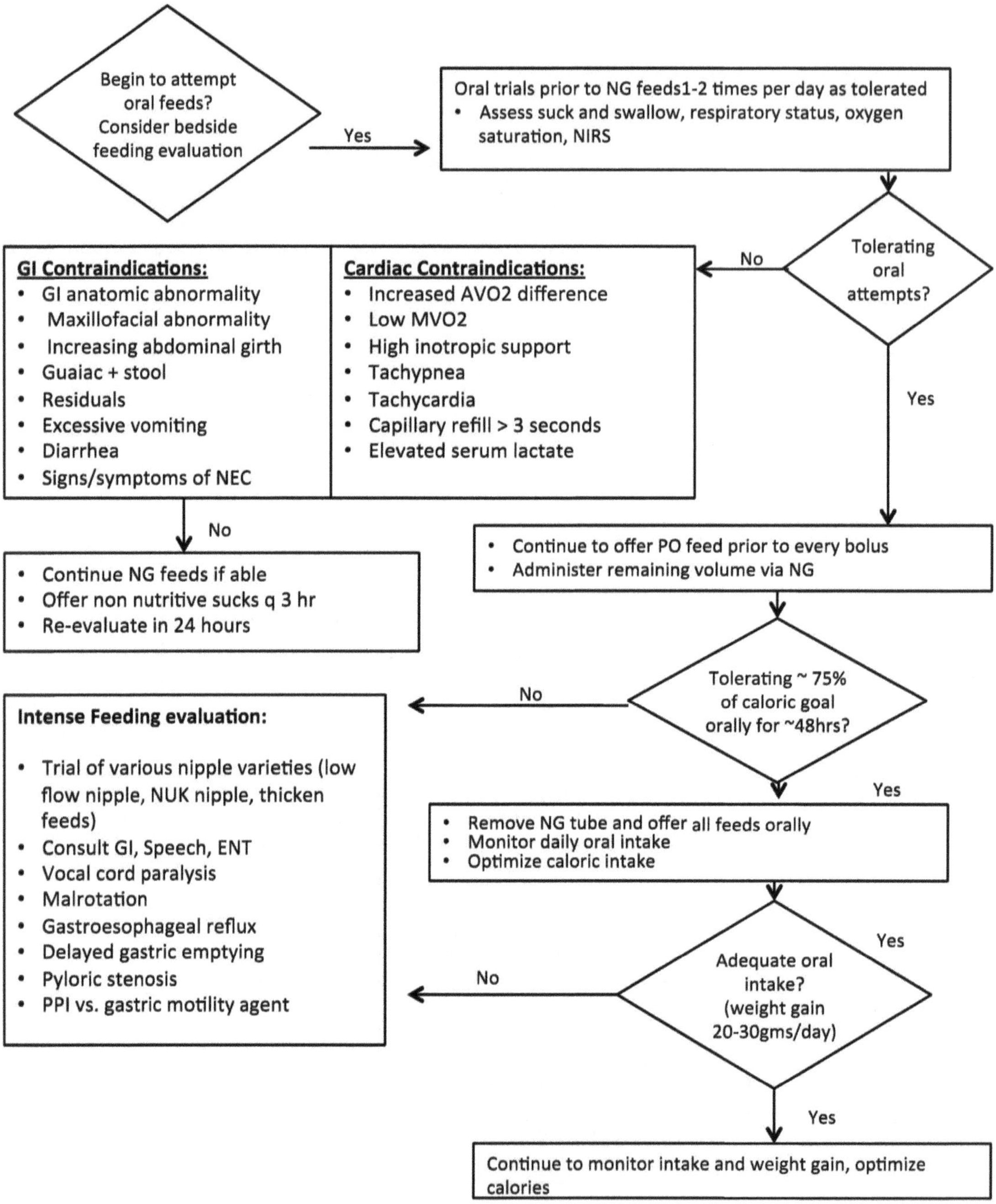

Fig. 11.5 Post operative oral feeding protocol

and children undergoing surgery for congenital heart disease [45]. Potential etiologies of chylothorax include thoracic duct injury, increased right-sided pressures and central vein thrombosis [46–48]. Chylous fluid consists of high levels of triglycerides, lymphocytes, and proteins including immunoglobulins and clotting factors [48]. Given the high nutrient content of the fluid, increased drainage puts patients at risk for protein-energy malnutrition, delayed initiation of enteral nutrition, electrolyte disturbances, coagulopathy, poor wound healing, impaired immune function, and respiratory complications due to required chest tube placement [49, 50].

Potential Adverse Events Secondary to Feeding

When feeding infants with congenital heart disease, even when following conservative guidelines, there are risks of adverse outcomes. The primary of these risks include the development of necrotizing enerocolitis and problems associated with feeding via a nasogatric tube. Infants with impaired systemic perfusion are at risk for necrotizing enterocolitis (NEC) [15]. Mortality in post-operative infants with congenital heart disease is significantly higher in those who develop NEC than those that do not [51]. Feeding intolerance can be the first indication of NEC, especially when associated with bloody stools. Any infant with concerns for NEC in the post-operative period should be fully evaluated with clinical examination, abdominal radiographs and appropriate consultation. Feeds should be immediately held during this evaluation period.

It is common to use a nasogastric tube to supplement feeding in infants with poor oral intake. This form of enteral feeding is used both in and out of the hospital setting [34]. While uncommon, one problem that has been associated with nasogastric tube feedings is misplacement of the tube and aspiration [52]. It is essential to educate caregivers of the potential risks of enteral feeding as well as the signs of problems with the nasogastric tube.

Future Work and Research Questions

While there has been improvement in our understanding of nutritional problems in infants and children with congenital heart disease, there are still aspects of this problem that require additional work. Standardization of feeding practices does improve overall patient growth but there is still a poor understanding of the etiology of growth problems in many forms of congenital heart disease. Several areas that may be addressed include actual energy expenditure, functional gastrointestinal perfusion studies, and biomarkers of nutritional problems. In addition to physiologic causes of poor growth, work should progress to understand the impact of the home environment on growth in these children with complex medical needs.

Finally, while it is important to continue to understand the causes of growth failure it is important for investigators to better understand the long-term problems associated with early struggles with growth, perhaps most importantly the role that early growth plays in neurodevelopment, neuro-recovery and plasticity and long term wellbeing.

Conclusions

Growth failure is well recognized and common in infants with complex congenital heart disease [5–7]. Adequate nutrition is essential for normal growth and development for infants and children. Growth problems in congenital heart disease can lead to both short and long term problems including an adverse effect on surgical outcomes and impairment of neurodevelopment. While the etiologies of growth problems in congenital heart disease are varied and multiple, much progress has been made in understanding these issues and determining interventions that mitigate this important problem. A multi-disciplinary approach to nutritional management and surveillance, and the use of standardized nutritional protocols, with the intention of early identification and mitigation of growth problems can improve growth in infants with congenital heart disease and further improve outcomes for these challenging patients.

References

1. Hui W, Grover G. Nutritional needs. In: Berkowitz BD, editor. Berkowitz's pediatrics: a primary care approach. Elk Grove Village: American Academy of Pediatrics; 2008. p. 63–9.
2. Steltzer M, Rudd N, Pick B. Nutrition care for newborns with congenital heart disease. Clin Perinatol. 2005;32(4):1017–30, xi.

3. Himes JH, et al. Parent-specific adjustments for evaluation of recumbent length and stature of children. Pediatrics. 1985;75(2):304–13.
4. Mascarenhas MR, Zemel B, Stallings VA. Nutritional assessment in pediatrics. Nutrition. 1998;14(1):105–15.
5. Forchielli ML, et al. Children with congenital heart disease: a nutrition challenge. Nutr Rev. 1994;52(10):348–53.
6. Gingell RL, Pieroni DR, Hornung MG. Growth problems associated with congenital heart disease in infancy. In: Lebenthal E, editor. Textbook of gastroenterology and nutrition in infancy. New York: Raven; 1981.
7. Greer F, et al. Cardiac disease. In: Kleinman R, editor. Pediatric nutrition handbook. Elk Grove: American Academy of Pediatrics; 2009. p. 981–99.
8. Anderson JB, et al. Lower weight-for-age z score adversely affects hospital length of stay after the bidirectional Glenn procedure in 100 infants with a single ventricle. J Thorac Cardiovasc Surg. 2009;138(2): 397–404.e1.
9. Anderson JB, et al. Poor post-operative growth in infants with two-ventricle physiology. Cardiol Young. 2011;21(4):421–9.
10. Anderson JB, et al. Low weight-for-age z-score and infection risk after the Fontan procedure. Ann Thorac Surg. 2011;91(5):1460–6.
11. Barton JS, et al. Energy expenditure in congenital heart disease. Arch Dis Child. 1994;70(1):5–9.
12. Davis D, et al. Feeding difficulties and growth delay in children with hypoplastic left heart syndrome versus d-transposition of the great arteries. Pediatr Cardiol. 2008;29(2):328–33.
13. Pillo-Blocka F, et al. Rapid advancement to more concentrated formula in infants after surgery for congenital heart disease reduces duration of hospital stay: a randomized clinical trial. J Pediatr. 2004;145(6):761–6.
14. Vogt KN, et al. Somatic growth in children with single ventricle physiology impact of physiologic state. J Am Coll Cardiol. 2007;50(19):1876–83.
15. Kelleher DK, et al. Growth and correlates of nutritional status among infants with hypoplastic left heart syndrome (HLHS) after stage 1 Norwood procedure. Nutrition. 2006;22(3):237–44.
16. Rogers EJ, et al. Barriers to adequate nutrition in critically ill children. Nutrition. 2003;19(10):865–8.
17. Kogon BE, et al. Feeding difficulty in newborns following congenital heart surgery. Congenit Heart Dis. 2007;2(5):332–7.
18. Kyle UG, Genton L, Pichard C. Hospital length of stay and nutritional status. Curr Opin Clin Nutr Metab Care. 2005;8(4):397–402.
19. Pichard C, et al. Nutritional assessment: lean body mass depletion at hospital admission is associated with an increased length of stay. Am J Clin Nutr. 2004;79(4):613–8.
20. Leite HP, et al. Serum albumin and clinical outcome in pediatric cardiac surgery. Nutrition. 2005;21(5):553–8.
21. Leite HP, et al. Nutritional assessment and surgical risk markers in children submitted to cardiac surgery. Sao Paulo Med J. 1995;113(1):706–14.
22. Goldberg C. Neurocognitive outcomes for children with functional single ventricle malformations. Pediatr Cardiol. 2007;28(6):443–7.
23. Mahle WT, et al. Neurodevelopmental outcome and lifestyle assessment in school-aged and adolescent children with hypoplastic left heart syndrome. Pediatrics. 2000;105(5):1082–9.
24. Marino BS, et al. Neurodevelopmental outcomes in children with congenital heart disease: evaluation and management: a scientific statement from the American Heart Association. Circulation. 2012;126(9):1143–72.
25. Mahle WT, Wernovsky G. Neurodevelopmental outcomes in hypoplastic left heart syndrome. Semin Thorac Cardiovasc Surg Pediatr Card Surg Annu. 2004;7:39–47.
26. Wernovsky G, et al. Cognitive development after the Fontan operation. Circulation. 2000;102(8):883–9.
27. Hoffman GM, et al. Systemic venous oxygen saturation after the Norwood procedure and childhood neurodevelopmental outcome. J Thorac Cardiovasc Surg. 2005;130(4):1094–100.
28. Bellinger DC, et al. Developmental and neurological status of children at 4 years of age after heart surgery with hypothermic circulatory arrest or low-flow cardiopulmonary bypass. Circulation. 1999;100(5):526–32.
29. Hovels-Gurich HH, et al. Long-term behavior and quality of life after corrective cardiac surgery in infancy for tetralogy of Fallot or ventricular septal defect. Pediatr Cardiol. 2007;28(5):346–54.
30. Grantham-McGregor S. A review of studies of the effect of severe malnutrition on mental development. J Nutr. 1995;125(8 Suppl):2233S–8.
31. Galler JR, Ramsey F, Solimano G. A follow-up study of the effects of early malnutrition on subsequent development. II. Fine motor skills in adolescence. Pediatr Res. 1985;19(6):524–7.
32. Grantham-McGregor SM, Walker S, Chang S. Nutritional deficiencies and later behavioural development. Proc Nutr Soc. 2000;59:47–54.
33. Schidlow DN, et al. Variation in interstage outpatient care after the Norwood procedure: a report from the Joint Council on Congenital Heart Disease National Quality Improvement Collaborative. Congenit Heart Dis. 2011;6(2):98–107.
34. Anderson JB, et al. Variation in growth of infants with a single ventricle. J Pediatr. 2012;161(1):16–21.e1; quiz 21 e2–3.
35. Marik PE, Zaloga GP. Early enteral nutrition in acutely ill patients: a systematic review. Crit Care Med. 2001;29(12):2264–70.
36. Braudis NJ, et al. Enteral feeding algorithm for infants with hypoplastic left heart syndrome poststage I palliation. Pediatr Crit Care Med. 2009;10(4):460–6.
37. Mehta NM, et al. Nutritional practices and their relationship to clinical outcomes in critically ill children–an international multicenter cohort study*. Crit Care Med. 2012;40(7):2204–11.
38. Medoff-Cooper B, Irving SY. Innovative strategies for feeding and nutrition in infants with congenitally malformed hearts. Cardiol Young. 2009;19 Suppl 2:90–5.

39. del Castillo SL, et al. Reducing the incidence of necrotizing enterocolitis in neonates with hypoplastic left heart syndrome with the introduction of an enteral feed protocol. Pediatr Crit Care Med. 2010;11(3):373–7.
40. Premji SS, McNeil DA, Scotland J. Regional neonatal oral feeding protocol: changing the ethos of feeding preterm infants. J Perinat Neonatal Nurs. 2004;18(4):371–84.
41. Skillman HE, Wischmeyer PE. Nutrition therapy in critically ill infants and children. JPEN J Parenter Enteral Nutr. 2008;32(5):520–34.
42. Slicker J, et al. Nutrition algorithms for infants with hypoplastic left heart syndrome; birth through the first interstage period. Congenit Heart Dis. 2013;8:89–102.
43. Connor JA, et al. Clinical outcomes and secondary diagnoses for infants born with hypoplastic left heart syndrome. Pediatrics. 2004;114(2):e160–5.
44. Skinner ML, et al. Laryngopharyngeal dysfunction after the Norwood procedure. J Thorac Cardiovasc Surg. 2005;130(5):1293–301.
45. Biewer ES, et al. Chylothorax after surgery on congenital heart disease in newborns and infants-risk factors and efficacy of MCT-diet. J Cardiothorac Surg. 2010;5:127.
46. Panthongviriyakul C, Bines JE. Post-operative chylothorax in children: an evidence-based management algorithm. J Paediatr Child Health. 2008;44(12): 716–21.
47. Pratap U, et al. Octreotide to treat postoperative chylothorax after cardiac operations in children. Ann Thorac Surg. 2001;72(5):1740–2.
48. Rosti L, et al. Octreotide in the management of postoperative chylothorax. Pediatr Cardiol. 2005;26(4): 440–3.
49. Nguyen DM, et al. The management of chylothorax/chylopericardium following pediatric cardiac surgery: a 10-year experience. J Card Surg. 1995;10(4 Pt 1):302–8.
50. Roehr CC, et al. Somatostatin or octreotide as treatment options for chylothorax in young children: a systematic review. Intensive Care Med. 2006;32(5): 650–7.
51. Jeffries HE, et al. Gastrointestinal morbidity after Norwood palliation for hypoplastic left heart syndrome. Ann Thorac Surg. 2006;81(3):982–7.
52. Johnstone JC, Leung JS, Friedman JN. Nasogastric tube misadventures. Clin Pediatr (Phila). 2011;50(10): 983–6.

Patients as Observers and Reporters in Support of Systems and Patient Safety

12

James W. Pichert and Gerald B. Hickson

Abstract

When patients and families observe and report their healthcare experiences, they can play important roles in promoting safety and improving quality. This chapter begins with the case of a busy, well regarded medical professional associated with a patient complaint. The complaint is a means by which patients and families can be "safety promoters". While barriers to this role exist, they may be reduced or eliminated when organizations commit to assessing their readiness to invite and address patient concerns, and build a robust infrastructure to support the effort. This chapter discusses our experience using unsolicited (voluntary) patient complaints to address unsafe systems and behaviors. We use the physician and the physician's practice group to illustrate implementation and outcomes of interventions designed to reduce unnecessary variation in healthcare professionals' behavior and performance that undermine a healthcare organization's culture of safety. The chapter concludes with guidance to hospital and healthcare systems on how best to develop, implement and sustain a patient and family experience program.

Keywords

Patient safety • Patient engagement • Patient empowerment • Patient activation • Patient centered care • Risk management • Professionalism • Professional conduct • Patient satisfaction • Patient complaints • Quality improvement

J.W. Pichert, PhD (✉)
Department of Medical Education and Administration, Center for Patient and Professional Advocacy, Vanderbilt University Medical Center, 2135 Blakemore Avenue, Nashville, TN 37212-3505, USA
e-mail: jim.pichert@vanderbilt.edu

G.B. Hickson, MD
Department of Quality, Safety & Risk Prevention, Center for Patient and Professional Advocacy, Vanderbilt University Medical Center, 2135 Blakemore Avenue, Nashville, TN 37212-3505, USA
e-mail: gerald.hickson@vanderbilt.edu

P.R. Barach, J.P. Jacobs, S.E. Lipshultz, P.C. Laussen (eds.),
Pediatric and Congenital Cardiac Care: Volume 2: Quality Improvement and Patient Safety,
DOI 10.1007/978-1-4471-6566-8_12,

Dr. Uro[1] is an experienced, busy, well-regarded urological surgeon and a valuable member of the large medical group affiliated with Celestial Medical Center. A patient has called Celestial's Office of Patient Relations (OPR) to complain about a visit earlier today with Dr. Uro. The patient reported: "My visit with Dr. Uro was only 5 min long. I felt Dr. Uro was rushed, and I wasn't able to get all my questions asked or answered." Does this patient complaint represent a problem? An anomaly? A patient with unrealistic expectations? Someone who simply underestimated the time Dr. Uro actually spent? Or something else?

[1] Dr. Uro and Dr. Uro's group are hypothetical, an amalgam of actual CPPA experiences and situations.

Patients and families are well positioned observers of their healthcare experiences, therefore they have a potential role to play in promoting safety and improving quality [1–4]. Drawing from literature on patient-centered care, engagement, empowerment (i.e., healthcare professionals' attempts to help patients discover and develop their capacity to be responsible for their healthcare [5]), and patient activation (i.e., patients' possession of skills and confidence for independently and actively engaging in their healthcare [6]), we review how patients and families can play a "safety promoter" role. We discuss the barriers to this role, a project planning readiness assessment, and elements of an infrastructure to ameliorate impediments. The chapter concludes with implications for practice.

Patients and Families as Observers

Patients see and experience things that concern them, including failures of professionals to:

- Practice hand hygiene consistently
- Arrive to appointments and show up for procedures on time
- Answer pages/cover call
- Communicate clearly and respectfully
- Practice evidence-based medicine
- Perform according to safety and quality protocols, and,
- Behave or perform in many other ways that threaten their own and others' safety [7–9].

Patients and visitors not only observe, but routinely make judgments about both "relational" and "functional" aspects of healthcare experiences [10], whether asked to share their observations or not. If patients share these and other observations, their concerns may be reliably coded [7, 11]. Relational aspects include:

- Providing emotional and psychological support: relieving fear and anxiety, demonstrating respect, kindness, compassion;
- Inviting patient participation in decision-making, and respecting patients' values and preferences;
- Involving family members and/or caregivers in decisions as needed and appropriate;
- Communicating clearly and honestly about available options, risks and benefits of treatments, and self-care procedures; and
- Disclosing unexpected adverse outcomes and errors.

Functional aspects include:

- Delivering evidence-based treatments;
- Managing physical symptoms in a timely and tailored fashion;
- Attending to physical needs and a clean, safe, comfortable environment; and
- Coordinating ongoing care and arranging smooth transitions from one care setting to another.

Patient Engagement

The Patient role in elevating the safety and quality of healthcare experiences have been described in terms of "patient activation" and "patient empowerment" and, more recently, as "patient engagement" in "patient-centered care" where they are recipients of "patient-centered communication" under the overarching term, "patient experience"[10, 12–18]. Put simply, patients are not merely observers or simple consumers, but are also producers or co-producers in their health and healthcare [19, 20].

However defined, described, and contrasted, activated/empowered/engaged patients are generally more likely to adhere to recommended healthcare behaviors and enjoy better health outcomes [18, 21–25], and they report better healthcare experiences [26–30]. Recent reports also suggest that activated and empowered patients may have lower healthcare-related costs [6, 18, 31, 32]. Finally, evidence continues to grow that patients can help promote both their own and institutional safety [33], and these findings appear to generalize across disadvantaged, ethnically diverse, and medically indigent populations. Moreover, the findings have been replicated in countries on four continents [6].

Patient Engagement in Safety

Patients can contribute to their own and health system safety in at least three ways [34–37]:

1. As "Choosers" who make informed decisions about where and from whom (which professionals and which payers for their circumstances) to receive care, share in making informed choices, and help assure their treatments are appropriate [38–43]. When patients perceive greater opportunity to be involved as choosers, they express greater confidence in their choices and in their professionals [41];
2. As "Co-producers" who help to promote their healing and wellness by partnering with healthcare professionals; monitoring whether treatments are delivered safely and as planned; attending and responding to educational materials, videos or posters that promote their confidence in asking questions; identifying safety issues; and speaking up with any concerns; and/or
3. As "Evaluators" or, as we conceptualize it, "promoters," of Safety and Quality, who provide data on systems and individual professionals' behavior/performance, participate in helping define personally meaningful elements of quality, help monitor behavior/performance, identify concerns and, if appropriate, help reduce problems and risks [33, 44–47].

Professionals who support these three roles are usually motivated by:

- realization that non-adherence is more likely when patients are not involved in treatment planning and decision-making [27];
- recognition that professional technical/content expertise can be supported or undermined by patient/family "expertise" (power) in carrying out choices and seeking care elsewhere, so the professional attempts to overcome perceived power differentials by engaging patients in tailoring recommendations when there are options [40];
- pressures related to increasing "consumerism," i.e., patient and payer expectations for care that is both kinder and safer [9, 12, 34, 39, 48, 49];
- democratization of knowledge with reduced knowledge gaps between professionals and many patients due to information available via the internet [50]; and
- effective advocacy of groups that promote patient involvement in safety and quality [51].

While the Chooser, Co-producer and Promoter roles are interrelated and each merits full attention, this chapter focuses on the third role, that of patients as active evaluators/promoters of safety and quality in partnership with their healthcare professionals and organizational leaders.

Barriers Exist, But Can Be Overcome

We acknowledge that many patients will feel uncertain or uncomfortable about sharing concerns. Many describe themselves as reluctant to appear to be challenging their healthcare professionals or health systems for fear of being categorized as "difficult" [52, 53]. An implication for practice is that organizations need strategies that affirm their desire to hear from patients, address common barriers, and support patients who speak up. They promote positive attitudes toward patient feedback among their healthcare team members, have systems and infrastructure in place to elicit/solicit patient involvement, use multiple media to ask for feedback, take patient feedback seriously, respond in a timely fashion to individual patient comments, compile and use aggregated feedback to promote improvement, and protect those who report their concerns from any retribution [9, 33].

The infrastructure usually requires third party "Patient Relations Representatives" because patients and families may feel more comfortable when they do not need to discuss concerns directly with their health professionals [53]. The attitudes and support of leadership, healthcare team members, and Patient Relations professionals can go a long way to make patients more willing and confident to speak up [47]. Fundamentally, the required attitudes and actions are based on the foundational concept of what it means to be a healthcare professional.

Professionalism Is the Foundation

Each professional on a healthcare team has made commitments to mastering specialized knowledge and technical skills, engaging respectfully with others in ways that promote teamwork and partnership, and giving and receiving feedback as a form of self- and group-regulation [9, 54–58]. Most medical specialty associations worldwide have issued definitions and standards regarding medical ethics and professional conduct in recognition of the responsibility for self-regulation. These statements uniformly include or allude to non-technical *behavioral* concepts such as altruism; respect; honesty and integrity; ethical standards; accountability; excellence; and duty/advocacy [59–66]. One review identified more than 90 characteristics [67] that patients may reasonably expect from medical professionals. Specific definitions aside [68–70], healthcare professionals, staff and patients alike know professionalism when we see it modeled, and when it is not [71].

In a medical culture that embodies professionalism and self-regulation, healthcare team members demonstrate willingness to report (and act) in support of safety and quality. They understand the need to report (and act) and do so in respectful ways. They also understand that failures to act threaten ongoing trust, an element critical to reliability and optimal team performance. But for professionals to share concerns, they must feel psychologically safe [72]. The same characteristics that promote willingness to report (and act) also apply to patients [73, 74]. In fact, Danis and Solomon [75] assert that true patient engagement obligates patients, professionals, healthcare organizations and delivery systems, insurers, and communities alike to hold one another accountable to raise safety concerns. For mutual accountability to occur, however, many persons will need support and reassurance that they can make reports in good faith without fear of retribution or retaliation [19].

How Patients Have Performed the Evaluator/Safety Promoter Role

The literature identifies both proactive and reactive means by which patients and family members have provided feedback to help promote patient safety. Proactive strategies include hospital rounding by patient relations specialists (ombudsmen) who ask inpatients about any concerns or fears they might have about their hospital stay [76, 77]; multidisciplinary rounding to uncover unmet needs [78]; and offering information to help patients identify and choose safe providers, involving patients in hand washing and other infection control processes, encouraging adherence to health promotion programs, offering patients access to their online medical records, encouraging patients to check their records and monitor their care processes, and advising patients to report adverse drug events [79, 80].

Reactive strategies for obtaining patient feedback include soliciting patient perceptions of their care. Surveillance tools have included retrospective surveys about safety events [81, 82], retrospective interviews [83, 84], incident reporting systems [85–88], various online multiple choice response tools [89], and most commonly standardized-item patient satisfaction questionnaires [90–96]. Summaries of strengths and limitations of these approaches include articles in the February 2013 theme issue of *Health Affairs* and The Health Foundation's January 2013 Evidence Scan on "Involving Patients to Improve Patient Safety" [33].

Best practices for employing these strategies include that the tool:

- Asks about interpersonal aspects and respectfulness of care [91];
- Asks about the quality of professionals' communications [94];
- Focuses on a specific visit [92];
- Is used within 48 hours to 6 weeks of the visit [93]; and
- Permits patients to express concerns about treatment, care coordination, engagement, and outcomes [90, 96].

Whatever the approach to involving patients in promoting safety, the impact depends on what is done with the information after it is collected. Significant improvements in safety therefore require an organizational infrastructure that supports a committed team that uses data to drive improvement efforts [9, 33]. We now turn our attention to an alternative to retrospective interviews and surveys: voluntarily offered (unsolicited) complaints.

Back to Dr. Uro

Dr. Uro's group uses signage, notices on billing statements, brochures and videos to invite patient compliments and concerns about their healthcare experience with group members. Over the past 18 months, Dr. Uro's patients have reported a number of concerns associated with Dr. Uro's practice and behaviors, including the following:

- "Dr. Uro is too hard to get in touch with. Dr. Uro never calls me back, and it takes months to get an appointment."
- "Dr. Uro was obviously in a hurry… took one look and told me to stop drinking so much and my bladder problems would be solved. It was totally insulting."
- "I had several questions. When I asked why I might be having so many UTIs, Dr. Uro just shrugged and said, 'I have no idea' and left."
- "Dr. Uro seemed to be distracted during my appointment. I wasn't sure Dr. Uro was really paying attention to anything I said…"

"Unsolicited" Patient Complaints

Unsolicited complaint narratives first and foremost offer patients the opportunity to give a full voice to their priorities and experiences, permitting descriptions of both chief complaints and ancillary issues. After all, complaint narratives indicate specific real or perceived deviation from anticipated behavior, performance, and/or outcome. Such complaints therefore offer important opportunities for specific, timely service recovery [45, 47, 97]. Second, as integral (and engaged) team members, patients in aggregate can signal markers of dysfunctional teams. Third, unsolicited complaints enjoy substantial research support. Results of multiple, independent studies of relationships between standardized patient satisfaction questionnaire scores and lawsuits, a marker for safety, do not find the results are sufficiently robust for supporting action [98–101]. In contrast, our team and the same independent researchers have repeatedly found significant, actionable relationships between unsolicited complaints and risk management activity [1, 98–105].

Although external regulations, like the Centers for Medicare and Medicaid Services (CMS) requirements, may motivate organizations to address complaints, the best programs are driven by three internal motivators [47]:

1. Moral motivation: Aims to "do the right thing";
2. Marketing motivation: Rebuilds patient/family confidence, defends against treatment nonadherence, retains loyalty, and reduces loss to follow-up. Numerous studies link patient nonadherence and dropout with patient dissatisfaction [27].
3. Monetary and margin motivation: May improve an organization's bottom line by reducing revenue loss and risk associated with dissatisfied patients and families because peer-delivered, peer-comparative, aggregated patient complaint-related feedback works to reduce subsequent complaints [106–108].

As Sage put it in an editorial following a study showing the relationship between patient complaints and lawsuit risk [1], "...healthcare organizations need to elicit patients' stories, capture information relevant to safety, and feed that information back to the professionals who organize and deliver care" ([109], p. 3004). Although Dr. Uro and other physicians might sometimes disagree with patients' perceptions, those patients' perceptions might signal potentially correctable systems issues and unsafe behavior/performance that undermines teamwork and safety [9]. So, consistent with the adage that "Data tell and stories sell" [110], we have spent nearly two decades turning patients' stories into actionable data, and using both as feedback to professionals whose complaint profiles indicate high risk of lawsuits. Unfortunately, until relatively recently, most healthcare organizations have not used unsolicited patient complaints to promote standards of care [111]. The next section summarizes our experience using unsolicited patient complaints as part of Vanderbilt's Patient Advocacy Reporting System® (PARS®). Details about the PARS tool and process are published elsewhere [3, 9, 106–108].

Using Unsolicited Patient Complaints to Promote Safety and Quality

Currently more than 50 healthcare systems and medical groups across the United States use PARS to identify physicians and other professionals associated with high numbers of unsolicited patient and family complaints [1, 9, 106–108]. PARS is designed to augment, not supplant, traditional peer review, aggregates patient/family complaint reports, codes embedded complaints, and transforms complaint data into peer-comparative local and national reports that peers share with high complaint (high risk) colleagues (described later in this chapter) [3, 9, 106–108, 112–114].

PARS intervention materials include a letter from a well trained peer "messenger" addressed to the at-risk, high-complaint physician. The letter describes the process and provides the physician with his/her numerical ranking among all medical group physicians (e.g., "You are number 3 of 387 physicians affiliated with Celestial Medical Center, and you rank second within your general field of surgery."). Feedback materials also include a "you-are-here" figure containing calculated Risk Scores for all of a physician group's members, a table that portrays the types of complaints voiced by patients and families (Table 12.1), and individual de-identified complaint narratives (for examples, see [3, 108]). Physicians see how their Risk Scores compare with the vast majority of physician peers who are associated with fewer complaints. For follow-up visits, a line graph shows changes in the physician's Risk Score over time relative to his/her area of practice and facility. Sharing the data in a non-directive, non-punitive way makes high risk physicians aware of their status. It gives them opportunities to reflect on what patients and families say, and respects their professionalism to address the comparatively high levels of dissatisfaction associated with their practices. Most professionals who receive feedback are subsequently associated with substantially fewer complaints, and the overall physician group risk declines [3, 9, 106–108, 115].

PARS is Employed by Dr. Uro's Organization

PARS was launched at Celestial Medical Center (the organization with which Dr. Uro's Department is affiliated) only after Vanderbilt's

Table 12.1 Distribution of types of patient complaints associated with Dr. Uro

Celestial Medical Center		
Complaint Type Summary		
Audit Period for Data in this Table		
Date 1 - Date 2		
Dr. Uro		
Complaint Type Categories	**Distribution of Complaints***	
	Your Complaints	**Average for Surgery**
Care & Treatment	29%	48%
Communication	33%	21%
Concern for Patient & Family	25%	9%
Accessibility & Availability	9%	14%
Money or Payment Issues Associated with Concerns About Care	4%	8%

*Complaint distribution figures are rounded to the nearest percent; therefore, totals may not equal precisely 100%.

Center for Patient and Professional Advocacy (CPPA) had established Celestial's readiness. We assess organization readiness for launching PARS (or any safety/quality improvement or risk reduction project) using a "Project Bundle" tool [9]. In brief, Celestial initiated the PARS program after key Celestial stakeholders/leaders and CPPA mutually judged that Celestial had sufficient (1) commitment from its people, and, (2) adequate organization-related supports, and (3) learning systems in place. Judgments were based on the following considerations:

1. Commitment from People
   (a) Celestial's leadership made public commitments to address the patient experience and address unnecessary variation demonstrated by Celestial-affiliated professionals with high PARS Risk Scores;
   (b) Two well-regarded Celestial-affiliated physicians agreed to Co-chair a PARS Messenger Subcommittee and become project champions, i.e., people who have the ability to motivate and hold others accountable to accomplish goals;
   (c) Celestial had an existing dedicated Patient Relations team to hear, address and document patient complaints. Celestial section leaders and department chairs nominated and the Co-chairs recruited peer physicians willing to receive training and deliver the data to high risk colleagues.
2. Organizational Supports
   (a) Alignment with goals: Celestial management set and disseminated goals to increase capture of patient complaints and provide prompt service recovery;

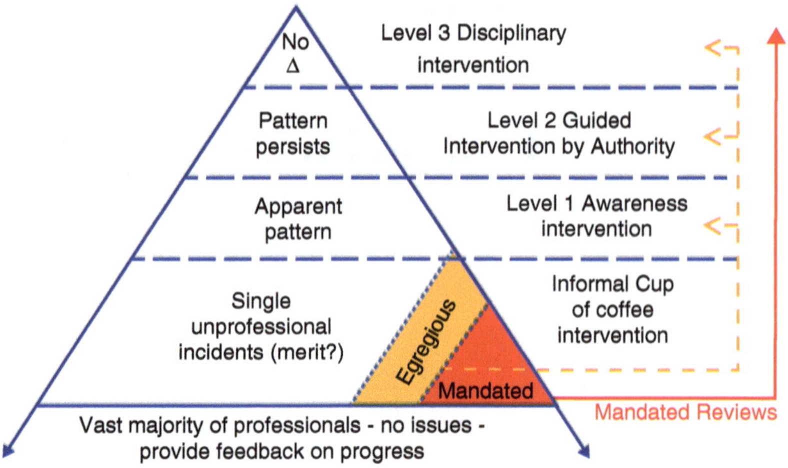

Fig. 12.1 Promoting reliability pyramid: a graduated intervention model for addressing behavior/performance that undermines a culture of safety (Adapted from Hickson et al. [105], with permission)

(b) Policies and procedures: Celestial reviewed and updated its professional conduct policy. Celestial also created and charged the Co-chairs and members of the PARS Messenger Subcommittee to implement the PARS program under the auspices of the Medical Executive Committee (to be consistent with state peer review statutes);

(c) Model for Planning and Interventions: Celestial Medical Center adopted the CPPA graduated intervention model for planning and for addressing high-complaint physicians (Fig. 12.1) (see [3, 105, 106] for details). At the pyramid's base and first level up, unless an allegation or incident is "egregious" or subject to mandated reviews (e.g., inappropriate touch, substance abuse), most professionals simply need encouragement or informal feedback to sustain professional conduct. But some physicians are associated with sufficient numbers of complaints that a pattern appears to have emerged. Consistent with individual and group self-regulation, high risk physicians deserve to be made "aware" of their standing (a Level 1 "Awareness Intervention") [3, 55, 105, 106, 108]. In this model, the well-trained peer-messengers share the data, encouraging high-risk physicians to consider etiologies for patient complaints, but not provide directive or corrective advice. Anticipating that some high risk physicians would be unable or unwilling to respond to peer-delivered messages, a Level 2 "Authority Intervention" provides the appropriate leader (chairman, chief medical officer, vice president of medical affairs) an opportunity to review the high risk physician's data, reflect upon other performance data, and then define an improvement plan (elements of which might range from coaching, a practice assessment, or a comprehensive mental and physical health screening). Level 2 interventions include ongoing tracking of complaint data with periodic updates provided to designated leaders. Level 3 interventions are reserved for individuals who fail to respond at Level 2 or who violate policy or legal boundaries (the small, colored triangle in Fig. 12.1, those complaints/events considered "most egregious") [116]. These persons are referred for appropriate investigative, corrective, or disciplinary action.

(d) Resources for teams: Celestial provided funding to support upgrades to an electronic complaint capture software program for use by Risk Management and the Office of Patient Relations.

3. Learning Systems
   (a) Measurement and surveillance tools: Celestial's upgraded software program enabled improved tracking of complaints and their resolution, and it provided safe, secure, easy routine transfer of complaint data for coding and aggregated analysis;
   (b) Process to review data: CPPA provides regular feedback regarding quantity and quality of patient complaint reports vs. agreed-upon benchmarks to Celestial's Office of Patient Relations. CPPA provides multiple reviews of complaint data for quality and consistency. The PARS Messenger Subcommittee Co-Chairs perform their own detailed review of the data prior to asking a Committee member to share the data with a particular colleague, and each Committee member performs reviews prior to agreeing to share the data with a colleague;
   (c) Multi-level training: The PARS tool and process were presented to Celestial's senior leaders for vetting and final approval, then described to the medical staff at group meetings and in Celestial's print and online communications. All Office of Patient Relations (OPR) staff were taught about their important role in PARS, and OPR staff participated in a course on best practices in service recovery and documentation [47]. All Messenger Subcommittee members engaged in 8 h of PARS messenger training. Finally, Celestial's senior leaders received coaching on how to address any high risk physician who attempted an "end around" in an attempt to be exempted from monitoring or interventions.

An Infrastructure for Ongoing Promotion of Reliability and Professional Accountability

The results of the Project Bundle planning assessment indicated that Celestial was ready to launch the PARS program, but actual, ongoing maintenance of any improvement project requires a fair, just, robust, and functioning organizational infrastructure to actually promote reliability and accountability. Ongoing tests of the infrastructure's functionality include the leadership's meaningful commitment and actions to address "unnecessary variation" in systems or individual behavior/performance, dissemination and enforcement of relevant institutional policies, use of relevant surveillance tools for obtaining observations or data (e.g., for PARS, complaint recording and delivery of complaint data), routine data reviews by leaders positioned to take action, post-training willingness of essential team members and Co-Chairs to perform "messenger" roles (for PARS, with high fidelity to PARS program training), and accountability to one another [9, 104, 105, 117, 118]. Again, we emphasize that the infrastructure's existence and ongoing reliability are driven by the organization's leadership and willingness to listen and take full advantage of their patients' experiences and stories of how they perceived their care.

Dr. Uro Qualified for a PARS "Awareness" Intervention

Dr. Uro's Risk Score was in the top 5 % of all Celestial-affiliated physicians and top 3 % of the 399 urologists in the national PARS database. A peer messenger (a surgeon practicing in a different surgical subspecialty) shared the data with Dr. Uro. The peer messenger completed a post-intervention debriefing report which included the messenger's perception that Dr. Uro was frustrated by the data and felt the complaints reflected systems and leadership issues, not his shortcomings. The messenger reported that Dr. Uro's specific comments included the following:

- Our area—our group—is terribly managed. You should be taking these complaints to Dr. ____ (Chair of Urology).
- I'm seeing increasing numbers of patients. It gets hectic because I don't have enough administrative support. None of us do in this department.
- The Chair gets all over me to produce… and see more patients and do more procedures. It's not me…it's the poor support.
- The system for turning over patients in the OR is especially poor. It would be more helpful for you to talk with the supervisor there.
- You could talk to our Department Chair, but frankly the problem is the lack of support we get in this department.
- And some of the patients are just unreasonable.

Dr. Uro's messenger reported to the Committee Co-Chairs her impression that Dr. Uro's systems-related explanations might have been rationalizations, but also might have merit. She had agreed to pass along the systems-related issues, but, consistent with her training, she had urged Dr. Uro to not only report any concerns up the chain of command, but help address them as well.

The Committee Chair notes that, in fact, several Celestial Medical Center urologists had Risk Scores above the PARS threshold that qualified them for initial awareness interventions (Fig. 12.2). According to several messengers' debriefing reports of their meetings, other urologists receiving awareness interventions cited similar system/management issues, although several of these messengers added that the physicians they visited took ownership: "some of these are my own doing…I will address these…" The Committee Chair also notes that no other Celestial Medical Center departments or physician "families" had a distribution similar to the one in Fig. 12.2; even in the largest departments, only 0–2 physicians qualified for awareness interventions.

The Co-Chairs de-identified the data presented in Fig. 12.2 and shared it at a messenger committee meeting a few weeks following initial interventions. The group recommended that the data (with the department identified) be shared with the Chief of Surgical Sciences and appropriate Celestial Medical Center leadership.

When the data were shared, the Medical Leadership:

- Were "not surprised" that Urology Department members are disproportionately associated with patient/family complaints;
- Expressed concerns that the group "does not appear to be functioning well." Observations included the following:
  - Patient and staff complaints appear to revolve around long waits, short visits, not listening/not answering patient questions, problems with timely follow-up
  - Access and communication complaints could be volume-related
  - Colleagues from other departments have mentioned a "tense environment"
  - Suggestions of jousting [69] with other departments and services

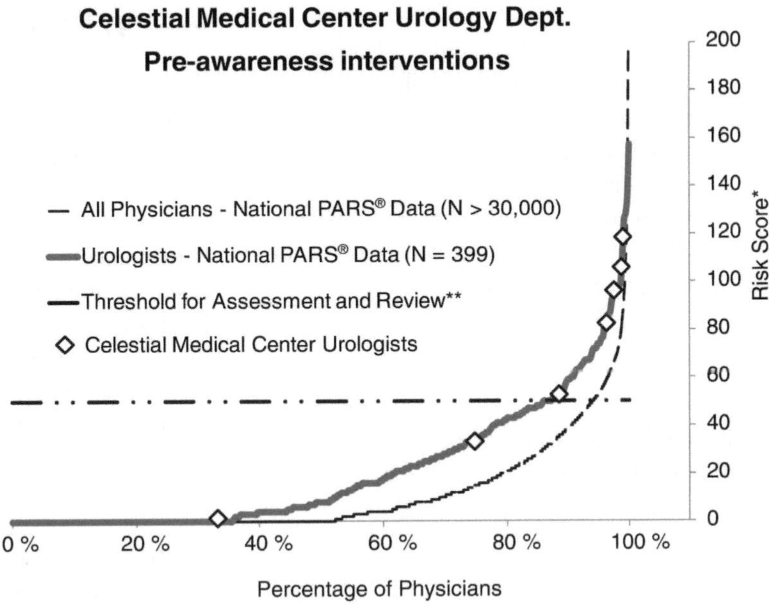

Fig. 12.2 Urology Department Physicians' Pre-Intervention PARS Risk Scores (*diamonds*) plotted over all physicians (*dashed line*) and all other urologists (*solid line*) in the PARS database. The horizontal line at the Risk Score of 50 indicates the PARS threshold for intervention pending assessment and review of an individual physician's underlying complaint data (*[112]; **[107])

- The Chair of Urology had been appointed from the 'ranks,' several department members were long-time colleagues, and the Chair appeared reluctant to hold them accountable. For example, the Chair was either unable or unwilling to address a long-time department colleague who exhibited abusive behavior towards junior staff and had three malpractice claims in the past 30 months
- The newest department members voiced concerns about what they perceived to be the Chair's lack of action in support of their work, and complained about the "unfair compensation package" that they believed sent "too much of our income" to the Chair and to the Department.

What was done? The leadership agreed that the Urology Department "family" of physicians stood out; no other departments exhibited a similar distribution of Risk Scores. Together the leadership reached consensus that, were it their department, they would want to know and have an opportunity to address the data. The Chief of Surgical Sciences agreed to meet with the Chair of Urology, express that the Chair was a valued member of the leadership team, share the data and leadership's concerns, and give the Chair the opportunity to "turn things around."

The Chair of Urology took several actions over the next 6–8 months:

- Enrolled in Celestial's leadership training on promoting reliability and accountability
- Added two advanced practice nurses to better manage volume
- Assigned the group manager to partner with Patient Relations and assist with internal service recovery

In addition, the Chief of Surgical Sciences did the following:

- Met over the course of the year with every department; shared quality, volume and complaint-related data; laid out clear expectations and goals; and described the plan for monitoring and feedback
- Adjusted all Surgical Department Chairs' incentives to more heavily weight Celestial's quality goals, and put less weight on service volumes.

Over the next year, total numbers of recorded patient complaints at Celestial Medical Center increased as a function of renewed efforts to let patients know "we want to hear from you." Complaints about urology began dropping, however, so several PARS messengers were able to deliver "good" news to their previously identified high risk urologists. Dr. Uro's Risk Score, however, was unchanged, and Dr. Uro's messenger reported that Dr. Uro responded with nothing except irritation about the process.

Urology Department 2 Years Later

Two years following the initial awareness interventions, the Risk Scores for all Department of Urology members except Dr. Uro fell below the intervention threshold (Fig. 12.3). Interventions were suspended for those below the threshold. Unfortunately, Dr. Uro had accumulated additional complaints. Consistent with Celestial Health System policies, Dr. Uro's messenger and the Messenger Committee Co-Chairs reviewed the data and agreed that Dr. Uro should progress to a Level 2 Authority intervention by the Department Chair.

The Department Chair agreed to meet with Dr. Uro, to affirm Dr. Uro's value to the department, review previous awareness interventions and new complaint reports, and mandate an improvement plan. In this case, the Chair directed Dr. Uro to undergo screening by a physician affiliated with a recognized Physician Wellness Program. Dr. Uro underwent individual assessment at a Health Professional Assessment Program. Deficits in team management skills and self awareness/personal insight regarding impacts of interactions with others were identified. Dr. Uro was mandated to participate in a program for "distressed" physicians [68, 119]. Dr. Uro grudgingly attended and grudgingly reported that the program had been "eye opening, helpful." Dr. Uro's complaints have since fallen.

Summary and Conclusions

We conclude, like the colleagues cited at the beginning of this chapter that patients can indeed play an important role in promoting safe medical care. Their unsolicited patient complaints provide a means for identifying high-claims physi-

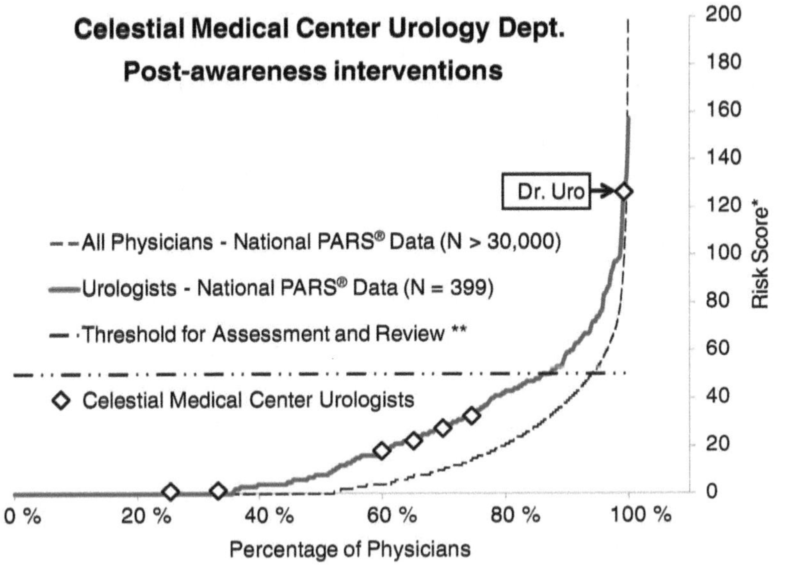

Fig. 12.3 Urology Department Physicians' PARS Risk Scores 2 years post initial awareness interventions. *Diamonds* represent individual urologists' Risk Scores, and Dr. Uro's high Risk Score is highlighted. The *dashed line* represents all physicians and the *solid line* all other urologists in the PARS database. The *horizontal line* at the Risk Score of 50 indicates the PARS threshold for intervention pending assessment and review of an individual physician's underlying complaint data (*[112]; **[107])

cians, making them aware (not to punish, at least initially), and offer them an opportunity to reduce their risk of claims. After all, it was patient complaints that, because Celestial medical center had an infrastructure to receive and address them, brought Dr. Uro to the attention of leadership. This increased safety and very likely saved his career. We believe the vast majority of physicians at high risk signaled by patient complaints are not aware that they stand out from their physician peers. Consider, if you were at high risk and could get a non-punitive "heads up," wouldn't you want to know? If physician colleagues are unaware, they are not likely to address risky or unsafe technical and interpersonal behaviors. Most physicians respond positively if those complaints are captured, reliably processed, and regularly communicated through a physician-driven feedback process.

Patient observations have limitations in promoting safety. Some leaders and colleagues may want to quibble with the evidence in support of these concepts that do not come from randomized controlled trials [120]. Some may cite studies that show patient engagement levels make no difference to outcomes, or the handful of studies that appear to link higher standardized patient experience survey scores to increased hospitalizations, higher costs, or mortality (none of which was methodologically superior to the majority with positive associations) (see the review by Doyle et al. [10]). Others may believe that engaged patients receive elective or unnecessary procedures and check a survey's "satisfied" boxes for the wrong reasons [90, 121, 122].

Of course, many patient complaints do not signal safety lapses. After all, many might seem to reflect mere annoyances (e.g., "The doctor never apologized for being 30 min late to my appointment." "The surgeon showed disrespect by using my first name.") rather than specific, valid observations of negligence or unsafe practices (e.g., "The doctor flew through my diagnosis and what it meant, she didn't listen to us, did not order some tests I later learned I needed, and wrote confusing discharge orders."). Nevertheless, we know that patients define medical errors more broadly than clinical mistakes, extending the concept to communication problems, lack of compassion, and responsiveness failures [77, 123], and these are associated with surgical complications and other adverse patient outcomes [103, 124, 125].

A related limitation is that the PARS process does not examine complaint validity. As we have argued previously [106], evaluating the validity of allegations requires exhaustive review beyond the resources available to most healthcare professionals and medical centers. Even when such evaluations occur, professional reviewers do not always agree [126, 127]. Nevertheless, aggregated complaints (allegations) are associated with risk management activity and identify a small proportion of physicians who stand out. There may be "noise" and "faulty perceptions" that contribute to Dr. Uro's high Risk Scores, but these patient/family expressions of concern drive lawsuits.

Implications and Reflections for Practice

1. Conduct Project Bundle and Infrastructure Assessments. If your organization is considering using (unsolicited) patient complaints to identify and systematically address service units and professionals associated with disproportionate numbers, the elements described above in the project bundle (people, organization supports, learning organization) can help establish readiness for successful implementation. If your organization already uses unsolicited complaints to promote safety and reduce unnecessary variation, what elements of the infrastructure described above might make their use more efficient and effective?
2. Employ proactive service recovery. Our work with more than 50 healthcare organizations reveals best practices for service recovery [47], some of which are summarized using the "HEARD" mnemonic:
   - Hear the person's concern(s)
   - Empathize with the person raising the issue
   - Acknowledge, express Appreciation to the person for sharing, and Apologize when warranted
   - Respond to the problem, setting timelines and expectations for follow-up
   - Document expressed concerns and responses/resolutions (or Delegate documentation of to an appropriate person).

   Note that the HEARD mnemonic emphasizes the importance of documenting patient complaints for purposes of tracking and trending in support of safety. In our experience documentation practices vary widely. Best practices in documentation should be part of standard orientation and training of Patient Relations professionals [47]. While proactive service recovery activity is important, it is not just about placating patients. Regular audits and feedback can help keep patients from becoming dissatisfied in the first place which, for many patients and families, signals concerns about their and others' safety. Therefore, attention to both individual and aggregated patient complaints is consistent with our collective commitments to professionalism and patient engagement, both of which help promote safety and improved outcomes.
3. Be prepared to promote patient activation, empowerment and engagement in support of patients as safety promoters/evaluators and the overall patient experience. Advocate for patients as the organization's eyes and ears on the basis of a commitment to professionalism, strong humanistic and moral reasons, strong theoretical backing (compelling logic model), and the impressive weight of evidence from the many studies that show patient engagement to be effective [10].
4. Make it easy and safe for patients/families to share concerns. Organizational characteristics

influence patient willingness and ability to be safety promoters. Hospitals, physician practices, Accountable Care Organizations, and healthcare systems encourage engagement by (1) asserting and demonstrating that patients' participation is critical to achieving mutually beneficial goals; (2) having supportive organizational policies [128–130]; and (3) promoting receptive patient–professional interactions around expressions of concern [19, 131]. When concerns are invited, taken seriously and acted upon, patients are reassured, but are otherwise discouraged from the safety promoter role [35, 132–137]. Finally, patients perceive more involvement when "we want to hear from you" is presented early and often, and the response is prompt and professional [40].

5. Patient engagement-related skills training may be necessary but not sufficient. Given the previous implications for practice, professionals need to be educated about and appreciate that involving patients in improving healthcare safety and quality outweigh any perceived disadvantages [138]. While training on patient engagement skills may help, it is hardly a cure-all [52, 131, 139, 140]. Creating and sustaining a safety culture that fosters improvement rather than retribution requires supportive systems and infrastructure [9].
6. Promote skills for managing patients' and professionals' expectations. Many patients bring expectations and make specific requests (demands) of physicians, and overall patient satisfaction correlates with fulfillment [141–146]. Some medical professionals may be tempted to "cave in," fearing *patient* retribution via low survey scores, especially if survey results impact compensation [144]. If true, such behavior would not always be consistent with evidence-based care and a commitment to professionalism. Physicians therefore need skills for educating patients and "agreeing to disagree agreeably" [90, 117, 147–149]. Without those skills, overemphasis on standardized assessments of patient satisfaction could have unintended adverse effects on healthcare utilization, costs of care, and outcomes [90]. Finally, managing patient expectations may require more time, at least in the short term [150], and some physicians may be reluctant or unwilling to give up a more authoritarian style [25]
7. Don't wait to see it in social media. Growing numbers of patients post online comments about their healthcare experiences. The availability of web-based, Yelp-like accounts offer another opportunity to obtain impressions of care quality data in the "cloud of patient experience" [50]. But wouldn't it be better to hear from dissatisfied patients directly, before they leave your facility, rather than from Angie's List, Consumer Reports, Health Grades or many other websites where you have little or no opportunity to use the postings to address individual patients' issues or demonstrate a pattern in carefully recorded aggregated data?
8. Read globally, act locally. Populations vary, so it's not surprising that patient complaints also vary [151, 152]. The data will be richer regardless of culture, if patients are asked to tell and organizations record and review their stories. Priorities for improvement should be developed locally.

References

1. Hickson GB, Federspiel CF, Pichert JW, Miller CS, Gauld-Jaeger J, Bost P. Patient Complaints & Malpractice Risk. JAMA. 2002;287(22):2951–7.
2. Vincent CA, Coulter A. Patient safety: what about the patient? Qual Saf Health Care. 2002;11(1): 76–80.
3. Hickson GB, Pichert JW. Identifying and Addressing Physicians at High Risk for Medical Malpractice Claims. In: Youngberg BJ, editor. Principles of Risk Management and Patient Safety. Sudbury: Jones and Bartlett Publishers, Inc; 2012. p. 347–68.
4. Vincent C, Davis R. Patients and families as safety experts. CMAJ. 2012;184(1):15–6.
5. Funnell MM, Anderson RM. Empowerment and self-management of diabetes. Clin Diabetes. 2004; 22(3):123–7.
6. Hibbard JH, Greene J. What the evidence shows about patient activation: better health outcomes and care experiences; fewer data on costs. Health Aff. 2013;32(2):207–14.
7. Hickson GB, Pichert JW, Federspiel CF, Clayton EW. Development of an Early Identification and Response Model of Malpractice Prevention. Law Contemp Probl. 1997;60(1):7–29.

8. Harbin T. Walking up blind – lawsuits over eye surgery. Blumenthal DR, editor. Minneapolis, MN: London Street Press; 2009.
9. Hickson GB, Moore IN, Pichert JW, Benegas Jr M. Balancing systems and individual accountability in a safety culture. In: Berman S, editor. From the front office to the front line: essentials issues for healthcare leaders. 2nd ed. Oakbrook Terrace: Joint Commission Recourses, Inc; 2012. p. 1–36.
10. Doyle C, Lennox L, Bell D. A systematic review of evidence on the links between patient experience and clinical safety and effectiveness. BMJ Open. 2013;3:e001570.
11. Pichert JW, Miller CS, Hickson GB, Hollo AH, Gauld-Jaeger J, Federspiel CF, Hickson GB. What health professionals can do to identify and resolve patient dissatisfaction. Joint Comm J Qual Improv. 1998;24(6):303–12.
12. Consuming health care. Lancet. 1994;344(8925): 763–5. [No authors listed].
13. Stewart M, Brown JB, Donner A, McWhinney IR, Oates J, Weston WW, et al. The impact of patient-centered care on outcomes. J Fam Pract. 2000;49(9): 796–804.
14. Epstein RM, Street Jr RL. Patient-centered communication in cancer care: promoting healing and reducing suffering. NIH Publ. 07:6225. Bethesda: National Cancer Institute; 2007.
15. Berwick DM. What 'patient-centered' should mean: confessions of an extremist. Health Aff. 2009;28(4): w555–65.
16. Epstein RM, Fiscella K, Lesser CS, Stange KC. Why the nation needs a policy push on patient-centered health care. Health Aff. 2010;29(8):1489–95.
17. Bertakis KD, Azari R. Patient-centered care is associated with decreased health care utilization. J Am Board Fam Med. 2011;24(3):229–39.
18. Greene J, Hibbard JH. Why does patient activation matter? An examination of the relationships between patient activation and health-related outcomes. J Gen Intern Med. 2012;27(5):520–6.
19. Annandale E, Hunt K. Accounts of disagreements with doctors. Soc Sci Med. 1998;46(1):119–29.
20. Allsop J. Two sides to every story: complainants' and doctors' perspectives in disputes about medical care in a general practice setting. Law Policy. 1994;16(2):149–83.
21. Remmers C, Hibbard J, Mosen DM, Wagenfield M, Hoye RE, Jones C. Is patient activation associated with future health outcomes and healthcare utilization among patients with diabetes? J Ambul Care Manage. 2009;32(4):320–7.
22. Rogvi S, Tapager I, Almdal TP, Schiøtz ML, Willaing I. Patient factors and glycaemic control—associations and explanatory power. Diabet Med. 2012;29(10):e382–9.
23. Terry PE, Fowles JB, Xi M, Harvey L. The ACTIVATE study: results from a group-randomized controlled trial comparing a traditional worksite health promotion program with an activated consumer program. Am J Health Promot. 2011; 26(2):e64–73.
24. Skolasky RL, Mackenzie EJ, Wegener ST, Riley LH. Patient activation and functional recovery in persons undergoing spine surgery. Orthopedics. 2011;34(11):888.
25. Dentzer S. Rx for the 'Blockbuster Drug' of patient engagement. Health Aff. 2013;32(2):202.
26. Hibbard JH, Stockard J, Mahoney ER, Tusler M. Development of the Patient Activation Measure (PAM): conceptualizing and measuring activation in patients and consumers. Health Serv Res. 2004;39(4 Pt 1):1005–26.
27. Glasgow RE, Wagner EH, Schaefer J, Mahoney LD, Reid RJ, Greene SM. Development and validation of the patient assessment of chronic illness care (PACIC). Med Care. 2005;43(5):436–44.
28. Mosen DM, Schmittdiel J, Hibbard J, Sobel D, Remmers C, Bellows J. Is patient activation associated with outcomes of care for adults with chronic conditions? J Ambul Care Manage. 2007;30(1):21–9.
29. Alexander JA, Hearld LR, Mittler JN, Harvey J. Patient-physician role relationships and patient activation among individuals with chronic illness. Health Serv Res. 2012;47(3 Pt 1):1201–23.
30. Maeng DD, Martsolf GR, Scanlon DP, Christianson JB. Care coordination for the chronically ill: understanding the patient's perspective. Health Serv Res. 2012;47(5):1960–79.
31. Begum N, Donald M, Ozolins IZ, Dower J. Hospital admissions, emergency department utilisation and patient activation for self-management among people with diabetes. Diabetes Res Clin Pract. 2011;93(2):260–7.
32. Shively MJ, Gardetto NJ, Kodiath MF, Kelly A, Smith TL, Stepnowsky C, et al. Effect of patient activation on self-management in patients with heart failure. J Cardiovasc Nurs. 2013;28(1):20–34.
33. The Health Foundation: involving patients in improving patient safety, London, January 2013 http://www.health.org.uk/public/cms/75/76/313/3998/Involving%20patients%20in%20improving%20safety.pdf?realName=sVAlBL.pdf. Last accessed 25 May 2013.
34. Guadagnoli E, Ward P. Patient participation in decision-making. Soc Sci Med. 1998;47(3):329–39.
35. Peat M, Entwistle V, Hall J, Birks Y, Golder S. Scoping review and approach to appraisal of interventions intended to involve patients in patient safety. J Health Serv Res Policy. 2010;15 Suppl 1:17–25.
36. Hibbard JH. Engaging health care consumers to improve the quality of care. Med Care. 2003;41(1): 1–61.
37. Bernabeo E, Holmboe ES. Patients, providers, and systems need to acquire a specific set of competencies to achieve truly patient-centered care. Health Aff. 2013;32(2):250–8.
38. Charles C, Gafni A, Whelan T. Shared decision-making in the medical encounter: what does it mean? (or it takes at least two to tango). Soc Sci Med. 1997;44(5):681–92.

39. Charles C, Gafni A, Whelan T. Decision-making in the physician–patient encounter: revisiting the shared treatment decision-making model. Soc Sci Med. 1999;49(5):651–61.
40. Burton D, Blundell N, Jones M, Fraser A, Elwyn G. Shared decision-making in cardiology: Do patients want it and do doctors provide it? Patient Educ Couns. 2010;80(2):173–9.
41. Fowler Jr FJ, Levin CA, Sepucha KR. Informing and involving patients to improve the quality of medical decisions. Health Aff. 2011;30(4):699–706.
42. Friedberg MW, Van Busum K, Wexler R, Bowen M, Schneider EC. A demonstration of shared decision making in primary care highlights barriers to adoption and potential remedies. Health Aff. 2013;32(2):268–75.
43. Légaré F, Witteman HO. Shared decision making: examining key elements and barriers to adoption into routine clinical practice. Health Aff. 2013;32(2):276–84.
44. The Joint Commission: facts about the joint commission's complaint process. http://www.jointcommission.org/GeneralPublic/Complaint/oqm.htm. Last accessed 26 May 2010.
45. Department of Veterans Affairs, Veterans Health Administration. Service Recovery in the Veterans Health Administration. 2004 [cited 2010 May 26]. Available from: http://www1.va.gov/vhapublications/ViewPublication.asp?pub_ID=433.
46. Society for Healthcare Consumer Advocacy (SHCA). In the name of the patient: consumer advocacy in health care. Chicago: SHCA (American Hospital Association); 2009.
47. Hayden AC, Pichert JW, Fawcett J, Moore I, Hickson GB. Best Practices & Advanced Skills in Healthcare Service Recovery Programs. Joint Comm J Qual Improv Patient Saf. 2010;26(7):310–8.
48. Reinhard EH. Medicine and the crisis in confidence. Pharos. 1974;37:117–23.
49. Haug MR, Lavin B. Public challenge of physician authority. Med Care. 1979;17(8):844–58.
50. Greaves F, Ramirez-Cano D, Millett C, Darzi A, Donaldson L. Harnessing the cloud of patient experience: using social media to detect poor quality healthcare. BMJ Qual Saf. 2013;22(3):251–5.
51. National Patient Safety Foundation. National Agenda for action: patients and families in patient safety. Nothing about me, without me. http://www.npsf.org/wp-content/uploads/2011/10/Nothing_About_Me.pdf. Last accessed 3 June 2013.
52. Frosch DL, May SG, Rendle KAS, Tietbohl C, Elwyn G. Authoritarian physicians and patients' fear of being labeled "difficult" among key obstacles to shared decision making. Health Aff. 2012;31(5):1030–8.
53. Donovan-Kicken E, Mackert M, Guinn TD, Tollison AC, Breckinridge B. Sources of patient uncertainty when reviewing medical disclosure and consent documentation. Patient Educ Couns. 2013;90:254–60.
54. Cruess SR, Cruess RL. The medical profession and self-regulation: a current challenge. Virtual Mentor. 2005;7(4). Available from: http://virtualmentor.ama-assn.org/2005/04/oped1-0504.html. Accessed 28 Feb 2014.
55. Hickson GB, Entman SS. Physicians influence the malpractice problem. Obstet Gynecol. 2010;115(4):682–6.
56. Leape LL, Shore MF, Dienstag JL, Mayer RJ, Edgman-Levitan S, Meyer GS, Healy GB. Perspective: a culture of respect, part 1: the nature and causes of disrespectful behavior by physicians. Acad Med. 2012;87(7):845–52.
57. Leape LL, Shore MF, Dienstag JL, Mayer RJ, Edgman-Levitan S, Meyer GS, Healy GB. Perspective: a culture of respect, part 2: creating a culture of respect. Acad Med. 2012;87(7):853–8.
58. Sawer G, Glendon MA, Alford WP. Legal profession. In: Encyclopædia Britannica. 2013. http://www.britannica.com/EBchecked/topic/334873/legal-profession/65821/Characteristics-of-the-profession. Accessed 16 Jan 2013.
59. Arnold L. Assessing professional behavior: yesterday, today, and tomorrow. Acad Med. 2002;77(6):502–15.
60. Accreditation Council for Graduate Medical Education (ACGME). Outcome project: general competencies. 1999. Available online at: http://www.acgme.org/outcome/comp/compFull.asp. Accessed 15 Jan 2013.
61. *Board of Regents, American College of Surgeons. Code of Professional Conduct. Approved June 2003. http://www.facs.org/memberservices/codeofconduct.html.
62. Canadian Medical Association. Code of ethics. Ottawa: Canadian Medical Association; 2004. http://policybase.cma.ca/dbtw-wpd/PolicyPDF/PD04-06.pdf. Accessed 3 Mar 2014.
63. Canadian Medical Association Conjoint Accreditation Services. Guiding principles for national entry-level competency profiles used in the Canadian Medical Association conjoint accreditation process. Ottawa: Canadian Medical Association; 2010. http://www.cma.ca/multimedia/CMA/Content_Images/Inside_cma/Accreditation/pdf/2010_guiding_principles_profile.pdf. Accessed 3 Mar 2014.
64. General Medical Council. Good medical practice. London: General Medical Council; 2013. http://www.gmc-uk.org/guidance/good_medical_practice.asp. Accessed 3 Mar 2014.
65. Royal College of Physicians. Medical professionalism and leadership. London: Royal College of Physicians; 2010. http://www.rcplondon.ac.uk/policy/physician-development/medical-professionalism-and-leadership. Accessed 3 Mar 2014.
66. Scottish Medical and Scientific Advisory Committee. Promoting professionalism and excellence in Scottish medicine. Edinburgh: Scottish Medical Association; 2009. http://www.scotland.gov.uk/Resource/Doc/275420/0082599.pdf. Accessed 3 Mar 2014.
67. Van De Camp K, Vernooij-Dassen MJ, Grol RP, Bottema BJ. How to conceptualize professionalism: a qualitative study. Med Teach. 2004;26(8):696–702.
68. Samenow CP, Swiggart W, Spickard Jr A. A CME course aimed at addressing disruptive physician behavior. Physician Exec. 2008;34(1):32–40.

69. Moran SK, Sicher CM. Interprofessional jousting and medical tragedies: strategies for enhancing professional relations. AANA J. 1996;64(6):521–4.
70. Phillips RL, Harper DC, Wakefield M, Green LA, Fryer Jr GE. Can nurse practitioners and physicians beat parochialism into plowshares? Health Aff. 2002;21(5):133–42.
71. Firth-Cozens J. Cultures for improving patient safety through learning: the role of teamwork. Health Care. 2001;10 suppl 2:ii26.
72. Edmondson A. Psychological safety and learning behavior in work teams. Adm Sci Q. 1999;44: 350–83.
73. Becker ER, Roblin DW. Translating primary care practice climate into patient activation: the role of patient trust in physician. Med Care. 2008;46(8): 795–805.
74. Fiscella K, Meldrum S, Franks F, Shields CG, Duberstein P, McDainel S. Patient trust: is it related to patient-centered behavior of primary care physicians? Med Care. 2004;42(11):1049–55.
75. Danis M, Solomon M. Providers, payers, the community, and patients are all obliged to get patient activation and engagement ethically right. Health Aff. 2013;32(2):401–7.
76. Garbutt J, Bose D, McCawley BA, Burroughs T, Medoff G. Soliciting patient complaints to improve performance. Jt Comm J Qual Saf. 2003;29(3): 103–12.
77. Burroughs TE, Waterman AD, Gallagher TH, Waterman B, Jeffe DB, Dunagan WC, et al. Medication safety: patients' concerns about medical errors during hospitalization. Jt Comm J Qual Patient Saf. 2007;33(1):5–14.
78. Gurses AP, Xiao Y. A systematic review of the literature on multidisciplinary rounds to design information technology. J Am Med Inform Assoc. 2006;13(3):267–76.
79. Coulter A, Ellins J. Effectiveness of strategies for informing, educating, and involving patients. BMJ. 2007;335(7609):24–7.
80. Stone S, Kontowski G, Gallagher R, Storr J, Teare L. Keeping hand hygiene high on the patient safety agenda. BMJ. 2013;346:f2699.
81. Haines S, Warren T. Staff and patient involvement in benchmarking to improve care. Nurs Manage. 2011; 18(2):22–5.
82. Daniels JP, Hunc K, Cochrane D, Carr R, Shaw NT, Taylor A. Identification by families of pediatric adverse events and near misses overlooked by health care providers. CMAJ. 2012;184(1):29–34.
83. Brown M, Frost R, Ko Y, Woosley R. Diagramming patients' views of root causes of adverse drug events in ambulatory care: an online tool for planning education and research. Patient Educ Couns. 2006; 62(3):302–15.
84. Schwappach DLB. "Against the silence": development and first results of a patient survey to assess experiences of safety-related events in hospital. BMC Health Serv Res. 2008;8(1):59.
85. Wallace LM, Spurgeon P, Benn J, Koutantji M, Vincent C. Improving patient safety incident reporting systems by focusing upon feedback – lessons from English and Welsh trusts. Health Serv Manage Res. 2009;22(3):129–35.
86. Gaal S, Hartman C, Giesen P, van Weel C, Verstappen W, Wensing M. Complaints against family physicians submitted to disciplinary tribunals in the Netherlands: lessons for patient safety. Ann Fam Med. 2011;9(6):522–7.
87. Millman EA, Pronovost PJ, Makary MA, Wu AW. Patient-assisted incident reporting: including the patient in patient safety. J Patient Saf. 2011;7(2):106–8.
88. de Feijter JM, de Grave WS, Muijtjens AM, Scherpbier AJ, Koopmans RP. A comprehensive overview of medical error in hospitals using incident-reporting systems, patient complaints and chart review of inpatient deaths. PLoS One. 2012;7(2):e31125.
89. Frost J, Okun S, Vaughan T, Heywood J, Wicks P. Patient-reported outcomes as a source of evidence in off-label prescribing: analysis of data from PatientsLikeMe. J Med Internet Res. 2011;13(1):e6.
90. Fenton JJ, Jerant AF, Bertakis KD, Franks P. The cost of satisfaction: a national study of patient satisfaction, health care utilization, expenditures, and mortality. Arch Intern Med. 2012;172(5):405–11.
91. Jha AK, Orav EJ, Zheng J, Epstein AM. Patients' perception of hospital care in the United States. N Engl J Med. 2008;359(18):1921–31.
92. Jayadevappa R, Schwartz JS, Chhatre S, Wein AJ, Malkowicz SB. Satisfaction with care: a measure of quality of care in prostate cancer patients. Med Decis Making. 2010;30(2):234–45.
93. Glickman SW, Boulding W, Manary M, Satelin R, Roe M, Wolosin R, et al. Patient satisfaction and its relationship with clinical quality and inpatient mortality in acute myocardial infarction. Circ Cardiovasc Qual Outcomes. 2010;3(2):188–95.
94. Boulding W, Glickman SW, Manary MP, Schulman KA, Staelin R. Relationship between patient satisfaction with inpatient care and hospital readmission within 30 days. Am J Manag Care. 2011;17(1):41–8.
95. Tehrani AB, Feldman SR, Camacho FT, Balkrishnan R. Patient satisfaction with outpatient medical care in the United States. Health Outcomes Res Med. 2011;2(4):e197–202.
96. Manary P, Boulding W, Staelin R, Glickman SW. The patient experience and health outcomes. N Engl J Med. 2013;17(368):201–3.
97. Bendall-Lyon D, Powers T. The role of complaint management in the service recovery process. Jt Comm J Qual Improv. 2001;27(5):278–86.
98. Stelfox HT, Gandhi TK, Orav EJ, Gustafson ML. The relation of patient satisfaction with complaints against physicians and malpractice lawsuits. Am J Med. 2005;118(10):1126–33.
99. Levtzion-Korach O, Frankel A, Alcalai H, Keohane C, Orav J, Graydon-Baker E, et al. Integrating incident data from five reporting systems to assess patient safety: making sense of the elephant. Jt Comm J Qual Patient Saf. 2010;36(9):402–10.

100. Fullam F, Garman AN, Johnson TJ, Hedberg EC. The use of patient satisfaction surveys and alternative coding procedures to predict malpractice risk. Med Care. 2009;47(5):553–9.
101. Cydulka RK, Tamayo-Sarver J, Gage A, Bagnoli D. Association of patient satisfaction with complaints and risk management among emergency physicians. J Emerg Med. 2011;41(4):405–11.
102. Hickson GB, Clayton EW, Githens PB, Sloan FA. Factors that prompted families to file malpractice claims following perinatal injuries. JAMA. 1992;267(10):1359–63.
103. Murff HJ, France DJ, Blackford J, Grogan EL, Yu C, Speroff T, Pichert JW, Hickson GB. Relationship between patient complaints and surgical complications. Qual Saf Health Care. 2006;15(1):13–6.
104. Hickson GB, Federspiel CF, Blackford JU, Gaska W, Merrigan MW, Miller CS. Patient complaints and malpractice risk in a regional healthcare center. South Med J. 2007;100(8):791–6.
105. Hickson G, Pichert JW, Webb LE, Gabbe SG. A complementary approach to promoting professionalism: Identifying, measuring, and addressing unprofessional behaviors. Acad Med. 2007; 82(11):1040–8.
106. Pichert JW, Hickson GB, Moore IN. Using patient complaints to promote patient safety: the patient advocacy reporting system (PARS). In: Henriksen K, Battles JB, Keyes MA, Grady ML, editors. Advances in patient safety: new directions and alternative approaches. Bethesda: Agency for Healthcare Research and Quality (AHRQ); 2008. p. 421–30.
107. Moore IN, Pichert JW, Hickson GB, Federspiel CF, Blackford J. Rethinking peer review: detecting and addressing medical malpractice claims risk. Vanderbilt Law Rev. 2006;59:1175–206.
108. Pichert JW, Moore IN, Karrass J, Jay JS, Westlake MW, Catron TF, Hickson GB. An intervention model that promotes accountability: Peer messengers and patient/family complaints. Jt Comm J Qual Patient Saf. 2013;39(10):435–46.
109. Sage WM. Putting the patient in patient safety: linking patient complaints and malpractice risk. JAMA. 2002;287(22):3003–5.
110. Sheppard F, Williams M, Klein V. Team STEPPS and patient safety in healthcare. J Healthcare Risk Manage. 2013;32(3):5–10.
111. Hsieh SY, Thomas D, Rotem A. The organisational response to patient complaints: A case study in Taiwan. Int J Health Care Qual Assur. 2005;18(4): 308–20.
112. Stimson CJ, Pichert JW, Moore IN, Dmochowski RR, Cornett MB, An AQ, Hickson GB. Medical malpractice claims risk in urology: an empirical analysis of patient complaint data. J Urol. 2010; 183(5):1971–6.
113. Mukherjee K, Pichert JW, Cornett MB, Yan G, Hickson GB, Diaz JJ. All trauma surgeons are not created equal: Asymmetric distribution of malpractice claims risk. J Trauma. 2010;69(3):549–56.
114. Pichert JW, Johns JA, Hickson GB. Professionalism in support of pediatric cardio-thoracic surgery: A case of a bright young surgeon. Prog Ped Card. 2011;32(2):89–96.
115. Hickson GB, Moore IN. Risk prevention, risk management, and professional liability. In: Rock JA, Jones III HW, editors. TeLinde's operative gynecology. 11th ed. Philadelphia: Lippincott Williams & Wilkins; 1991 (in press).
116. The Joint Commission. Behaviors that undermine a culture of safety. Sentinel event alert #40. Oakbrook Terrace: The Joint Commission; 2008.
117. Pichert JW, Hickson GB, Vincent C, Pinto A. Communicating about unexpected outcomes and errors. In: Carayon P, editor. Handbook of Human Factors and Ergonomics in Healthcare and Patient Safety. 2nd ed. Boca Raton, FL: CRC Press; 2012. p. 401–22.
118. Reiter CE, Pichert JW, Hickson GB. Addressing behavior and performance issues that threaten quality and patient safety: What your attorneys want you to know. Prog Ped Card. 2012;33(1):37–45.
119. Samenow CP, Worley LL, Neufeld R, Fishel T, Swiggart WH. Transformative learning in a professional development course aimed at addressing disruptive physician behavior: a composite case study. Aca Med. 2013;88(1):117–23.
120. Smith RC, Dwamena FC, Grover M, Coffey J, Frankel RM. Behaviorally defined patient-centered communication – a narrative review of the literature. J Gen Intern Med. 2011;26(2):185–91.
121. Roseman D, Osborne-Stafsnes J, Amy CH, Boslaugh S, Slate-Miller K. Early lessons from four 'aligning forces for quality' communities bolster the case for patient-centered care. Health Aff. 2013;32(2):232–41.
122. Bechel DL, Myers WA, Smith DG. Does patient-centered care pay off? Jt Comm J Qual Improv. 2000;26(7):400–9.
123. Kuzel AJ, Woolf SH, Gilchrist VJ, Engel JD, LaVeist TA, Vincent C, et al. Patient reports of preventable problems and harms in primary health care. Ann Fam Med. 2004;2(4):333–40.
124. Taylor BB, Marcantonio ER, Pagovich O, Carbo A, Bergmann M, Davis RB, et al. Do medical inpatients who report poor service quality experience more adverse events and medical errors? Med Care. 2008;46(2):224–8.
125. Catron TF, Guillamondegui OD, Karrass J, Cooper WO, Martin BJ, Dmochowski RR, Pichert JW, Hickson GB. Surgical risk moderates the relationship between patients' observations of care and surgical outcomes. Manuscript submitted for publication.
126. Entman SS, Glass CA, Hickson GB, Githens PB, Whetten-Goldstein K, Sloan FA. The relationship between malpractice claims history and subsequent obstetric care. JAMA. 1994;272(20):1588–91.
127. Hickson GB, Clayton EW, Entman SS, Miller CS, Githens PB, Whetten-Goldstein K, et al. Obstetricians' prior malpractice experience and patients' satisfaction with care. JAMA. 1994;272(20):1583–7.

128. Carman KL, Dardess P, Maurer M, Sofaer S, Adams K, Bechtel C, et al. Patient and family engagement: a framework for understanding the elements and developing interventions and policies. Health Aff. 2013;32(2):223–31.
129. Maurer M, Dardess P, Carman KL, Frazier K, Smeeding L (American Institutes for Research, Washington, DC). Guide to patient and family engagement: environmental scan report [Internet]. Rockville: Agency for Healthcare Research and Quality; 2012 [cited 2013 Jan 8]. Available from: http://www.ahrq.gov/qual/ptfamilyscan/ptfamilyscan.pdf.
130. Johnson B, Abraham M, Conway J, Simmons L, Edgman-Levitan S, Sodomka P, et al. Partnering with patients and families to design a patient- and family-centered health care system: recommendations and promising practices. Bethesda: Institute for Patient and Family-Centered Care, Institute for Healthcare Improvement; 2008. http://www.ipfcc.org/pdf/PartneringwithPatientsandFamilies.pdf. Accessed 25 May 2014.
131. Tamblyn R, Abrahamowicz M, Dauphinee D, Wenghofer E, Jacques A, Klass D, et al. Physician scores on a national clinical skills examination as predictors of complaints to medical regulatory authorities. JAMA. 2007;298(9):993–1001.
132. Entwistle VA, McCaughan D, Watt IS, Birks Y, Hall J, Peat M, et al. Speaking up about safety concerns: multi-setting qualitative study of patients' views and experiences. Qual Saf Health Care. 2010;19(6):e33.
133. Schwappach DLB, Wernli M. Chemotherapy patients' perceptions of drug administration safety. J Clin Oncol. 2010;28(17):2896–901.
134. Schwappach DL, Hochreutener MA, Wernli M. Oncology nurses' perceptions about involving patients in the prevention of chemotherapy administration errors. Oncol Nurs Forum. 2010;37(2):E84–91.
135. Schwappach DLB, Frank O, Davis RE. A vignette study to examine health care professionals' attitudes towards patient involvement in error prevention. J Eval Clin Pract. 2012;19:840–8.
136. Longtin Y, Sax H, Leape LL, Sheridan SE, Donaldson L, Pittet D. Patient participation: current knowledge and applicability to patient safety. Mayo Clin Proc. 2010;85(1):53–62.
137. Mira JJ, Guilabert M, Pérez-Jover V, Lorenzo S. Barriers for an effective communication around clinical decision making: An analysis of the gaps between doctors' and patients' point of view. Health Expect. 2012; doi: 10.1111/j.1369-7625.2012.00809.x.
138. Davis RE, Sevdalis N, Jacklin R, Vincent CA. An examination of opportunities for the active patient in improving patient safety. J Patient Saf. 2012;8(1): 36–43. Epub 2012 Jan.
139. Jordan JE, Briggs AM, Brand CA, Osborne RH. Enhancing patient engagement in chronic disease self-management support initiatives in Australia: the need for an integrated approach. Med J Aust. 2008;189(10):9–S13.
140. Levinson W, Lesser CS, Epstein RM. Developing physician communication skills for patient-centered care. Health Aff. 2010;29(7):1310–8.
141. Kravitz RL, Epstein RM, Feldman MD, Franz CE, Azari R, Wilkes MS, et al. Influence of patients' requests for direct-to-consumer advertised antidepressants: a randomized controlled trial. JAMA. 2005;293(16):1995–2002.
142. Macfarlane J, Holmes W, Macfarlane R, Britten N. Influence of patients' expectations on antibiotic management of acute lower respiratory tract illness in general practice: questionnaire study. BMJ. 1997;315(7117):1211–4.
143. Marple RL, Kroenke K, Lucey CR, Wilder J, Lucas CA. Concerns and expectations in patients presenting with physical complaints: frequency, physician perceptions and actions, and 2-week outcome. Arch Intern Med. 1997;157(13):1482–8.
144. Pham HH, Landon BE, Reschovsky JD, Wu B, Schrag D. Rapidity and modality of imaging for acute low back pain in elderly patients. Arch Intern Med. 2009;169(10):972–81.
145. Kravitz RL, Cope DW, Bhrany V, Leake B. Internal medicine patients' expectations for care during office visits. J Gen Intern Med. 1994;9(2): 75–81.
146. Kravitz RL, Bell RA, Azari R, Krupat E, Kelly-Reif S, Thom D. Request fulfillment in office practice: antecedents and relationship to outcomes. Med Care. 2002;40(1):38–51.
147. Deyo RA, Diehl AK, Rosenthal M. Reducing roentgenography use. Can patient expectations be altered? Arch Intern Med. 1987;147(1):141–5.
148. Peck BM, Ubel PA, Roter DL, Goold SD, Asch DA, Mastat ASJ, et al. Do unmet expectations for specific tests, referrals, and new medications reduce patients' satisfaction? J Gen Intern Med. 2004;19(11): 1080–7.
149. Pfifferling JH. The myth of telling patients "No." Protector. Spring 2012, http://www.medpro.com/the-myth-of-telling-patients-no.
150. Audet AM, Davis K, Schoenbaum SC. Adoption of patient-centered care practices by physicians: results from a national survey. Arch Intern Med. 2006; 166(7):754–9.
151. Carroll KN, Cooper WO, Blackford JU, Hickson GB. Characteristics of families that complain following pediatric emergency visits. Ambul Pediatr. 2005;5(6):326–31.
152. Papanicolas I, Cylus J, Smith PC. An analysis of survey data from eleven countries finds that 'satisfaction' with health system performance means many things. Health Aff. 2013;32(4):734–42.

13 Failure to Rescue and Failure to Perceive in Pediatric Cardiac Surgery: Lessons Learned from Aviation

Edward J. Hickey, Glen S. Van Arsdell, and Peter C. Laussen

Abstract

Failure to rescue is now a commonly used term in healthcare, and describes the likelihood and ability of a team or providers to recover a patient from actual or impending harm. It can be used as a metric of performance for clinical teams and individual clinicians, but does require robust benchmarking to determine acceptable standards of care and expectations, as well as risk adjustment for patient populations, procedures and complexity. The key principles of effective threat and error management are *anticipation, recognition and recovery.* As outlined here, high-stakes industries with exemplary safety records exhibit a preoccupation with possibility of failure. They promote a culture of continuous vigilance, communication and problem-solving, and expect personnel to make errors but embrace non-punitive reporting to understand the root cause of threats and errors. They train their workforce to predict and prevent *loss of situational awareness.* We propose that a more meaningful metric of the performance of teams and providers is one that describes the *failure to perceive* an evolving clinical state, in addition to the ability to rescue patients once an event has occurred.

Keywords

Threat and error management • Human factor • Error • Failure to Rescue • Crew resource management

E.J. Hickey (✉)
Division of Cardiac Surgery,
The Hospital for Sick Children,
555 University Avenue, Toronto,
ON M5G 1X8, USA
e-mail: edward.hickey@sickkids.ca

G.S. Van Arsdell
Division of Cardiac Surgery,
The Hospital for Sick Children,
University of Toronto, Toronto, ON, Canada
e-mail: glen.vanarsdell@sickkids.ca

P.C. Laussen, MBBS, FCICM
Department of Critical Care Medicine,
The Hospital for Sick Children, Toronto, ON, Canada

Department of Anaesthesia, University
of Toronto, 555 University Avenue,
Toronto, ON M5G 1X8, Canada
e-mail: peter.laussen@sickkids.ca

P.R. Barach, J.P. Jacobs, S.E. Lipshultz, P.C. Laussen (eds.),
Pediatric and Congenital Cardiac Care: Volume 2: Quality Improvement and Patient Safety,
DOI 10.1007/978-1-4471-6566-8_13,

Introduction

In August 2013, a captain and first officer on a British long-haul commercial airliner reported that they had both unintentionally – and simultaneously – fallen asleep mid-flight [1]. The *systems approach* of the airline industry to human error encourages such reporting and the pilots involved did so freely and without repercussion. The commercial airline industry currently functions beyond the 6-σ level[1] – approximately 2.6 incidents per million takeoffs and landings [2]. The stakes are high though: every one of these rare incidents that does occur potentially leads to mass casualties and therefore captures global headlines. Other high-stakes industries – nuclear power, military aircraft carriers and air traffic control, for example – have also acquired 6-σ safety [3], through a philosophy towards human error akin to that of commercial aviation: (1) all have developed a pre-occupation with failure and therefore engrain a culture of systemic vigilance, (2) all have endorsed and promoted mechanisms for blame-free reporting, and (3) all accept that human error is both ubiquitous and inevitable. These industries, therefore, have all embraced a *systems approach* to error by focusing on preventing, predicting, recognizing and rescuing the errors that they anticipate will occur.

Human Error in Medicine – The "Personal Approach"

The medical profession has, instead, been obstinate in its approach to human error. Historically, there has been reluctance to acknowledge the occurrence of errors, or their impact [4]. When errors are exposed, there is frequently a general resistance to transparency regarding the details and circumstances. The reasons for this stem from the fact that the medical profession has generally adopted a *personal approach* to human error [3]. Accordingly, error is considered a shortcoming of a person or small group of individuals with whom responsibility is therefore deemed to rest. Consequently, *blame* is implied, if not stated. This personal approach to human error is satisfying in many respects: failures are "contained" and accounted for. It provides easy and direct causation for colleagues, patients and their families. Naming, blaming and shaming have seemingly provided a sense of gratification for patients, and also makes for fantastic sensationalist journalism.[2] Competitive medical specialties, too, seem to feed off the *personal approach* to human error; conventional "morbidity and mortality" sessions may often be adversarial or even vitriolic. A fundamental flaw of the *personal approach* to understanding human error is that it ignores contributing causal factors beyond the individual perpetrator. There is therefore a high likelihood of error recurrence.

Failure to Rescue

The frequency of an adverse event, such as preventable cardiac arrest, healthcare acquired infection or specific complications after a procedure, may reflect the capabilities and skills of a team or provider and the systems and culture in place to support that team or provider. Fundamental systems- and human-engineering factors continue to be studied in detail to ameliorate these events and prevent harm. No question, this is important. *Failure to rescue* is now a commonly used term in healthcare, and describes the likelihood and ability of a team or providers to recover a patient from actual or

[1] For confusing reasons that relate to long-term process iteration models, 6σ actually correlates statistically to 4.5 standard deviations and hence 3.4 events per million, or an event rate of 0.00034 %. Commerical aviation exceeds this quality metric. The top paediatric heart surgery centres currently function at ~3.5σ in terms of patient mortality (about 3 %).

[2] The press seems comfortable with the phrase and concept of "pilot error" as a frequent factor in air accidents. Simple online searches for surgical error lead to national newspaper headlines describing "scandals" of "bungling surgeons", "botched operations" and "baby killers".

impending harm. Based on the original report by Silber et al, studying hospital and patient characteristics associated with death after surgery, a low failure to rescue rate for a particular adverse event implies preventable harm occurred, and that this is often a reflection of systems failure [5]. A failure to rescue can be used as a metric of performance for clinical teams and individual clinicians, but does require robust benchmarking to determine acceptable standards of care and expectations, as well as risk adjustment for patient populations, procedures and complexity.

Failure to Perceive

Clinical decision making in highly complex and intense environments, such as the intensive care unit or operating room, is both *analytic*, based on the input directly from physiologic data and knowledge, and *intuitive* based on experience, and plausible outcomes. The sheer volume and complexity of data can oftentimes be overwhelming, difficult to integrate and subject to variable interpretation among clinicians. The introduction of the electronic medical record and addition of new monitoring technology has only made the environment more complex. To support patients and staff in these ever more complex environments, it is essential the volume, velocity and variability of patient data now available is simplified, integrated and understandable. The aim should be to allow clinicians to move from prescriptive and intuitive decision making to one that is predictive and analytic (Fig. 13.1). A more meaningful metric of the performance of teams and providers therefore is one that describes the *failure to perceive* an evolving clinical state, in addition to the ability to rescue patients once an event has occurred.

Failure to perceive is grounded within resilience engineering, which provides a new way of thinking about safety. Complex socio-technical systems are inherently risky. Rather than considering a system or organization to be inherently safe by following a set procedure or rules, safety is something that people in complex environments *create*, by understanding competing demands and variations in conditions.

Lessons form the Flightdeck – Vigilance and Communication

In the cockpit, *error* is a human action or inaction that leads to a deviation from the intended or expected circumstance that then leads to a reduction in safety margin and increased probability of adverse event [6]. They are common, ubiquitous and, in accordance with the systems approach, can be considered inevitable [7]. Fly-on-the-wall assessments of >3,500 commercial airline flights by trained observers conclude that 80 % contain error [8]. Fortunately, during routine workload, few crews perform "poorly" and instead 75–80 % crews are graded as either "good" or "outstanding". However, during high-intensity scenarios, there is a significant increase in the number of crews performing "poorly" [9], but also a significant increase in the number of crews who perform "outstandingly". Understanding the working patterns high-functioning crews is central to understanding effective threat and error management.

Crews that excel in crisis situations are highly vigilant and highly communicative. Review of >10,000 utterances has revealed that during abnormal situations, the number of utterances increases on average by a factor of twofold. The proportion increase in number of utterances during these periods of stress correlates significantly with increased performance, fewer errors and – especially – with fewer *consequential errors* [10]. Importantly, the number of *problem-solving utterances* – a surrogate for vigilance – is highly linked to highly performing crews. Irrespective of workload complexity, outstanding captains devote one third of all utterances to problem solving – even in routine, low-intensity flight segments. This is in contrast to crews performing poorly or with mid-proficiency, where 5–10 % of utterances related to problem solving [10]. During both high- and low-intensity situations,

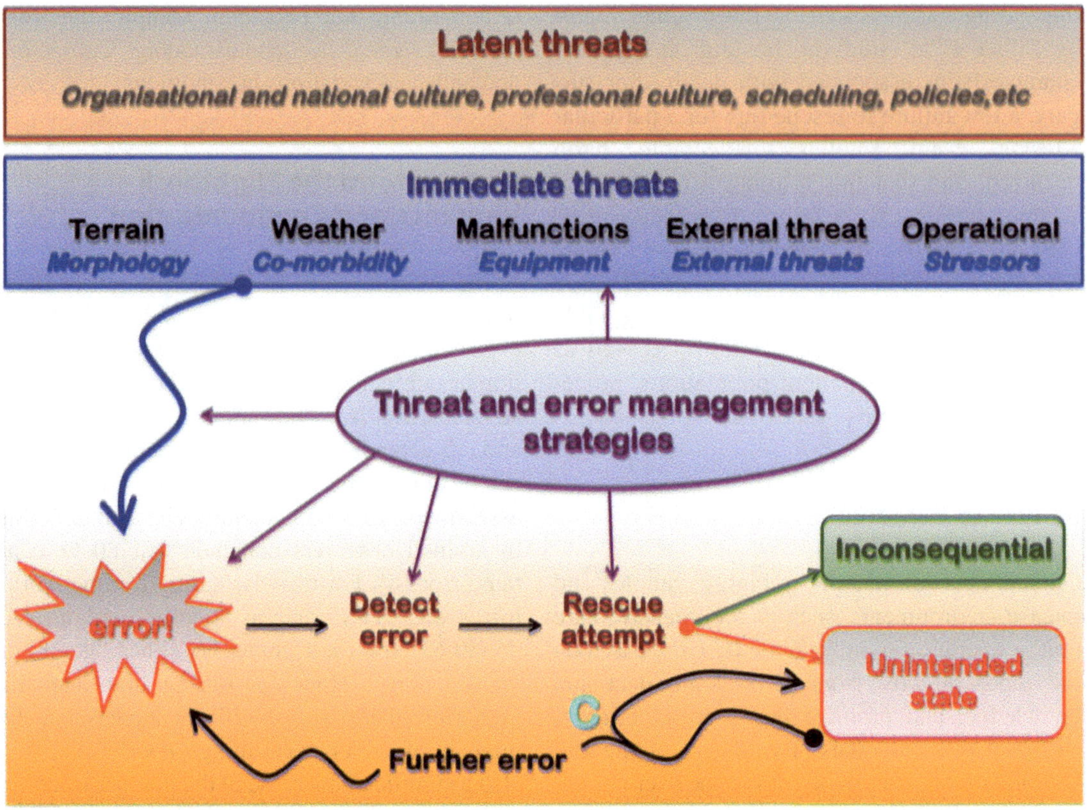

Fig. 13.1 Threat and error model proposed by Helmreich [8]. Immediate threats are factors outside the control of the cockpit crew that act to increase the complexity of the situation and therefore predispose to error occurring. Errors must necessarily be recognized in order for a rescue attempt to correct for the error. The rescue may completely mitigate the error (*inconsequential error*). On the other hand, a *consequential error* is one that leads to an *unintended state* (either ineffective or mismanaged rescue attempt, or a completely unrecognized but important error). The unintended state may not itself be dangerous, but serves as a threat for *cycles ("C")* of additional error or unintended states. It is these cycles that serve as the stage for amplification of the situation and potential catastrophe. Over-arching organizational and cultural factors may serve as *latent threats*. We propose that the same model holds true in high-stakes medical specialties. Aviation threats have corollaries in medicine (blue), as do error types. Threat and error management strategies, such as *crew resource management* serve to: (1) predict and manage threats, (2) minimize human error, (3) increase error recognition, (4) improve team coordination and resource utilization during rescues, (5) maximize safety margins during unintended states and (6) recognize and break cycles of error-unintended states

the outstanding captains vocalize problem-solving more than poorly functioning captains by a factor of 7–8 [10]. Problem-solving communications had consequently become the centre of modern threat and error management techniques. To quote Robert Helmreich [10], "it is not that effective communication can overcome inadequate technical flying proficiency; rather, good rudder and stick skills cannot overcome the adverse effects of poor communication."

Threats May Prompt Error

To paraphrase an Australian pilot: "a threat is anything that takes you away from the ideal day." Errors may occur completely unprompted, but often occur as a result of a mismanaged threat. Strictly speaking, threats are external influences that increase the operational complexity of the planned procedure or journey [6]. They are the risk factors, therefore, for errors occurring.

Table 13.1 Classification and prevalence of threat and error subtypes observed during simulator studies and direct observation of >3,500 commercial airline flight segments [8]

Threats		Errors	
Aviation	Medicine	Aviation	Medicine
Terrain – 58 %	*Morphology*	Violation of SOP – 54 %	*Non-adherence to guidelines, SOP*
Weather – 28 %	*Co-morbidity*	Procedural – 28 %	*Procedural*
Aircraft malfunctions – 15 %	*Equipment*	Communication – 7 %	*Communication*
External errors – 8 %	*External factors*	Proficiency – 6 %	*Proficiency, knowledge or skill*
Air traffic control, ground crew	*Ward, admin, etc*		
Operation pressures – 8 %	*Operational stressors*	Decision error – 7 %	*Decision or judgment*
Fatigue, crew stresses	*Fatigue, scheduling, etc*		

All have corollaries in medicine, as indicated in italics

Understanding and mitigating threats are central to the systems approach of threat and error management. In the airline cockpit, threats tend to fall into one of five distinct categories [8] (Table 13.1). The most common relate to terrain or adverse weather. Observational data from commercial airline cockpits indicate about ~75 % flights face one or more threat (range 0–11; median 2) and approximately 10 % of these threats are mismanaged, therefore leading to an error.

Latent threats are a particularly important type of threat from a system error management perspective. They are operational, management or training conditions which indirectly lead to circumstances that exacerbate the risk of error [11]. Their importance lies in the fact that unless they are addressed, it is highly likely that errors will recur. To use James Reason's analogy [3]: active failures are like mosquitos – they can be swatted one by one, but keep coming. A better remedy is to drain the swamps from which they breed. The swamps represent the latent conditions from which many of the active threats breed.

Categories of Error

In the airline cockpit, errors tend to fall into one of five category types [8] (Table 13.1). By far the most frequent type of error documented during in-flight cockpit observation is violation of a "standard operating procedure" [8]. This is most commonly intentional non-compliance, for example knowingly omitting or abbreviating a standard checklist. Whilst such non-compliance may reflect a cavalier work ethic, contempt for controlling regulations or misperceptions of personal invulnerability (which, like surgeons, pilots have been shown to exhibit [12]) it should be recognized that over-enthusiastic introduction of protocols will in itself breed non-compliance and disdain for the philosophy of systemic error control. Procedural errors reflect a true "mistake" in the execution of a certain task (often termed "lapses"), for example touching the wrong key when entering coordinates, or reading the wrong line of data from a chart. "Proficiency" errors are the least comforting, as the name implies a personal deficiency in skill level. Perhaps, though, they are the most important to acknowledge: denial of failures in proficiency (a tendency in medicine) is to completely ignore the huge innate fallibility of humans.

Unperceived Failure: Unrecognized or Ignored Errors

An error may be actively ignored or not even be recognized. Of course, errors that are either ignored or unrecognized cannot be managed successfully; they will only be inconsequential either because they are genuinely trivial, or through pure luck. Conceptually, therefore, unperceived errors are perhaps among the most important target for error management, as error recognition is a pre-requisite of error rescue. In certain situations, humans may have reasonable judgment regarding when an error can be ignored. However investigations into intentional non-compliance (by definition ignored errors) in the aviation industry errors raise serious doubts about this general assumption. More than 40 % of approach and landing accidents involve intentional non-compliance of a standard operating procedure [8]. Perhaps more importantly, pilots who commit intentional non-compliance errors are 25 % more prone to other types of error than pilots who adhere to standard operating procedures [8]. Therefore, non-adherence represents a general propensity to err.

Error Rescue and Unintended States

For those errors that are recognized and not ignored, there is by definition some attempt made to *rescue* or *contain* the error. These error rescue actions may lead to: (1) no change in the situational circumstances (inconsequential error), or otherwise (2) an unintended state (consequential error). Importantly, an unintended state may not itself be a danger at all (for example a perfectly safe, but different, flying configuration in an aircraft). However, a central premise of the threat-error model described by Helmreich [8] is that an *unintended state* is itself an important *threat* that significantly increases the propensity for further errors and additional unintended states occurring.

In commercial airline cockpits, 25 % of errors are considered *consequential:* 19 % lead to an unintended state, whereas 6 % of errors lead directly to a second error [8]. This *cycle* of unplanned circumstances and errors is considered to be the stage for a catastrophe (Fig. 13.1). Recognition of the error-unintended state cycle requires extreme *vigilance*, as each unintended state may itself not seem dangerous or unfamiliar. Essentially, the gradual *deviation away from the planned or expected journey* should indicate that an error-unintended state cycle might be occurring. The over-arching goal in these circumstances should first be to *maximize safety margins* and then to problem-solve. It should be noted that unintended states might not necessarily be preceded by an error; they may be simply a consequence of appropriate crew actions in response to various threats (weather, terrain, external errors, for example). A third of all flights contain unintended states, and 5 % of landing approaches are considered to be frankly unstable [12]. One third of all unintended aircraft states are considered to be the end result of a chain from threat leading to error leading to unintended state [12].

Extreme Stress

The most dangerous and extreme form of unintended state is *loss of situational awareness*, which is frequently evident to air accident investigators from cockpit voice recordings. The 2009 disaster of Air France flight 447 is an excellent example of this [13]: complete loss of situational awareness led a crew of three pilots stall a completely functional aircraft at 38,000 ft.[3] When loss of situational awareness occurs, the absolute priority is to *maximize safety margins* via coordinated use of all available resources ("crew resource management"). Problem solving then takes a second priority. Sensory and cognitive senses become highly distorted in situations of extreme stress or fear and behavior becomes quite unpredictable [14]; it is for these reasons that skills such as role allocation, task prioritization and resource utilization need to be taught and rehearsed [12]. In Air France 447, standard operating procedures and checklists were ignored for the initial upstream problem [13]. Role allocation was poor and attention of all pilots

[3] Icing of a pitot tube led to brief and transient loss of air speed data and autopilot disengagement. The crew responded with some inappropriate manual flight control inputs which led to an escalation of unintended states, errors and increasingly unstable flying configurations. The crew became increasingly confused and disbelieving of the instruments. Task-sharing and coordination of roles was poor and even at the point of impact two pilots were attempting to make opposite manouvres with the side-sticks.

turned to problem solving rather than initially maintaining a safe flight envelope. The fully functional aircraft hit the Atlantic Ocean belly first, with a forward velocity of only 107 knots.

Effective Integration of Crewmembers

Effective integration between cockpit members of different rank appears to be an important aspect of crew effectiveness, especially during high workload situations. The use of first person plural (we, our, us) versus singular (I) is associated with better performance and fewer errors [10]. This finding probably has two facets – firstly crew familiarity, and secondly power-distance. Cockpit members who are unfamiliar with one another seem to be less effective in high-intensity situations, perhaps because of social unease. In fact, fatigued crews whose members are known to each other perform better than well-rested crews who are unfamiliar [15]. Analysis of aviation accidents has revealed that ~75 % occur on the first day of an initial crew pairing (versus 7–30 % of all flights) [15]. Power-distance relates to the likelihood of a subordinate questioning their superior, and the receptiveness of a superior to such questioning [12, 16].[4] A large power-distance implies wider divides between ranks (more autocratic), whereas a small power-distance implies more discussion and collective decision-making between ranks (more democratic). The latter is considered safer, and is a key facet of crew resource management.

Crew Resource Management

The aim of *crew resource management* (CRM) is to train people to perform effectively in degraded situations [12]. During training, emphasis is placed on four behavioural indicators: ability to cooperate, management and leadership, situational awareness and decision-making [12]. Crews develop effective cross-checking and support capabilities that reduces confusion and enhances task allocation. Since its inception at a NASA/Industry workshop in 1979 [9], CRM has become a mandatory and core component of commercial cockpit training. Whilst the efficacy of CRM is difficult to prove, the vast expenditure of energy and resources on CRM training by commercial and military aviation is some testament to value [17, 18]. Analysis of recent near-catastrophes has demonstrated exemplary CRM skills by cockpit crew and serves as anecdotal support of its merit.[5] Comparable training has been developed for medical and surgical teams in pediatric cardiac surgery and critical care in an effort to learn to function with maximal effectiveness in highly degraded and stressful circumstances, but the impact of such training is hard to measure [19].

Human Error in High-Stakes Medicine – Pediatric Heart Surgery Experience

Investigating Mortality – "Accident Investigation"

In the same way that early lessons in the aviation industry were gleaned from investigating catastrophic accidents, we too have explored the role of error leading up to patient deaths after pediatric heart surgery [20]. In a retrospective analysis of

[4] In 1977, Captain Veldhuyzen van Zanten – KLM's most senior captain – powered up his 747 and trundled down the runway at Tenerife without ATC clearance. The young engineer in the cockpit realised that a taxiing Pan Am 747 may still be on the runway, and asked rhetorically whether clearance had been given. The captain cut him short and asserted that things were fine. They were not fine; the two planes collided with what remains to this day the biggest loss of life in any air accident. Ironically, Captain van Zanten was held in such high regard as a pilot by KLM's executive that upon hearing about the crash they immediately sought him to lead their investigation, only to discover that he was the captain involved. The Tenerife disaster was one of a number of high profile air crashes in the 1970s and 1980s that highlighted the dangers of a traditional steep hierarchy.

[5] US Airways flight 1549 successfully landed in the Hudson River after a double bird strike shortly after take-off. British Airways flight 38 lost thrust on both engines at an altitude of 720 ft during the final approach to Heathrow and crash-landed 890 ft short of the runway. There was no loss of life in either accident and both crews were praised for their CRM skills during the crises.

Fig. 13.2 Actuarial survival of 191 infants (2000–2011) with hypoplastic left heart syndrome that underwent stage-1 (S1) palliation, stratified by whether or not they were exposed to a post-operative clinical error in management. In risk-adjusted models, post-operative errors were associated with significant decrements in survival. Other risk factors included morphology of double inlet left ventricle (DILV) and longer cardiopulmonary bypass duration (CPB min)

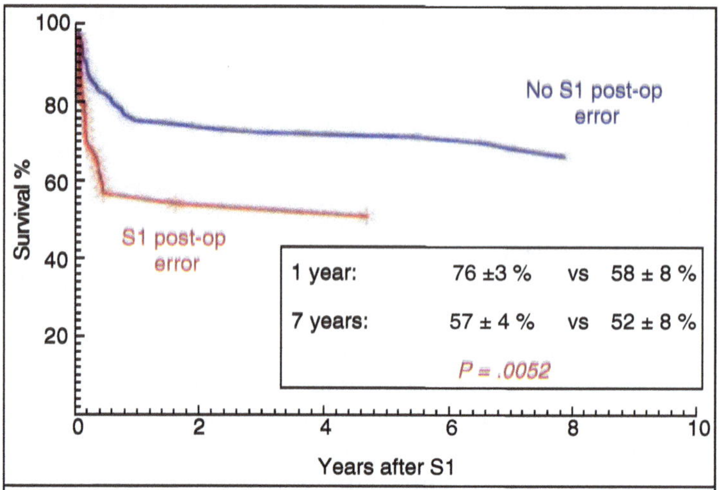

Risk factors for death/transplant

Risk factor	P	Reliability
DILV	.0036	84 %
CPB min	.0169	81 %
Any post-operative error	.0034	67 %

all 261 deaths spanning a decade at our institution, over 50 % had identifiable errors evident in clinical management leading up to their death. Children with the most complex anatomy and physiology who required complex neonatal surgery (e.g. single ventricle palliation) exhibited the highest incidence of errors (~70 %), and errors were significantly more common during the intra-operative and post-operative periods, which have high-intensity workloads. This pattern is exactly analogous to the situation in the aircraft cockpit, where the error rate more than doubles during periods of high workload, e.g. approach and landing (~40 % of all cockpit errors) [8]. Cardiovascular deaths were very significantly associated these errors made during the intra-operative and intensive care windows (*P~.005*). When causality between error and death was explored, approximately 40 % of all deaths were linked to an identifiable upstream error. Of these upstream errors, ~85 % were considered to be mismanaged errors that could have been prevented or contained [20].

Retrospective Insights into High-Risk Patients

As a next iteration, we chose to concentrate on the highest risk patient group: those with hypoplastic left heart syndrome who underwent single ventricle palliation via either a Norwood or hybrid approach. Only 20 % of children had error-free hospital admissions; 80 % instead experienced one or more error at some point during their care (median 2) [21]. The clinical phase with the highest prevalence of errors was again during the periods of highest workload intensity – the intra-operative surgical window and the post-operative intensive care period. Although no direct link between errors and unintended states (or complications) was made during this retrospective investigation, children whose post-operative journeys contained one or more identifiable error exhibited long-term survival decrements ~15 % below those who were error-free (Fig. 13.2).

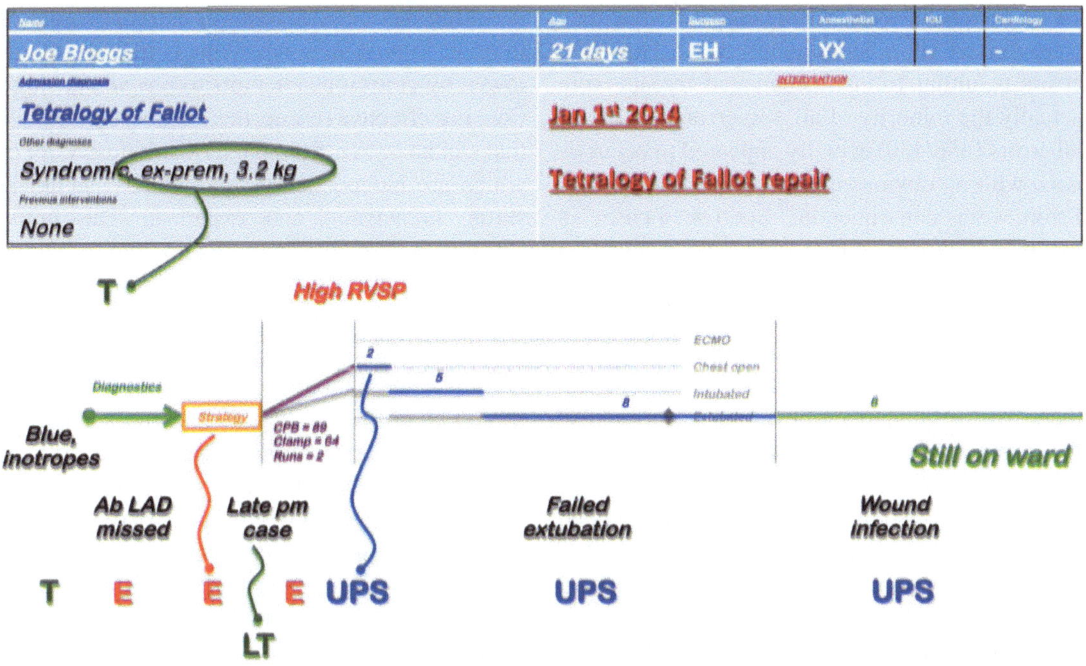

Fig. 13.3 Representative illustration of a patient "flight". Children are tracked from the point of admission, during which investigations are undertaken to confirm diagnosis. Management strategies are then decided before an operation is undertaken, usually involving cardiopulmonary bypass (*purple*). Longer CPB duration is considered to represent greater risk for the patient. When the patient arrives on intensive care (*blue*), the child will gradually pass through reducing stages in risk: the highest being on artificial heart-lung machines (ECMO) and the lowest being extubated and simply on medications. The child will then transfer to the ward (*green*), prior to being discharged. Risk is the y-axis, and time is the *x*-axis. Various threats (*T*), latent threats (*LT*), errors (*E*) and unintended patient states (*UPS*) are tracked on the graphs, and linked together if related. Permanent outcomes (persisting complications) and deaths are also indicated and linked to upstream UPS or E

"Fly-on-the-Wall" Insights in Patients' Journeys

In order to gain further insight into the role of error across all patients (including the ~97 % majority who survived), we have instigated a real-time assessment of patient care in order to identify errors and their interplay with perceived threats. This is not directly representative of fly-on-the-wall line audit assessments of airline cockpit crew [6, 22], but instead involves continuous scrutiny of every patient's clinical care by a third party, which is then reviewed weekly in an open forum to gain consensus. Prior to every operation, each child has a "flight plan" published, which details potential threats and stipulates the operative intentions. We then model the patient's path through their operative and post-operative course, until the point of discharge from hospital, in a graphic broadly representative of an aircraft's flight (Fig. 13.3). We term their in-hospital journey a "flight". Risk is depicted on the y-axis, and time proceeds along the x-axis. In reviewing the classification of threats and errors used by Helmreich's group [8], it was immediately apparent that threat and errors in the aviation industry have direct correlations in the surgical specialties (Table 13.1), and we therefore use these classifications. As the child passes along their operative and post-operative journey, threats and errors can be marked on their graphic, together with unintended states and the final outcome.

Of 524 consecutive patient "flights", the operative team had to manage 761 identifiable threats in 364 (70 %) patients [23]. Of all 761 threats,

14 % (N = 105) were mismanaged in that they were linked to a subsequent error. However, errors resulting from mismanaged threats were actually the minority of all 430 errors – 82 % of all errors (356/430) actually appeared to occur *de novo* with no obvious upstream threat identified. Errors were "consequential" in 66 % of cases, in that they led to an unintended state – a deviation from the expected path for that particular child. These unintended deviations from the preoperative plan are not necessarily dangerous in themselves, and indeed in 40 % of cases no further error or unintended deviation occurred: i.e. the situation did not escalate and the original error was *rescued or contained.* However, in 60 % of consequential errors, the unintended patient state led to a further error and/or a further unintended deviation: i.e. the situation escalated and a *cycle of errors/unintended states was occurring.* Exactly in accordance with the threat and error model developed by the NASA-Ames research teams and University of Texas, these *cycles of error and unintended states are dangerous.* They can easily amplify and lead to catastrophe and therefore need to be rescued. Indeed in our model of pediatric cardiac surgery, such cycles were highly significantly associated with residual haemodynamic lesions, end-organ injury and death (all $P < .0001$) [23]. Deaths were almost always preceded by upstream cycles of error and unintended patient states in 85 % of cases, which is remarkably similar to the proportion of commercial air accidents that have identifiable cycles of human error and unintended aircraft states upstream [23].

Summary

In our initial investigations outlined above, exactly 50 % of all patient "flights" contained at least one error somewhere during their care, and two-thirds of these errors were "consequential", leading to an unintended state. Of these consequential errors, 60 % then led to *cycles of error-unintended state*. Therefore, an alarming 104/524 (20 %) of all patient flights contained such cycles, which we now understand to be dangerous. Breaking these cycles requires extreme *vigilance* in order to *recognize* when one is in a cycle, followed by conscious attempts to *rescue* the situation. For effective rescue, there are certain lessons that can be drawn from the airline industry, all of which are independent of individuals' technical skills, knowledge and expertise. The initial actions should all be aiming to maximize the safety margins for the patient. Only subsequently, once the safety margins have been increased, should problem-solving attempts be made. During rescue attempts, all available resources should be utilized to best effectiveness using the principles of *crew resource management.* Clear role allocation leads to effective task-sharing and allows individuals to focus on discrete tasks. The rapid increase in workload during a dangerous or confusing situation can rapidly lead to degradation in the quality of communication and coordination between pilots in a cockpit, and the same is true during the medical emergencies.

Our performance rounds provide a forum to debrief and learn from cycles of error-unintended states. Possible and real errors across the flight path, the continuum of care for each patient, are gathered and displayed for each patient. The interrelation between errors becomes clear, with open and multidisciplinary input enabling frank discussion about preventative measures and potential changes in management paradigms. Importantly, these conversations serve as a platform for gathering a central memory to avoid repetitive errors.

Key Principles of Effective Crisis Management

The key principles of effective threat and error management are *anticipation, recognition and recovery.* As outlined here, high-stakes industries with exemplary 6-σ safety records exhibit "chronic unease" and a preoccupation with possibility of failure. They promote a culture of continuous vigilance, communication and problem-solving. They expect personnel to make errors, and embrace a systems approach by encouraging non-punitive reporting to understand the root cause of threats and errors. They train their workforce to predict and recognize errors. They plan and rehearse recovery from dangerous situations. When deviations from the planned circumstances occur, however seemingly benign, heightened vigilance for cycles of error and further deviations helps to contain the situation and prevent *loss of situational awareness.* However, when the latter does occur, emphasis is placed on:

- **Recover first, analyze later**
- **Initial priority to *maximize safety margins***
- **Task allocation**
- **Adherence to standard procedures or guidelines**
- **Clear communication and cross-checking**
- **Verbally acknowledge and review all available data**
- **Problem-solve only once initial safety maximized**

References

1. Silverman R. Airline pilots asleep in the cockpit during long-haul flight. In: The Telegraph, London, 2013.
2. Organization ICA. State of global aviation safety – evolving toward a risk-based aviation safety strategy. 2013.
3. Reason J. Human error: models and management. BMJ. 2000;320:768–70.
4. Bristol Royal Infirmary. The report of the public inquiry into children's heart surgery at the Bristol Royal Infirmary 1984–1995: learning from Bristol. Edited by Kennedy I. Bristol, 2001.
5. Silber JH, Williams SV, Krakauer H, Schwartz JS. Hospital and patient characteristics associated with death after surgery. A study of adverse occurrence and failure to rescue. Med Care. 1992;30:615–29.
6. Merritt A, Klinect J. Defensive flying for pilots: an introduction to threat and error management. University of Texas Human Factors Research Project. The LOSA Collaborative; 2006.
7. Reason J. Human error. New York: Cambridge University Press; 1990.
8. Helmreich RL. Culture, threat, and error: assessing system safety. In: Safety in Aviation: the management commitment. London; 1999.
9. Ruffell Smith HP. A simulator study of the interaction of pilot workload with errors, vigilance, and decisions. NASA Tech Memo. 1979;78482:1–54.
10. Sexton JB, Helmreich RL. Analyzing cockpit communications: the links between language, performance, error, and workload. Hum Perf Extrem Environ. 2000;5:63–8.
11. Helmreich RL. On error management: lessons from aviation. BMJ. 2000;320:781–5.
12. Helmreich RL. Culture, error, and crew resource management. In: Salas E, Bowers CA, Edens E, editors. Improving teamwork in organizations: applications of resource management training. Mahwah: Lawrence Erlbaum Associates, Inc; 2001.
13. civile BBdEedAplsdla. Final report: accident of Air France flight 447. Edited by: BEA; 2012. p. 1–223.
14. Sinnett S, Spence C, Soto-Faraco S. Visual dominance and attention: the Colavita effect revisited. Percept Psychophys. 2007;69:673–86.
15. Helmreich RL, Sexton JB. Using language in the cockpit: relationships with workload and performance. In: Dietrich R, Von Feltzer T, editors. Communication in high risk environments. Hamburg: Helmut Buske Verlag; 2003. p. 57–73.
16. Sexton JB, Thomas EJ, Helmreich RL. Error, stress, and teamwork in medicine and aviation: cross sectional surveys. BMJ. 2000;320:745–9.
17. Helmreich RL. How effective is cockpit resource management training? Flight safety foundation: flight safety digest. 1990. p. 1–17.
18. Helmreich RL. Whither CRM? Future directions in Crew Resource Management training in the cockpit and elsewhere. In: International symposium on aviation psychology. Vol. 1 and 2. Columbus; 1993. p. 543–48.
19. Allan CK, Thiagarajan RR, Beke D, Imprescia A, Kappus LJ, Garden A, Hayes G, Laussen PC, Bacha E, Weinstock PH. Simulation-based training delivered directly to the pediatric cardiac intensive care unit engenders preparedness, comfort, and decreased anxiety among multidisciplinary resuscitation teams. J Thorac Cardiovasc Surg. 2010;140:646–52.
20. Jacques F, Honjo O, Moga M, Grasso F, Baba K, Hickey EJ, Humpl T, Schwartz S, Caldarone CA, Redington AN, et al. Improving survival by targeting error. In: American College of Cardiology scientific sessions, Chicago; 2012
21. Jacques F, Anand V, Hickey EJ, Kotani Y, Yadava M, Alghamdi A, Caldarone CA, Redington AN, Schwartz S, Van Arsdell GS. Medical errors: the performance gap in hypoplastic left heart syndrome and physiologic equivalents? J Thorac Cardiovasc Surg. 2013;145:1465–73; discussion 1473–5.
22. Klinect J, Murray P, Merritt A, Helmreich RL. Line operation safety audits (LOSA): definition and operating characteristics. In: 12th international symposium on aviation psychology, Dayton; 2003. p. 663–8.
23. Hickey EJ, Nosikova Y, Pham-Hung E, Gritti M, Caldarone CA, Redington AN, Van Arsdell GS. NASA "threat and error model" applied to pediatric cardiac surgery: error cycles precede ~85% of patient deaths. J Thorac Cardiovasc Surg. 2014; (in press).

Quality Improvement in Noninvasive Imaging: Present and Future Initiatives

14

Leo Lopez

Abstract

Indicators of quality services in pediatric and congenital echocardiography include structural, process, and outcome factors. Structural indicators involve the available resources related to the facility, the equipment, and the staff. Process indicators relate primarily to the activities and tasks associated with echocardiography, and these include patient selection as well as study performance, interpretation, and reporting. Outcome indicators involve the results of quality services and are intimately related to quality improvement activities as well as quality metrics. Current quality improvement activities in the field of pediatric and congenital echocardiography include development of the accreditation process for sonographers, physicians, and echocardiography laboratories; evaluation of productivity standards within echocardiography laboratories; identification of appropriate use criteria specific to pediatric and congenital echocardiography; and establishment of a robust database of normal reference values for cardiovascular measurements in children. Candidate quality metrics currently in development involve reporting of critical results, adverse events with sedated studies, variability of echocardiographic measurements, diagnostic errors, study completeness, and image quality.

L. Lopez, MD, FASE, FACC, FAAP
Department of Pediatrics, Albert Einstein College of Medicine, Children's Hospital at Montefiore, 3415 Bainbridge Avenue, Rosenthal 1, Bronx, NY 10467, USA
e-mail: llmd@llmd.net

P.R. Barach, J.P. Jacobs, S.E. Lipshultz, P.C. Laussen (eds.),
Pediatric and Congenital Cardiac Care: Volume 2: Quality Improvement and Patient Safety,
DOI 10.1007/978-1-4471-6566-8_14, © Springer-Verlag London 2015

Keywords
Pediatric echocardiography • Congenital echocardiography • Quality improvement • Structure indicators • Process indicators • Outcome indicators • Quality metrics • Productivity standards • Appropriate use criteria • Pediatric reference values

Introduction

Echocardiography (echo) is the primary noninvasive diagnostic modality for patients with acquired and congenital heart disease (CHD). Quality improvement (QI) efforts in echo have become crucial components in the delivery of health care to these patients [1, 2]. According to recommendations for quality echo laboratory operations published by the American Society of Echocardiography (ASE), quality "can be measured as adherence to established guidelines for the use of a technology to ensure patient satisfaction and outcomes" [2]. Hence, QI initiatives must necessarily involve quantifiable changes in *structure* and *process* in order to effect changes in *outcome* with the following goals: to decrease variations in practice, provide appropriate care, and diminish waste in terms of technical and human resources, thereby optimizing results [3].

The use of echo in children has increased tremendously over the past several decades, mostly because of advances in imaging technology and improved understanding of cardiovascular pathophysiology. However, QI initiatives in this population have been limited, especially in comparison to similar activities in adult echo. Historically, the wide variation in terminology and methodology and the absence of standard performance and reporting practices have precluded the establishment of quality standards in children. Efforts by the ASE, the European Association of Cardiovascular Imaging (EACVI), the Intersocietal Accreditation Commission (IAC), the American College of Cardiology (ACC), the American Heart Association (AHA), the Pediatric Heart Network (PHN), and the International Society for the Nomenclature of Paediatric and Congenital Heart Diseases (ISNPCHD) have created frameworks to identify QI indicators and develop quality metrics in pediatric and congenital echo. This chapter will evaluate structure, process, and outcome indicators for quality in the pediatric and congenital echo lab (Table 14.1) and focus on current and future QI initiatives, including the development of quality metrics specific to the pediatric and congenital population (Table 14.2).

Table 14.1 Quality indicators in pediatric and congenital echocardiography

1. Structure
(a) Facility
(b) Equipment
(c) Staff
2. Process
(a) Patient selection
(b) Study performance
(c) Study interpretation
(d) Study reporting
3. Outcome
(a) Death
(b) Disease
(c) Discomfort
(d) Disability
(e) Dissatisfaction

Table 14.2 Quality initiatives in pediatric and congenital echocardiography

1. Accreditation
(a) Sonographers
(b) Physicians
(c) Echocardiography laboratories
2. Productivity standards
3. Appropriate use criteria
4. Normal reference values
5. Quality metrics
(a) Reporting for critical results
(b) Adverse events with sedated echocardiograms
(c) Variability in pediatric echocardiographic measurements
(d) Diagnostic errors
(e) Study completion
(f) Image quality

Structural Indicators

Structural indicators refer to the type and amount of resources needed to provide quality echo services [3], specifically in terms of the *facility*, the *equipment*, and the *staff*.

Facility

Determinants of quality services within the facility include the physical space, availability of patient privacy, patient volume, and daily workflow. How big is the echo lab? How many examination rooms are available? Does the physical space account for patient privacy? How much time is allotted for each study? How many patients can the facility accommodate at any time? How many patients are evaluated in the echo lab every year? What happens when studies are being performed? How is supervision provided to sonographers and fellows within the facility's physical space and daily workflow? Where and how are the studies reviewed?

Equipment

Equipment maintenance, software, and safety practices certainly play important roles in the provision of quality services. How many echo machines does the facility have? Are the machines old or new? Is all the necessary software for the machines and for the digital echo system updated to the most recent version? Are all the machines and other equipment compliant with standards from The Joint Commission? Are they compliant with IAC standards?

Staff

Lastly, staffing indicators involve individual responsibilities and workload in the context of established benchmarks. Are the clinical and administrative responsibilities clearly delineated within the echo lab? Who manages the workflow? Who provides supervision? Are there system checks to assure that workload is not excessive and not associated with increased errors? Does the echo lab meet established benchmarks in terms of staffing responsibilities and workload?

Process Indicators

Process indicators involve the activities and tasks needed to provide quality echo services [3]. The components of an echo that serve as indexes of quality include *patient selection*, *study performance*, *study interpretation*, and *study reporting* [1].

Patient Selection

Quality assessment as it pertains to patient selection necessarily involves the reported indication and its appropriateness. In 2007, the ACC Foundation, ASE, and five other subspecialty societies published a report on appropriate use criteria (AUC) for transthoracic and transesophageal echo studies in adults organized by indication categories and based on specific methodology developed by the RAND Corporation and researchers from the University of California, Los Angeles [4]. Only 4 years later, the same group along with three additional organizations drafted a revised AUC document to include criteria for stress echo, to account for changes in clinical practice and test utilization patterns, and to address deficiencies in the original publication [5]. Combining evidence-based medicine and practice experience data during the vetting process, the new document lists over 20 categories and almost 100 indications for transthoracic echo, each one categorized as appropriate, inappropriate, or uncertain criteria, and it has become an important component of the IAC guidelines and standards for adult echo. A similar document does not exist for pediatric echo, mostly because of the potential for a significantly extensive list of indications, especially if the criteria need to be specific for each CHD. Interestingly, the 2011 document lists 7 indications for adult CHD with only 4 being labeled as appropriate.

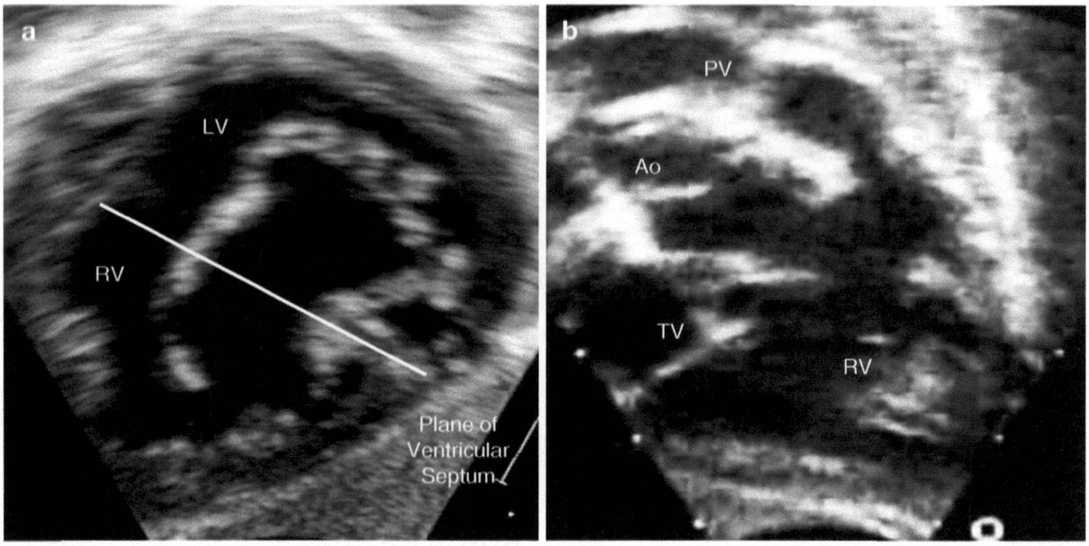

Fig. 14.1 Non-standard echocardiographic views for specific lesions: (**a**) "en face" or "in-between" view in subcostal windows of a complete atrioventricular canal depicting a cross-section en face view of the common atrioventricular valve, usually obtained at a plane between the long-axis and short-axis subcostal view; (**b**) right axial oblique view in subcostal windows of tetralogy of Fallot depicting the right ventricular inflow and outflow as well as the anterior deviation of the conal septum, usually obtained with counterclockwise rotation of the probe from the standard long-axis subcostal view (*Ao* aorta, *LV* left ventricle, *PV* pulmonary valve, *RV* right ventricle, *TV* tricuspid valve)

Study Performance

Another important indicator involves study performance, which is determined primarily by established guidelines and standards, individual lab protocols, and sonographer knowledge. Publications outlining recommendations based on expert consensus certainly provide a framework in which to assess study performance quality. Over the last 4 years, the ASE has published over 15 guidelines documents encompassing such topics as diastolic function [6], prosthetic valves [7], right heart evaluation [8], cardiac mechanics [9], and 3-dimensional echo [10], but all of these documents pertain only to studies performed in adults. Nevertheless, the ASE has published 5 pediatric documents since 2004 establishing recommendations pertaining to the performance of a pediatric echo [11], quantification methods during a pediatric echo [12], performance of a pediatric transesophageal echo [13], performance of a fetal echo [14], and targeted studies in the Neonatal Intensive Care Unit [15].

Study performance within an echo lab is dependent on protocols that are based on published guidelines and standards, but the specific contents of the protocols must be established in the context of local culture, clinical practice, and experience. Many centers have developed lesion-specific echo protocols in an effort to prevent sonographers from forgetting the most important aspect of each lesion during the performance of a study, definitely contributing to quality echo services.

General and local algorithms for study performance enhance sonographer knowledge, but this knowledge also depends on experience and education. It definitely requires experience to know when non-standard views are needed to evaluate specific lesions, such as complete atrioventricular canal defects or tetralogy of Fallot (Fig. 14.1). From an education standpoint, all sonographers must attend ultrasound school, but only a few schools have established a specific pediatric or congenital curriculum. Hence most sonographers begin working in a pediatric echo lab with minimal knowledge and experience, and

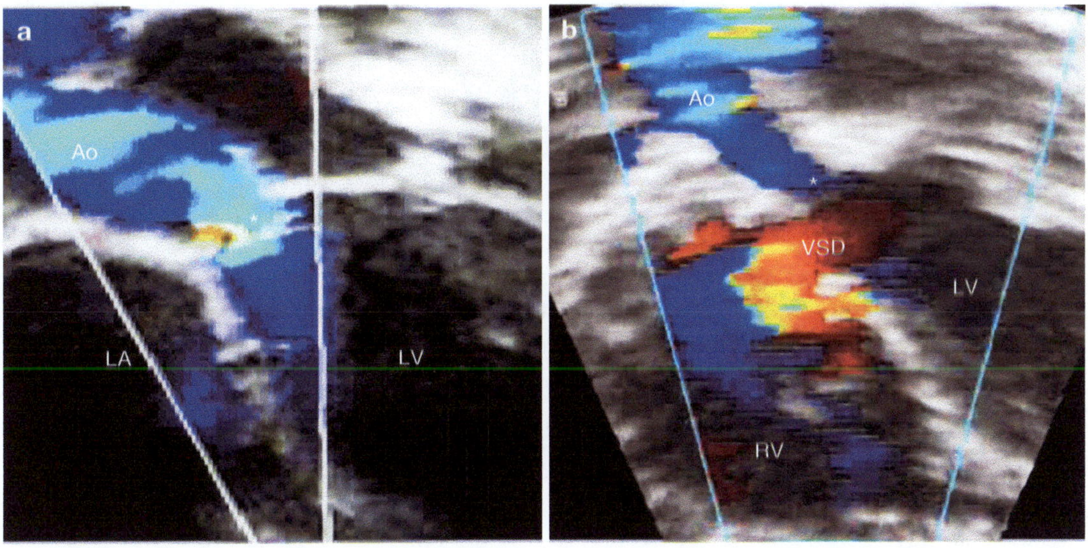

Fig. 14.2 Variable echocardiographic presentation of subvalvar aortic stenosis based on the pathophysiology and associated anomalies: (**a**) isolated subvalvar aortic stenosis (*star*) revealing turbulence in flow along the area of obstruction; (**b**) subvalvar aortic stenosis (*star*) in association with a ventricular septal defect, an interrupted aortic arch, and a large patent ductus arteriosus (the last two lesions are not shown) revealing absence of turbulence along the subaortic region because of left-to-right flow at the ventricular septal defect and right-to-left flow at the patent ductus arteriosus; in this instance, there is still significant obstruction along the subaortic region despite the absence of turbulence because of the pathophysiology of the associated lesions (*Ao* aorta, *LA* left atrium, *LV* left ventricle, *RV* right ventricle, *VSD* ventricular septal defect)

their improvement is usually dependent on learning from senior sonographers and physicians. In addition, the infrastructure must ensure continuing education with regular didactic sessions at the center as well as at local, regional, and national conferences.

Study Interpretation

Physician knowledge is the most crucial determinant of quality interpretation of studies. As with sonographer knowledge, this is dependent on education and experience. The Accreditation Council for Graduate Medical Education (ACGME) is fairly specific in terms of the body of knowledge needed during the training of pediatric cardiology fellows [16]. In addition, the ACC Foundation, AHA, and American Academy of Pediatrics (AAP) have established training guidelines for pediatric noninvasive cardiac imaging with very specific goals for core and advanced imaging skills [17]. In fact, many of the major clinical centers in North America have developed 4th year advanced imaging fellowships for trainees who want to focus specifically on echo or some other aspects of noninvasive imaging.

The role of experience in developing physician knowledge cannot be stressed enough. Experience allows one to understand how variants of abnormal physiology can have different effects on abnormal morphology, such as the presentation of subaortic stenosis as a solitary lesion or in association with a ventricular septal defect and an interrupted aortic arch (Fig. 14.2). Experience is crucial in the diagnosis of rare anomalies such as a persistent 5th arch or a retro-aortic innominate vein (Fig. 14.3). In fact, the ACGME as well as the IAC and other regulatory bodies are quite specific in terms of the target number of studies for trainees prior to graduating from a fellowship program and for echo physicians as part of the echo lab accreditation process [1, 16, 18].

The quality of study interpretation is also determined by validation activities within an

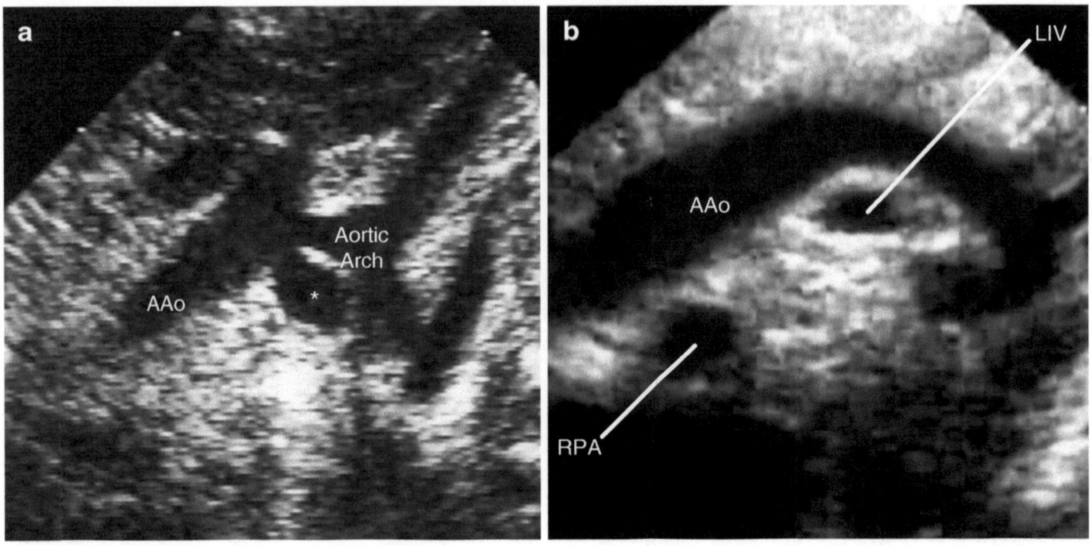

Fig. 14.3 Rare anomalies: (**a**) persistent 5th aortic arch (*star*) revealing two aortic arches coursing from right to left (in contrast with a double aortic arch where one arch courses to the right and the other to the left); (**b**) retro-aortic innominate vein which courses behind the ascending aorta and is seen as two vessels in cross-section below the aortic arch in suprasternal long-axis views (the second vessel is the right pulmonary artery) (*AAo* ascending aorta, *LIV* left innominate vein, *RPA* right pulmonary artery)

echo lab to evaluate the accuracy and repeatability of echo findings and measurements. Many reports have been published comparing echo diagnoses with data from other modalities (such as cardiac magnetic resonance imaging, computed tomography imaging, and cardiac catheterization) as well as findings in the operating room during surgery [19–22]. More recently, other publications have evaluated multi-acquisition, intra-observer, and inter-observer variability for echo measurements and have shown that some measurements are more prone to poor repeatability than others, even with multiple heart beat averaging [23]. The IAC has developed specific recommendations for quarterly correlation assessments (to compare echo findings in specific instances with results from other modalities and from the operating room) and variability assessments (to evaluate the repeatability of specific measurements performed during an echo) [18].

Study Reporting

The reporting of echo findings has certainly been fraught with problems, particularly in terms of the inconsistent terminology and coding systems for CHD. Controversies in nomenclature originate partly from the different approaches used to describe the morphology of cardiac malformations and their variants, such as seen with heterotaxy syndrome [24]. In the current era of digital echo, individual diagnoses and procedures are coded within the structured reporting platform of each system, and the organization of codes is usually customizable and frequently based on consumer preference. Therefore, although databases of echo diagnoses have been established at individual institutions, the ability to share data between centers can be quite limited, especially if each center uses a different digital echo vendor and creates its own customized structured reporting platform. The varied and heterogeneous coding systems that are currently in use include multiple American and European codes created by pediatric cardiology or cardiac surgical organizations, codes from the 9th, 10th, or 11th revision of the International Classification of Diseases (ICD-9, ICD-10, or ICD-11) developed by the World Health Organization, and the Current Procedural Terminology (CPT) codes established by the American Medical

Association. Efforts by the ISNPCHD to cross-match these codes have resulted in the International Pediatric and Congenital Cardiac Code, which now provides a framework in which to establish a common diagnostic and procedural coding system [25, 26].

Another issue relevant to quality reporting involves the standardization of reports within an institution, usually involving a description of relevant positive and negative findings organized in a segmental fashion, a list of all measurements along with reference values based on the patient's age and body size, a summary of the patient's clinical history, and a hierarchical summary of the important findings during the evaluation. In addition, local standards must be established in terms of turnaround time (time from study completion to report completion), reporting of critical findings to relevant health care providers, automatic distribution of reports to appropriate physicians and inpatient locations within the institution, and their incorporation into the medical records. Again the IAC has developed specific recommendations and guidelines for study reporting that are important components of the accreditation process for an echo lab [18]. Lastly, reports should provide recommendations if other modalities are needed to establish or confirm a diagnosis, thereby functioning as the 1st step in deciding what interventions if any are needed for a specific patient.

Outcome Indicators

Outcome indicators evaluate the states of health or events resulting from quality echo services, and these generally refer to death, disease, discomfort, disability, and dissatisfaction [3]. The QI initiatives must follow caveats established by the Institute of Medicine, specifically that they are safe, effective, patient-centered, timely, efficient, and equitable [27]. Current QI initiatives in pediatric and congenital echo have involved *certification*, *productivity standards*, *AUC* for pediatric echo, *pediatric reference values* for standard echo measurements, and *quality metrics* specific to pediatric echo.

Certification

The process of assessing competency as well as adherence to established standards in pediatric and congenital echo has been addressed for sonographers, physicians, and echo labs. The two major organizations involved with sonographer certification in the United States are the American Registry for Diagnostic Medical Sonography and Cardiovascular Credentialing International. Both have recognized that the skills and knowledge necessary to be a congenital sonographer are different than those necessary in adult echo, thereby establishing distinct and specific registry requirements for those practicing pediatric and/or congenital echo. In addition, both organizations have developed qualifying examinations using rigorous psychometric methodology to certify congenital sonographers.

A similar certification process exists for physicians interpreting adult echo studies with a qualifying examination developed by the National Board of Echocardiography. However, a similar certification examination does not exist for physicians involved with pediatric echo in the United States. Interestingly, the EACVI has developed a CHD certification involving a written examination testing standard knowledge of pediatric and congenital echo as well as individual documentation of cumulative clinical experience with CHD [28]. Over the past 7 years, 90 registrants have been certified in CHD after passing the examination (which has a pass rate of approximately 75 %), submitting a logbook of CHD cases and direct observation reports of procedural skills.

The major organization involved with certification of echo labs in North America has been the IAC. Since its creation in 1996, it has developed and established minimum standards for accreditation of pediatric echo labs in terms of instrumentation; facility; procedure volume; indications, ordering, and scheduling; techniques; study components; interpretation and reporting; and quality assurance [18]. IAC statistics at the end of 2012 reveals over 3,000 accredited echo labs and almost 5,000 accredited sites, with 190 labs certified for pediatric transthoracic echo, 59 for pediatric transesophageal echo, and 98 for fetal echo.

Because of the successes of its own physician certification process as well as the work done by the IAC, the EACVI has recently established its own lab accreditation process, now having certified over 35 labs since 2009. However, an accreditation application for pediatric echo labs has not yet been established at this time.

Productivity Standards

Structural quality indicators include knowledge of benchmarks in terms of echo lab staffing responsibilities and workload. The IAC has required that each pediatric transthoracic echo study be allotted 45–60 min from patient encounter to departure [18], but data regarding optimal time allotment for study performance and interpretation are lacking. Recent efforts by members of the ASE Pediatric and CHD Council have involved a survey of North American pediatric echo labs and analysis of the data to establish productivity standards for centers caring for children with acquired and CHD. These standards include daily and annual data on sonographer and attending physician productivity as well as equipment and technological needs based on the total number of studies done at each site per year, findings that will be published in the near future.

Appropriate Use

Given the absence of AUC in pediatric echo and the potentially overwhelming challenge of creating a comprehensive list of lesion-specific indications, a recent initiative from the ACC AUC Task Force has focused on the more manageable task of identifying AUC for pediatric echo studies in the outpatient setting. Utilizing the RAND methodology and working in conjunction with the ASE, Society of Pediatric Echocardiography, and AAP, the writing group for this initiative has established indication categories, definitions, and assumptions involved with drafting the AUC. Indication categories include symptoms and signs such as palpitations, syncope, chest pain, and murmurs as well as family history and systemic disorders with cardiovascular manifestations. The list of indications, definitions, and assumptions is currently undergoing several rounds of review by an external expert panel, and the manuscript will be published in 2014. Once published, the document will serve as a framework for the development of other AUC in pediatric echo.

Reference Values

Study interpretation also involves the ability to distinguish normal measurements from abnormal ones, especially since many disease states can have a significant effect on the sizes of cardiovascular structures. However, the sizes of cardiovascular structures in children are affected by body size, age, gender, and race [29–31], and measurements should be adjusted for the effects of these confounders in order to determine normal reference values. A common tool used to present normal data involves Z-scores, which represent the number of standard deviations a measurement value is from the mean value for a particular parameter or set of parameters (such as body surface area, age, gender, and/or race). Currently available reference values have been established at single centers [32, 33] and are limited by relatively small sample sizes and a paucity of neonatal data [34], and most databases do not account for the effects of gender and race. In fact, Z-scores for a particular measurement and body size can vary significantly, dependent on which Z-score database one uses [34]. In an effort to address these limitations, the PHN, a multicenter program funded by the National Institutes of Health to evaluate issues in pediatric cardiology and cardiac surgery, has utilized the pediatric quantification guidelines [12] to develop a large multicenter database of measurements from normal children. This initiative will then establish universally available normal reference values (Z-scores) adjusted for the effects of body size, age, gender, and race.

Quality Metrics

The ACC has recently established a task force to measure QI in all aspects of pediatric cardiology, including a subgroup team to develop and define quality metrics in noninvasive imaging. The team has identified six areas in noninvasive imaging where quality assessment would be quite valuable, and the specifications for each metric are currently being drafted. The first metric involves comprehensive quantification of diagnostic echo errors within an institution using a recently published taxonomy system to categorize pediatric echo errors based on type, severity, preventability, and cause [35]. Most centers establish periodic QI meetings to discuss errors identified ad hoc during a specified period of time without a standard approach, and this quality metric should help centers organize the data. The other quality metrics include timing to report critical findings, adverse events during a sedated echo, variability in common echo measurements, study completeness, and image quality. Challenges to this initiative have included the paucity of published data and the fact that methodologies and technology are both evolving, often resulting in changes in the measurable parameters. The biggest issue for all metrics is feasibility: no one will use a metric which requires an unreasonable amount of time and manpower, especially in this era of limited resources. Lastly, each metric must be meaningful (the sample size must be big enough to represent the center's level of quality) and tied to outcomes.

Conclusions

There have been few QI initiatives in pediatric cardiac noninvasive imaging despite the significant attention that QI has received in the field of adult echocardiography. However, recent efforts by multiple pediatric and congenital organizations and societies (including the ASE, EACVI, ACC, and PHN) have resulted in increased QI activities. Quality indicators can be categorized as structural, process, or outcome indicators. Structural indicators involve components of the facility, equipment, and staff. Process indicators are related to patient selection as well as study performance, interpretation, and reporting. Current QI initiatives in pediatric and congenital echo fall in the realm of evaluating and addressing outcome indicators, and some of the more important ones include work with accreditation, productivity standards, AUC, normal reference values, and the development of quality metrics specific to pediatric and congenital noninvasive imaging.

References

1. Popescu BA, Andrade MJ, Badano LP, Fox KF, Flachskampf FA, Lancellotti P, et al. European Association of Echocardiography recommendations for training, competence, and quality improvement in echocardiography. Eur J Echocardiogr. 2009;10(8):893–905. Epub 2009/11/06.
2. Picard MH, Adams D, Bierig SM, Dent JM, Douglas PS, Gillam LD, et al. American Society of Echocardiography recommendations for quality echocardiography laboratory operations. J Am Soc Echocardiogr. 2011;24(1):1–10. Epub 2010/12/22.
3. Mainz J. Defining and classifying clinical indicators for quality improvement. Int J Qual Health Care. 2003;15(6):523–30. Epub 2003/12/09.
4. Douglas PS, Khandheria B, Stainback RF, Weissman NJ, Brindis RG, Patel MR, et al. ACCF/ASE/ACEP/ASNC/SCAI/SCCT/SCMR 2007 appropriateness criteria for transthoracic and transesophageal echocardiography: a report of the American College of Cardiology Foundation Quality Strategic Directions Committee Appropriateness Criteria Working Group, American Society of Echocardiography, American College of Emergency Physicians, American Society of Nuclear Cardiology, Society for Cardiovascular Angiography and Interventions, Society of Cardiovascular Computed Tomography, and the Society for Cardiovascular Magnetic Resonance. Endorsed by the American College of Chest Physicians and the Society of Critical Care Medicine. J Am Soc Echocardiogr. 2007;20(7):787–805. Epub 2007/07/10.
5. Douglas PS, Garcia MJ, Haines DE, Lai WW, Manning WJ, Patel AR, et al. ACCF/ASE/AHA/ASNC/HFSA/HRS/SCAI/SCCM/SCCT/SCMR 2011 appropriate use Criteria for echocardiography. A eport of the American College of Cardiology Foundation Appropriate Use Criteria Task Force, American Society of Echocardiography, American Heart Association, American Society of Nuclear Cardiology, Heart Failure Society of America, Heart Rhythm Society, Society for Cardiovascular Angiography and Interventions, Society of Critical Care Medicine, Society of Cardiovascular Computed Tomography, Society for Cardiovascular Magnetic Resonance American College of Chest Physicians. J Am Soc Echocardiogr. 2011;24(3):229–67.
6. Nagueh SF, Appleton CP, Gillebert TC, Marino PN, Oh JK, Smiseth OA, et al. Recommendations for the evaluation of left ventricular diastolic function by echocardiography. J Am Soc Echocardiogr. 2009;22(2):107–33.

7. Zoghbi WA, Chambers JB, Dumesnil JG, Foster E, Gottdiener JS, Grayburn PA, et al. Recommendations for evaluation of prosthetic valves with echocardiography and doppler ultrasound: a report From the American Society of Echocardiography's Guidelines and Standards Committee and the Task Force on Prosthetic Valves, developed in conjunction with the American College of Cardiology Cardiovascular Imaging Committee, Cardiac Imaging Committee of the American Heart Association, the European Association of Echocardiography, a registered branch of the European Society of Cardiology, the Japanese Society of Echocardiography and the Canadian Society of Echocardiography, endorsed by the American College of Cardiology Foundation, American Heart Association, European Association of Echocardiography, a registered branch of the European Society of Cardiology, the Japanese Society of Echocardiography, and Canadian Society of Echocardiography. J Am Soc Echocardiogr. 2009; 22(9):975–1014; quiz 82–4.
8. Rudski LG, Lai WW, Afilalo J, Hua L, Handschumacher MD, Chandrasekaran K, et al. Guidelines for the echocardiographic assessment of the right heart in adults: a report from the American Society of Echocardiography endorsed by the European Association of Echocardiography, a registered branch of the European Society of Cardiology, and the Canadian Society of Echocardiography. J Am Soc Echocardiogr. 2010;23(7):685–713; quiz 86–8. Epub 2010/07/14.
9. Mor-Avi V, Lang RM, Badano LP, Belohlavek M, Cardim NM, Derumeaux G, et al. Current and evolving echocardiographic techniques for the quantitative evaluation of cardiac mechanics: ASE/EAE consensus statement on methodology and indications endorsed by the Japanese Society of Echocardiography. J Am Soc Echocardiogr. 2011;24(3):277–313.
10. Lang RM, Badano LP, Tsang W, Adams DH, Agricola E, Buck T, et al. EAE/ASE recommendations for image acquisition and display using three-dimensional echocardiography. J Am Soc Echocardiogr. 2012;25(1): 3–46.
11. Lai WW, Geva T, Shirali GS, Frommelt PC, Humes RA, Brook MM, et al. Guidelines and standards for performance of a pediatric echocardiogram: a report from the Task Force of the Pediatric Council of the American Society of Echocardiography. J Am Soc Echocardiogr. 2006;19(12):1413–30.
12. Lopez L, Colan SD, Frommelt PC, Ensing GJ, Kendall K, Younoszai AK, et al. Recommendations for quantification methods during the performance of a pediatric echocardiogram: a report from the Pediatric Measurements Writing Group of the American Society of Echocardiography Pediatric and Congenital Heart Disease Council. J Am Soc Echocardiogr. 2010;23(5):465–95; quiz 576–7.
13. Ayres NA, Miller-Hance W, Fyfe DA, Stevenson JG, Sahn DJ, Young LT, et al. Indications and guidelines for performance of transesophageal echocardiography in the patient with pediatric acquired or congenital heart disease: report from the task force of the Pediatric Council of the American Society of Echocardiography. J Am Soc Echocardiogr. 2005;18(1):91–8. Epub 2005/01/08.
14. Rychik J, Ayres N, Cuneo B, Gotteiner N, Hornberger L, Spevak PJ, et al. American Society of Echocardiography guidelines and standards for performance of the fetal echocardiogram. J Am Soc Echocardiogr. 2004;17(7):803–10. Epub 2004/06/29.
15. Mertens L, Seri I, Marek J, Arlettaz R, Barker P, McNamara P, et al. Targeted Neonatal Echocardiography in the Neonatal Intensive Care Unit: practice guidelines and recommendations for training. Writing Group of the American Society of Echocardiography (ASE) in collaboration with the European Association of Echocardiography (EAE) and the Association for European Pediatric Cardiologists (AEPC). J Am Soc Echocardiogr. 2011; 24(10):1057–78.
16. ACGME. ACGME program requirements for graduate medical education in pediatric cardiology. Accreditation Council for Graduate Medical Education website; 2007.
17. Sanders SP, Colan SD, Cordes TM, Donofrio MT, Ensing GJ, Geva T, et al. ACCF/AHA/AAP recommendations for training in pediatric cardiology. Task force 2: pediatric training guidelines for noninvasive cardiac imaging endorsed by the American Society of Echocardiography and the Society of Pediatric Echocardiography. J Am Coll Cardiol. 2005;46(7): 1384–8.
18. IAC. The IAC standards and guidelines for pediatric echocardiography accreditation. Intersocietal Accreditation Commission website; 2013.
19. Margossian R, Schwartz ML, Prakash A, Wruck L, Colan SD, Atz AM, et al. Comparison of echocardiographic and cardiac magnetic resonance imaging measurements of functional single ventricular volumes, mass, and ejection fraction (from the Pediatric Heart Network Fontan Cross-Sectional Study). Am J Cardiol. 2009;104(3):419–28.
20. Soriano BD, Hoch M, Ithuralde A, Geva T, Powell AJ, Kussman BD, et al. Matrix-array 3-dimensional echocardiographic assessment of volumes, mass, and ejection fraction in young pediatric patients with a functional single ventricle: a comparison study with cardiac magnetic resonance. Circulation. 2008;117(14): 1842–8.
21. van den Bosch AE, Ten Harkel DJ, McGhie JS, Roos-Hesselink JW, Simoons ML, Bogers AJ, et al. Surgical validation of real-time transthoracic 3D echocardiographic assessment of atrioventricular septal defects. Int J Cardiol. 2006;112(2):213–8.
22. Sadagopan SN, Veldtman GR, Sivaprakasam MC, Keeton BR, Gnanapragasam JP, Salmon AP, et al. Correlations with operative anatomy of real time three-dimensional echocardiographic imaging of congenital aortic valvar stenosis. Cardiol Young. 2006; 16(5):490–4.

23. Colan SD, Shirali G, Margossian R, Gallagher D, Altmann K, Canter C, et al. The ventricular volume variability study of the Pediatric Heart Network: study design and impact of beat averaging and variable type on the reproducibility of echocardiographic measurements in children with chronic dilated cardiomyopathy. J Am Soc Echocardiogr. 2012;25(8):842–54 e6.
24. Cohen MS, Anderson RH, Cohen MI, Atz AM, Fogel M, Gruber PJ, et al. Controversies, genetics, diagnostic assessment, and outcomes relating to the heterotaxy syndrome. Cardiol Young. 2007;17 Suppl 2:29–43. Epub 2008/02/23.
25. Franklin RC, Jacobs JP, Tchervenkov CI, Beland MJ. Bidirectional crossmap of the Short Lists of the European Paediatric Cardiac Code and the International Congenital Heart Surgery Nomenclature and Database Project. Cardiol Young. 2002;12(5):431–5. Epub 2005/03/19.
26. Franklin RC, Jacobs JP, Krogmann ON, Beland MJ, Aiello VD, Colan SD, et al. Nomenclature for congenital and paediatric cardiac disease: historical perspectives and The International Pediatric and Congenital Cardiac Code. Cardiol Young. 2008;18 Suppl 2:70–80. Epub 2008/12/17.
27. IOM. Crossing the quality chasm: a new health system for the 21st century. Institute of Medicine website; 2001.
28. Mertens L, Miller O, Fox K, Simpson J. Certification in echocardiography of congenital heart disease: experience of the first 6 years of a European process. Eur Heart J Cardiovasc Imaging. 2013;14(2):142–8. Epub 2012/06/28.
29. Sluysmans T, Colan SD. Theoretical and empirical derivation of cardiovascular allometric relationships in children. J Appl Physiol. 2005;99(2):445–57.
30. Sarikouch S, Peters B, Gutberlet M, Leismann B, Kelter-Kloepping A, Koerperich H, et al. Sex-specific pediatric percentiles for ventricular size and mass as reference values for cardiac MRI: assessment by steady-state free-precession and phase-contrast MRI flow. Circ Cardiovasc Imaging. 2010;3(1):65–76. Epub 2009/10/13.
31. Lamers L, Ensing G, Pignatelli R, Goldberg C, Bezold L, Ayres N, et al. A prospective assessment of myocardial contractility in young African Americans: does ethnicity impact the wall stress-heart rate-corrected velocity of circumferential fiber shortening relationship? J Am Soc Echocardiogr. 2005;18(7):743–8. Epub 2005/07/09.
32. Zilberman MV, Khoury PR, Kimball RT. Two-dimensional echocardiographic valve measurements in healthy children: gender-specific differences. Pediatr Cardiol. 2005;26(4):356–60.
33. Pettersen MD, Du W, Skeens ME, Humes RA. Regression equations for calculation of z scores of cardiac structures in a large cohort of healthy infants, children, and adolescents: an echocardiographic study. J Am Soc Echocardiogr. 2008;21(8): 922–34.
34. Cantinotti M, Scalese M, Molinaro S, Murzi B, Passino C. Limitations of current echocardiographic nomograms for left ventricular, valvular, and arterial dimensions in children: a critical review. J Am Soc Echocardiogr. 2012;25(2):142–52.
35. Benavidez OJ, Gauvreau K, Jenkins KJ, Geva T. Diagnostic errors in pediatric echocardiography: development of taxonomy and identification of risk factors. Circulation. 2008;117(23):2995–3001. Epub 2008/06/04.

Improving Clinical Outcomes in Pediatric Cardiology

15

Shakeel A. Qureshi and Thomas Witter

Abstract

Quality in pediatric cardiology is in an evolving process where clinicians and researchers have access to large registries and databases allowing them to understand and develop more effective cardiac procedures, whilst monitoring outcomes. It is important that the information relating to outcomes is published and shared to ensure that this evolution continues and we learn from the shared international experiences. It is important that we incorporate the views and experiences of the patient and the families firmly into our quality measures and quality improvement program.

Keywords

Pediatric Cardiology • Quality • Clinical outcomes • Patient safety • Congenital heart disease

Introduction

Over the last 30 years, we have witnessed vast clinical improvements in patients with congenital heart disease. Many of these areas are discussed in more detail in other chapters, however, we will touch on them briefly, as improving clinical outcomes in pediatric cardiology is centred on bringing together each of these advances and applying them to patient care.

Clinical knowledge is one of the key elements of improving the outcomes of patients with congenital heart disease (CHD). The work done by morphologists in expanding our knowledge and

S.A. Qureshi, MBCHB, FRCP (✉)
Department of Congenital Heart Disease, Evelina London Children's Hospital, Westminster Bridge Road, London SE1 7EH, UK
e-mail: shakeel.qureshi@gstt.nhs.uk

T. Witter, RN (Child)
Department of Congenital Heart Disease, Evelina London Children's Hospital, Guy's and St Thomas' NHS Foundation Trust, Westminster Bridge Road, London SE1 7EH, UK
e-mail: thomas.witter@gstt.nhs.uk

P.R. Barach, J.P. Jacobs, S.E. Lipshultz, P.C. Laussen (eds.),
Pediatric and Congenital Cardiac Care: Volume 2: Quality Improvement and Patient Safety,
DOI 10.1007/978-1-4471-6566-8_15, © Springer-Verlag London 2015

understanding of congenital cardiac morphology has meant that operations and procedures are performed nowadays with less mortality, morbidity and fewer complications than previously. A vast number of case studies, series and original research articles have been produced over the last few decades and this research has covered topics from basic science through to longitudinal studies of disease cohorts. All have contributed to the wealth of knowledge, which is shared and used on a daily basis to deliver the best care for our patients.

Role of Databases and Registries

Collecting data on the outcome measures is a major undertaking and can only be supported with the use of databases and registries. Many countries around the world have national procedural databases or registries, which are fairly well developed and continue to develop with input from clinicians. They reflect the improvements in clinical outcomes over time and across nations. Some examples are data collected by the Society of Thoracic Surgeons [1] (STS) database in the United States or the EACTS [2], (European Association of Cardiothoracic Surgeons). The United Kingdom has a fully validated congenital procedural database, National Congenital Heart Disease Audit (NCHDA), which has been in place since 2000. The output of this database has been in the public domain and the information generated has led to improvements in pediatric cardiology. This can be seen as more resources have been allocated to antenatal diagnosis. More children and infants, who require surgery in the first year of life, are now diagnosed antenatally. This great improvement however, is not uniform across the whole of United Kingdom [3] (Fig. 15.1).

A funnel plot showing performance by UK regions suggests that the London region is performing better but in actual fact there are pockets of large quality variation and uneven detection as seen in Fig. 15.2. When we look at improving quality, there is a clear target for our energy and limited resources to drive improvements in a more focussed way.

The major limitation of many of these databases is that they focus only on those patients, who have operative or interventional procedures. Most nations do not have comprehensive congenital heart disease registries. This information is often held in local unit systems only, as a result of which we lack a true understanding of the real disease burden. This issue has a real impact as it

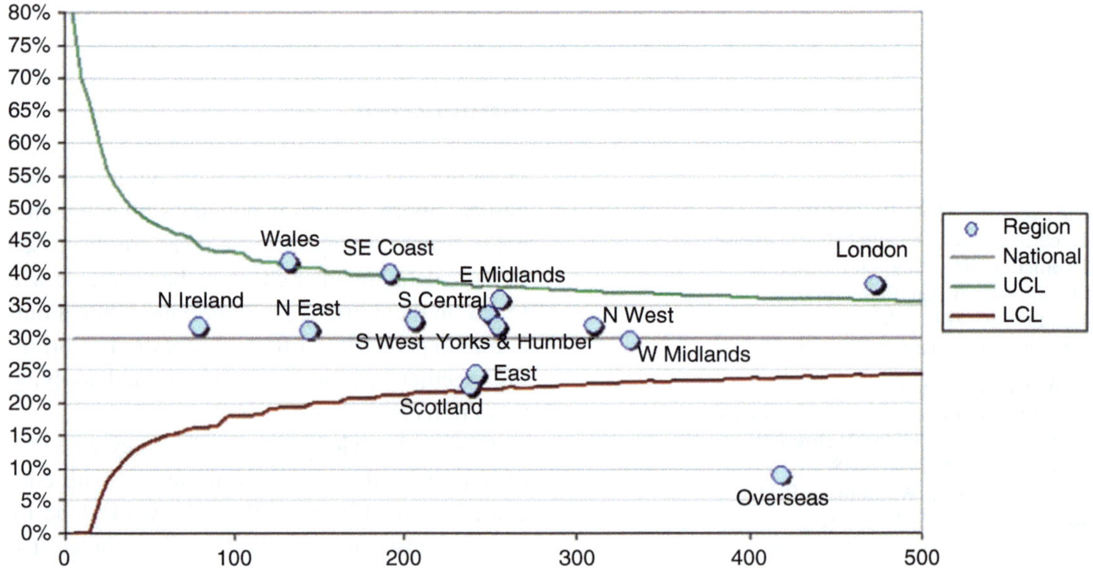

Fig. 15.1 Antenatal Funnel plot by UK region for the financial year 2010–2011

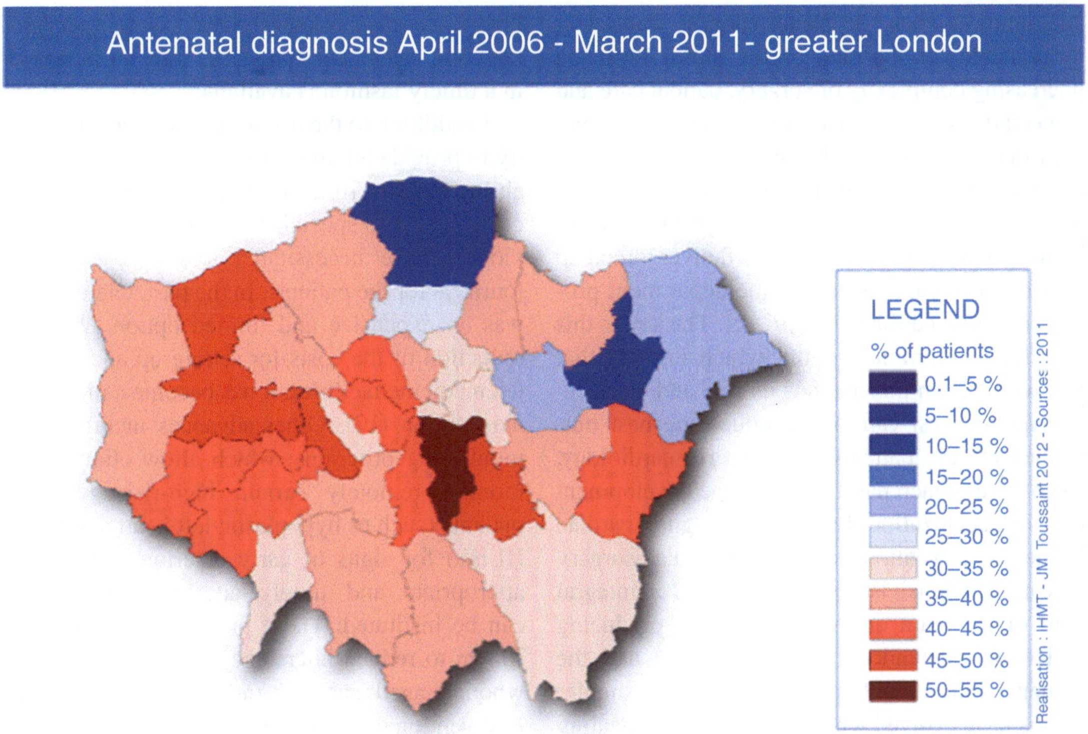

Fig. 15.2 Antenatal diagnosis in greater London between 2006 and 2011. This figure demonstrates the variation of antenatal diagnosis in Greater London

limits our understanding of the true epidemiology of the congenital heart disease and the impact over the patient lifetime. Sweden acknowledged this deficiency a few years ago and amended its registries for GUCH (Grown-up Congenital Heart Disease) and surgery, to include all children with congenital heart disease (Swedcon) [4] to answer the questions about lifelong illness and its burden. In its annual report in 2011, the Swedcon registry identified 35,974 patients in its registry, 6,125 patients, who should have been seen in a GUCH centre, but had not done so. This represents 17 % of the total in the Swedcon registry. This information is of vital importance in ensuring ongoing good quality of care [5]. No information is available, on how many of these patients may have moved overseas or who may have died in the period during transition.

Clinicians have recognized the need for standard nomenclature for both surgical and diagnostic coding. During the early part of the last decade, clinicians worked together to cross-map and define a common coding set, which combined several European and North American nomenclatures into one which is the International Pediatric and Congenital Cardiac Code (IPCCC) [6, 7]. This harmonisation has allowed international collaborators from STS, EACTS and NCHDA to work on comparing outcomes for surgical and interventional procedures [8].

In-hospital care has significantly changed since the 1980s. These changes have delivered improvements for patients in pediatric cardiology based around three key areas:

- Teamwork
- Technology
- Quality of Care

Care in hospitals is delivered to the patients by many teams from different specialities, all working together to deliver excellent healthcare. Gone are the days when one doctor/surgeon was solely responsible for the care of the child. With the increasing complexity of surgery, patient care and expectations, the success stories are in no small part due to the comprehensive and co-ordinated working of many different specialities. It is common practice in major units for **multidisciplinary teams** to meet, discuss, plan and deliver joined up co-ordinated care, as can by the department profiles of major cardiac units [9–12]. The key to this is effective communication, which ensures that the whole team understands its role and works to deliver the best care and produce the best outcomes for the patients. In pediatric cardiology, such an approach has also led to the development of subspecialization. Experts in imaging, cardiac catheter interventions, congenital cardiac surgery & cardiac intensivists have all become an integral part of the team delivering care and producing outcomes demanded by the regulators and the patients. Indeed, within each subspecialty, smaller teams have evolved who become adept at dealing with more rare defects. In parallel, there has been the development of clinical skills within the nursing teams, whose roles are often developed through specific university courses and clinical based competencies.

Improvement in **technology** has occurred almost hand in hand with the development of multidisciplinary team working. Technology influences every aspect of the delivery of care. Over the last 30 years, major advances have been seen in imaging. Currently, three-dimensional echocardiography, magnetic resonance imaging and computerized tomography are routinely used and are rapidly replacing the need for cardiac catheterisations for the purposes of diagnosis in many units. Surgeons in particular and interventional cardiologists have achieved greater understanding from these imaging modalities of the complex defects they treat. Furthermore, image storage has moved from videotapes to CD/DVD technology and digital server based archiving, which ensures that images are available, whenever and wherever they are needed. In the internet age, for the clinicians in the United Kingdom, the ability to share secure images through the National Health Service (UK) Image Exchange Portal, a secure transfer portal via an encrypted network, has meant that secure transfer of images in a timely fashion is available.

In addition to the use of the internet is the ability to provide telemedicine. Telemedicine has the ability to allow rural communities and local clinicians access to specialist advice, which may previously have necessitated long and expensive journeys for the patients. In the past, telemedicine was an expensive and limited option. With the reduction of the costs for setting up and running telemedicine facilities, it has become a more realistic option [13]. Other advances include home monitoring programs, which allow clinicians to monitor remotely certain high-risk group of patients (such as hypoplastic left heart syndrome, HLHS) for signs of early deterioration, so that appropriate and timely admission/intervention can be instituted. These programmes have been shown to reduce interstage mortality in cases in whom staged surgical management is needed. Interventional cardiology was in its infancy 30 years ago. With technological advances, all types of devices, in different shapes and sizes, are available to treat many cardiac defects. Cardiac pacemakers have developed over a similar period with improvements in their battery life and size, resulting in the ability to treat more patients from an earlier age. In the last decade, other advances such as hybrid procedures have allowed the highest risk patients to undergo palliative combined surgical/interventional procedures with lower associated risks. Transcatheter valve implantation is a clear improvement in quality of care, by reducing the number of open heart procedures a patient may have over the lifetime and by avoiding the need for anticoagulation therapy, with its associated complications.

Videoconferencing technology has become a mainstream tool and has allowed clinicians to connect and discuss patients with all of the information and many of the commercial systems available incorporate content sharing. Obtaining a second opinion of a patient can now be done in the virtual presence of colleagues anywhere in the world. This has to be to the greater benefit of the patients and to the increasing expertise and learning of experts.

Quality of Care

When looking at quality improvements, many of us think of outcomes in terms of mortality from the procedures and this is a well-established marker nationally and internationally. However due to differences in the datasets, comparisons between international cohorts may be more difficult. The UK national database is the only one in the world, which has an annual validation of the complete procedural activity. Work aimed at harmonising and collaborating across international borders is in its infancy. Technological advances have led to the ability to treat more severe and serious defects, but at a cost both to the healthcare services and to families. Over the last two decades, healthcare providers have been forced to deliver higher quality services within an ever decreasing healthcare budget. Length of hospital stay has a significant impact as longer lengths of stay may mean an increased risk of hospital-acquired infections, in addition to an increase in costs. Low rates of hospital acquired infections such as methicillin resistant staphylococcus aureus (MRSA) may be seen as a gross marker of good quality.

Similar analogies may be applied within pediatric cardiology to post-operative complications, such as the rates of surgical site infections and readmission to intensive care units after previous treatment. We are still faced with the global issue of consensus of how to measure these critical quality measures and to obtain sufficient data to deliver continued improvements in this speciality. Registries such as CCISC and IMPACT in USA form the beginning of this work [14, 15].

International registries help to provide the global answers to the outcomes and complications but most units have their own adverse incident reporting systems. These systems and internal audit systems form the backbone of the governance structures, which will deliver local changes and improvements. Therefore, it is important that pediatric cardiac units have sufficient access to resources to analyse outcomes locally. The analysis should be reported to the clinical teams on a regular basis and any adverse trends must be scrutinised in a more formal and structured way. Fundamental to this type of governance is the willingness and commitment of the team to learn from processes of care and to do things differently.

Local initiatives may focus on the way congenital services are delivered eg, single-plane catheter laboratories have been displaced by biplane laboratories and more and more are being replaced by hybrid laboratories. These changes may at least indirectly have contributed to reduction in procedure times and radiation exposure, which over the life of these patients with congenital heart defects may be of considerable importance.

National quality initiatives are much more difficult to implement, as these are often aimed at the rationalisation or centralisation of services. Long standing efforts to centralise pediatric cardiac care in Sweden have successfully reduced the number of surgical centres to two. Following a formal process in 2008, these units have a 5 year license to perform surgery and are required to submit annual reports, including medical data and indicators of quality of care [16, 17]. It may be too early to tell if this has led to a sustainable improvement in the quality of care. In the UK, a similar rationalisation has been recommended several times in the last 20 years and a further attempt has been underway again since 2009, with the aim to make all of the units in the UK safe and sustainable [18]. At the time of writing, this process has been replaced with a new review looking at joined up care from the fetus through to adult congenital heart services [19].

Quality outcomes in pediatric cardiology should not be limited to the patients experience, whilst receiving treatment in our institutions, but to the experience throughout the whole of their life. The quality of life the patients achieve should be a major source of information, which should help to deliver the quality of services required. It is vital that improvements in care are delivered by the use of learned knowledge, technology and with the crucial input of patients and parents, thus ensuring that their voice and the issues that are at the heart of their everyday life are not forgotten. This can be done by ensuring that patients are asked for their opinions on how to improve their care and the use of focus groups and patient or parent questionnaires. Clinicians around the world have developed systems to determine the quality of life of the patients [20] and these will continue to provide new information, which will help to inform clinicians and families about the risks posed from certain diagnosis and procedures [15, 21–23].

Conclusions

Quality improvement firmly embedded into the current healthcare services. The use of registries and databases ensure that lessons can be shared on both national and international scales. Technology, so long at the heart of congenital service delivery, continues to change the way services are provided, with more minimally invasive procedures available, remote monitoring, better imaging, all to the benefit of patients, The challenge ahead is delivering on issues that matter to the patients. The use of patient questionnaires and feedback will influence the design and delivery of services. Improvement in quality over the last 30 years are vast, as more children survive cardiac surgery and interventions and live longer and healthier lives than ever before, but now is not the time to sit back on our laurels, as the quality journey has only just begun.

References

1. The Society of Thoracic Surgeons. Quality, research & patient safety. Available at: http://www.sts.org/quality-research-patient-safety. Accessed 28 May 2014.
2. European Association for Cardio-thoracic Surgery. EACTS congenital database. Available at: http://www.eactscongenitaldb.org/index.php?LANG=en&level=1&struct=1. Accessed 28 May 2014.
3. National Institute for Cardiovascular Outcomes Research. Antenatal diagnosis. Available at: https://nicor4.nicor.org.uk/CHD/an_paeds.nsf/vwContent/Antenatal%20Diagnosis?Opendocument. Accessed 26 Aug 2013.
4. Swedcon. Årsrapporter. Available at: http://www.ucr.uu.se/swedcon/index.php/arsrapporter. Accessed 21 Aug 2013. [Translations courtesy of Dr PetruLiuba, Lund.]
5. Sanders SP. Quality in paediatric cardiology. Paediatr Child Health. 2009;19 Suppl 2:S96–7.
6. Franklin RCG, Jacobs JP, Tchervenkov CI, et al. The International Nomenclature Project for Pediatric and Congenital Heart Disease: Bidirectional crossmap of the short lists of the European Paediatric Cardiac Code and the International Congenital Heart Surgery Nomenclature and Database Project. Cardiol Young. 2002;12:431–5.
7. Gaynor JW, Jacobs JP, Jacobs ML, et al. Congenital heart surgery nomenclature and database project: update and proposed data harvest. Ann Thorac Surg. 2002;73(3):1016–8.
8. Jacobs J, Jacobs M, Austin III E. Quality measures for congenital and pediatric cardiac surgery. World J Pediatr Congenit Heart Surg. 2012;3(1):32–47.
9. Joy BF, Elliot E, Hardy C, et al. Standardized multidisciplinary protocol improves handover of cardiac surgery patients to the intensive care unit. Pediatr Crit Care Med. 2011;12:304–8.
10. UAB Medicine. Congenital heart disease overview. Available at: http://www.uabmedicine.org/conditions-and-services/heart-disease-congenital-overview. Accessed 10 Apr 2014.
11. Cedars-Sinai. Pediatric cardiothoracic program. Available at: http://cedars-sinai.edu/Patients/Programs-and-Services/Heart-Institute/Centers-and-Programs/Pediatric-Cardiothoracic-Program/. Accessed 10 Apr 2014.
12. All Childrens Hospital. The All Children's Hospital Heart Center: multidisciplinary care. Available at: http://www.allkids.org/heartsurgeon_new.cfm?id=1861. Accessed 10 Apr 2014.
13. Building Better Healthcare. Telemedicine revolutionises surgical care at London hospital. Available at: http://www.buildingbetterhealthcare.co.uk/news/article_page/Telemedicine_revolutionises_surgical_care_at_London_hospital/95573. Accessed 10 Apr 2014.
14. Martin GR, Beekman RH, Ing FF, et al. The IMPACT registry: improving pediatric and adult congenital treatments. Semin Thorac Cardiovasc Surg Pediatr Card Surg Annu. 2010;13(1):20–5.
15. Holzer R, Qureshi S, Ghasemi A, et al. Stenting of aortic coarctation: acute, intermediate and long-term results of a prospective multi-institutional registry – Congenital Cardiovascular Interventional Study Consortium (CCISC). Catheter Cardiovasc Interv. 2010;76:553–63.
16. Socialstyrelsen. National Specialised Medical Care. Available at: http://www.socialstyrelsen.se/national-specialisedmedicalcare. Accessed 10 Apr 2014.
17. Hanseus K. Heart of the matter. Available at: http://horizon2020projects.com/sc-health-profile/heart-of-the-matter/. Accessed 10 Apr 2014.
18. NHS Specialised Services, Safe and Sustainable. A new vision for children's congenital heart services in England. Available at: http://www.webarchive.org.uk/wayback/archive/20130325152925/http://www.specialisedservices.nhs.uk/library/30/Safe_and_Sustainable___A_New_Vision_for_Childrens_Congenital_Heart_Services_in_England_Consultation_Document_1.pdf.
19. NHS England. New review of congenital heart services. Available at: http://www.england.nhs.uk/wp-content/uploads/2013/07/180713-item13.pdf. Accessed 28 May 2014.

20. Marino BS, Shera D, Wernovsky G, et al. The development of the pediatric cardiac quality of life inventory: a quality of life measure for children and adolescents with heart disease. Qual Life Res. 2008;17(4):613–26.
21. Pagel C, Uttley M, Crowe S, et al. Real time monitoring of risk-adjusted paediatric cardiac surgery outcomes using variable life-adjusted display: implementation in three UK centres. Heart. 2013;99:1445–50. Epub 2013 Apr 5.
22. NICOR. Congenital heart disease website. Available at: https://nicor4.nicor.org.uk/CHD/an_paeds.nsf/vwContent/home?Opendocument. Accessed 28 May 2014.
23. Mavroudis C, Mavroudis CD, Jacobs JP, et al. Procedure-based complications to guide informed consent: analysis of Society of Thoracic Surgeons Congenital Heart Surgery Database. Ann Thorac Surg. 2014;97(5):1838–51. pii: S0003-4975(14)00020-4. doi: 10.1016/j.athoracsur.2013.12.037.

The Impact of Continuous Quality Improvement on Pediatric Cardiac Surgery

16

Erle H. Austin III

Abstract

The recognition that outcomes in pediatric cardiac surgery were in need of closer assessment became evident in the early 1990s. The courageous disclosure by a prominent congenital heart surgeon of a cluster of surgical failures and the forced closure of two separate pediatric heart surgery programs suggested that more vigilance was required for this highly specialized area of surgery. The development of registry databases in Europe and North America for congenital heart surgery patients is described. The maturation of these databases and the development of a common nomenclature and risk stratification scheme are also reviewed. Now that pediatric cardiac surgery outcomes are being tracked reliably, significant variation in these outcomes within and between centers has become evident, especially with higher risk procedures. Strategies to address this variation and to improve the quality of pediatric heart surgery are discussed.

Keywords

Quality improvement • Pediatric • Congenital • Cardiac surgery • Heart surgery • Bristol report • Manitoba affair • Databases • Nomenclature • Risk stratification • Variation • Learning collaboratives

Assessing Quality

Quality improvement begins with accurate quality assessment. The concept of assessing medical quality goes back as far as Florence Nightingale in the 1850s when she proposed evaluating outcomes of war casualties in the Crimean War [1]. In 1913 Earnest Codman a surgeon at the Massachusetts General Hospital recognized the importance of tracking outcomes of surgical

E.H. Austin III , MD
Department of Surgery, Kosair Children's Hospital, Louisville, KY, USA

Department Cardiothoracic Surgery, University of Louisville, 201 Abraham Flexner Way, Suite 1200, Louisville, KY 40202, USA
e-mail: eaustin@louisvilleheartsurgery.com

P.R. Barach, J.P. Jacobs, S.E. Lipshultz, P.C. Laussen (eds.),
Pediatric and Congenital Cardiac Care: Volume 2: Quality Improvement and Patient Safety,
DOI 10.1007/978-1-4471-6566-8_16, © Springer-Verlag London 2015

procedures and introduced the "End Result Idea" [2]. Unfortunately his colleagues not only did not embrace his ideas but actually got him fired and run out of town. Few medical providers followed the concept of regularly measuring outcomes. Whether this disinterest in monitoring results was because variability in outcomes was not suspected or because some providers feared exposure of poor outcomes is not clear. Nevertheless, it was not until the mid-1960s that Avedis Donabedian, a physician at the University of Michigan, rekindled interest in medical outcomes. Donabedian introduced the field of health systems research and recommended that health care quality be evaluated in terms of structure, process, and outcomes.

Assessing Quality in Cardiac Surgery

Almost simultaneously with the development of health systems research, the field of cardiac surgery arose. In the early days of heart surgery, procedures were relatively few and mortality as high as 100 %, consistent with the often desperate conditions of those patients. Good outcomes were hoped for but uniformly unexpected. The emphasis at the time was more on achieving survival than on measuring quality. The field of cardiac surgery did mature, however, with improving results in adults with valve and coronary artery disease and in children with uncomplicated congenital heart defects. As the practice of cardiac surgery improved, the number of procedures increased significantly. Coronary artery bypass grafting became one of the most commonly performed surgical procedures in the world. As heart surgery became commonly accepted practice it was recognized that a reliable measure of quality was the ability of the patient to survive the operation. Whether a patient lives or dies after an operation is clearly definable with limited subjectivity [3, 4]. This measure can be compared to the same measure at other institutions or to an overall benchmark. In the 1970s and 1980s cardiac surgery centers would typically monitor their own mortality rates to assure "acceptable" outcomes. Unfortunately those subjective outcome reports were rarely shared between centers and often only disclosed in the form of a publication when a center was proud of exceptionally good results. Such mortality rates were unlikely to be representative of the majority of centers performing heart surgery and individual centers were uncertain of what an "acceptable" mortality should be. In 1987 the Health Care Financing Administration published the mortality rates for Medicare recipients undergoing coronary artery bypass surgery. A striking variation in mortality was revealed and many heart surgery programs were embarrassed [5]. Cardiac surgeons began to recognize with this public release of sensitive information from individual centers the importance of keeping track of their results. The Society of Thoracic Surgeons began to develop an Adult Cardiac Surgery Database. The purpose was to invite centers to submit their own data confidentially in a way that each center could assess its own outcomes and compare them to the outcomes of the other submitting centers. This form of registry data more accurately represented outcomes across multiple centers and permitted the setting of realistic benchmarks and outcome targets.

Lessons Learned in Pediatric Cardiac Surgery

Although many cardiac surgeons in the late 1980s performed both adult and pediatric heart surgery, the emphasis in pediatric cardiac surgery at that time was more related to achieving survival in some of the smallest patients with complex life threatening heart defects than to the overall assessment of quality. Outcomes were highly variable and complex malformations almost uniformly had bad outcomes. The concept of continuous quality assessment that was beginning to take hold for adult cardiac surgery had not taken hold in the world of pediatric heart surgery.

That attitude began to change with a courageous presentation by Marc de Leval at the 1993 meeting of the American Association for Thoracic Surgery. At that meeting de Leval presented an "Analysis of a cluster of surgical

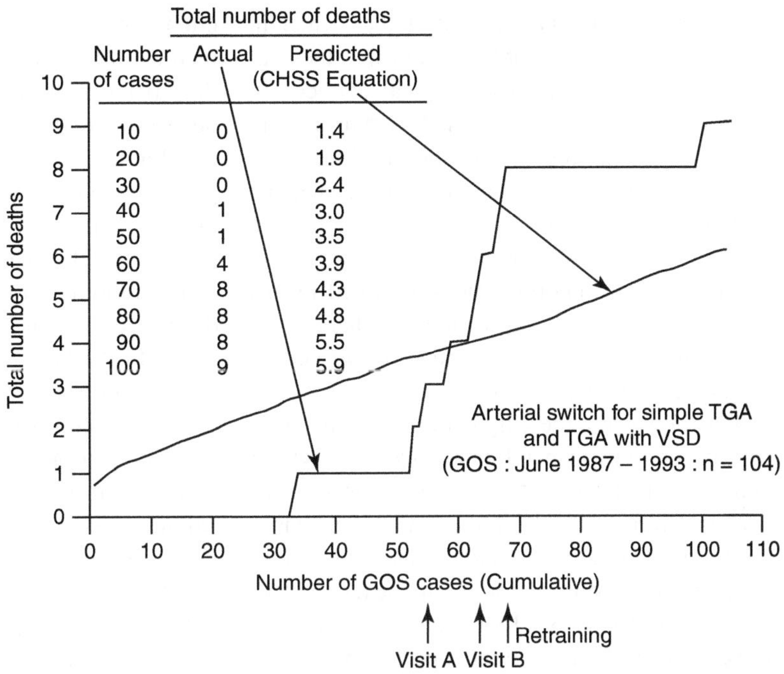

Fig. 16.1 Figure taken from de Leval et al., 1994, demonstrates cumulative sum (CUSUM) technique charting deaths as they occurred with comparison to a predicted rate determined by the Congenital Heart Surgeons' Society (CHSS). If this type of continuous monitoring had been in place at Great Ormand Street (GOS) during this experience the abrupt change in failure rate would have been recognized earlier (*Abbreviations*: *TGA* transposition of great arteries, *VSD* ventricular septal defect) (Reprinted from de Leval et al. [6], with permission from Elsevier)

failures" in which he described his own experience with the neonatal arterial switch operation [6] (Fig. 16.1). Having experienced only one death in his first 52 arterial switch procedures, he was troubled by the occurrence of seven deaths in 16 subsequent cases. After losing patient no. 53 and no. 55 he "instinctively" sensed concern and visited another center known for low mortality in an effort to derive insights into his unanticipated significant change in outcomes. After losing patient no. 59, no. 63, and no. 64 he revisited the same institution. After patient no. 67 and no. 68 died, he ceased performance of the procedure at his own institution and did not resume it until he had retrained at a third institution. Upon resumption at his own institution he experienced only one death in his next 35 arterial switches. His retrospective "analysis" examined the full experience of 104 consecutive arterial switch operations in an effort to determine if the "cluster of failures" could have occurred by chance alone, and, if not, could the unfavorable trend have been detected earlier. In his manuscript, de Leval describes two techniques for identifying worrisome trends: the CUSUM procedure (cumulative sum) [7] and comparison to benchmarks derived from multicenter data [8]. Looking retrospectively with those techniques he indicated that had "a mechanism of continuous monitoring…been in place" at his institution the decision to retrain would have been reached sooner. By bravely divulging his own experience with failure and proposing techniques to detect failure early, de Leval deserves the credit for introducing quality assessment and quality improvement into the cloistered world of pediatric cardiac surgery.

Pediatric cardiac surgery is a complex and challenging endeavor that requires more than the deft surgical skills of a single individual. Successful cardiac surgery programs employ a teamwork approach with collaboration between surgeons, cardiologists, anesthesiologists, intensivists, nursing staff, other hospital staff, and hospital administrators. When a highly functional team is not established or breaks down because of poor communication or failed leadership, patients die unnecessarily. Around the time that de Leval was sensing his "cluster of failures" with the arterial switch operation, concerns were arising about the outcomes of infants undergoing heart surgery at the Bristol Royal Infirmary in Bristol, England [9]. Those concerns reached the point where infant heart surgery was discontinued at that center in 1995. A retrospective public inquiry into the adequacy of pediatric cardiac surgical services in Bristol was led by Sir Ian Kennedy and resulted in an extensive final report published in 2001. This thorough and incisive document delineates the multiple systemic and individual factors that resulted in excessive mortality at that center over that period. An important factor revealed in this report was the lack of a systematic mechanism for monitoring the clinical performance of the pediatric cardiac surgery program.

Bristol was not the only pediatric cardiac surgery program to suspend its services in 1995. In February of that year the pediatric cardiac surgery program at the Winnipeg Health Sciences Centre in Manitoba, Canada ceased providing children's heart surgery following the death of 12 children in 1994. An Inquest was initiated in December 1995 and a final report published in 2000 [10–12]. This retrospective evaluation discovered problems in leadership, teamwork, communication, mentorship, and decision-making. Of primary importance was a failure to collect and analyze group data to track trends and to compare results with other programs. Less publicized but similar situations at centers providing pediatric heart surgery in the United States also occurred during and since. Because of the inherent vulnerability of the patient population and the complexity required to integrate resources and disciplines, pediatric cardiac surgery programs are especially sensitive to breakdowns. All three of the referenced situations point to the importance of collecting and tracking outcomes as well as the need to implement a human factors and safety systems approach to improving pediatric cardiac surgical outcomes.

Development of Multi-institutional Pediatric Cardiac Surgery Databases

While surgeons and programs may have monitored their own results, the assessment of those results was limited by the lack of agreed standards for comparison. If any standards were cited, they were derived from publications in the medical literature of exceptional results. Real data from multiple institutions was required to determine realistic standards. Thus began the development of databases in pediatric heart surgery. The first multi-institutional database for this group of patients was initiated in the upper Midwest of the United States to derive data to justify funding for children with congenital heart disease for the state of Minnesota and surrounding states. In 1982 the Northern Great Plains Regional Cardiac Program (NGPRCP) was begun under the leadership of Dr. James Moller of the University of Minnesota [13]. Initially data was collected from five centers: the Mayo Clinic, Minneapolis Children's Medical Center, the University of Iowa, the University of Nebraska, and the University of Minnesota. Other centers outside of the upper Midwest began to voluntarily join the program. In 1990 the name was changed to the Pediatric Cardiac Care Consortium (PCCC) and the number of programs submitting data exceeded 40 by the year 2000. The database focused on two outcomes: death and length of hospital stay. Data was submitted to a central center with trained coders and was kept confidential with de-identified patient information. Annual center specific reports were made available to each submitting center permitting a comparison to aggregate data from the other participating centers. The PCCC was truly the first database providing data from multiple centers performing pediatric heart surgery allowing realistic information regarding mortality rates for a variety of pediatric cardiac surgical procedures. Benchmarks for mortality of individual operations could now be realistically derived [14].

Another database for patients with congenital heart defects was introduced in 1985 by the Congenital Heart Surgeons' Society (CHSS). Two members of this group of pediatric heart surgeons, Dr. John Kirklin and Dr. Eugene Blackstone, proposed the pooling of data from the members' institutions to assess the management outcomes of specific cardiac malformations. This database differed from the PCCC in that only select congenital heart lesions were tracked and each patient was followed annually. The first lesion to be studied was transposition of the great arteries. This was a timely choice that provided useful feedback permitting comparison of atrial redirection operations (Mustard and Senning procedures) to the newly introduced arterial switch operation. Data derived from the CHSS database provided valuable evidence favoring the latter procedure facilitating the pediatric surgical community's transition to the newer operation for newborns with complete transposition [8]. Other cardiac lesions addressed by the CHSS Database have been pulmonary atresia with intact ventricular septum, pulmonary stenosis, interrupted aortic arch, coarctation of the aorta, critical aortic stenosis, aortic atresia, and tricuspid atresia. The CHSS database continues to serve as a repository of important data from which longer-term outcomes of rare congenital heart anomalies can be determined.

The PCCC and CHSS Databases are representative of the two forms of databases that have become valuable in the assessment of pediatric heart surgery outcomes [15]. The PCCC Database is a *registry* database in which some data is collected for all of the patients. The amount of data collected on each case is limited to a predetermined set of identifiers and early outcomes. This minimal dataset must be clearly assessable and easily and reliably entered for each patient. Registry databases like the PCCC help determine standard of care references from which benchmarks can be developed. The CHSS Database is an *academic* database in which "all of the data" is collected on some of the patients. Academic databases investigate specific populations or subgroups of patients to generate new knowledge. An academic database is much more amenable to longitudinal follow-up than a registry database and allows much more detailed studies. Both forms of databases continue to be important in the assessment and improvement of pediatric cardiac surgery quality.

In 1990 an informal group of European congenital heart surgeons (later formalized into what is presently the European Congenital Heart Surgeons Association (ECHSA)) recognized the importance of collecting data from all of the operations performed at their respective centers. This collaboration led to the birth of the European Congenital Heart Defects Database (ECHDD) in 1992, which began under the direction of Dr. Martin Elliot at Great Ormond Street Hospital for Children in London, England. By 1995 31 centers from 18 countries were submitting data. In 1998 the ECHDD relocated to the Children's Memorial Health Institute in Warsaw, Poland under Dr. Bohdan Maruszewski as director. As congenital data was being collected in the ECHDD, the European Association for Cardio-Thoracic Surgery (EACTS) was developing the European Cardio-Thoracic Surgical Registry (ECSUR). In 1999 it was decided that the ECHDD would be part of the ECSUR. Initially termed the Pediatric ECSUR this registry database would soon be known as the EACTS Congenital Heart Surgery Database. By 2001 84 programs from 34 countries were represented. By 2012 the number of European centers had risen to 265 representing 36 countries. By that time another 147 centers outside of Europe from 43 countries all over the world had been added. Today, these databases include data from over 100,000 patients and 125,000 operations.

Contemporarily with what was happening in Europe, the US Society of Thoracic Surgeons was developing its own registry database for congenital heart surgery in North America. Dr. Constantine Mavroudis at Children's Memorial Hospital in Chicago, Illinois was responsible for the initial development of the STS Congenital Heart Surgery Database. Centers began joining in 1994 and by 1997 24 North American centers had provided data that included mortality and length of stay derived from over 8,000 patient records. In the late 1990s Dr. Jeff Jacobs of St. Petersburg, Fl. assumed the Chairmanship of the STS Congenital Heart Surgery Database Task Force and has been responsible for the continued maturation and growth of this database [16]. By the end of 2011 there were over 100 participating centers representing more than 80 % of all congenital heart programs in the United States. Data from over 200,000 operations have been submitted from 1994 to today.

The key to the successful development of the congenital databases in Europe and North America was the establishment of a common language or nomenclature to describe the large number of disease entities treated and procedures performed. In addition, it was necessary to determine the minimal set of data required to allow valid linkage with other databases. In 1998 the EACTS and STS collaboratively initiated the International Congenital Heart Surgery Nomenclature and Database Project. By 2000 a minimum dataset was agreed upon and updated in 2001 [17, 18]. In the next few years the International Society for Nomenclature of Paediatric and Congenital Heart Disease (ISNPCHD) was created including surgeons, pediatric cardiologists, and congenital cardiac morphologists. By 2005 the nomenclature working group of the ISNPCHD had cross-mapped the nomenclature of the International Congenital Heart Surgery Nomenclature and Database Project of the STS and EACTS with the European Paediatric Cardiac Code (EPCC) of the Association for European Paediatric Cardiology (AEPC) creating the International Paediatric and Congenital Cardiac Code (IPCCC). With this common language and an agreed upon minimum dataset, the EACTS and STS Databases were up and running and able to combine information from two very large experiences in pediatric heart surgery. Furthermore, the stage was set for linkage with databases from other parts of the world, from other medical disciplines, and even with some administrative databases.

In pediatric cardiac surgery there is a broad spectrum of complexity and risk. The mix of cases at one institution may consist of simple low risk cases whereas the mix at another institution may contain more complex cases subject to significantly higher risk. Comparing the overall mortality of the two institutions would provide a misleading assessment of outcomes. Thus to provide fairer comparisons between centers, stratification schemes were developed. The first scheme (the Risk Adjustment in Congenital Heart Surgery-1 (RACHS-1) method) consisted of six risk categories for surgical procedures. This stratification, which was developed and championed by Dr. Kathy Jenkins at Boston Children's Hospital, was derived from a consensus of pediatric cardiologists and cardiac surgeons [19]. The application of RACHS-1 to the PCCC dataset for the year 1996 confirmed a spread of mortality rates across RACHS-1 categories with category 1 having a mortality of 0.4 % and category 6 having a mortality of 41.5 %. Another approach to risk stratification, fostered by Dr. Francois Lacour-Gayet who worked at the Eppendorf University Hospital in Hamburg, Germany, applied scores and levels to each operation based on the perceived risk of mortality, morbidity, and the technical difficulty of the procedure [20, 21]. These values were referred to as Aristotle basic complexity (ABC) scores and levels. As with RACHS-1 the ABC scores were derived from expert opinions of experienced clinicians. The Aristotle approach was incorporated in the reports from the EACTS and STS Congenital Databases beginning in 2002 and the RACHS-1 stratification was added to the reports in both databases in 2006. Both approaches provided reasonable risk stratification, but the Aristotle levels classified more operations than did RACHS-1, whereas RACHS-1 provided more discrimination at the higher end of complexity [22]. By 2008 enough data had been collected in both the EACTS and STS Congenital Databases to permit an objective determination of risk from actual surgical outcomes. This new stratification scheme resulted in five "STS-EACTS Mortality Levels" which demonstrated better predictive value for mortality than the RACHS-1 or Aristotle systems [23]. This objectively derived system, now referred to as STAT Mortality Categories, has become the preferred stratification protocol for congenital heart operations and is currently incorporated in all EACTS and STS Congenital Database reports.

Now with an accepted nomenclature and means for risk stratification the EACTS and STS registry databases provide useful quality assessment for centers willing to participate. The formats of these databases continue to evolve to further improve the value of the information collected and analyzed. Periodically data fields are added and subtracted as experience with the information accrues and clinical questions increase and decrease in importance. The validity of the data in the databases must be assured with regular audits and other forms of data verification [24]. Measurement of outcomes has focused mostly on hospital or 30 day mortality. Mortality data alone, however, is insensitive to quality issues experienced by low risk procedures and says little about process failures that may lead to near misses and harm but not death. The hospital length of stay is available in these databases and has served as a proxy for the morbidity of pediatric cardiac surgical procedures. Other measures of morbidity are now being tracked in these databases including unplanned reoperations, postoperative renal failure, and postoperative complete heart block [25–27]. Hopefully tracking these measures will provide a more thorough assessment of process and outcomes for these patients. How these patients do after the initial 30 days following an operation is also important. Although registry databases are poorly suited for longitudinal follow-up, efforts are in progress to create Health Insurance Portability and Accountability Act (HIPAA)-compliant unique patient identifiers that would permit tracking of patients through a series of operations and for longer-term follow-up [28]. As many pediatric cardiac surgical conditions require staging of surgical procedures, the ability to keep track of the same patient through more than one procedure is important in assessing the outcomes of such sequenced approaches for individual patients. HIPAA-compliant unique patient identifiers may also permit linkage with administrative databases to enable assessment of costs or other nonclinical information or to assist with data verification regarding death, length of hospital stay, or other demographics [29].

From Quality Assessment to Quality Improvement

Pediatric cardiac surgery centers have the ability now to participate in highly developed multi-institutional databases such as the STS and EACTS Congenital Databases, with each center having the ability to compare its own outcomes with those of other database members. For the STS Congenital Heart Surgery Database each center's outcomes are kept confidential but can be compared to the outcomes experienced in the aggregate of the other centers. In addition, graphical depictions are provided such that an individual center can visualize its outcomes in comparison with those of the other centers in a de-identified manner (Fig. 16.2). Outcome information is provided at a reasonable interval (every six months for the STS Congenital database) to each center who can continuously monitor its outcomes. Of course, not every center will feel assured, as its outcomes may not be satisfactory for every procedure. In fact, analysis of data from the STS Congenital Database has revealed that there is significant variation in outcomes among institutions providing pediatric heart surgery [30, 31]. The degree of variation in terms of mortality is minimal for low risk procedures, but tends to be as high

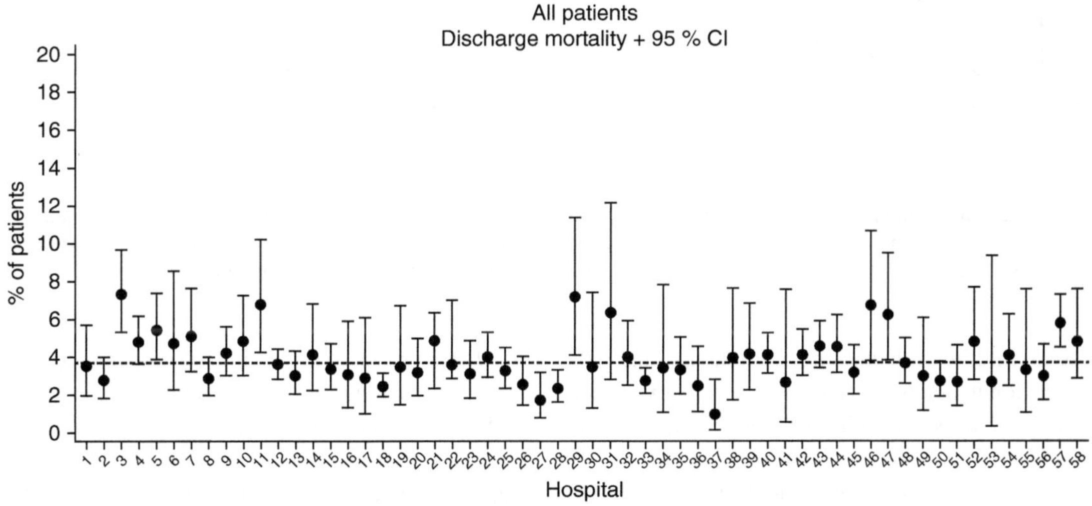

Fig. 16.2 Example of the graphical presentation of discharge mortality from a semiannual report from the Society of Thoracic Surgeons Congenital Heart Surgery Database. Each hospital, identified only to itself, can compare its results with the other unidentified hospitals. Similar graphical presentations are provided for each strata of risk (*Abbreviation*: *Cl* confidence limits)

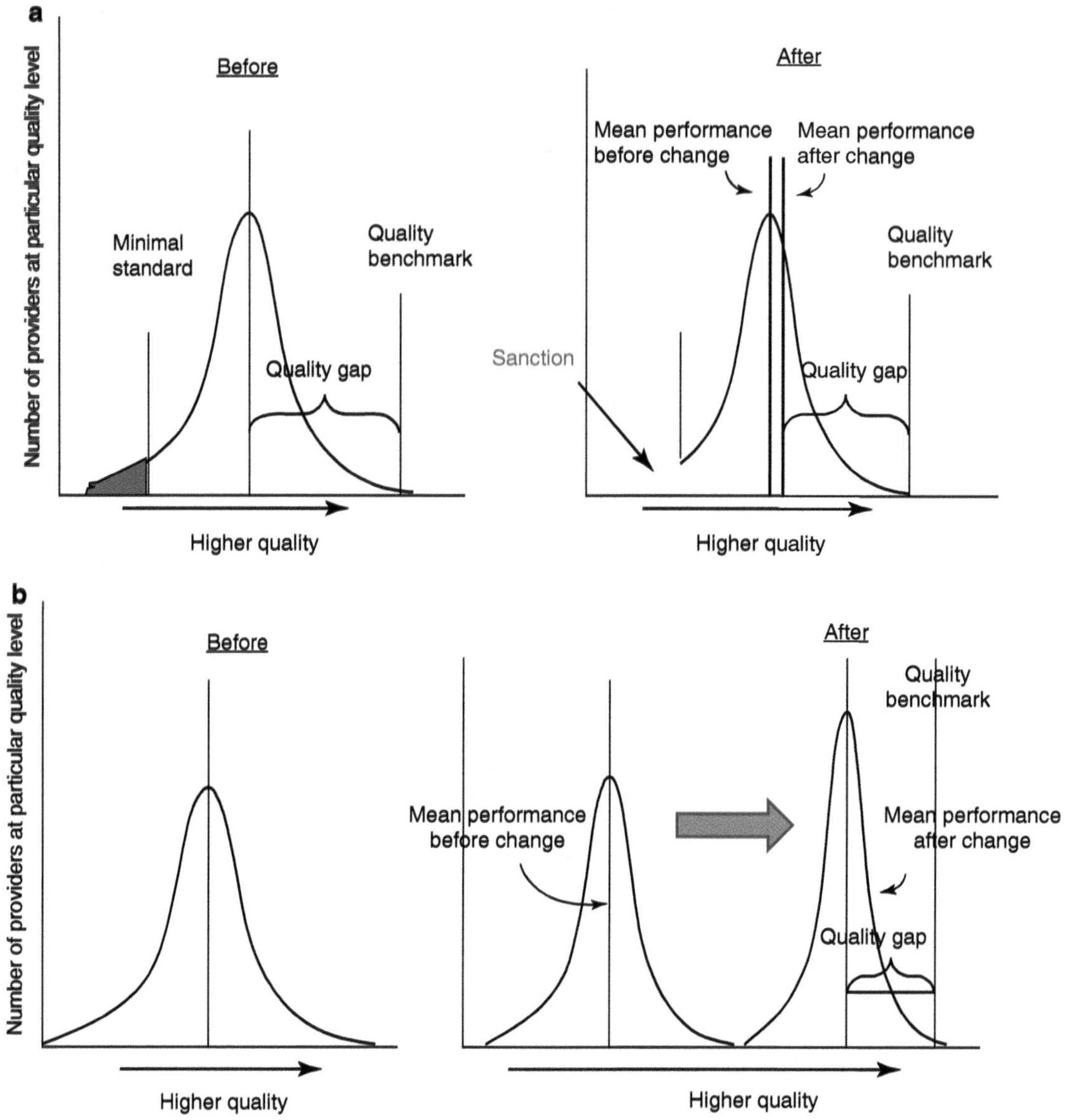

Fig. 16.3 (**a**) Removing poor performing providers has minimal effect on improving overall quality (From Miles [48]). (**b**) Applying a quality improvement initiative to all providers reduces variation among providers and improves overall quality (Reprinted from Miles [48]. Reproduced by permission of the American Board of Family Medicine)

as sixfold with increasing complexity and risk. Variation in outcomes is not only seen between centers but can occur within the same institution and with different surgeons with good results for one operation and much less satisfactory results for another operation [32]. These analyses indicate a spectrum of performance among and within programs providing pediatric cardiac surgery. These findings indicate a need for some programs to reevaluate their performance as a whole or for particular procedures.

One approach to improving the overall outcomes in pediatric cardiac surgery is to identify the lowest performers and eliminate them, such as occurred in the cases of Bristol and Winnipeg, in the UK and Canada, respectively. A graphical depiction of this approach presented by the American Board of Pediatrics [33] is demonstrated in Fig. 16.3a. In this graphic variation in quality of care is represented as a bell shaped curve. When the tail of the curve (lower 5 % of performers) is eliminated, the improvement in quality realized by the system as a whole is only

Table 16.1 Quality measures for congenital and pediatric cardiac surgery

1.	Participation in a National Database for Pediatric and Congenital Heart Surgery
2.	Multidisciplinary rounds involving multiple members of the health care team
3.	Availability of institutional pediatric extracorporeal life support (ECLS) program
4.	Surgical volume for pediatric and congenital heart surgery: total programmatic volume and programmatic volume stratified by the five STAT Mortality Categories
5.	Surgical volume for eight pediatric and congenital heart benchmark operations
6.	Multidisciplinary preoperative planning conference to plan pediatric and congenital heart surgery operations
7.	Regularly Scheduled Quality Assurance and Quality Improvement Cardiac Care Conference, to occur no less frequently than once every two months
8.	Availability of intraoperative transesophageal echocardiography (TEE) and epicardial echocardiography
9.	Timing of antibiotic administration for pediatric and congenital cardiac surgery patients
10.	Selection of appropriate prophylactic antibiotics for pediatric and congenital cardiac surgery patients
11.	Use of an expanded preprocedural and postprocedural "time-out"
12.	Occurrence of new postoperative renal failure requiring dialysis
13.	Occurrence of new postoperative neurological deficit persisting at discharge
14.	Occurrence of arrhythmia necessitating permanent pacemaker insertion
15.	Occurrence of paralyzed diaphragm (possible phrenic nerve injury)
16.	Occurrence of need for postoperative mechanical circulatory support (IABP, VAD, ECMO, or CPS)
17.	Occurrence of unplanned reoperation and/or unplanned interventional cardiovascular catheterization procedure
18.	Operative mortality stratified by the Five STAT Mortality Categories
19.	Operative mortality for eight benchmark operations
20.	Index cardiac operations free of mortality and major complication
21.	Operative survivors free of major complication

Reprinted from Jacobs et al. [34]
Abbreviations: *IABP* intra-aortic balloon pump, *VAD* ventricular assist device, *ECMO* extracorporeal membrane oxygenation, *CPS* cardiopulmonary support system

modest. On the other hand, if strategies for improvement are applied across all institutions, the variation between institutions can be significantly diminished (a narrower bell) and overall quality improved (bell moved to the right) (Fig. 16.3b). One such strategy is the application of standardized structures and processes to all programs.

In 2007 under the leadership of its president at the time, Dr. John Mayer, the Society of Thoracic Surgeons created a task force to develop a list of quality measures for pediatric and congenital heart surgery. By 2011 this task force, which consisted of pediatric and congenital heart surgeons, had developed a set of 21 Quality Measures which was further vetted by four other STS committees and approved by the Executive Committee of the Society of Thoracic Surgeons. In the same year the same set of Quality Measures was reviewed and endorsed by the Congenital Heart Surgeons' Society. This set of quality measures is listed in Table 16.1 and follows Donabedian's principles for quality with five measures related to structure, six related to process, and ten different outcome measures. These Quality Measures for Pediatric and Congenital Heart Surgery were published in early 2012 where the details of each measure are described [34]. Most of these quality measures were derived from the experience and expert opinions of the STS task force and will require further evaluation in terms of reliability, validity and scientific acceptance. The STS Congenital Heart Surgery Database has added a Quality Module that will help determine if these measures are indeed associated with improved outcomes. The National Quality Forum, which also reviewed these measures, agreed that more data is required before it could support most of these measures, but it did endorse three measures: (1) participation in a national database, (2) measurement of total programmatic volume and programmatic volumes stratified by the five STAT mortality categories, and (3) operative mortality stratified by the five STAT mortality categories.

Minimizing variation in patient outcomes and improving the overall quality in pediatric heart surgery requires more than adoption and adherence to a set of quality measures. The Society of

Thoracic Surgeons and the Congenital Heart Surgeons' Society have both been instrumental in making quality improvement a priority for their members. The STS Congenital Heart Surgery Database has been the foundation for quality assessment and improvement in North America. The STS has also created separate workforces dedicated to Congenital Heart Surgery, Surgical Treatment of Adults with Congenital Heart Disease, and Peer Review and Evaluation. The Congenital Heart Surgeons' Society has created the Committee on Quality Improvement and Outcomes to address these issues and to serve as a resource for centers seeking assistance.

Several areas of clinical research will prove valuable in improving the outcomes and minimizing variation. Studies in human factors, team performance, and the complex interactions required of a team providing pediatric heart surgery may lead to a substantial decrease in the number of errors that result in untoward outcomes [35–39]. The technical aspects of complex pediatric cardiac operations themselves are now being carefully assessed and are revealing a significant effect on results [40–42]. The ability to grade each operation with a Technical Performance Score will be valuable to surgeons who can use that feedback to hone their surgical skills [43]. Improvement in team dynamics and interactions as well as improvement in the performance of individual team members is expected to further improve the quality of pediatric heart surgery.

One other area that has promise for the field of pediatric heart surgery is the concept of learning collaboratives. Learning collaboratives involve the sharing of processes, approaches, and outcomes with other institutions. This approach was pioneered by a group of adult cardiac surgery programs in northern New England. When these hospitals noted that their outcomes for coronary artery surgery were unacceptable, they decided to collaborate rather than compete with each other [44]. The collaboration consisted of feedback of outcome data, training in continuous quality improvement techniques, and round robin site visits to each other's institution. Site visiting teams consisted of surgeons, anesthesiologists, perfusionists, nursing staff, and others considered important to the delivery of coronary artery surgery at each institution. By observing practices at the other sites variation in processes diminished and variation in outcomes improved with a 24 % decrease in operative mortality for the programs as a whole [44]. Similar learning collaboratives have been successfully applied in other regions of the United States for the delivery of adult cardiac surgery [45, 46]. Such a learning collaborative coupled with a robust continuous quality improvement framework has yet to be attempted in pediatric cardiac surgery, but could result in substantial quality improvement for those centers courageous enough to participate in such a venture [47].

References

1. Huxley E. Florence Nightingale. London: Weidenfeld and Nicolson; 1975. p. 186.
2. Neuhauser D. Ernest Amory Codman, M.D., and end results of medical care. Int J Technol Assess Health Care. 1990;6:307–25.
3. Jacobs JP, Mavroudis C, Jacobs ML, Maruszewski B, Tchervenkov CI, Lacour-Gayet FG, et al. What is operative mortality? Defining death in a surgical registry database: a report of the STS Congenital Database Taskforce and the Joint EACTS-STS Congenital Database Committee. Ann Thorac Surg. 2006;81(5):1937–41. PubMed PMID: 16631716.
4. Williams W. Defining operative mortality: it should be easy, but is it? Ann Thorac Surg. 2006;81(5):1557–60. PubMed PMID: 16631634.
5. US Dept of Health and Human Services. Medicare Hospital Mortality Information, 1986. Washington, DC: US Dept of Health and Human Services; 1987. DHHS publication No. 01–002.
6. de Leval MR, Francois K, Bull C, Brawn W, Spiegelhalter D. Analysis of a cluster of surgical failures. Application to a series of neonatal arterial switch operations. J Thorac Cardiovasc Surg. 1994;107(3):914–23; discussion 23–4, PubMed PMID: 8127123.
7. Williams SM, Perry BR, Schlup MMT. Quality control: an application of the CUSUM. BMJ. 1992;304:1359–61.
8. Kirklin JW, Blackstone EH, Tchervenkov CI, Castaneda AR. Clinical outcomes after the arterial switch operation for transposition: patient, support, procedural, and institutional risk factors. Congenital Heart Surgeons' Society. Circulation. 1992;86:1501–15.
9. Kennedy I. The report of the Public Inquiry into children's heart surgery at the Bristol Royal Infirmary 1984–1995. July 2001. http://webarchive.nationalarchives.gov.uk/+/www.dh.gov.uk/en/Publicationsandstatistics/Publications/PublicationsPolicyAndGuidance/DH_4005620.

10. Sinclair CM. The report of the Manitoba Pediatric Cardiac Surgery Inquest: an inquiry into twelve deaths at the Winnipeg Health Sciences Center in 1994. 1994:XXV–XXVII. http://www.pediatriccardiacinquest.mb.ca.
11. Sinclair CM. The report of the Manitoba Pediatric Cardiac Surgery Inquest: an inquiry into twelve deaths at the Winnipeg Health Sciences Center in 1994. 1994:325–75. http://www.pediatriccardiacinquest.mb.ca.
12. Sinclair CM. The report of the Manitoba Pediatric Cardiac Surgery Inquest: an inquiry into twelve deaths at the Winnipeg Health Sciences Center in 1994. 1994:465–502. http://www.pediatriccardiacinquest.mb.ca.
13. Moller JH, Hills CB, Pyles LA. A multi-center cardiac registry. A method to assess outcome of catheterization intervention or surgery. Prog Pediatr Cardiol. 2005;20(1):7–12.
14. Moller JH, Powell CB, Joransen JA, Borbas C. The pediatric cardiac care consortium – revisited. Jt Comm J Qual Improv. 1994;20(12):661–8.
15. Williams WG, McCrindle BW. Practical experience with databases for congenital heart disease: a registry versus an academic database. Semin Thorac Cardiovasc Surg Pediatr Card Surg Annu. 2002;5:132–42. PubMed PMID: 11994873.
16. Jacobs JP, Maruszewski B, Tchervenkov CI, et al. The current status and future directions of efforts to create a global database for the outcomes of therapy for congenital heart disease. Cardiol Young. 2005;15 suppl 1:190–7.
17. Mavroudis C, Jacobs JP. Congenital Heart Surgery Nomenclature and Database Project: overview and minimum dataset. Ann Thorac Surg. 2000;69 (4 Suppl):S2–17. PubMed PMID: 10798411.
18. Maruszewski B, Tobota Z. The European Congenital Heart Defects Surgery Database experience: Pediatric European Cardiothoracic Surgical Registry of the European Association for Cardio-Thoracic Surgery. Semin Thorac Cardiovasc Surg Pediatr Card Surg Annu. 2002;5:143–7. PubMed PMID: 11994874.
19. Jenkins KJ, Gauvreau K, Newburger JW, Spray TL, Moller JH, Iezzoni LI. Consensus-based method for risk adjustment for surgery for congenital heart disease. J Thorac Cardiovasc Surg. 2002;123(1):110–8.
20. Lacour-Gayet F. Risk stratification theme for congenital heart surgery. Semin Thorac Cardiovasc Surg Pediatr Card Surg Annu. 2002;5:148–52. PubMed PMID: 11994875.
21. Lacour-Gayet F, Clarke DR, Aristotle C. The Aristotle method: a new concept to evaluate quality of care based on complexity. Curr Opin Pediatr. 2005;17(3): 412–7. PubMed PMID: 15891437.
22. Jacobs JP, Maruszewski B, Kurosawa H, Jacobs ML, Mavroudis C, Lacour-Gayet FG, et al. Congenital heart surgery databases around the world: do we need a global database? Semin Thorac Cardiovasc Surg Pediatr Card Surg Annu. 2010;13(1):3–19. PubMed PMID: 20307856.
23. O'Brien SM, Clarke DR, Jacobs JP, Jacobs ML, Lacour-Gayet FG, Pizarro C, et al. An empirically based tool for analyzing mortality associated with congenital heart surgery. J Thorac Cardiovasc Surg. 2009;138(5):1139–53. PubMed PMID: 19837218.
24. Maruszewski B, Lacour-Gayet F, Monro JL, Keogh BE, Tobota Z, Kansy A. An attempt at data verification in the EACTS Congenital Database. Eur J Cardiothorac Surg. 2005;28(3):400–4; discussion 5–6, PubMed PMID: 16054826.
25. Lacour-Gayet F, Jacobs ML, Jacobs JP, Mavroudis C. The need for an objective evaluation of morbidity in congenital heart surgery. Ann Thorac Surg. 2007;84(1):1–2. PubMed PMID: 17588371.
26. Jacobs JP, Jacobs ML, Mavroudis C, Maruszewski B, Tchervenkov CI, Lacour-Gayet FG, et al. What is operative morbidity? Defining complications in a Surgical Registry Database. The Society of Thoracic Surgeons (STS) Executive Committee, The STS Council on Quality, Research and Patient Safety, The STS Workforce on National Databases, and The STS Congenital Database Task Force have all reviewed this manuscript and approved this article for submission to The Annals of Thoracic Surgery as an official publication of The STS Congenital Database Task Force. Ann Thorac Surg. 2007;84(4):1416–21.
27. Jacobs ML, O'Brien SM, Jacobs JP, Mavroudis C, Lacour-Gayet F, Pasquali SK, et al. An empirically based tool for analyzing morbidity associated with operations for congenital heart disease. J Thorac Cardiovasc Surg. 2013;145(4):1046–57.e1. PubMed PMID: 22835225.
28. Jacobs JP, Haan CK, Edwards FH, Anderson RP, Grover FL, Mayer Jr JE, et al. The rationale for incorporation of HIPAA compliant unique patient, surgeon, and hospital identifier fields in the STS database. Ann Thorac Surg. 2008;86(3):695–8. PubMed PMID: 18721549.
29. Pasquali SK, Li JS, Jacobs ML, Shah SS, Jacobs JP. Opportunities and challenges in linking information across databases in pediatric cardiovascular medicine. Prog Pediatr Cardiol. 2012;33(1):21–4. PubMed PMID: 23671377, Pubmed Central PMCID: 3651671.
30. Jacobs JP, O'Brien SM, Pasquali SK, Jacobs ML, Lacour-Gayet FG, Tchervenkov CI, et al. Variation in outcomes for benchmark operations: an analysis of the Society of Thoracic Surgeons Congenital Heart Surgery Database. Ann Thorac Surg. 2011;92(6):2184–91. PubMed PMID: 22115229, Pubmed Central PMCID: 3263755, discussion 91–2.
31. Jacobs JP, O'Brien SM, Pasquali SK, Jacobs ML, Lacour-Gayet FG, Tchervenkov CI, et al. Variation in outcomes for risk-stratified pediatric cardiac surgical operations: an analysis of the STS Congenital Heart Surgery Database. Ann Thorac Surg. 2012;94(2):564–71; discussion 71–2, PubMed PMID: 22704799.
32. Karamlou T, McCrindle BW, Blackstone EH, Cai S, Jonas RA, Bradley SM, et al. Lesion-specific outcomes in neonates undergoing congenital heart surgery are related predominantly to patient and management factors rather than institution or surgeon

experience: a Congenital Heart Surgeons Society Study. J Thorac Cardiovasc Surg. 2010;139(3):569–77.e1. PubMed PMID: 19909989.
33. Miles P. The future of maintenance of certification: a reaction to the paper by Kevin B. Weiss, MD. Jour Am Bd. Fam Med. 2010;23:S42–5.
34. Jacobs JP, Jacobs ML, Austin EH, Mavroudis C, Pasquali SK, Lacour-Gayet FG, et al. Quality measures for congenital and pediatric cardiac surgery. World J Pediatr Congenit Heart Surg. 2012;3(1):32–47.
35. Carthey J, de Leval MR, Reason JT. The human factor in cardiac surgery: errors and near misses in a high technology medical domain. Ann Thorac Surg. 2001;72(1):300–5. PubMed PMID: 11465216.
36. Galvan C, Bacha EA, Mohr J, Barach P. A human factors approach to understanding patient safety during pediatric cardiac surgery. Prog Pediatr Cardiol. 2005; 20(1):13–20.
37. ElBardissi AW, Wiegmann DA, Dearani JA, Daly RC, Sundt 3rd TM. Application of the human factors analysis and classification system methodology to the cardiovascular surgery operating room. Ann Thorac Surg. 2007;83(4):1412–8; discussion 8–9, PubMed PMID: 17383348.
38. Catchpole KR, Giddings AE, de Leval MR, Peek GJ, Godden PJ, Utley M, et al. Identification of systems failures in successful paediatric cardiac surgery. Ergonomics. 2006;49(5–6):567–88. PubMed PMID: 16717010.
39. Barach P, Johnson JK, Ahmad A, Galvan C, Bognar A, Duncan R, et al. A prospective observational study of human factors, adverse events, and patient outcomes in surgery for pediatric cardiac disease. J Thorac Cardiovasc Surg. 2008;136(6):1422–8. PubMed PMID: 19114184.
40. Bacha EA, Larrazabal LA, Pigula FA, Gauvreau K, Jenkins KJ, Colan SD, et al. Measurement of technical performance in surgery for congenital heart disease: the stage I Norwood procedure. J Thorac Cardiovasc Surg. 2008;136(4):993–7, 7.e1–2. PubMed PMID: 18954641.
41. Shuhaiber J, Gauvreau K, Thiagarjan R, Bacha E, Mayer J, Del Nido P, et al. Congenital heart surgeon's technical proficiency affects neonatal hospital survival. J Thorac Cardiovasc Surg. 2012;144(5):1119–24. PubMed PMID: 22421402.
42. Karamichalis JM, Colan SD, Nathan M, Pigula FA, Baird C, Marx G, et al. Technical performance scores in congenital cardiac operations: a quality assessment initiative. Ann Thorac Surg. 2012;94(4):1317–23; discussion 23, PubMed PMID: 22795058.
43. Karamichalis J, Barach P, Henaine R, del Nido P, Bacha E. Assessment of surgical competency in pediatric cardiac surgery. Prog Pediatr Cardiol. 2012;33:115–20.
44. O'Connor GT, Plume SK, Olmstead EM, Morton JR, Maloney CT, Nugent WC, et al. A regional intervention to improve the hospital mortality associated with coronary artery bypass graft surgery. The Northern New England Cardiovascular Disease Study Group. JAMA. 1996;275(11):841–6. PubMed PMID: 8596221.
45. Prager RL, Armenti FR, Bassett JS, Bell GF, Drake D, Hanson EC, et al. Cardiac surgeons and the quality movement: the Michigan experience. Semin Thorac Cardiovasc Surg. 2009;21(1):20–7. PubMed PMID: 19632559.
46. Speir AM, Rich JB, Crosby I, Fonner Jr E. Regional collaboration as a model for fostering accountability and transforming health care. Semin Thorac Cardiovasc Surg. 2009;21(1):12–9. PubMed PMID: 19632558.
47. Winlaw DS, d'Udekem Y, Barach PR. Where to now for paediatric cardiac surgery? ANZ J Surg. 2011; 81:659–60.
48. Miles PV. Collaborative Improvement Networks and Physician Accountability. https://www.abp.org/abp-website/moc/collabimp/Paul%20Miles.pdf

17 Leadership and Quality Improvement

Robert Campbell and Larry Mohl

Abstract

A leader can be defined as a teacher or person of influence. Leaders of teams need to collaborate and negotiate change. Change is occurring rapidly in healthcare and in our profession of pediatric cardiac services. Therefore, leadership has now become a critical new area of subspecialty expertise within pediatric cardiology divisions, practices, and service lines.

This chapter deals with identification of potential leaders possessing natural aptitude, as well as strategies around which to develop leadership competencies. Leadership of teams requires collaboration and negotiation to be effective; these teams may require interaction between physician and administrative leaders, which in our current system of medicine have not always been the most natural of partners.

Roles for leaders and leadership teams, and measures of leadership competency, are discussed. Potential opportunities to provide leadership for our profession are discussed.

Keywords

Leader • Leadership Teams • Health Care • Collaboration • Service Line • Quality

R. Campbell, MD (✉)
Department of Pediatrics, Emory University School of Medicine, Children's Healthcare of Atlanta Sibley Heart Center, 2835 Brandywine Road, Suite 300, Atlanta, GA 30341, USA
e-mail: campbellr@kidsheart.com

L. Mohl, BS EE, MS EE
Performance Inspired, Inc., Jamstir Inc., 5130 Crayln Court, John's Creek, GA 30097, USA
e-mail: larry.mohl@performanceinspired.tv

Leaders establish the vision for the future and set the strategy for getting there; they cause change. They motivate and inspire others to go in the right direction and they, along with everyone else, sacrifice to get there. John Kotter[1]

[1] John P. Kotter, Leading Change, 2012.

P.R. Barach, J.P. Jacobs, S.E. Lipshultz, P.C. Laussen (eds.),
Pediatric and Congenital Cardiac Care: Volume 2: Quality Improvement and Patient Safety,
DOI 10.1007/978-1-4471-6566-8_17, © Springer-Verlag London 2015

Introduction

Leadership and Quality Improvement

As recently as three decades ago, pediatric cardiology was simpler. A "triple threat individual" – the best clinician, best researcher, and best teacher in the division – was usually designated as Director of the division, or "the Chief". In our current more complex world of higher patient volumes, increased patient acuity, advanced technology, more stringent research consents and study designs, decreased research funding, and now healthcare reform, a triple threat individual just won't suffice. Our new normal requires additional business alignment and leadership expertise. No one individual is likely to possess expertise in all five of these categories, nor the bandwidth to perform all these tasks. Therefore, we need "quintuple threat organizations" that provide comprehensive expertise in all five domains, with collaboration among multiple individuals to direct the efforts and achieve sustainable results.

Leadership now becomes a new area of subspecialty within pediatric cardiology divisions, practices, and service lines. In this chapter we will describe the evolving need and role for pediatric cardiac leaders, the skills and behaviors of these leaders, and strategies around which to enhance leader competencies. The ultimate success of our pediatric cardiac profession may depend upon our new leaders and their new and evolving competencies.

The Need for Leaders

Change is occurring to our profession. Leading change becomes one of the ultimate measures of success of any leader. A leader is best defined as a teacher or a person of influence. Leaders need to collaborate and negotiate change successfully, often with new and unexpected partners. We will need to negotiate rapid change in healthcare reform which has introduced new terms such as accountable care organizations and clinically integrated networks. Healthcare now requires a focus on business metrics such as quality, outcomes, and value (quality/cost). Our profession is expected to provide more (better care, improved outcomes, greater distribution, advanced technologies) at lower cost. It is no longer good enough to state that you have excellent outcomes, since data now must validate results, preferably with national benchmarked references. Transparency with data and charges will soon be the standard expectation, as evidenced by the recent CMS disclosure of sharing of hospital charges and impending physician charges.

As reimbursement for physician performance decreases, and simultaneously the expense to deliver greater technology to more and sicker patients increases, the business revenue margin will be reduced. Pediatric cardiac services, like the rest of the medical profession, will likely slowly transition from a fee-for-service world (pay based on procedures) to a more value-based payment scheme, a reimbursement strategy that places more emphasis on health and population management rather than per procedure episodes of care [1].

Many adult cardiologists have now become hospital-employed physicians, partnered with hospital administration and systems, in order to adapt to the changing medical reimbursement landscape. Whereas physicians and hospital administrators in the past may have experienced a more siloed and sometimes adversarial relationship, leadership (physician and administrative) and collaboration becomes the formula for success, helping to navigate complex changes in the business world.

Identifying Leadership Aptitude

In past years, physician leaders were often chosen based upon recognized clinical excellence or academic credentials. However, clinical and/or research competencies are not necessarily translated into the new world leadership competencies. Just as not all cardiothoracic surgeons want to specialize in the world of congenital heart disease surgery, not all pediatric cardiologists choose to specialize in intensive care management, electrophysiology, or interventional catheterization. Identifying physician candidates with an aptitude for leadership is a key first step.

Through many years of medical education, clinical training, and competitive grading, physicians have been selected for certain skills and behavior that may help with clinical or research expertise. Physicians are very competitive, seeking top class rank, highly desired but limited high profile internship or residency positions, and/or clinical or research opportunities at premier institutions. These competitive instincts, honed over years, may help to develop critical thinking, decision-making, and directing action, especially in emergency situations. However, leadership requires a different focus; collaboration, negotiation, excellent communication, and team building become key performance metrics.

In order to identify potential administrative physician leaders, Children's Healthcare of Atlanta uses a leadership potential checklist (Table 17.1) developed by Development Dimensions International. The demonstration of passion and promise to lead is a critical criterion. Following his or her passion, a new physician leader will quickly demonstrate accountability for mastering leadership skills, and implementing these in the day to day decision making of a complex pediatric cardiac organization. Other leadership assessment tools including the DISC [2], StrengthsFinder 2.0 [3], the Hogan [4], and the Birkman [5] are used to identify personal aptitude, inclination, and characteristic tendencies. In the end the desire to become a leader is a choice that has implications at the level of a physician's identity. One of the first signs is when a physician starts to speak about his/her desire to move from improving the outcomes of a single patient to improving the system of care. This type of conversation indicates that a physician is in the midst of navigating their changing identity in terms of values, role, and future impact. It is a critical point at which physician leaders and administrators can challenge and support these emerging leaders to take on leadership responsibilities and develop their capabilities.

Table 17.1 CHOA Center for Leadership Strategies leadership potential checklist

Passion and Promise to Lead
Brings Out the Best in People
Authenticity
Receptivity to Feedback
Learning Agility
Culture Fit
Adaptability
Conceptual Thinking
Navigates Ambiguity
Passion for Results

The transition from clinician with a recognized technical expertise to a leader is a journey, not a specific destination endpoint. Clinicians typically have the responsibility for a distinct service area, whereas the leader or leadership team requires a cross-disciplinary vision of the entirety of the service line or hospital system (Fig. 17.1). For the leader this will likely require a 'we" rather than "me" perspective. The author Ken Blanchard writes about "servant leadership" [6]

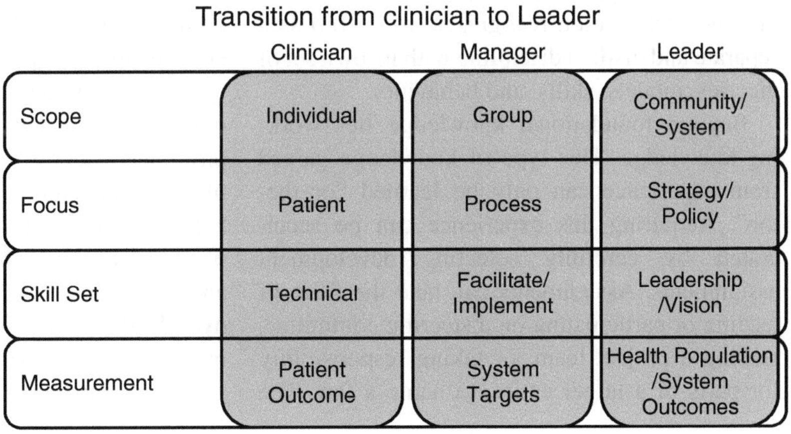

Fig. 17.1 The transition from clinician to manager to leader

in which leaders realize their main role is to help people and organizations achieve collective goals. This requires an emphasis on communication and vision.

Leadership Development

Physician leaders may seek to gain leadership expertise through several avenues, the first, a formal process of a Master's of Business Administration (MBA) or Public Health (MPH) degree. These programs offer curricula including, but not limited to, accounting, business strategy, economics, finance, human resources, marketing management, manufacturing and production, operations management, statistics and technology, and information systems. An MBA degree augments leadership but does not guarantee effectiveness. To succeed within the co-management model for healthcare administration, the physician manager should be conversant and knowledgeable in these business metrics. Another option is the Cardiovascular Leadership Institute, developed by the American College of Cardiology [7]. This process assists cardiovascular professionals as they develop into effective and visionary leaders. A third choice is by way of the American College of Physician Executives, which offers formal classroom and on-line education courses to advance physician business and operational knowledge. Gaining the foundational knowledge of leadership principles and practices is extremely important. Spending time and money on this type of development demonstrates that the organization recognizes leadership as a separate and distinct discipline with its own set of theories, models, skills, and behaviors.

Beyond foundational knowledge lies working knowledge. This type of knowledge gained from experience can only be learned "on-the-job". Acquiring this experience can be accelerated by carefully selecting development assignments. Assignments can take the form of leading or participating on a steering committee, leading a project team, or taking responsibility for parts of a larger entity, to name a few. The role of coaching and mentoring as an accelerator cannot be overstated. Emerging leaders need people they can turn to when they are confronted with organizational and operational challenges they have never faced before. These coaches and mentors should go beyond "giving advice" to a model that encourages physicians to reflect on and frame what they are experiencing. Once they have done this critical step they can move toward generating ideas and solutions they feel they can own and implement. The opportunity to develop as a leader, on the job under the guidance of a physician leader as mentor, may rapidly accelerate competency within the culture of the organization.

Leadership Collaboration

A physician leader must see administrative managerial responsibilities and the interface with hospital or practice administration as legitimate important responsibilities, not simply a time filler between patient encounters. Administrative leaders (practice and/or hospital) face a cultural challenge, meeting with physician and non physician leaders to define strategy and operations. Physician and administrator (or nursing) co-leaders assume accountability and credit for their respective areas of expertise within the whole of the enterprise and they collectively succeed or fail. A dyad management model for integrated health systems (Fig. 17.2) defines the relationship between qualified physician and non-physician leadership partners. These two co-managers provide unique perspectives, different skillsets and specialized expertise that should synergistically define strategy, clinical performance, and business metrics. The key role of the physician leader is to define clinical vision and to manage physician teams' performance and behavior. The administrative partner is primarily more focused on operations, business, staffing, and support systems and services. Together these dyad leaders define mission, vision, values, culture, overall performance, internal organization relationships, and finally strategy.

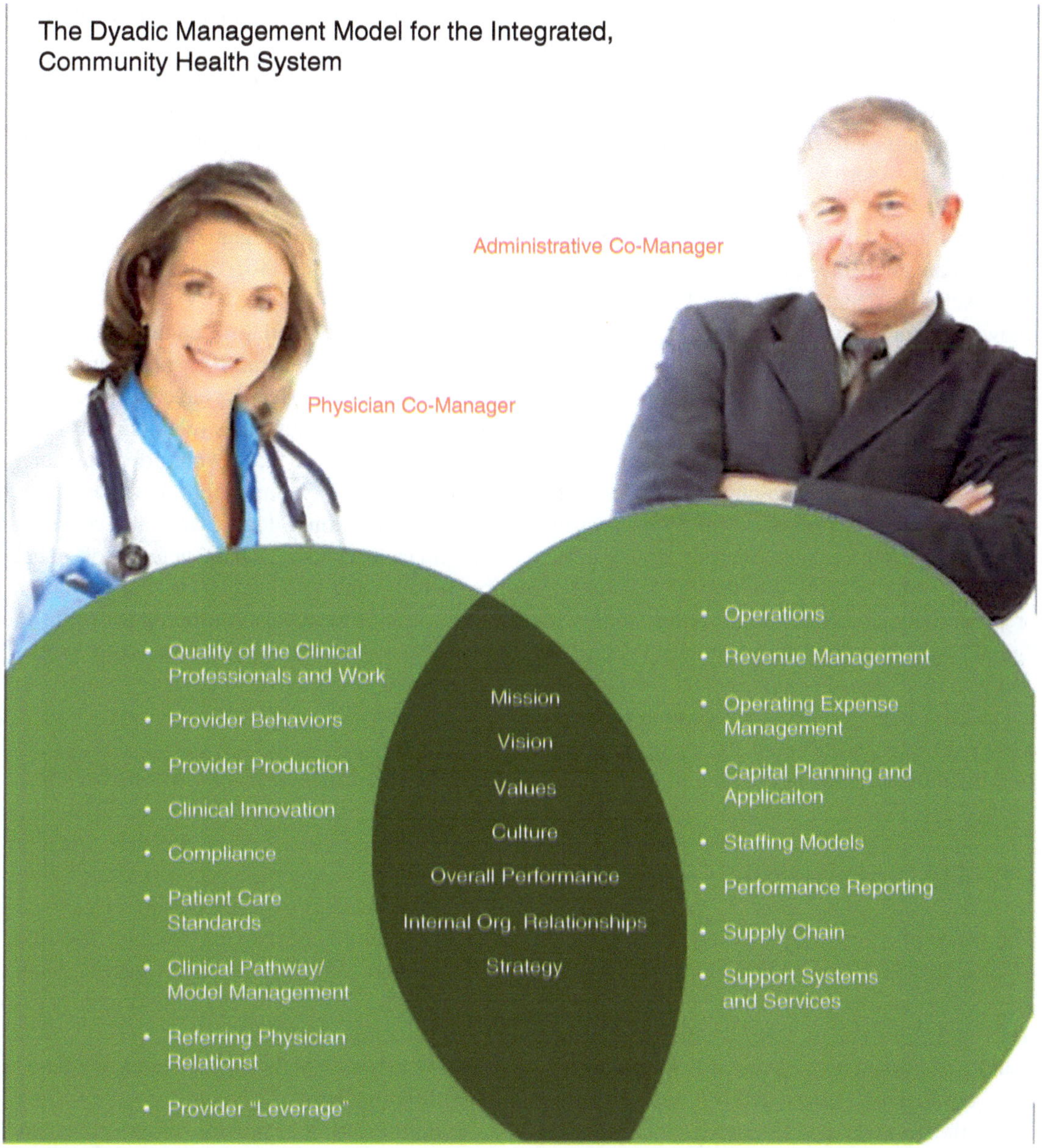

Fig. 17.2 Roles for physician and admin co-managers within the dyad management model (Image used with permission from ACPE.org – Zismer DK, Brueggemann J. Examining the "Dyad" as a Management Model in Integrated Health Systems. PEJ. January*February/2010)

Leadership Teams

In contrast to classic physician training, which often emphasizes the physician as an independent operator, this new leadership role by necessity requires participation as part of a high performing team. Being one part of a larger team is not a value set or skillset generally nurtured during medical school or residency, nor may it be of particular interest for clinical or academic practicing physicians. In Patrick Lencioni's book *The Five Dysfunctions of a Team* [8], the strategy around which teams either fail or succeed is well described. The role of the leader, or in the case of the dyad model the co-leaders, is to develop team performance. The best teams will demonstrate vulnerability-based trust, clarity, constructive confrontation, and a focus on productive discussions and decisions and team outcomes. Communication within teams becomes even more important during discussions and decisions. Teams need to know in advance how decisions will be made: consensus, majority vote, or by executive decree. Regardless, team members need to support group decisions. Physician leaders would be well advised to direct much of their leadership development time on enhancing communications. Books such as *Crucial Conversations* [9] provide simple, but powerful, strategies for enhancing discussions involving negotiations or potentially confrontational discussions with "good physicians with bad behavior". Lencioni believes that the role of the leader, or the dyad leadership, is to "go first". Leaders must model trust with one another and the team and skillfully lead discussions in a vulnerable fashion.

Defining Organizational Culture

The role of organizational culture in which to develop physician and administrative leaders cannot be underestimated. Culture can be described as a set of shared attitudes, values, goals and practices. Successful organizations take care to define values and behaviors that constitute the desired culture in order to achieve their stated vision. Physician behavior is at the core of either reinforcing or undermining the culture in a practice, and thus "culture fit" is one of the most, if not the most, important aspect of hiring new physicians with leadership potential and identifying internal high potential physicians.

Hirschfield and Moss [10] suggest that to reduce the chances of a culture clash, it is imperative to identify leaders on both sides who can provide models of behavior that represent the new desired culture. A multi-step process to ensure culture alignment may include:

1. develop a compelling and measurable vision for the organization,
2. listen well to understand perspectives of leadership, staff, patients, and providers,
3. develop a transparent organization that implements communication to clarify vision and strategic initiatives,
4. use leadership in organizational surveys to solicit "weigh-in" for opinions, helping to ensure "buy-in".

Realizing the potential for culture clash within the physician-administrator dyad is important. Managers and physicians have diverse backgrounds and even languages (e.g., clinical versus financial) and will be faced with different primary responsibilities. Administrators have an operational organizational focus, and are concerned with financial budgets, management of patient populations, and even the fiscal survival of an organization. Physicians, on the other hand, find themselves with a clinical focus, with primary responsibility for survival of the individual patient.

Measuring Leadership Competency

The Healthcare Leadership Alliance [11] has recently created a competency directory (www.healthcareleadershipalliance.org) to measure current and future healthcare leaders regarding potential and experience to meet the challenges of leadership in healthcare. This directory surveys five competencies:

1. Knowledge of the healthcare environment;
2. Professionalism;
3. Communication of relationship management;
4. Business skills and knowledge; and
5. Leadership.

Within the fifth category, physicians will be evaluated for leadership skills and behavior, organizational climate and culture, communicating vision, and managing change. The Children's Healthcare of Atlanta Center for Leadership Strategies has developed a leadership competency checklist (Table 17.2). Leaders can be graded on competencies that include, but are not limited to, delivering operational excellence, championing innovation and change, building

Table 17.2 CHOA Center for Leadership Strategies leadership competency checklist

Delivers Operational Excellence
Acts Strategically
Focuses on the Customer
Builds Capability
Champions Innovation and Change
Builds Productive Relationships
Demonstrates Personal Mastery
Communicates and Influences Effectively

productive relationships, and effective communication and influence. Assessment against this set of competencies forms the basis of development actions aimed at leveraging strengths and shoring up weaknesses.

Dowling [12] has described the principles of transformational leadership to address the need to improve access, produce better outcomes, and reduce cost for healthcare in the United States. Dowling believes that transformational leaders in healthcare will succeed through seven principles (similar to competencies) and four practices.

Dowling's Seven **Principles** [12]:

1. Manage and promote change
2. Create a purpose and a mission
3. Pursue sustainable change over time
4. Build capabilities
5. Manage paradox
6. Act as savvy politicians
7. Manifest optimism and passion, instilling confidence and trust

In order to operationalize these principles, these leaders should focus on four **practices**:

1. Focus on the customer
2. Define the reality that the organization faces
3. Set the moderate and long-term direction for the organization
4. Invest in your followers

Several other tools are available for assessing leadership competencies. The CHOA Center for Leadership Strategies employs a more formal 360° evaluation process to provide peer and direct report feedback to help leaders identify areas of greatest strengths and weaknesses. Individual coaches and mentors may be used in a more one-on-one session, targeting specific areas of need.

The author Marshall Goldsmith describes the use of a "feedforward" [13] process that differs distinctly from feedback. This feedforward process employs a distinctly different philosophy applicable for either process or behavioral improvement. In order for this feedforward process to be successful, the leader must identify an area of need, own the change process, and provide sincere effort and follow through to improve. Another model, described as the "dyad assessment of the dyad" [14], allows for continuing review and reinforcement of leadership competencies between co-managers themselves.

Perhaps the greatest measure of success as a physician leader is demonstration of true alignment with hospital administration and leadership team members, as evidenced by organizational health. As Lencioni wrote in "The Advantage" [15], organizational health is defined as minimal politics, minimal confusion, high morale and productivity, and low turnover, manifesting a culture of productivity and communication. Smart businesses excel in terms of strategy, marketing, technology, and finance, but those truly healthy organizations outperform in terms of efficiencies and competitive advantage.

Leading Change

Given all the pressures that healthcare systems around the world now face, perhaps change implementation is the number one leadership role. Physician leaders or dyad leaders, or leadership teams lead change continuously. A seven-step change implementation template (Fig. 17.3) outlines key steps, in order, for successful change implementation. The role of a physician leader is to recognize physician inertia and resistance (step 1) and to build a case for change (step 2) through a strong guiding team (step 3) is critical. The guiding team should represent all facets of practice or hospital business, and collectively guide teams by creating a compelling vision and action plan. The action plan must be financially sound and well-communicated to engage the entire organization. Quick wins build momentum, and then the work begins to spread change

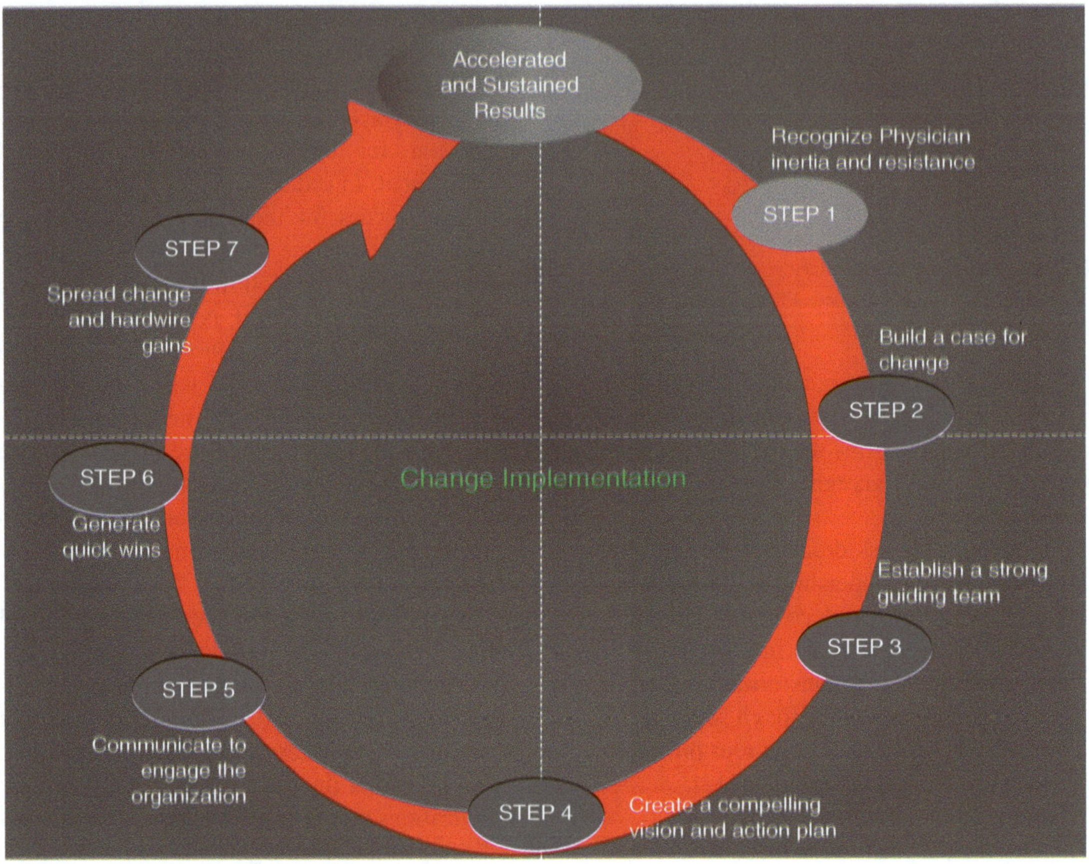

Fig. 17.3 A step change implementation template outlines key steps, in order, for successful change implementation

and hardwire gains that lead to enhanced financial and operational efficiencies. Successful change implementation will be best achieved by teams that have invested in the lessons from Pat Lencioni's "Five Dysfunctions of a Team" [8]. Teams that manifest organizational trust, leading to vulnerable discussions and "best choice" decisions, will lead change not only at the hospital level but also for the profession of pediatric cardiac services. Significantly, if there is limited or no trust between management and providers, there will not be engagement and thus improvement will occur only at the margins. Current examples of change opportunity include the development of appropriate use criteria and quality metrics, which define evidence-based physician performance. The collaboration among national centers to define core databases and registries, with ultimately the generation of national benchmark data, will allow institutions to objectively measure performance at a local level. Cost management strategies, including elimination of unnecessary variability and physician orders and procedural/device choices, will permit hospital systems then to define value (outcomes/cost). All of these steps involve change, and will require strong physician and administrative leadership to be successful.

Avoiding Leadership Dysfunction

Not all emerging leaders will find the leadership role enjoyable or successful; some leaders will fail and others burn out. Likewise, some team members fail to integrate successfully into the team and may need replacement. If organizational vision and culture has been successfully defined and defended throughout, then the use of a leadership competency checklist, 360° process, or one-on-one coaching may identify leaders who need to change or leave. Jim Collins, in his book *Good to Great* [16], defines the need to place "the right people on the right bus", meaning that to function as a leader, or as a leadership team member, trumps title alone. Dysfunction among leadership teams can paralyze organizations faced with the need to make important, and timely, change. The role of the leader to define leadership and performance competencies objectively is crucial towards advancement toward the desired change end point. Failure to hold individuals, and especially leadership team members, accountable might be regarded as one of the greatest failures of a team leader. The use of techniques and strategies described in the book *Crucial Conversations* [9] can help leaders become more competent, and thus comfortable, with the difficult conversations to address substandard physician performance or "good physicians with difficult behaviors".

Valuing Physician Leaders

Just as individual physicians must show passion for their new leadership role, likewise hospital systems need to demonstrate appreciation for the value of physician leadership and expertise by appropriating time and money for education and training of physician leaders, as well as compensating them for leadership time. Administrative time and expertise needs to be fairly compensated, to offset the loss in clinical income earning opportunity.

Conclusions

Successful integrated healthcare systems depend upon new physician leadership roles. Ultimately the best leaders may prove to be those who are internally passionate about this new role and realize the added value to the system provided by their dedication to perfecting leadership competencies. These leaders partner well with others who have differing opinions to work towards solutions which can be supported on the journey to more efficient healthcare in the future.

References

1. Porter M. What is value in health care? N Engl J Med. 2010;363:2477–81.
2. DiSC Profile Test. Illinois: Inscape Publishing. Available at http://onlindiscprofile.com.
3. StrengthsFinders. Available at http://www.strengthsfinder.com.
4. Hogan Assessment Systems. Available at http://www.hoganassessments.com/content/we-predict-performance.
5. The Birkman Method. Available at http://www.birkman.com/birkmanMethod/whatIsTheBirkmanMethod.php.
6. Blanchard K. Leading at a higher level. Upper Saddle River: FT Press; 2007.
7. ACC Cardiovascular Leadership Institute. Information available at http://www.cardiosource.org/ACC/Cardiovascular-Leadership-Institute.aspx.
8. Lencioni P. Five dysfunctions of a team: teamwork solutions. Lafayette: The Table Group; 2002. Available at http://www.tablegroup.com/books/dysfunctions.
9. Patterson K, Grenny J, McMillan R, et al. Crucial conversations: tools for talking when the stakes are high. New York: McGraw-Hill; 2002.
10. Hirschfield M, Moss R. Culture clash: the impact of culture on physician-hospital integration. HFM: 2011. Accessed online at: http://www.hfma.org/Publications/hfm-Magazine/Archives/2011/July/Culture-Clas--he-Impact-of-Culture-on-Physician-Hospital-Integration.
11. The Healthcare Leadership Alliance. HLA competency directory available at: www.healthcareleadershipalliance.org.
12. Dowling MJ. Transformational leadership: the key to success. In: Shore DA, editor. Forces of change. San Francisco: Josey-Bass; 2012. p. 35–48.
13. Goldsmith M. What got you here won't get you there. New York: Hyperion; 2007.
14. Spanier GB. Measuring dyadic adjustment: new scales for assessing the quality of marriage and similar dyads. J Marriage Fam. 1976;38(1):15–28.
15. Lencioni P. The advantage. San Francisco: Josey-Bass; 2012.
16. Collins J. Good to great: why some companies make the leap… and others don't. New York: HarperCollins Publishers; 2001.

18 The Role of the Federal Government in the Improvement of Healthcare Quality and Reduction of Costs in the United States

John E. Mayer Jr.

Abstract

Improving both the quality and costs of healthcare has become a major focus for the US Federal Government in its role both as a payor and as the source of healthcare policy. A series of initiatives have been undertaken since the mid-1990s culminating in the Accountable Care Act. There is a continued need to engage the medical profession in both quality improvement and wise allocation of society's healthcare resources, and the profession must advocate for this role in its interactions with the Federal Government.

Keywords

Healthcare Policy • Medical Profession • Accountable Care Act • Healthcare Quality

The quality of healthcare that is delivered to patients now represents a major focus for the governments of most Western democracies. Glenn Hackbarth, as chair of the United States Government's Medicare Payment Advisory Commission (MedPAC), succinctly described the reasons for this governmental focus as follows: "U.S. healthcare is too expensive and the quality is too inconsistent" [1]. However, this US Federal governmental focus on healthcare quality has existed since the Clinton Administration as reflected in the report of a Presidential Commission entitled Quality First [2]. Subsequent US Institute of Medicine reports entitled "To Err is Human" [3] and "Crossing the Quality Chasm" [4] further raised the issue of the quality of care delivered by the US healthcare system and led to an even greater focus on healthcare quality. It has been frequently observed that the United States expends 50–100 % more than other Western democracies on healthcare and has a lower life expectancy [5]. Recent data also show that governmental sources now account for at least 45 % of the total healthcare expenditures in the US [5]. Since Federal and state governments are providing such a significant fraction of the payments for healthcare and represent the people of the US who have an obvious interest in

J.E. Mayer Jr., MD
Department of Cardiac Surgery, Children's Hospital, Boston, Harvard Medical School, 300 Longwood Avenue, Boston, MA 02115, USA
e-mail: john.mayer@cardio.chboston.org

P.R. Barach, J.P. Jacobs, S.E. Lipshultz, P.C. Laussen (eds.),
Pediatric and Congenital Cardiac Care: Volume 2: Quality Improvement and Patient Safety,
DOI 10.1007/978-1-4471-6566-8_18,

the quality of the healthcare that is provided, it is not surprising that this major payor has continued to make efforts to improve both the cost and quality of healthcare.

One of the first steps that the Federal Government undertook to attempt to improve healthcare quality began with the National Technology and Transfer Advancement Act 1995. As a result of this act and based on recommendations from the Presidential Commission on Consumer Protection and Quality in the Health Care Industry, the National Quality Forum (NQF) was established as a voluntary, consensus standards setting body for quality measures. A rigorous, evidence-based review of proposed quality measures through a formal consensus development process was established, and the NQF has now become the gold standard for healthcare performance measures. Importantly, governmental agencies were obligated under this Act to use NQF measures quality measures that were adopted through the NQF process rather than each developing their own measures. Funding for the NQF continues to come from grants provided by government and not for profit foundations, and from member dues and government contracts. Membership is currently over 300 healthcare institutions, health insurers, government agencies, and professional organizations. The current missions of the NQF include (1) Building consensus on national priorities and goals for performance improvement, (2) Endorsing national consensus standards for measuring and publicly reporting on performance, and (3) Promoting the attainment of national goals through education and outreach programs. The Society of Thoracic Surgeons was one of the first physician organizations to propose a set of quality measures for surgical coronary artery revascularization procedures which were adopted through this NQF process. Subsequently, the STS also proposed a series of measures for congenital heart surgery, and many of these were adopted as well.

The most important Federal action in the healthcare sector has clearly been the Affordable Care Act which became law in 2010. Several sections of this legislation were drafted in an attempt to achieve the dual goals of cost reduction and improvement of quality and patient access to healthcare, and these were summarized by Kocher and Sahni in 2010, who also noted that 10 % of patients account for 64 % of all US healthcare costs [6]. A key goal of this legislation was to achieve coordination of care among various providers of healthcare, and the legislation provided for the formation of "accountable care organizations" which would receive payments for the management of populations rather than individual patients but would also have to meet quality goals that would be established. These accountable care organizations would be allowed to share in the savings that occurred through the coordinated efforts of physicians, hospitals, and other providers in these accountable care organizations. These savings were anticipated to result from the development or redesign of care processes to achieve both high-quality and high efficiency. Kocher and Sahni also noted that a key question was whether physicians or hospitals would control the ACO's, and noted that whoever controls the ACO's will capture the largest share of any savings [6]. Initially, 65 quality measures in the 5 domains of patient experience, care coordination, patient safety, preventive health, and the health of "at risk" and frail elderly populations were adopted. In addition, the ACA also provided for funding of "medical homes", which were to be community based, interdisciplinary, interprofessional teams that support primary care practices. An additional provision of the ACA directed at incentivizing more coordinated and less costly care were bundled payment programs for standard surgical procedures. These bundled payment programs were proposed as pilot programs for procedures such as coronary artery bypass surgery and hip replacement surgery. An additional provision was directed at reducing hospital readmissions by reducing the payments to hospitals for the care delivered to patients who were readmitted within 30 days of hospital discharge with the rationale that these reduced payments would motivate hospitals to engage with care coordinators to organize better delivery systems for post-hospital care. Reductions in payments were also mandated for "hospital acquired conditions" to provide hospitals an incentive to standardize protocols and procedures to reduce hospital-acquired conditions such as urinary tract infections and pneumonias. The impacts of the implementation of the ACA on healthcare quality and costs are still being acquired, but the results of the Physician Group Practice Demonstration, which began as a medical home demonstration project prior to the enactment of the ACA have been mixed [7]. Additional funding was provided to increase the use of electronic health records to further improve the coordination of care across providers and sites of care. An additional Executive Branch initiative, under the leadership of Dr. Donald Berwick during his tenure as acting administrator of the Centers for Medicare and Medicaid Services, was the formation of the "Partnership for Patients", which aimed to save 60,000 lives by stopping preventable injuries and complications in patient care. This initiative gathered pledges of support from 4,500 organizations and included a $500 M demonstration project focused on Community-Based Care Transitions and the development of a CMS Innovation Center, which was designed as a mechanism by which hospital systems could spread best practices to reduce hospital-acquired infections. The outcomes of all of these provisions of the ACA directed at improving quality and reducing costs remain unknown.

One observation regarding the ACA legislation is that there were relatively few provisions that directly engaged physicians, other than those in primary care specialties, in addressing the cost and quality goals of the legislation. The commonly cited conventional wisdom is that physicians either control or significantly influence as much as 70 % of the healthcare expenditures in the US through provision of services and through ordering of diagnostic tests, drugs, and procedures. However, professions are expected to serve the societal interests by not only providing care, but also through the wise allocation of societal resources [8]. Throughout much of modern history, the physician has had two roles, "healer of the sick" and "member of a profession" [8]. Although the distinction between these two roles has not been commonly appreciated, these roles have different historical origins and involve different activities [8]. Professions were created by and exist for the benefit of the general society as a means of organizing the delivery of complex services which society requires, including that of the healer. Characteristics of a profession include (1) an occupation whose core element is work based upon mastery of a complex body of knowledge and skills (2) knowledge or practice of a knowledge-based art that is used in the service of others, (3) governance by codes of ethics, (4) commitments to competence, integrity and morality, and (5) altruism and promotion of the public good [9]. The relationship between society and a profession has been described as a "social contract" with implied prerogatives and responsibilities for each profession [8]. Among the most important of these professional responsibilities is the expectation that the profession will act in the societal interest and not its own [10]. Other responsibilities articulated by a number of different individuals and organizations include (1) maintaining, advancing, and disseminating a body of knowledge, (2) setting and enforcing its own standards and values, i.e. self-regulation, (3) cherishing performance above personal reward, (4) placing patients' interests above their own, and (5) fairly distributing finite medical resources [9]. An important prediction made by Kocher and Sahni was that if hospital systems dominated accountable care organizations, physicians' incomes and status as independent professionals will decline [6].

Viewed from this context, quality improvement is a fundamental responsibility of the medical profession, and databases and registries, created and maintained by professional groups that are focused on patient outcomes, are a critically important tool by which quality improvement can occur. These databases foster the two of the most important functions of a profession, in particular, dissemination of knowledge and mastery of a complex body of knowledge. These registries can also be an important vehicle for setting and enforcing standards and evaluating performance. Ultimately these databases and registries could serve as a mechanism for the wise allocation of societal resources for healthcare, provided that both government and private payors will provide the resource utilization data. Database/registry participation, careful review of the resulting outcomes data, and active attempts to improve are thus fundamental to both being better "healers of the sick" and responsible "members of a profession." In this regard, Federal legislation has now been passed that establishes "qualified registries" which can at least serve as reporting vehicles under the Physician Quality Reporting Program establish in earlier "pay for reporting" quality legislation. Continuing efforts are underway to allow these "qualified registries" to be eligible to also receive resource utilization data from governmental sources. The technical feasibility of this merging of clinical outcomes and resource utilization data has been demonstrated in the ASCERT trial in which both resource utilization data and long-term survival information from the Medicare claims dataset has been able to be linked with the STS National Database and the American College of Cardiology's interventional catheterization database [11].

This author would argue that it is the merging of these clinical and resource utilization databases that will provide the best prospects for both improving the quality of care and reducing the costs of that care. In this way, the medical profession can fulfill both of its responsibilities to be healers of the sick and wise stewards of society's healthcare resources. Federal support of both the formation of professional registries and provision of access to the extensive resource utilization datasets maintained by the Federal Government could prove to be a wise investment of resources to further advance the goals of improved quality and more effective use of resources. It remains to be seen whether the formation of accountable care organizations will succeed and whether the role of the medical profession in improving the quality of health care will evolve in ways that allow truly professional activity to continue.

References

1. Hackbarth G, Boccuti C. Transforming graduate medical education to improve health care value. N Engl J Med. 2011;364:693–5.
2. Quality first: better healthcare for all Americans. Report of the Presidential Commission on Quality in Health Care; 1998.
3. Kohn LT, Corrigan JM, Donaldson M, editors. Committee on Quality of Health Care in America, Institute of Medicine Report. To err is human: building a safer health system. Washington DC: National Academy of Sciences; 2000. ISBN 0-309-06837-1.
4. Committee on Quality of Health Care in America. Crossing the quality chasm: a new health system for the 21st century. Washington, DC: Institute of Medicine: 2001. ISBN 0-309-07280-8.
5. Fuchs VR, Milstein A. The $640 billion question – why does cost-effective care diffuse so slowly? N Engl J Med. 2011;364:1985–7.
6. Kocher R, Sahni NR. Physicians versus hospitals as leaders of accountable care organizations. N Engl J Med. 2010;363:2579–82.
7. Igelehart JK. Assessing an ACO Prototype-Medicare's Physician Group Practice demonstration. N Engl J Med. 2011;364:198–200.
8. Creuss RL, Creuss SR. The Osler Fellows Program: physicianship, professionalism, and medicine's social contract with society. www.medicine.mcgill.ca/physicianship/Presentations/IntrotoProfessionalismforOslerFellows.
9. Mayer Jr JE. Is there a role for the medical profession in solving the problems of the American Health Care System? Ann Thorac Surg. 2009;87:1655–61.
10. Krause EA. Death of the guilds. New Haven: Yale University Press; 1995. p. 29–49.
11. Weintraub WS, Grau-Sepulveda MV, Weiss JM, O'Brien SM, Peterson ED, Kolm P, Zhang Z, Klein LW, Shaw RE, McKay C, Ritzenthaler LL, Popma JJ, Messenger JC, Shahian DM, Grover FL, Mayer JE, Shewan CM, Garratt KN, Moussa ID, Dangas GD, Edwards FH. Comparative effectiveness of revascularization strategies. N Engl J Med. 2012;366:1467–76.

19 Lessons Learned from the Public Inquiry into Children's Heart Surgery at the Bristol Royal Infirmary and the English Safe and Sustainable Cardiac Review

Martin Elliott

Abstract

This chapter discusses the consequences of an episode in Bristol, UK in the 1980s and 1990s, in which there was an unacceptably high mortality in children undergoing open heart surgery. A major public inquiry followed and amongst many other recommendations, it was suggested that UK cardiac surgical services should be concentrated in a smaller number of centers. Subsequent service reviews came to the same conclusion. It did not happen. Eventually, a process called Safe and Sustainable Cardiac Surgery was established by the Department of Health, building on agreement of all centers to attempt once again to reduce the number of centers, using a standards-based approach. This chapter outlines, from the personal perspective of one lead care center involved, the process, its complexity, the scale of investment, the massive public consultation and, the final analysis that led to its ultimate failure. It contains salutary lessons for all those involved in pediatric cardiac service reform.

Keywords

Pediatric cardiac surgery • Service reform • Health service management • Bristol • Safe and Sustainable

Introduction

There is a classic golfing quote, attributed to many, but mostly Gary Player who, when speaking to a journalist after a low score round beset by many lipped putts, said "the more I practice, the luckier I get!". Cardiac surgeons know that is largely true for them, as it is for anyone carrying out a practical skill. The more you do the better you get. This principle underpinned a recent review of surgery for congenital

The author was a member of both the Safe and Sustainable Cardiac Surgery Standards Group and the Steering Group

M. Elliott, MD, FRCS
Paediatric Cardiothoracic Surgery,
University College London, Gresham College,
London, UK

The Great Ormond Street Hospital for Children NHS
Foundation Trust, London WC1N 3JH, UK
e-mail: martin.elliott@gosh.nhs.uk

P.R. Barach, J.P. Jacobs, S.E. Lipshultz, P.C. Laussen (eds.),
Pediatric and Congenital Cardiac Care: Volume 2: Quality Improvement and Patient Safety,
DOI 10.1007/978-1-4471-6566-8_19, © Springer-Verlag London 2015

heart defects in England,[1] called 'Safe & Sustainable Children's Cardiac Services' [1]. The aim of this review was to reorganize services in England to deliver care through a smaller number of bigger centers, themselves at the center of a rational geographic network of peripheral units staffed by general pediatricians with cardiology training. Each unit should have enough cases to ensure expertise of surgeons, and enough surgeons to provide cross cover and long term, sustainable staffing. The process of the review was standards based, complex and time-consuming for all involved. It also proved to be the biggest public consultation in the history of the National Health Service (NHS). It had the support of all the Royal Colleges, national patients groups, the Commissioners (the purchasers in the NHS model) and initially all the cardiac units in the UK. Many senior NHS managers experienced in health service change regarded *Safe and Sustainable* as the best process they had seen for achieving large scale service reconfiguration. Despite all this support, the process failed under a waterfall of litigation, process challenge, mixed publicity, 'nimby'ism, and bad timing, occurring in the middle of the biggest reorganization of the NHS in its history.

I have to own up to being personally bruised by these events. I have striven over years to pursue excellence in cardiac care, and that was the underlying driver behind our involvement in this review. I am sorry that it did not proceed immediately, and hope that quality will not suffer. Yet another review has been commissioned and I hope that it does not lie in the political long grass since service redesign should be the very benefit of a state run health system, free at the point of delivery. This chapter summarizes the history of the process and lists some of the lessons learned.

Background

As in most countries throughout the 1950–1970s, pediatric cardiac surgery sprang up in places where there existed talented risk-taking surgeons, innovative and brave cardiologists and a hospital management team keen to put their institution on the map. They were usually sited in reasonably large pediatric hospitals or in single-organ specialist units. They were rarely designed from the bottom up as a networked service. It was a classic alpha-male environment with a work-all-hours ethic and highly competitive between institutions and especially between surgeons. New operations were being developed, and the age at which they could be performed fell rapidly as new technology developed, and results from pioneering units became known. Each surgeon, and each unit, became 'tested' by their willingness to adopt and their ability to deliver these new operations. By the mid-1980s the transition to neonatal surgery was firmly established and there were preliminary attempts at reporting of results through voluntary registries. Then came Bristol.

Bristol

Bristol is a large city in the west of England with a proud history, a good University and a well-established children's hospital. In 1975, it had a small cardiac center, doing just over 100 cases per year when Mr. James Wisheart was appointed as a pediatric cardiac surgeon. The regional management team invested in the service and by 1985 the unit was performing 435 cases per year. That expansion required another surgeon to be hired, and Janardan Dhasmana was appointed as a junior colleague, and soon (1988) introduced the arterial switch procedure, by now the operation by which units were judged. He carried out 38 switches in all, with 20 deaths, way above the mortality rate anywhere else.

In 1988, Steve Bolsin was appointed as an anesthesiologist and immediately noticed that operations were taking very much longer than he was used to during his training in London. He became worried about the quality of the surgical results. And this was not helped in the years 1990–1994 when James Wisheart had a mortality rate of 9/15 AVSD repairs, prompting Bolsin to write to the Clinical Director of the hospital, John Roylance, later to be replaced by James Wisheart himself. Steve Bolsin kept his own audit of outcomes.

[1] Paediatric congenital cardiac services were also reviewed separately at the two other units in the United Kingdom, in Scotland in 2011 and Northern Ireland in 2012.

I should add here that I was approached by Bristol in 1990 to apply for the Chair of Cardiac Surgery and to develop the pediatric practice. I turned down the offer, stating in writing that the way the unit was organized (multi-site, patchy cover, adult cardiac juniors covering pediatrics, ECHO on another site) was ineffective, inefficient and potentially dangerous.

Bolsin's story reached the press, via the satirical magazine Private Eye whose MD column is written by a GP, Dr. Phil Hammond [2]. Finally various official bodies, including the Royal College of Surgeons, reviewed the unit, but the College decided not to withdraw the license to carry out surgery, and its president was quoted in a later BBC documentary as suggesting the surgeons 'needed to get more practice'. In 1993 Bolsin's audit was completed and despite a limited circulation, revealed a mortality rate considerably higher than was expected from the voluntary national register that the UK cardiac surgeons kept.

Dhasmana stopped doing switches that year, but was persuaded to do another on Joshua Loveday in 1995. Joshua died on the table. It emerged that a senior NHS official, Peter Doyle, had advised the hospital not to let the procedure go ahead because of previous poor results. An external review by Professor Marc de Leval (Great Ormond Street and University College London) and Stewart Hunter (a senior cardiologist from Newcastle-upon-Tyne) concluded that Bristol *was* a high risk unit and that there were excessive deaths. A patients' group called the Bristol Action Group was established to campaign both to learn more and improve services to other children.

In 1996, Bolsin felt his position untenable and he emigrated to Australia. Wisheart stepped down as medical director, stopped operating and retired in 1997. The General Medical Council (GMC) launched an investigation and the BBC broadcast a damning documentary in its Panorama series [3]. The GMC struck Roylance and Wisheart off the register, and suspended Dhasmana. In 1999, a huge public inquiry began, chaired by Sir Ian Kennedy, a prominent lawyer with a specialist interest in health ethics.

His extensive, thorough and damning Inquiry made 198 recommendations for change, too many to cover here, but it is worth giving you some quotes from his press release; they form the core of why *Safe and Sustainable* developed:-

> Sir Ian said Bristol was a hospital that had "over-reached itself", where clinicians only had "limited experience" at the time it became a regional center.
> "Clinicians were ambitious to expand – the ambitions were too ambitious."
> "The management of the hospital was flawed – too much power was in too few hands."
> "There was a club culture where it was hard to raise matters of concern and harder to get anything done."
> And he said wider problems in the NHS were also to blame.
> "There were no agreed national standards as to what amounted to good quality care for paediatric cardiac surgery – no agreed measure or benchmark."
> "Bristol was awash with data … [but] there was confusion in the NHS from top to bottom as to where responsibility lay for monitoring the quality of paediatric cardiac surgery."

NHS Inquiries are frequent and fraught with implementation difficulties [4]. However, Sir Ian's view, expressed clearly in his report, was that there were too many centers in the UK, that complex surgery should be done in centers of excellence and that the whole process of care should be both standards-based and thoroughly monitored. *Safe and Sustainable* was thus 'unfinished business.'

Safe and Sustainable

The Bristol scandal highlighted appalling lapses in the care of children with congenital heart defects. In 2001, Kennedy explained the need for children to have heart surgery in fewer specialist centers. His report concluded:

> …standards should stipulate the minimum number of procedures which must be performed in a hospital over a given period of time in order to have the best opportunity of achieving good outcomes for children. Paediatric cardiac surgery must not be undertaken in hospitals which do not meet the minimum number of procedures. Considerations of ease of access to a hospital should not be taken into account in determining whether PCS should be undertaken at that hospital.

In 2003, a review group led by the late lamented Professor James Monro, then President of the Society of Cardiothoracic Surgeons, recommended that surgical centers should do no fewer than 300 open heart procedures per year. That would have meant that at the time, about half the centers should have closed. Action was not taken by government Ministers at the time who, no doubt mindful of the political storm inherent in moving hospital services (regardless of the strength of professional consensus), justified their inaction on the grounds that the review had not unearthed concrete evidence of unsafe practice in any particular unit.

Concerns persisted; in 2006 a national workshop of experts chaired by Professor Roger Boyle (a cardiologist and national cardiac 'Tsar') and Dr. Sheila Shribman (who held a similar role for pediatrics) concluded that the current configuration of services was unsustainable. All the surgical units sent representatives to this meeting to discuss rationalization, and they agreed that the number of units should be reduced, probably to about 7 from the 11 that were then open. Each unit was challenged with the argument that the consequence of rationalization might be that their own unit would be scheduled for closure. They all agreed on the need for change.

In 2007, the Royal College of Surgeons of England called for the concentration of surgical expertise into fewer, larger specialist centers [5]. A year later, Professor Sir Bruce Keogh, NHS medical director and himself a cardiac surgeon, instigated the *Safe and Sustainable* (S&S) review, which began in 2008. His frank public warning was that failure to re-organize pediatric cardiac services this time round would be "a stain on the soul of the specialty".

It was a response to the long-standing concerns of NHS clinicians, their professional associations, national parent groups and NHS commissioners about the sustainability of the service configuration then extant. Surgeons were thought to be spread too thinly across surgical centers (31 congenital cardiac surgeons spread over 11 surgical centers), leading to concerns around lack of 24/7 cover in smaller centers and the potential for sudden closure or suspension of smaller centers because of illness, burn out or diminished performance.

Sir Bruce had at the front of his mind the warnings made by the two previous reviews in 2000 and 2003 about the risk of something going wrong again in one of the English units. The case for change seemed unarguable when the pediatric congenital surgical service in Oxford (the smallest unit in England) was suddenly suspended in March 2010 after a number of deaths of babies following heart surgery. The NHS has very good experience of concentrating highly specialized services in the interests of quality and excellence; in our field these were ECMO (3 units), transplantation (2), tracheal surgery (1) and pulmonary hypertension (1). These units were producing world-leading results at low cost, concentrating expertise and delivering research output. The argument seemed clear.

The S&S review was managed by the National Specialised Commissioning Team (NSC Team), on behalf of the 10 Specialised Commissioning Groups (SCGs) in England and their constituent Primary Care Trusts.[2]

Governance Arrangements

It may seem boring to cover the governance arrangements, but this was bound to be a controversial piece of work, and great care was taken to ensure appropriate governance and attempt to get both top down and bottom up support, as well as strong political and professional leadership and lay involvement. The lessons we learned need to take into account the immense consideration that was put into this phase of the project.

Steering Group

A Steering Group was convened in January 2009, chaired by Dr Patricia Hamilton CBE, Director of Medical Education for England and Immediate Past President of the Royal College of Paediatrics and Child Health. The Steering Group comprised representatives of relevant professional and lay

[2] At the time, NHS health care budgets were held by Primary Care Trusts for the majority of conditions, with some money being top-sliced from the NHS budget for Nationally Commissioned Highly specialized services such as ECMO, transplantation, tracheal surgery and pulmonary hypertension. These budgets were monitored and distributed by Commissioners as indicated.

associations. The role of the Steering Group was advisory and it had no role in decision making:

- Develop and communicate the clinical 'Case for Change'
- Consider the available research evidence around the relationship between larger surgical centers and clinical outcomes
- Develop designation criteria that surgical centers must meet in the future
- Develop a proposed model of care for regional pediatric cardiology networks
- Oversee stakeholder engagement and communication
- Endorse the process for the assessment of the current surgical centers

There was much debate early in the meetings of the Steering Group about whether it was right to consider pediatric cardiac surgery in isolation from adult congenital surgery. There was disagreement on the group about this and it was referred 'upwards', and the group was given clear guidance from the Department of Health that it should limit its scope to pediatrics. Thus, the scope of the S&S review *excluded* the designation of surgical services for adults with congenital heart disease, for which a separate designation process would be led later by individual SCGs once the pediatric review had concluded. However, the S&S review and the pediatric clinical standards gave prominence to the importance of *transition* to adult services.

Standards Group

Also in 2009, a pediatric cardiac surgery standards group was established, chaired by Mr. William Brawn, then President of the British Congenital Cardiac Association. Once again, this group had wide membership from professional organizations (cardiology, surgery, intensive care, adult CHD etc.), as well as commissioners. This group met regularly to define and publish standards of care and service to achieve excellence. In other words, the minimum standards a unit must have in order to be designated by the NHS as a suitable provider of care. The group consulted widely on the draft standards, including with the surgical units themselves. The finished standards are too detailed to present here, but are available at http://www.specialisedservices.nhs.uk/document/paediatric-cardiac-surgery-standards. They are clear and comprehensive and were widely supported as an outcome of public consultation.

Decision Making

Somebody had to make some tough decisions though and at the time it was clear that – in law – the only bodies which had legal powers for consulting on proposed changes to the number of units and for eventual decision making were the 152 Primary Care Trusts in England who commissioned secondary healthcare services. In July 2010, the Secretary of State endorsed a recommendation made by the National Specialised Commissioning Group (December 2009) to establish a joint committee of PCTs with delegated powers for consultation and decision-making. Each PCT Board in England accepted this recommendation via formal resolution after discussion at one of their own board meetings (this in itself conveys a sense of the scale of this program).

The joint committee of PCTs (JCPCT) comprised the Chair (or PCT Chief Executive Nominee) of each SCG in England and the Director of National Specialised Commissioning. They were thus very senior NHS managers, highly experienced in matters of service reconfiguration and implementing service change. It was chaired by Sir Neil McKay the Chief Executive of the East of England Strategic Health Authority – an experienced NHS career manager (this region does not have a pediatric cardiac surgical service within its borders, and so he was 'neutral'). It should also be remembered that Wales, Scotland and Northern Ireland, whilst in Britain, are devolved administrations so this review only covered England. Thus, representatives of the devolved administrations were present at the meetings.

However, there were as an important caveat to the arrangements for decision making that proved incredibly problematic to the smooth running of the review process, and arguably proved to be fatal to its success. Democracy is a complex and untidy business.

Whilst in law it was clear that only the JCPCT had legal authority to make a "final" decision in the first instance, other legislation enabled local Health and Overview Scrutiny Committees (of which there are hundreds in England at local Council level) to challenge the decision by way of referral to the Secretary of State for Health. These committees have a very local focus, and it was apparent from the start that no committee (made up of elected councilors with no particular expertise in health matters) would dare incur the wrath of the local electorate by supporting the closure of its own local heart unit. A challenge by a scrutiny committee was therefore inevitable at some point, and it was thus an "open secret" from the start of the process that the final decision would ultimately rest with the Secretary of State for Health himself – as it did in 2003 with the disregarded Monro report.

The likely success of a challenge to the JCPCT's decision by this route depended on the relevant scrutiny committee being able to demonstrate that the decision making process had been flawed – hardly an incentive for local politicians and local campaign groups to engage positively with the review team to achieve a good process. It also meant that campaigners realized early on that the way to influence government Ministers was to make the review a very public and controversial issue – and the various ensuing campaigns of misinformation and propaganda were quite extraordinary, resulting in a number of Ministerial debates in the House of Commons and House of Lords. In these debates government Ministers were always very careful to note the professional consensus on the need for change, but never actually gave a commitment to make changes. Instead, the role of the JCPCT as decision-maker was emphasized, along with a nod-and-a-wink to the likely role of the Secretary of State for Health once the JCPCT's eventual decision had been challenged.

In April 2010, the extensive professional and lay support was crystallized in a document called 'The Need for Change' [6]. This need can be summarized as follows:-

- Children's heart surgery was becoming increasingly complex
- Services had developed on an ad hoc basis; there was a need for a planned approach for England and Wales
- Surgical expertise (31 surgeons) was spread too thinly over 11 surgical centers
- Some centers were reliant on one or two surgeons and could not deliver a safe 24 h emergency service
- Smaller centers are vulnerable to sudden and unplanned closure
- Current arrangements were inequitable as there was too much variation in the expertise available from centers
- Fewer surgical centers were needed to ensure that surgical and medical teams were seeing a sufficient number of children to maintain and develop their specialist skills
- Available research evidence identified a relationship between higher-volume surgical centers and better clinical outcomes
- Having a larger and varied caseload would mean that larger centers are best placed to recruit and retain new surgeons and plan for the future
- The delivery of non-surgical cardiology care for children in local hospitals was inconsistent; strong leadership was thought to be required from surgical centers to develop expertise through regional and local networks
- Increasing the national pool of surgeons was not considered the answer, as this would result in individual surgeons performing fewer surgical procedures and increase the risk of occasional surgical practice

The ***benefits*** of the proposed change were predicted to be as follows:-

- Better results in the surgical centers with fewer deaths and complications following surgery
- Better, more accessible diagnostic services and follow up treatment delivered within regional and local networks
- Reduced waiting times and cancelled operations
- Improved communication between parents and all of the services in the network that see their child
- Better training for surgeons and their teams to ensure the sustainability of the service
- A trained workforce expert in the care and treatment of children and young people with congenital heart disease

- Centers at the forefront of modern working practices and innovative technologies that are leaders in research and development
- A network of specialist centers collaborating in research and clinical development, encouraging the sharing of knowledge across the network

Who could argue with those benefits? However, there was still much to do and, because of the massive public interest in the Bristol case, the potential important political decisions that need to be made, and the fact that the whole population could potentially be affected, a very complex and wide ranging process of evidence gathering, consultation and debate was set in train by the JCPCT.

The standards defined by the Standards Group morphed into designation criteria, of which the core ones were:-

- A minimum of four full-time congenital cardiac surgeons in each surgical center
- A minimum volume of 400 pediatric surgical procedures per year in each surgical center and ideally 500 pediatric surgical procedures
- 24/7 cover in each surgical center
- Co-location of surgical centers with interdependent services (e.g. intensive care, otorhinolaryngology, renal medicine etc.) as described in the Critical Interdependencies Framework [7].
- Development of pediatric cardiology networks via the proposed model of care

The importance to everyone of networks emerged during debate. Patients groups expressed very clearly that they would like informed follow up as close as possible to their homes. There was general acceptance about the rationale for concentrating deeply specialist services, but the need for local pediatricians and nurses trained in pediatric cardiology was strongly stated. Additional local community support via primary care and out into schools was also considered deficient. Thus there grew up the idea that the specialist center might be at the center of a network that it managed, guaranteeing quality throughout the geographic area.

This created a new *Model of Care* [8], built around the network concept, the features of which would be:-

- strengthened arrangements for the delivery of non-interventional diagnostic and follow-up care in local hospitals
- formal pathways from antenatal screening to the transition to adult services
- formal protocols agreed by the surgical center with local services
- delivered in local settings
- development of the role of Pediatricians with Expertise in Cardiology across the networks
- strengthened Cardiac Liaison Teams

Thus, more and more people and issues became incorporated into the debate. Everyone had a view, about everything. It was clear reconfiguration of the service was going to be very challenging. The Secretary of State had laid down four generic criteria which had to be fulfilled if a reconfiguration was to be allowed:-

1. Support from GP commissioners
2. Strong public and patient engagement
3. A clinical evidence base
4. Developed and supported patient choice.

Most of this was straightforward, but the public and stakeholder consultation was an enormous exercise, which began first with support from all relevant professional bodies (British Congenital Cardiac Association, Children's Heart Federation, Paediatric Intensive Care Society, Royal College of Nursing, Royal College of Paediatrics and Child Health, Royal College of Surgeons of England, Society for Cardiothoracic Surgery in Great Britain and Ireland, Specialised Healthcare Alliance). In retrospect, getting all these groups to agree was a wonderful thing.

The JCPCT launched public consultation on four options for configuration. No preferred option was stated, but options were scored against a number of criteria. A number of units immediately felt threatened through their own reading of the JCPCT's direction of travel – in particular in Leeds, Leicester, Oxford, Southampton and the Royal Brompton Hospital in London. The campaigns "for and against" had started in earnest.

A string of public meetings were held, and everyone was asked for their view, via a wide range of communication methods. In October 2009, a national partnership event was attended by 200 people from across the country. The outcome of this event informed the development of the clinical standards and the clinical case for change. There were also further local partnership engagement events, held throughout England in 2010. Partners were kept informed of the review's progress via quarterly newsletters, publication of all relevant papers on the NSCT website and presentations at patient group conferences.

The process of public consultation was huge in scope and delivery. It ran for 4 months between March and July 2011. A 7-min video was produced and published on the web to provide background and to encourage people to "have their say". A comprehensive public consultation document which ran to 234 pages was published [9] together with an "easy read" version for children and young people that provided details of how responses could be sent by text message. In Leeds alone a petition was signed by 600,000 people supporting retention of surgery in the city.

Town-hall style consultation events were held with the public, and focus groups were held with children and young people; with parents of children with congenital heart disease; and with members from Black and Minority Ethnic groups. In total, thousands of people attended over 50 consultation events, workshops and focus groups held in major cities across England and Wales.

It was important that stakeholders were reassured about the independence of the process, so Ipsos Mori, the international market research company, was commissioned to design a questionnaire survey, and to analyse the responses and report the outcome [10].

Around 75,000 responses were received, including from interested professionals in Europe, North America, the Middle East, Asia and Australia. Responses were also provided by: Members of Parliament representing their local constituents; professional bodies; local and national charities; various NHS bodies representing the pathway between antenatal screening to adult congenital services; health scrutiny committees; London Assembly members; patients, parents of patients and members of the public. Media interest was significant, and the public consultation become a regular item for national and local media (TV, radio and print).

No stone was left un-turned, it seemed. When the Royal Brompton Hospital complained that the impact of losing pediatric cardiac work would fatally jeopardize its respiratory service, the JCPCT responded by convening an international panel of respiratory experts, including from Toronto Children's Hospital, to spend a week in London in the autumn of 2011 visiting the Royal Brompton and three other hospitals in London that provide respiratory medicine. The panel advised the JCPCT that respiratory services at the Royal Brompton would remain viable but this did not convince the Royal Brompton to desist in making its claims.

In addition to this public and stakeholder work, each center had to apply for designation as a pediatric cardiac center, reporting against their ability to meet the agreed Standards, or with plans as to how to meet them. In May and June of 2010, and expert and senior team led by Sir Ian Kennedy (who, remember, chaired the Bristol Inquiry) and including Professor James Monro, visited all the units and scored them against the proscribed standards. These scores were used in the final decision process but were not determinative.

In his introduction to the panel's report to the JCPCT [11] Sir Ian wrote:

> During the current assessment process I and my colleagues on the panel found many examples of commendably high commitment and dedication by talented NHS staff delivering congenital cardiac services. But we found exemplary practice to be the exception rather than the rule. Mediocrity must not be our benchmark for the future.

To the panel's data were added extensive demographic research, transport time data and other complex modeling, all helped by external professional consultants. The resultant "Decision Making Business Case" [12] was submitted to the JCPCT for consideration and a formal, webcast and media-heavy Board meeting was held on 4th July 2012. The JCPCT decided to reduce the numbers of centers from 11 to 7, and they would be at Newcastle, Liverpool, Birmingham, Bristol, Southampton, Great Ormond Street and Guy's/St Thomas'. The units earmarked for de-designation were The Royal Brompton Hospital in London, Leicester, Leeds and Oxford.

A few days later *The Times* newspaper printed a letter signed by the presidents of the relevant royal colleges of medicine that congratulated the

JCPCT and welcomed its decision as one that would improve outcomes and save the lives of more children in the future.

Unsurprisingly, and despite their agreements to abide by the outcome in 2006, the units earmarked for change were far from happy and used all the tools at their disposal to both influence public opinion and, where possible, to take legal or procedural proceedings against the JCPCT process. There was much media coverage and in the summer of 2012 the streets of Leeds city center were closed to make way for an organized march by thousands of demonstrators. Bitter arguments between senior clinicians played out in the media, including claims by supporters of Leeds that children would die on the "road to death" to Newcastle. Both the Prime Minister, David Cameron, and Deputy Prime Minister, Nick Clegg, were door-stepped by journalists asking questions about the review. The JCPCT asked the clinicians on the steering group to front up to the media, not to defend the decision but to explain for lay-people the clinical rationale for change. Perhaps predictably, given the extent of negative campaigning by disaffected units, much of the debate became heated and personal rather than objective and cool. Social media and blog sites did not make pleasant reading for many of us who were involved.

The primary mode of attack in the courts was via Judicial Review of the whole JCPCT decision-making process. Such review was first launched by the Royal Brompton & Harefield NHS Foundation Trust[3] in 2010, who won the first round but lost on appeal, and later by a campaign group based in Leeds called Save our Surgery Ltd in 2012.

It is important to bear in mind that the Courts were not interested in whether the JCPCT had made the *correct decision* (the Court recognizes that it has no expertise in this regard) but whether the JCPCT had followed a proper and lawful *process*. The Royal Brompton's challenge was brought in March 2010 – some two years before the JCPCT actually made a decision. The Royal Brompton objected to the process of public consultation (held between March and July 2011) on a number of grounds: that the public consultation was a sham as the JCPCT members had secretly pre-determined the outcome; that the proposal for two units in London, rather than three, was irrational; bias within the steering group in favour of certain units[4]; misinformation in the consultation document; and a failure properly to consider the knock-on impact of ceasing pediatric cardiac surgery to the hospital's respiratory services. The Court rejected all of these challenges but upheld the hospital's challenge that the JCPCT's process for assessing the hospitals against one of the assessment criteria (research and innovation) had been flawed. This ruling paralyzed *Safe and Sustainable* because it meant that the entire process of a 4-month public consultation (the largest ever national consultation held by the NHS) was now null and void. The decision was over-turned by the Court of Appeal in March 2012 and the process was back on track – but the damage had been done by way of delay to the process and adverse publicity. It had made very public the inter-unit animosity that was infecting the process, including between clinicians who had previously regarded themselves as colleagues and friends. The total cost of legal fees incurred by the NHS on this case alone was around two million pounds of tax-payers money.

The second legal challenge was brought in October 2012 after the JCPCT's decision to reduce the number of units. It was brought by a campaign group called Save our Surgery (SoS) Ltd, formed to promote the pediatric cardiac service based at Leeds Teaching Hospitals NHS Trust and whose directors included clinicians working in the Leeds cardiac service. This challenge was

[3] To the consternation of many commentators, this was the first time that one NHS body had brought legal challenge against another, which was now possible by NHS hospitals who had attained quasi-independence through Foundation Trust status. It is current government policy to increase the number of Foundation Trust hospitals in England.

[4] I was named in the case made by the Royal Brompton has someone who used their influence in committee to suggest closure of the unit. This is not true, and the judge made clear that there were no grounds to support a suggestion of bias.

brought on the narrow ground that the JCPCT had failed to publish 450 sub-scores generated by the panel. The group argued that, by only publishing a limited number of headline scores, respondents to public consultation had been denied the opportunity to make a more informed judgement about the quality of the service in Leeds (the service in Leeds had received the second lowest score – out of 11 units – by Sir Ian Kennedy's panel against the assessment of standards). This challenge once again highlighted the acrimony between units, to the extent that the Newcastle-upon-Tyne Hospitals NHS Foundation Trust felt obliged to join the legal proceedings against SoS Ltd to counter what it perceived to be unfair and improper attacks made by the Leeds group in pursuance of its campaign to keep surgery in Leeds at the expense of Newcastle. The JCPCT argued, with the support of Sir Ian Kennedy, that the sub-scores were irrelevant to the process of consultation and decision making, and that even had they been published they could not have been used by respondents to second-guess the Kennedy panel's eventual conclusions – which had been reached using subjective expert judgment based on written and oral evidence submitted by the units to which respondents had no access. The judge, Mrs Justice Nicola Davies, found in favour of SoS Ltd in March 2013. She said that "*as the scores were relevant to the assessment, the breakdown of the scoring should have been disclosed to the centers whether or not the JCPCT proposed to look at it …if there is a public law duty to make information available to a consultee, disclosure cannot be denied simply because one party does not wish to look at that information.*" On that narrow ground, the entire process of consultation and decision making between 2009 and 2012 was declared unlawful.

The JCPCT prepared to challenge this ruling in the Court of Appeal, as it had successfully done with the previous Brompton ruling, citing strong legal advice that a successful appeal was likely. But this course of action proved to be politically impossible following intervention by the Secretary of State for Health in April 2013 in response to challenges made against the JCPCT's decision by health and overview scrutiny committees in Leeds and Leicester. The established procedure, upon receipt of such a challenge, allowed the Secretary of State to ask a body called the *Independent Reconfiguration Panel* (IRP) to review the JCPCT's decision and processes and to advise him as to whether the JCPCT's decision would lead to "safe and sustainable" pediatric cardiac services in the future. It would then be for the Secretary of State to decide the fate of the JCPCT's conclusions based on the advice of the IRP. Although chaired by a past president of the Royal College of Surgeons, the IRP did not comprise experts in the specialty but rather experts in hospital configuration, NHS managers and public engagement specialists. The IRP carried out a 5-month review, visiting every pediatric cardiac unit, interviewing those involved in the process, local campaign groups and took evidence from members of the public similar to a public consultation. This did not help to mitigate against the increasing sense of consultation fatigue within the specialty.

To many of us involved over the years, the resulting report by the IRP appeared to lack substance, insight or understanding of the issues when compared to the detailed analysis of the Safe and Sustainable process [13]. But it was sufficiently critical of the JCPCT's process to allow the Secretary of State for Health, Jeremy Hunt, to inform the House of Commons in April 2013 that:-

> The IRP report also concludes that the outcome of the Safe & Sustainable review was based on a flawed analysis of the impact of incomplete proposals, and leaves too many questions about sustainability and implementation.[5] This is clearly a serious criticism of the Safe & Sustainable process. I therefore accept their recommendation that the proposals cannot go ahead in their current form and am suspending the review today.

He said the consultation, which has already cost more than £6 million, did not have the confidence of the public with some feeling the decision was predetermined. He said choosing which hospitals provided surgery was one of the most

[5] Much of this and the next couple of paragraphs are drawn from an excellent piece by the BBC's science correspondent, James Gallagher, on 12/06/13.

flawed areas of the review, but added "we need to get on with this" as the original argument for improving care was unchanged.

The IRP's report said: "The Panel's advice addresses the weaknesses in the original proposals, but it is not a mandate for either the status quo or going back over all the ground in the last five years."

Lord Ribeiro (a former president of The Royal College of Surgeons), the chairman of the IRP, said access to services was one of the panel's main concerns, thereby overturning Sir Ian Kennedy's previous recommendation in the Bristol Inquiry that issues of access and convenience should *not* be a consideration in any future process to decide the number and location of surgical units, and contrary to what partners had told the JCPCT during the Safe and Sustainable process.

It is not the role of the IRP to offer an actual solution to the configuration of pediatric cardiac services, and Mr. Hunt was certainly not going to offer one. Instead he set NHS England, which has taken over the responsibilities of the Joint Committee of Primary Care Trusts, a deadline of the end of July 2013 to come up with the next step in the process.

The fate of children's heart surgery would now be considered alongside changes to adult congenital heart surgery.

So NHS England, the overarching management body for the NHS after the massive reforms implemented by Jeremy Hunt's predecessor, Andrew Lansley, has committed itself to a further review chaired by its own Chairman, Sir Malcolm Grant and with Sir Bruce Keogh on the panel. As at January 2014 the new review is once again reviewing quality standards and developing a process for change. Concerns persist at the planning blight and low morale amongst staff, exacerbated by consultation fatigue and an entrenched culture of review without actual change. Despite the IRP's assurances that its recommendations were not intended to prolong the status quo we are back to square one, 23 years after the Bristol report. However, almost without exception, people have agreed with the core recommendation that there should be a reduction in the number of centers. In view of the continuing public interest, and the comments of the IRP that some views were not heard (despite the extensive consultation), absolutely everything this new group does, says, hears or reads is made public, and can be read on line via this blog: http://www.england.nhs.uk/2013/06/28/john-holden/. The process goes on and it will be another year before we hear the next set of options, which will no doubt themselves be subject to judicial review and appeal.

Lessons Learned

This is a personal chapter, and the views are mine. However, I have spoken to many people who were involved in this process and I hope I reflect their opinions, at least to some extent. There is no ducking the fact that health is a political issue, especially when played out on a national stage. Obamacare and recent NHS reforms exemplify this. Political careers can be made or lost over it, and views are strong. Politics also get played out locally, by physicians, patients, hospitals *and* local politicians. This reflects that everyone cares, but also that often they put more weight on local issues than national. This is prominent in the lessons learned.

There are so many lessons, and feeling the need to organize them, I looked for others who had analysed policy decisions and implementations. Luckily, as I prepared this, an outstanding book had just been published which did just that, it is "*Anthony King and Ivor Crewe; The Blunders of our Government: 2013; Oneworld Publications, Bloomsbury, London, UK*". This book should be compulsory reading for anyone in a large organisation who finds themselves responsible for change. Errors are repeated generation after generation, and the characteristics of such failure are clearly not learnt. King and Crewe have listed some common themes of failure of big programmes. They are; Cultural Disconnect; Group Think; Prejudice and Pragmatism; Operational Disconnect: and Panic, Symbols and Spin. I have chosen to test the Safe and Sustainable process against those criteria. I have added some other lessons and taken note of an essay by Sir Ian Kennedy *"Learning from Bristol: are we?"* [14]

Cultural Disconnect

King and Crewe define cultural disconnect as 'the failure of those making the plans to empathize with the users of the product of the plan'. In other words, perhaps the planners simply cannot understand what happens on the shop floor because they have never been there. I do not think this was so relevant in the case of Safe and Sustainable. Most of the members of the steering group and the standards group either worked in the specialty or had had children treated in them. However, there was a need for some element of disconnection, in the sense of being dispassionate. If too much consideration had been given to the stories told by parents, the resulting emotions would have caused paralysis in the process. Most of us thought it was better to take on board any objective information from parents, and focus on a belief that the professionals had got it right in advising the concentration of expertise they needed to save more lives and improve outcomes. It seems to me that there was a balance to be achieved, and it is clear that all the members of this review were trying hard to keep the patient at the center of their thinking. This is reflected in the various discussions in the JCPCT documentation.

Group Think

Group-think exists *when members of a group feel under pressure to maintain the groups cohesion, and often happens when outside people are regarded as hostile.* Could this have applied to safe and Sustainable in the context of failing to get real opponents to be really engaged and thus better challenge any case being argued in committee? Specifically, is it possible that we all convinced ourselves that the argument over the number of operations or surgeons a center should have was really the only argument and we 'group thought' our way into believing that?

This is possible, but at the outset it was felt that argument and advice would be more effective if advisors and committee members were selected, not on the basis of the center they came from, but as a representative of the relevant professional or lay society to which they belong, e.g. cardiac surgeons, anaesthetists, intensivists, nurses, parent support group and so on. If one takes such a representative view, it is possible that significant opposition could occur from a unit that did not have a representative on the committees, effectively by accident. That was the case with the Royal Brompton, and perhaps we should have invited them directly to criticize.

The problem with this approach is how to be sure those who oppose are really going to engage in a meaningful way. Even if they had wanted to, how could a local councilor / MP / cardiologist / parent risk incurring the wrath of the local community by engaging with the reform process in a meaningful way? An unwritten code seemed to develop amongst them that appeared to encourage and reward behavior meant to undermine the whole process and damage the reputation of those engaged in it. This bubbled over into actual threats on occasions (on Facebook for example when a local parent dared to question the local campaign group).

Usually though, the review team went out of its way to engage with those opposed to it, and the many public meetings were meant to do just this. However, they may have had the opposite effect as I describe later.

Prejudice and Pragmatism

Prejudice & pragmatism were defined as '*An unquestioning belief that some kinds of policies can be counted on to work better than others'.* King and Crewe also describe these as prejudgments or even hunches. It has been argued that the fundamental premise upon which this programme was based (that surgeons should do a large number of operations, but in a supported team environment, and that this meant, because of the total number of operations done that there must therefore be fewer centers) was predetermined. To some extent it was. I have yet to meet a cardiac surgeon who doesn't believe that the more he or she does, the better the outcomes [15].

In giving evidence to a recent *inquiry* I made the point that 'data make change,' (and one of the key problems with making the case was the fact that the Central Cardiac Audit Database information (based on validated mortality data) showed outstanding results across the board, and no English center fell outside the confidence intervals, implying they were all safe and of good quality. There were no data about complications, other morbidity or quality of life that could be used as a comparator. Each unit was able to say that it was safe and that its mortality was not significantly different from the best performing centers, even if case volume was disconcertingly low. But differences did exist and were given little weight. For example in the published record are data which show that, for equivalent case mix, units had wide ranging lengths of stay, ranging from 9.3 days to 24 days (who would you buy care from?). These data were not used to make or challenge the case.

The IRP amongst others took the view that the whole pathway of care from prenatal to adult should have been reviewed. It was difficult enough getting consensus amongst the pediatric cardiac centers; imagine how hard it is going to be when one adds in maternity and adult service across a whole country. It may simply become impractical and permanently in the long-grass.

One could reasonably argue that the IRP process is equally subject to such risks, and its appropriateness, fairness and effectiveness as a process deserve separate challenge.

Operational Disconnect

Operational Disconnect was defined as '*Disconnecting those who make the policy from those who have to implement it.*' It relates to the whole concept of doability. Is what is proposed able to work at all? King and Crewe reveal many examples of this, especially in relation to large IT projects, but in Safe and Sustainable, the people who would have had to carry out the policy were also the ones designing it. In a sense the policy was widely agreed…reduce the number of centers. It wasn't the implementation of the policy that was a problem, it was the choices of centers to lose their designation.

Of course, as the decision approached, and individuals began to realize that there was a real possibility that something might actually happen, they began to think about what might happen to them, and to their families. New homes? New schools? New town? One can easily understand the anxiety, and there was little open debate about what compensation might be available. This may have hardened opposition, but only at the end.

Panic, Symbols and Spin

This is harder to define in the context of Safe and Sustainable, since it usually refers to Ministers. Here is the definition: '*The response of ministers (usually) to media and public outcry. They need to decide something must be done in response [to media pressure, especially if from their core support newspapers], they are often under intense pressure to act or respond quickly and to be seen to respond, and often they blunder under these circumstances'.*

The whole of Safe and Sustainable was played out, deliberately, in the public eye. It was recognized from the start that many of the issues were contentious, and everyone involved realized that the process could become a model for reconfiguration of services in many other parts of the NHS, indeed neurosurgery was next up. Public awareness and 'stakeholder' involvement were seen as critical to long-term success. A cynical view might be that the NHS was required to carry out *excessive* public consultation, driven by legal precedent, but was motivated internally by risk aversion and fear of criticism. Having been involved, I certainly don't buy the cynical view. All the people I met were motivated to deliver the very best for the patient, and the overriding principle was the delivery of excellence, measured against global benchmarks. Mediocrity was never on the table.

For someone new to open debate of decisions, the 'psychology' behind campaigning was very interesting. With others, I have noticed that all public campaigns (NHS or otherwise) have a similar *modus operandi* in terms of language used and stances adopted. The allegation of predetermination is consistently used to attack a process, second only to "we are being ignored". The lesson learned is this – no matter how well you explain the clinical case for change and describe a professional consensus, campaigners who oppose you will be deaf to what you have to say; and (in this case) the better organized the NHS was in managing the review and getting its message out, the more organized the campaign group became because of a genuine fear that it could all be pulled off.

Massive sums were spent on public consultation to ensure that all views were taken into account and the process was 'fair'. But public consultation in the traditional sense appears dead in this age of social media. What's the point of the NHS spending lots of money responsibly to communicate a message, or question when postings by anonymous people on social media are capable of building up a head of steam that undermines the process? Why are campaigners more susceptible to believing an anonymous posting than something said by an expert such as Sir Roger Boyle? Maybe it is because they want to – and they pass it on to friends and family who want to believe also, and before long the mistruth is so well established that it appears in speeches by MPs in parliament and in an (independent) IRP report, set up 'to hear all views'. How do we respond to Mr. or Ms. Anonymous? What became very difficult to bear was that we had to remain professional, polite and balanced with no such obligation on the other side (including from some clinicians it seemed).

The public meetings themselves were very difficult. They were big, town hall meetings with aggressive questioning and high emotions. The expert panels were not prepared for the abuse they received. The original intention in 2010 was to hold interactive workshops rather than townhall meetings, but it was quickly apparent that the units and local groups would not allow this because they wanted an opportunity for heated public debate. It was in their interests so to do.

Each local team presented highly emotive, individual cases, with the child and its family often present, and arguing in favour of the unit. Sometimes this clearly exposed poor treatment masquerading as great care because of a long time spent in the intensive care unit (ICU). It was especially upsetting to hear repeatedly from parents of certain units (but not others) how good was the bereavement support care.

Several senior clinicians, myself included, were put up to the media as spokespeople for the programme. As a result, we got a great deal of flak from colleagues and support groups in the areas scheduled for de-designation of services. It became very personal and quite difficult. For a while I was very angry and upset, and thought putting us up for this was a mistake, and protecting the back of the NHS administrators who sat on the JCPCT. Now however, I have become convinced that there was no one better to put across the voice of reason. Who else would the public trust? We were not asked to defend the decision – we were asked to explain the case for change etc. What is the lesson learned here? Is it that no matter how credible and respected the spokesman, the media will cheat by portraying him or her as the decision maker just for good TV? That as soon as a heavyweight and respected clinician dares to defend a process those clinicians on the other side will quickly break ranks and resort to attacking him or her personally? Or perhaps that, despite all appearances to the contrary the professional consensus on the need for change was never really there? It was all a lie. Clinicians in potentially threatened units had no option but publicly to back the case for change at the outset in the knowledge that change would happen "over their dead bodies".

The final decision-making meeting of the JCPCT was held in public, broadcast on the web from a room full of stakeholders and journalists. TV cameras were waiting outside to interview whoever was most affected. It was rolling news in action. There was criticism at the time that the process was stage managed, largely because people were polite and argument mild. In my experience that is how good committees work, but that cut no ice with critics. The work had indeed been done in advance, but the decision *was* made in public.

We had stepped into the world of the public politician, and had to live that life or a while. The pressure on our families was immense. We had started by really wanting to provide optimum care for children in the UK, and had ended up being vilified. It was a salutary experience and required patience and fortitude to survive. Panic, symbols and spin were well in play in this saga.

Some Final Lessons

In no particular order, here are some final points I hope will be of interest.

- The process has taken way too long, and is still incomplete
- Consultative decision making is horribly expensive (staff costs, including opportunity costs incurred by NHS clinicians acting as advisors; management support; communications support; public consultation; legal fees)
- Problems with the definition of quality in the scoring system used by the JCPCT. As the Kennedy team travelled the country to review the individual centers were scored on a number of criteria, including quality. The team understood what it meant by quality, namely the ability of the center to meet, either now or in the near future, the agreed standards. However, the widespread clinical and lay interpretation of quality related to the *clinical outcomes* of the units, and only mortality was available for comparison. The reason for the JCPCT choosing this definition of quality was that there was no statistically significant difference in mortality between units, but it was obvious to them at least that quality was different. The centers scheduled for de-designation were thus really upset either if their quality scores were low, or, as in the case of the Brompton, quality was scored fairly high, but still de-designation followed. Clarity of terms or the choice of a different word to describe 'quality' would have been helpful.
- Too much focus may have been placed on travel times, given that England is geographically quite small and with excellent transport links. Kennedy had suggested in 2001 that travel times should be disregarded, and that the focus should be on creating centers of excellence. The stakeholders advised that travel times were important to them, and they became hugely contentious, yet Canada and Australia clearly demonstrate that travel per se is no longer a risk factor for outcome. This was an argument about convenience.
- ECMO, transplantation and tracheal surgery were nationally commissioned services carried out in only one or two of the cardiac units. All of these services were internationally recognized and successful, and the maintenance of the teams involved became an issue because of the potential knock on impact to other services. This was especially important in the face off between Leeds and Newcastle, and Leicester and Birmingham (cities in close proximity).
- Local politicians will always defend their local service ... 'any center but mine'.
- Legal challenge is inevitable, and whatever the cost, it must be prepared for from the start. But everyone must be taught to expect it. Hopes and expectations rose and fell in line with legal process. It became exhausting and emotional.
- Rationally to decide about where services should be provided, we need more outcomes than just mortality and we need to know in real time what our customers want. Data really do count, and we have a moral obligation to acquire the right information and make available, if we want to advance quality. We need as a profession to get on with this, as other chapters in this book make quite clear.
- There were wider issues about overall capacity in the system, especially in relation to intensive care beds in feeder and down-stream units. I do not think these were given sufficient attention. There were fears, often poorly expressed, that closure of units may result in excess pressure on the survivors.
- No matter how well a message is put across, or how persuasive it is in terms of professional sign-up, local people will always be more persuaded in a debate by a local clinician supporting the *status quo,* no matter how inaccurate or bizarre their message is.
- In a public debate there is never a persuasive response to a parent who opens by saying "my child would have died under your proposals".

Local parents remain surprisingly supportive of a unit, even when it has been assessed by experts as providing a 'dangerously poor service', (as was the case in Oxford in 2010 when a review by the local Strategic Health Authority suspended the service). How should one engage meaningfully with such devoted people at the same time as showing empathy and emphasizing quality?

- The lessons of the English civil war were not appreciated. The possibility that politicians and the media would use the process to play out regional differences was under estimated. These regional differences were often deep rooted and historical. The Newcastle v. Yorkshire skirmish was particularly disturbing, with real vitriol amongst members of the public at the Leeds consultation event. MPs relished the opportunity to defend their own constituencies. Safe and Sustainable should perhaps have avoided where possible references in its literature to cities, as this provoked local 'patriotism' amongst people with no previous connection to the review (Southampton v. Bristol; Leicester v. Birmingham; London v. Southampton). Honesty created division, and it is difficult to find the correct balance.

Conclusions

Whenever I travel to other countries, and discuss organisation of pediatric cardiac services, I have been struck by the admiration of my peers for the English system of care delivery. This system is characterized by (generally) regional services, a limited number of centers and a commitment to open presentation of (limited) outcomes to the public. And the English results are rather good. Those same peers were almost unified in their support for the underlying principles behind the Safe and Sustainable process, namely 'the more you do the better you get', and that concentration of services would permit better training, subspecialization and succession planning, as well as delivering a better quality of life to all staff, and particularly surgeons. I was proud to be part of that process.

It turns out that some people were of the view that the process was flawed, and that has brought it to its knees and we must start again. That there remains an appetite to do this within the NHS is a tribute, I think, to the quality of the underlying idea. So why is it taking so very long, when the logic is so widely supported and has been so for over 20 years?

The detailed lessons listed above reflect the importance to health and children to communities, local and national, and the unavoidable link between health care and politics. In England, the various governments have attempted to place the NHS into arms-length organisations, currently exemplified by NHS England. But when push comes to shove, every secretary of state for health is under pressure from party and constituents to apply local rules to national issues. The media love a good fight, and fan the flames of local disputes.

One might argue that one could let the market decide, but that can only work if there is a true market, and in none of our systems is that really the case. In the USA, where market forces have been dominant for several years, the expenditure on health is more than twice the percentage of GDP as Europe, and results are not better for the population. In the UK, where there is artificial competition via an internal market (the purchaser:provider split), it seems that local or regional pressures trump competition in the end. In Scandinavia, rationalization has occurred, and results are excellent, costs low, and data collected nationally and well over the course of patients' lives. Michael Porter [16] has long argued that what really matters is the *Value* of health care interventions over life, dividing the outcome of the intervention (over life) by the cost (over life). We need to know the outcomes and reduce cost. Rationalization of services in large, efficient centers has to be part of that process. However painful and bruising it has been so far, we must not give up now.

References

1. http://www.specialisedservices.nhs.uk/safe_sustainable/childrens-congenital-cardiac-services/
2. Dr. Phil Hammond [website]. Available at: http://drphilhammond.com/. Accessed 11 Apr 2014.
3. BBC News. Panorama: broken hearts. Available at: http://news.bbc.co.uk/1/hi/health/latest_news/104197.stm. Updated 14 Sept 1998. Accessed 11 Apr 2014.
4. Walshe K. Inquiries: learning from failure in the NHS. BMJ. 2002;325:895–900.
5. Children's Surgical Forum. Surgery for children: delivering a first class service. London: The Royal College of Surgeons of England; 2007. Available at: http://www.rcseng.ac.uk/publications/docs/CSF.html. Accessed 13 Apr 2014.
6. http://www.specialisedservices.nhs.uk/document/children-s-heart-surgery-in-england-need-change.
7. Department of Health. Commissioning safe and sustainable specialised pediatric services: a framework of critical inter-dependencies [PDF download]. London: Department of Health; 2008. p. 9. Available at: https://www.bspar.org.uk/DocStore/FileLibrary/PDFs/Commissioning%20Safe%20and%20Sustainable%20Specialised%20Paediatric%20Services.pdf. Accessed 13 Apr 2014.
8. http://www.specialisedservices.nhs.uk/document/developing-model-care
9. http://www.specialisedservices.nhs.uk/images/pdf-section/downloads/section11.pdf
10. http://www.specialisedservices.nhs.uk/library/30/Safe_and_Sustainable_Review_of_Childrens_Congenital_Heart_Services_in_England_Report_of_the_public_consultation.pdf
11. http://www.specialisedservices.nhs.uk/library/30/Appendix_K1___Reports_of_the_Independent_Expert_Panel_Chaired_by_Professor_Sir_Ian_Kennedy_1.pdf
12. http://www.specialisedservices.nhs.uk/document/safe-sustainable-review-children-s-congenital-cardiac-surgery-decision-making-business-case
13. Independent Reconfiguration Panel. Advice on safe and sustainable proposals for children's congenital heart services [PDF download]. London: Independent Configuration Panel; 2013. Available at: http://www.irpanel.org.uk/lib/doc/000%20s&s%20report%2030.04.13.pdf. Accessed 13 Apr 2014.
14. Kennedy I. Learning from Bristol: are we? 2011. Available from www.healthcarecommission.org.
15. Elliott M. The role of information in ensuring quality and patient safety [PDF download]. London: The Mid Staffordshire NHS Foundation Trust; 2011. Available at: http://www.midstaffspublicinquiry.com/sites/default/files/uploads/Martin_Elliot_paper.pdf. Accessed 13 Apr 2014.
16. Porter ME. What is value in health care? N Engl J Med. 2010;363(26):2477–81.

Lean in the Cardiac Intensive Care Unit

20

Howard E. Jeffries, Jerry J. Zimmerman,
J. Elaine-Marie Albert, and Silvia M. Hartmann

Abstract

Lean management principles have been used extensively in manufacturing for decades and are increasingly being utilized in healthcare settings over the last 10 years. Lean principles, developed as part of the Toyota Management System, their simultaneous focus on waste reduction and customer satisfaction are vital for healthcare to reach its potential. Lean begins with mapping process flow and then applying lean tools and techniques to optimize the current state, including waste removal, inventory optimization through kanban (signal) systems and standard work. The translation of this manufacturing philosophy to healthcare involves the use of huddles in order to optimize situational awareness and develop clinical standard pathways to ensure that patients with similar pathophysiological abnormalities are treated in a similar fashion.

Keywords

Lean healthcare • Process improvement • Lean process improvement • Clinical standard work

H.E. Jeffries, MD, MBA (✉)
Department of Pediatric Critical Care,
Seattle Children's Hospital, 4800 Sandpoint Way,
NE, MB.6.550, Seattle, WA 98105, USA
e-mail: howard.jeffries@seattlechildrens.org

J.J. Zimmerman, MD, PhD
Pediatric Critical Care Medicine, Department
of Pediatrics, Seattle Children's Hospital,
University of Washington School of Medicine,
4800 Sand Point Way NE, Seattle, WA 98105, USA
e-mail: jerry.zimmerman@seattlechildrens.org

J.E.-M. Albert, MD, MHA
Pediatric Intensive Care Unit, Department
of Pediatric Critical Care Medicine,
Seattle Children's Hospital, 4800 Sand Point Way,
NE, M/S MB.10.620, Seattle, WA 98105, USA
e-mail: elaine.albert@seattlechildrens.org

S.M. Hartmann, MD
Department of Critical Care Medicine,
Seattle Children's Hospital, 4800 Sand Point Way
NE, Seattle, WA 98105, USA
e-mail: silvia.hartman@seattlechildrens.org

P.R. Barach, J.P. Jacobs, S.E. Lipshultz, P.C. Laussen (eds.),
Pediatric and Congenital Cardiac Care: Volume 2: Quality Improvement and Patient Safety,
DOI 10.1007/978-1-4471-6566-8_20,

Introduction

Lean management principles have been used extensively in manufacturing industries for many years, most notably by Toyota. The primary principles that underpin Lean thinking are the removal of waste in order to make work as value added as possible, and a laser-like focus on the customer. Lean has spread from manufacturing to all manners of service, governmental and many other sectors over the last 20 years. While there are fundamental differences in healthcare to these other industries, the transformative impact of Lean thinking on healthcare has been no different. The pioneer healthcare institutions began adopting these principles around the year 2000 and their success has led to their adoption by numerous other hospitals and health systems and its endorsement by the Institute for Healthcare Improvement [1]. The focus on increasing value for patients or customers, the bedrock of this philosophy, gives Lean both its power and its relevance.

Much of Lean thinking has been associated with the Toyota Production System (TPS). This system moved managers from a focus on mass inspection, to improving the production process and building quality and worker engagement into the product the first time. In healthcare, this can be translated into "No waiting" and "No harm". "No waiting" refers to doing things "Just in Time", giving the right service in the right amount at the right time in the right place. "No Harm" refers to "Built-in-Quality" where system vulnerabilities are made visible, never passing along defects and stopping the line when there is a quality concern.

There are numerous examples of the power of Lean in healthcare. From dramatic improvements in patient flows in emergency departments [2], inventory savings [3], improvements in lab turnaround times [4] to financial savings with a Seattle Children's capital project. In addition, there have been recent efforts to improve the practice of pediatric critical care utilizing Lean methods [5]. Leadership engagement has been crucial to these efforts. Leadership must be knowledgeable, tenacious, present and patient in order to achieve these results.

Mapping the Process Flow

Mapping out the flow of the work process under consideration facilitates an understanding as well as an improved design of a particular process. This is a useful tactic for any quality improvement activity. For the purpose of illustration (Fig. 20.1), the activity of mechanical ventilation in the cardiac intensive care unit will be referenced. When undertaking the process mapping, it is useful to summarize the requirements for process flow:

1. **Standardize the sequence of work or activities as well as the physical layout of the process.** For mechanical ventilation as any other process, there exists initiation, maintenance, and termination phases. Each of these nodes of activity need to be carefully scrutinized. Standard physical layout of a cardiac intensive care unit (CICU) room ensures that the appropriate mechanical ventilator and supplies are always present for a scheduled or emergency admission. Electronic order sets for each phase of mechanical ventilation help ensure standard work (see below) for each aspect of the process. In terms of mechanical ventilation, although the maintenance aspect of ventilator support typically comprises the largest duration of time, intubation and extubation actually represent the most dangerous time for critically ill patients, particularly those with cardiovascular disease [6–8]. Accordingly, as part of the process flow of mechanical ventilation in the CICU, it would be prudent to include team huddles at both initiation and termination of mechanical ventilation to consider worst case scenarios and how to respond to them [9].
2. **Implement standard work for all elements of the process with explicit methods.** This requirement is considered in detail in another portion of this chapter. However, with respect to flow, standard work will define the expected clinical pathway or trajectory for the process. There can be no measured improvement without standard work because in its absence nuisance variables typically obscure any meaningful process change [10]. In developing standard work it is useful to scrutinize the work where it is actually performed and the way it

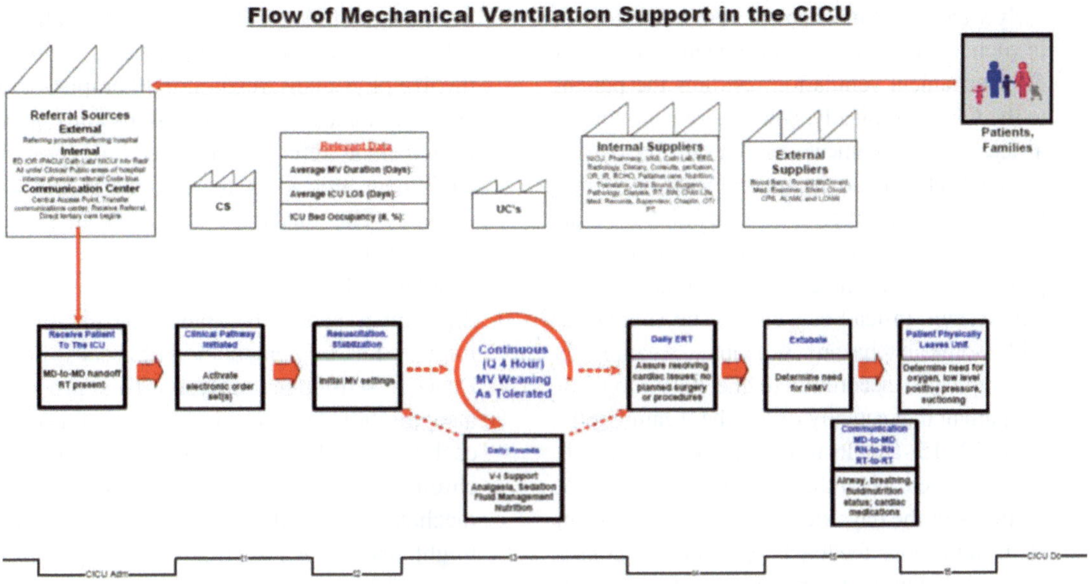

Fig. 20.1 Process flow of mechanical ventilation (MV) support in the CICU. Duration of MV is frequently the rate-limiting process in terms of duration of stay in the CICU. The process of MV is mapped from admission to the CICU, through initiation of MV, weaning MV support and discontinuation of MV and tracheal extubation. Cycle times for each aspect of the flow is displayed along the bottom. *CS* central supply, *UC* unit clerk, *V-I* vasoactive-inotropic, *MD* physician, *RN* nurse, *RT* respiratory therapist. Most of the waste in the process occurs in the interval t3, when weaning of MV is safely physiologically possible, but not undertaken for a variety of reasons

is actually done. Standard work provides the infrastructure for process flow and continuous improvement. Along the process flow, standard work should be evidence-based as possible and consensus-based where evidence is not available. In the case of mechanical ventilation, standard work can be composed for emergent, hypoxemic, acute respiratory failure and various management aspects of pediatric acute respiratory distress syndrome as well as management of the post-operative surgical patient [11]. It should be stressed that in distinction to a reliability method, standard work involves a time component as will be illustrated for mechanical ventilation. Decision support tools mandating scheduled assessments provide this time component [12].

3. **Keep pace with customer (patient) demand.** Within the current context this concept refers to recognition of physiologic prompting by the patient that will enable to pull off the flow process. Administratively this may also refer to administrative load-levelling. For example, a surgical schedule that is balanced and extends over the course of the entire week ensuring that the CICU is not overloaded some days of the week and underloaded during other days of the week.
4. **Ensure flexibility of the system.** This characteristic relates to responding to variation in demand. In the case of mechanical ventilation, proper process flow would dictate continuous, deliberate weaning around the clock (24/7/365). In the case of mechanical ventilation, flexibility also particularly relates to dynamics of the patient's cardiovascular status, analgesic and sedative needs, nutritional status and input, as well as fluid balance. All of these will influence the process flow along the trajectory of a patient's mechanical ventilation course.
5. **Pull the flow.** In the quality improvement literature this characteristic refers to the notion of pulling the flow rather than pushing it [13]. Specifically for mechanical ventilation, the practice of scheduled assessments to facilitate

early weaning of mechanical ventilation results in such a pull system [14]. Frequently, the need for mechanical ventilation restrains the patient to the CICU. Typically, when there is no longer a need for mechanical ventilation, the patient can be discharged to the general ward or even to home. Weaning mechanical ventilation typically encumbers the majority of time that the patient spends on mechanical ventilation. In a pull system, instead of weaning the ventilation with some haphazard schedule, weaning is accomplished according to the physiology of the patient that actually drives the weaning process [12, 15–18]. In this scenario, weaning is accomplished when the patient is ready and at all times of the day. Ideally, there is some form of instantaneous feedback regarding the consequences of a particular pull on the process flow. In the case of mechanical ventilation, the CICU provides multiple monitoring signals of the success or not of a particular weaning step. Computerized decision support tools to pull the mechanical ventilation weaning process may prove to be useful in the future. Such tools utilize so-called time-based kanban signalling for assessment and possible weaning interventions. For mechanical ventilation, input variables may include ventilatory rate, $PaCO_2$ or end tidal carbon dioxide, and SpO_2 or PaO_2. Output variables that may be suggested include changes in peak inspiratory pressure, tidal volume, positive end expiratory pressure or fraction of inspired oxygen concentration. Such decision support tools prompt proactive, scheduled pull of the process flow, in this case weaning of mechanical ventilation. Such process flow tools have been shown to decrease the duration of both mechanical ventilation and intensive care unit (ICU) length of stay [12, 15–18].

Tools Used to Achieve Process Flow

A number of quality improvement tools are available to facilitate design of the process flow including:

1. **Process quantity analysis.** This key activity involves stakeholder analysis of both the type and quantity of work. In the case of mechanical ventilation these discussions should involve physicians, respiratory therapists and bedside nurses [14]. The discussions may also include reference to specific types of equipment and when these items would be utilized. The analysis would also include determination of cycle times for mechanical ventilation for specific disease processes as these times should be able to be iteratively improved by implementation of process flow.
2. **Process sequence analysis.** This process, also multidisciplinary in nature, considers each node of the process flow, ensuring synchronization with all process steps. For mechanical ventilation, such discussions might also include alternative starting points along the mechanical ventilation process flow including non-invasive mechanical ventilation, conventional mechanical ventilation, high-frequency oscillatory ventilation or airway pressure release ventilation and event extracorporeal life support.
3. **Standard work analysis**. This activity is typically recognized as the proverbial spaghetti diagram. For mechanical ventilation, this analysis might include the respiratory coverage patterns in the CICU. Such an analysis should ultimately lead to more efficient work and flow assignments.
4. **5S analysis. 5S** is the name of a workplace organization method that uses a list of five Japanese words: *seiri, seiton, seiso, seiketsu,* and *shitsuke.* Transliterated or translated into English, they all start with the letter "S". The list describes how to organize a work space for efficiency and effectiveness by identifying and storing the items used, maintaining the area and items, and sustaining the new order. Included here is analysis of the process flow and identification of any obstacles or monuments that will require change-out or workaround in order to achieve consistent process flow.
5. **Waste removal.** Both 5S and waste removal are considered in detail later in this chapter. In the case of mechanical ventilation in the CICU, it is important to identify value-added

steps in the process while eliminating waste as possible. As with most processes, much of mechanical ventilation might be viewed as non-value-added, particularly if the patient's mechanical ventilator support could be weaned but was not. For mechanical ventilation, the largest waste is waiting, and eliminating this wasted time during weaning by employing decision support tools is an ideal intervention for process flow improvement.

6. **Time observation form.** For mechanical ventilation, this analysis might involve monitoring cycle times for duration of mechanical ventilation for the most common causes of pulmonary failure encountered in the CICU. This might include the post-operative setting for various surgeries for congenital heart disease or alternatively, times of mechanical ventilation for various types of cardiac medical admissions.
7. **Work balance form.** Load leveling in the CICU in terms of surgery scheduling can result in a steady velocity of patients and process flow, avoiding both over and under utilization and activity of the care team, both potential safety issues.
8. **Kanban (signal) to facilitate pull.** As indicated above, such signalling may relate not only to supply–demand issues but also to the actual processes.
9. **Cross-training and contingency planning.** Establishing a float pool for both CICU nurses as well as respiratory therapists will ensure flow through the CICU even when demand is heavy.
10. **Visual clues.** The use of visual tools and graphics coupled with the support of computerized decision support tools to facilitate weaning of mechanical ventilation. These conspicuous, scheduled assessments of the patient's pulmonary status leverages a forcing function that literally adds pull to the process flow of mechanical ventilation weaning.
11. **Build in safety and quality.** Here the emphasis relates to eliminating opportunities for error so they don't reach the patient. Poka-Yoke or mistake-proofing should be incorporated along the process flow whenever possible. In the case of mechanical ventilation, for example, sedation is a delicate balancing act to at once ensure patient comfort and provide modulation of the stress response, while at the same time not over sedating and thus impairing natural weaning of mechanical ventilation or alternatively increasing the risk for accidental extubation.

Maintaining the Flow

As in all quality improvement efforts, sustainability represents the greatest challenge. Ideally, a mapped process flow can be iteratively redesigned and adapted to maximize efficiency and safety of the process [19]. This requires ongoing maintenance that will include education for a large staff with frequent change over, as well as incorporation of new evidence as it emerges. In the case of pediatric mechanical ventilation, there should perhaps be additional scrutiny of interventions to avoid ventilator-associated lung injury [20]. Prone positioning may turnout to be beneficial in some settings but its inherent dangers need to be considered [21, 22]. Faster weaning of mechanical ventilation support utilizing electronic decision support tools could decrease the rate of ventilator-associated, hospital-acquired pneumonia [23] and tracheitis [24].

A champion for a particular process and its flow is invaluable in terms of maintaining a burning platform and sharing success of the quality improvement effort with others. In the case of designing a flow for mechanical ventilation support in the CICU, the benefits include improved quality, enhanced delivery of a particular service, lowered cost and improved safety, ultimately with the focus on the patient, facilitated by engagement of a coordinated care team supporting the process flow. When flow is well established and pull drives the flow, ultimately, patient care can be viewed as either on-flow or off-flow for a particular disease process. Rounds then should concentrate on identifying patients with abnormal flow trajectories and developing a plan to reestablish the patient in a particular flow process.

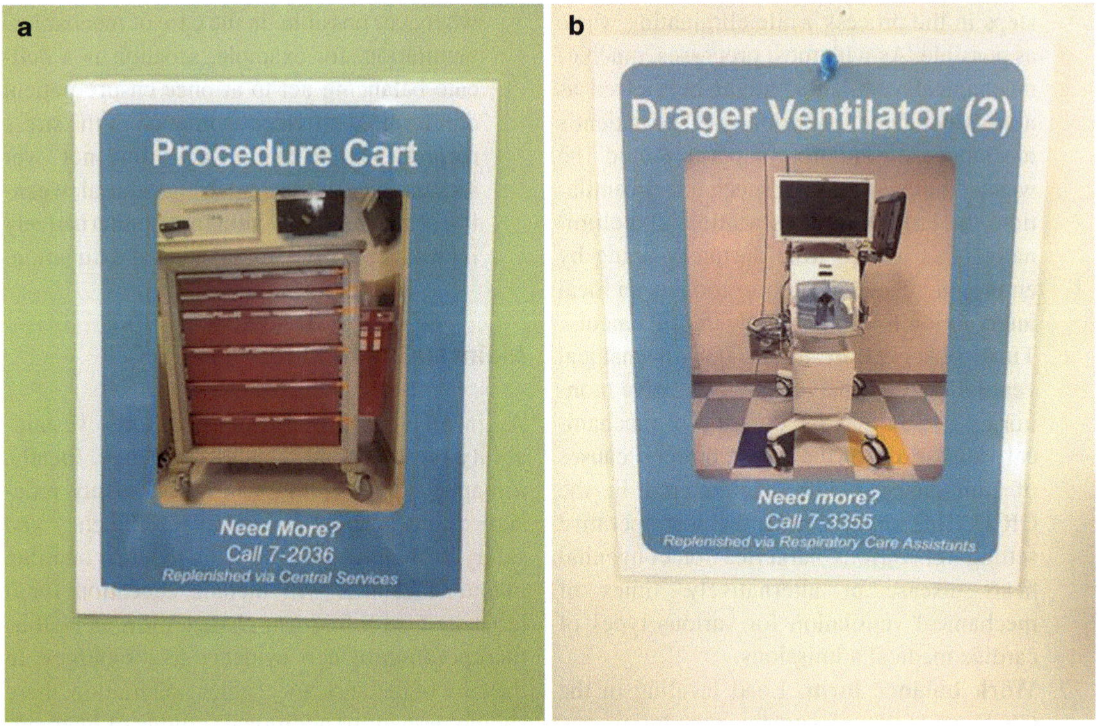

Fig. 20.2 Visual communication tells personnel where items are located, how many should be there, and who is responsible for maintaining them (**a**) Card depicting location of ICU based procedure cart. (**b**) Card depicting location of two ventilators

Waste

Waste (muda) is a key concept in the Toyota Production System and in Lean. Waste refers to anything that does not add value to the delivery of health care to the patient. The goal of Lean is to identify waste and eliminate it. There are seven types of waste in healthcare, as there are in manufacturing and include:

- *Inventory:* stockpiling of clinical supplies
- *Transportation:* refers to damage to items and transaction costs associated with moving them
- *Movement:* RNs looking for items that should be clearly labeled or having to walk a distance to retrieve commonly used supplies
- *Waiting:* Staff waiting for supplies to be delivered or for a patient to be admitted
- *Over-processing*
- *Over-production*
- *Defects*

5S

The 5S process tackles several types of waste: excessive movement, waiting, and inventory management. Inventory often accumulates in hospitals and can become excessive and obsolete if not evaluated on a regular basis. While waiting can be a necessary part of clinical care, how often is staff waiting for supplies that are not readily available to them? Or how often is an OR case canceled because the right implants were not ordered? Finally, excessive movement is a less recognized form of waste in healthcare. 5S can reduce the amount of "walk time," increase the amount of productive time by placing supplies near where there will be used, and be used to designate places for commonly used items. For example, if the bedside procedure cart or ventilator are always returned to their labeled locations (Fig. 20.2); the provider will not have to spend several minutes walking around the unit looking for it. In short, 5S is a way of organizing the workplace to make it function more effectively.

The 5S process is carried out by small teams of ICU staff who work to get supplies closer to the point of care and organized and labeled to facilitate care with the least amount of wasted time and materials. The 5S's are sort, simplify, sweep, standardize, and sustain.

- *Sort:* Go through all supplies, materials, etc. at the bedside and in the ICU work area. Eliminate what is not required. If in doubt, throw it out. Keep only essential items in readily accessible locations.
- *Simplify:* Everything should have a place or point of use (POU). Items should be arranged according to how frequently they are used. Visual cues (i.e. photographs of equipment) and labels should be used to call out the POU for item.
- *Sweep:* Keep the workplace clean and organized using visual and physical checks. Everything should be at its POU. The 5S plan calls out how frequently a sweep will occur and who will do it, i.e. the charge nurse at the end of every shift.
- *Standardize:* The work groups create standards that describe how the work will be done. These standards are communicated to everyone involved in the work process.
- *Sustain:* Ensure disciplined adherence to rules and procedures to prevent backsliding. This is the most difficult and, arguably, most important "S" of the process. The work groups should also create a plan of how they will sustain the gains made with the first 4S's.

Creating Demand Flow

One of the key principles of the Lean methodology is to use "pull" systems to avoid overproduction and streamline flow. In a "pull" system, an upstream process replaces what the downstream consumer has used. The ICU is a highly variable, dynamic and consumptive environment. The need for supplies varies with patient census, acuity, and diagnosis. Furthermore, ICU staff often need supplies in a highly time-sensitive manner. The ICU is not a place where the staff can wait to provide care because the "parts are on order." ICU staff members need to know that supplies will be where they want them, when they want them. Missing supplies can, quite literally, be the difference between life and death in the ICU. ICU is the embodiment of the "just in time" (JIT) mantra from Lean methodology.

How do members of the ICU team respond to variability in the supply delivery chain? They hoard the supplies they need and keep them close by. Ask any ICU team member why they do this and they will say "Well, I know I'll have what I need when I need it." How can this behavior be changed? What can organizations do to ensure timely delivery of and access to supplies? The typical answer is to have a large warehouse or central supply area that holds a great deal of inventory; this ensures that every product one might need is maximally represented, but is expensive.

The experience of the Toyota Company demonstrated that this approach does not work well and actually leads to the "hoarding" behavior described earlier. Using the Lean methodology, Toyota modeled a delivery system based on supermarket delivery systems in the United States. Grocery owners know that goods are sold at different rates. If bananas sell much faster than kumquats, does it make sense to buy the same volume of both? The store wastes kumquats and loses money if it buys as many kumquats as it does bananas; conversely, the store will run out of bananas very quickly and lose customers, if it buys them at the kumquat rate. The solution is to buy small volumes of each fruit and restock the shelves at the rate the fruit is being sold. The same logic can be applied to medical supplies. Alcohol wipes are used at an infinitely higher rate than dialysis catheters. It doesn't make sense to restock both at the same volume or rate; however, this is what most hospitals do.

This practice is further supported by the fact that most hospitals lack standards around supply and storage. For example, regarding supplies, hospitals often purchase a large variety of items to meet provider preferences or to achieve volume discounts. Three surgeons doing the same procedure may use three different sets of supplies and surgical kits, leading the hospital to purchase and maintain more items. Further, if the supplies are not stored in an orderly manner, they accumulate in hidden areas or are lost, leading to more purchasing. These behaviors adversely affect the hospital's revenue by tieing up capital in excess inventory and space.

At Seattle Children's Hospital, we created a process called Demand Flow (DF) to ensure that correct supplies are delivered to the right location, at the appointed time, in the necessary quantity. DF is based on the use of *kanban* in Lean. *Kanban,* which means "a visual signal," automatically signal when a new product or supply is needed & is based on the "pull" system. It is a key part of JIT production which is essential in eliminating waste in a system. DF creates a reliable method for supply replenishment. As the name suggests, as the customer needs supplies (demand), they are replaced as needed (flow). The DF process started with a comprehensive review of the supply needs of our ICUs. What supplies did we use with greater frequency? What supplies languished on our shelves for months? What supplies did nurses and doctors hoard? This review yielded information on what supplies the ICU used and at what volume and velocity.

Each supply is assigned to a *kanban* or, at Seattle Children's, a blue bin that is sized to hold 5 days' worth of supplies. Our team determined that the par-level for our supplies should be 5 days. Par level is the level of supplies or items considered necessary to have at all times. The blue bins are then placed on shelving in the unit's supply area. The bins are labeled with a barcode that contains information about the item itself, the number if items in the bin, and the bins' location.

Seattle Children's uses a "2-bin" *kanban* system (Fig. 20.3). In the 2-bin system, each blue bin has a duplicate, containing the same item, behind it. When the first bin is empty, it is pulled from the shelf and put in an empty bin container. The duplicate bin is moved to the front of the shelf. The first bin, after has been refilled, is placed behind the bin that is currently in use. Inventory technicians from Central Supply check the empty bin container several times per day and return empty bins to the DF staging area in Central Supply. Here the bins are scanned, refilled, and returned to the ICUs DF area. Our 2 bin system doesn't rely on a central warehouse for supplies; in a unique process, order information is transmitted directly to our distributors and manufacturers. The scanning process allows Central Supply to track the frequency with which bins are refilled on hour to hour basis. This allows them to increase the par-level of commonly used items and decrease or eliminate items that are being used less frequently.

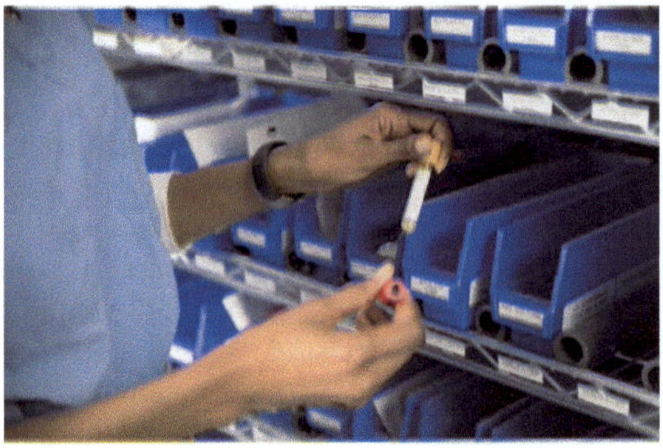

Fig. 20.3 Supply chain demand flow node

DF worked so well in our supply areas that nurses thought the same principle could be applied to our bedside carts. In the ICUs, bedside carts contain items that nurses and respiratory therapists need to have at their fingertips, i.e. alcohol swabs, syringes, and suction catheter. Nurses and other staff were frequently going to the unit DF to replenish supplies in the bedside carts; they were now hoarding at the bedside. The flow of work was often disrupted to go and get supplies. Hence, a work group of ICU RNs and RTs replicated the entire DF process with the bedside carts. They determined what supplies were needed and what the par-levels should be. The group designed special bedside cart that could support a two bin *kanban* system. The DF principles are the same; however, when the bin is empty, it is placed in the "empty bin spot" in each room. It is restocked by our ICU techs that check each room every few hours, more frequently if needed. The techs restock from the unit's DF area; thus the information about supply use is still communicated to Central Supply.

DF has allowed reducing waste by creating an organized and visual delivery supply system, reducing excess and obsolete supplies, eliminating storage space in warehouses and in clinical areas, and improving just in time access to supplies. It has also changed the culture of our providers who no longer have to hoard and have learned to trust that the equipment they need will be available for them when they need it. All of this adds up to improvements in the delivery of quality patient care, a trusting culture and financial savings.

Huddles/De-Briefs

Several years ago, the number of ICU beds and, hence, the number of staff had grown considerably; the complexity of our patient population had also increased dramatically. Huddles were created as a way to improve situational awareness and communication between team members. Situational awareness is an understanding of the current environment and the ability to accurately anticipate future problems, thus enabling effective actions to be taken [25]. Simply, it is the shared knowledge of what is happening in the ICU (Fig. 20.4). Which RN has the sickest patient? Who will be traveling to CT?

Every day prior to the start of each shift, a huddle occurs in the CICU next to the patient status board. Each member of the team introduces herself and states her role on the team, i.e. "I'm Debi Newberry and I'm the CICU attending today." The charge nurse then goes on to update the team on admissions, discharges, patients on support devices (ECLS or CRRT), "active" patients, and who will be traveling of the unit. The whole process takes from 5 to 7 min; the entire CICU staff now knows what's going on in the unit.

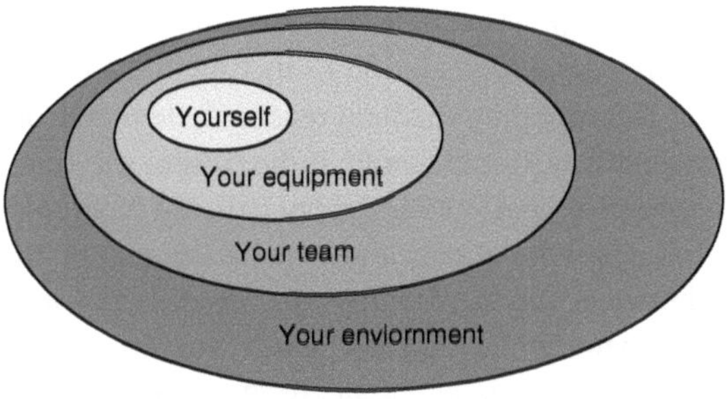

Fig. 20.4 Situational awareness depiction

The success of the twice daily shift huddles led the team to implement huddles following both admissions to the ICUs and major events (i.e. code blues). These huddles are very similar in function and purpose to After Action Reviews used by the military [26]. After Action Reviews are structured short debriefs that occur to analyze a complex process. Huddles that occur following admissions are brief reviews of why the patient is in the ICU, what the plan is for next hour or two, and whom to contact with questions. During the post-event huddles, the team discusses what happened, why it happened, and how the process could have been done better/differently. These reviews create a culture of accountability and drive the team to improve.

Bedside Catheter-Associated Bloodstream Infection Reviews

Central venous catheters (CVCs) are used extensively in the ICU for the delivery of vasoactive and/or high-osmolarity medications, monitoring of intravascular status, and removal of blood for laboratory evaluation. More than five million patients in the US alone required central venous access in 2010 [27, 28]. As central line venous catheters have become more common, so have the many complications that are associated with them. The most common complications are infectious and thrombotic; both of which are associated with increased length of ICU and hospital stay, increased medical costs, and increased morbidity and mortality. By far the most common adverse result of CVC use in the ICU is catheter line-associated bloodstream infection (CLA-BSI). CLA-BSIs, in addition to being significantly detrimental to the health of patients, are expensive and often difficult to treat.

In an effort to reduce CLA-BSIs, our ICU formed a committee to track all infections and implement practice changes. The committee is comprised of all members of the ICU team and infection prevention officers. The committee proposed and implemented standardized CVC insertion and maintenance bundles. The number of days without a CLA-BSI was tabulated and posted in a central location for staff and families to see. In 2009, we implemented a bedside root cause analysis team to review all infections. Within 48 h of the identification of a BSI, the ICU Clinical Nurse Specialist, the ICU infection prevention officer, and an ICU physician convene at the patient's bedside to discuss the BSI. The bedside RN and the parents join the discussion. The goal is to determine if there were any risk factors for infection and what, if anything, could have prevented the infection. This process supports a culture of accountability to our patients, involved families in transparent and authentic manner, and identifies areas for improvement and process change.

Standard Work

Standard work is a common method for treating a particular population of patients that all providers at an institution are expected to adhere with the aim of reducing variability of care. When possible, standard work methods are based on published evidence and guidelines for diagnosis and management. When published literature is absent for a particular question, multidisciplinary providers involved in the care for this population of patients comes to a consensus regarding the best approach to treatment. Standard work in the clinical setting may be implemented in a variety of forms that includes algorithms, checklists, computerized alerts, and electronic ordersets. A single person, the process owner, is responsible for receiving feedback regarding the treatment methods and implementation tools. The consistent approach to treating a group of patients serves as a basis for improvement. Outcome measures are followed and evaluated with the intent of future modifications to improve patient care based on institutional experience and the advent of new published literature. The following example is meant to illustrate one way these concepts have been used in our clinical setting.

In August of 2012, Seattle Children's Hospital began to use a standard pathway to treat neonates with ductal dependent systemic blood flow admitted to the cardiac intensive care unit during the pre-operative period. The specific population addressed by the pathway included patients greater than 35 weeks gestational age with ductal dependent systemic blood flow that was not secondary to an isolated coarctation of the aorta or obstructive pulmonary venous return. Patients presenting in septic or cardiogenic shock were excluded. Similarly, patients with significant comorbidities outside of cardiac disease and those with plans for comfort care or withdrawal of life-sustaining support were also not included. This pathway included management recommendations for pre-hospital care, initial evaluation, preferred intravenous access, and a step-wise approach to pulmonary overcirculation based on severity. The pathway was operationalized in the form of an algorithm (Fig. 20.5) and electronic order set. For example, a neonate born with prenatally diagnosed hypoplastic left heart syndrome would be started on alprostadil at a rate of 0.03 mcg/kg/min prior to transportation to Seattle Children's Hospital in accordance with the pathway. However, suppose the infant has periods of apnea after admission to the cardiac intensive care unit. Based on previous consensus, the first step in treating this patient would be to decrease the rate of alprostadil to 0.01 mcg/kg/min. If this intervention proved ineffective, then high flow nasal cannula would trialed before continuous positive airway pressure (CPAP), and prior to intubation. The expectation is to adhere to this planned escalation of therapy unless there was a compelling medical reason to deviate from the pathway. For example, if the patient was diagnosed postnatally with hypoplastic left heart syndrome and the ductus arteriosus was small on the admission echocardiogram, then a provider may choose to initiate high flow nasal cannula as a first step to treat episodic apnea rather than decrease the dose of alprostadil. The algorithm is rapidly

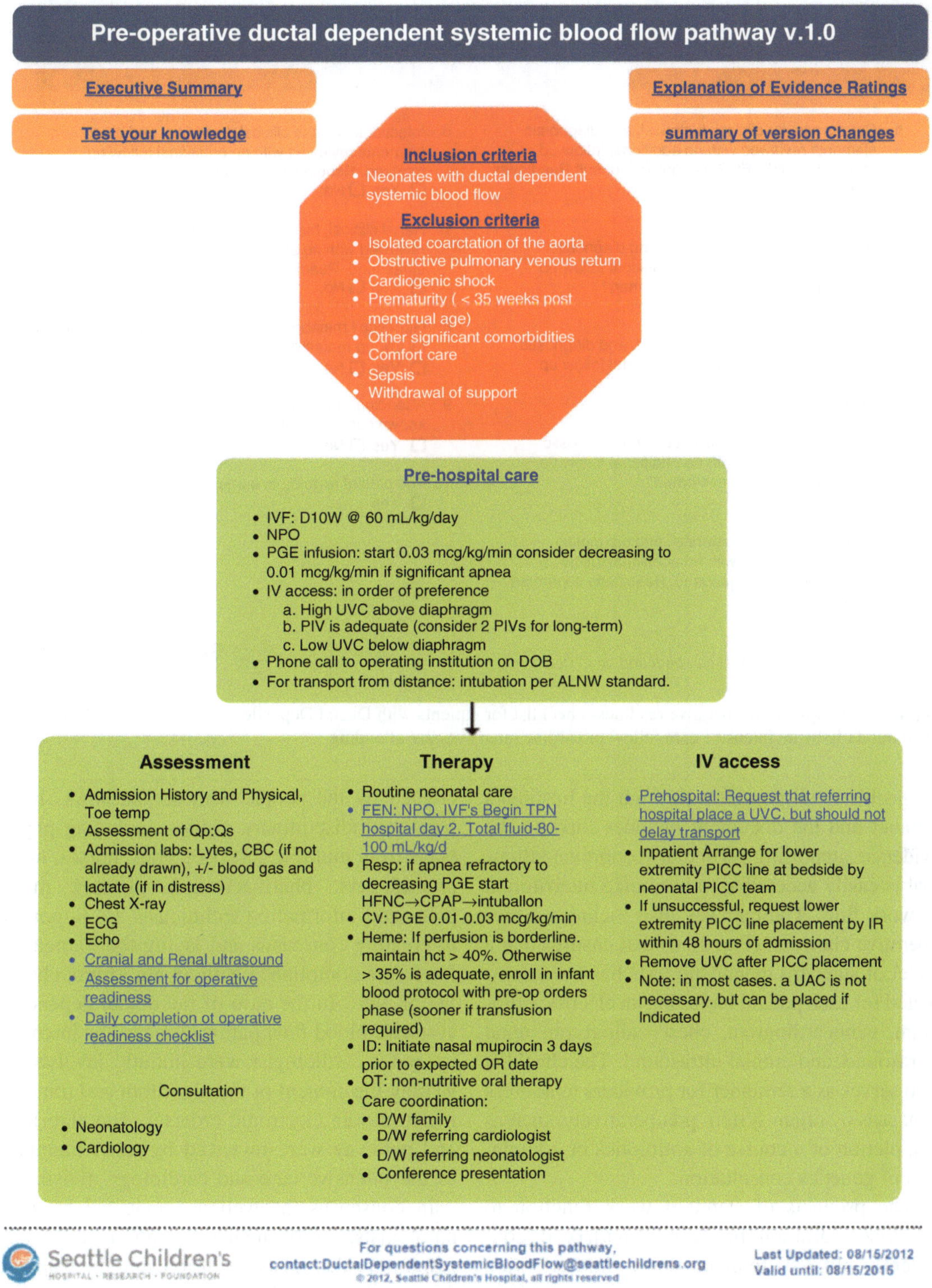

Fig. 20.5 A sample of the Ductal Dependent Systemic Blood Flow pathway at Seattle Children's Hospital. Links to the rationale behind the pathway and to summaries of the evidence behind recommendations are easily accessed through the diagram. Feedback or questions can be easily directed to the appropriate personnel through e-mail contacts listed at the bottom of each page of the pathway

Operative Readiness Checklist (Cont'd)

1. Cardiovascular clinical, historical, and diagnostic elements reviewed with no additional follow up required: ECHO, ECG, cardiology consult Readiness confirmed?
   ☐ Yes ☐ No:

2. Respiratory clinical, historical, and diagnostic elements reviewed with no additional follow up required: CXR. Readiness confirmed?
   ☐ Yes ☐ No:

3. Gastrointestinal clinical, historical, and diagnostic elements reviewed with no additional follow up required. Readiness confirmed?
   ☐ Yes ☐ No:

4. Hematologic clinical, historical, and diagnostic elements reviewed with no additional follow up required. Readiness confirmed?
   ☐ Yes ☐ No:

5. Neurologic clinical, historical, and diagnostic elements reviewed with no additional follow up required: Cranial ultrasound. Readiness confirmed?
   ☐ Yes ☐ No:

6. Infectious disease clinical, historical, and diagnostic elements reviewed with no additional follow up required. Readiness confirmed?
   ☐ Yes ☐ No:

7. Renal clinical, historical, and diagnostic elements reviewed with no additional follow up required: Renal ultrasound. Readiness confirmed?
   ☐ Yes ☐ No:

8. Genetics I metabolic issues reviewed with no additional fol low up required. Readiness confirmed?
   ☐ Yes ☐ No:

9. Attending Attestation: All elements reviewed with no known contraindications to proceed with surgery.
   ☐ Yes ☐ No:

10. The patient is going to surgery now.
    ☐ Yes

Copies of this checklist can be found on CHILD here.

Seattle Children's
HOSPITAL • RESEARCH • FOUNDATION

Fig. 20.6 A copy of the operative readiness checklist for patients with Ductal Dependent Systemic Blood Flow that is filled out daily by an intensive care fellow or cardiac intensive care attending

accessible to all providers through the hospital's intranet and the document includes links to the evidence supporting particular recommendations that is easily accessible to minimize interruption in work flow. The pathway also includes a preoperative checklist (Fig. 20.6) that ensures that a panel of standard diagnostic tests has been completed for each patient including an electrocardiogram, echocardiogram, chest radiograph, renal ultrasound, and cranial ultrasound. The checklist also serves as a reminder for providers to address concerns by organ system preoperatively, such as completion of a course of antibiotics or completion of genetics consultation.

The products of standard work function to minimize variation between providers if consistently utilized. Implementation and adoption of standard work relies on creating consensus or getting "buy-in" from the various groups of people involved in patient care. Standard work processes generally function best when they are created by the people who do the work. Input from multidisciplinary groups, including physicians from multiple subspecialities, nurses, nurse practitioners, pharmacists, respiratory therapists, and information technicians are important in creating consensus and laying the foundation for future compliance with an algorithm, checklist or alert. In the case of the ductal dependent systemic blood flow pathway, a cardiac intensivist and a cardiologist were initially involved in writing the content of the algorithm and translating it into an electronic orderset. The algorithm and pathway were reviewed by other members of the intensive care and cardiology division to gain consensus, as well as, reviewed by neonatologists, nurse managers, pharmacists and respiratory therapists. Prior to using the pathway for patients, providers who work in the cardiac intensive care unit learned about the elements of the ductal dependent systemic blood flow pathway and orderset through a mandatory online educational module. The module reviewed the evidence and level of evidence for management decisions. Recommendations that were derived from local consensus were also noted. Providers were required to complete a series of questions pertaining to content of the pathway. As providers began to use the order set for admission of neonates with ductal dependent systemic circulation and follow management recommendations, feedback could be given to the process owner.

The metrics for improvement of patient care were determined prior to the implementation of the pathway. For this particular pathway, the metrics included median hospital length of stay and preoperative length of stay, the number of patients who meet criteria for the pathway who had the orderset utilized, average hospital charges per patient, and daily operative readiness checklist completion. Data was collected and regularly reviewed by the clinical standard work group to ensure adequate implementation of the existing pathway. The content of the pathway is planned to undergo periodic review every 3 years to incorporate new evidence-based medicine and experience of the providers with the current management strategy.

Concerns that the implementation of standard work processes will diminish the "art of medicine" have arisen. Clinical standard work in its many forms does not replace the need for clinical experience and assessment skills, but rather is useful to expedite work flow in a busy hospital environment by allowing similar types of patients to receive necessary tests and interventions and avoiding unnecessary expenses. Information about patient outcomes should be used to further refine standard work processes in an iterative fashion to continually improve the quality of patient care.

Conclusions

Lean management techniques have found an important place in quality and process improvement in hospitals and ICUs. In order for this methodology to continue to gain acceptance, hospitals must prove that it adds value and can stand the test of time and effort. The most difficult aspect of any improvement technique is sustaining and lean is no different. However, with the incorporation of management systems that require continual reevaluation of process outcomes, lean should have the staying power that has eluded earlier methods.

References

1. Institute for Healthcare Improvement. Going Lean in Health Care. IHI Innovation Series white paper. Cambridge, MA: Institute for Healthcare Improvement; 2005. (Available on www.IHI.org).
2. Holden RJ. Lean thinking in emergency department: a critical review. Ann Emerg Med. 2011;57(3):265–78.
3. Hintzen BL, Knoer SJ, Van Dyke CJ, Milavitz BS. Effect of lean process improvement techniques on a university inpatient pharmacy. Am J Health Syst Pharm. 2009;66(22):2042–7.
4. Buesa RJ. Adapting lean to histology laboratories. Ann Diagn Pathol. 2009;13(5):322–33.
5. Vats A, Goin KH, Villareal MC, Yilmaz T, Fortenberry JD, Keskinocak P. The impact of a lean rounding process in a pediatric intensive care unit. Crit Care Med. 2012;40(2):608–17.
6. Mekontso-Dessap A, de Prost N, Girou E, et al. B-type natriuretic peptide and weaning from mechanical ventilation. Intensive Care Med. 2006;32(10):1529–36.
7. Chien JY, Lin MS, Huang YC, et al. Changes in B-type natriuretic peptide improve weaning outcome predicted by spontaneous breathing trial. Crit Care Med. 2008;36(5):1421–6.
8. Foster CB, Spaeder MC, McCarter RJ, et al. The use of near-infrared spectroscopy during an extubation readiness trial as a predictor of extubation outcome. Pediatr Crit Care Med. 2013;14(6):587–92.
9. Quality AfHR. Pocket guide: TeamSTEPPS: US Department of Health and Social Services; 2008.
10. Ohno T. Toyota production system: beyond large-scale production. Portland: Productivity Press; 1988.
11. Newth CJ, Venkataraman S, Willson DF, et al. Weaning and extubation readiness in pediatric patients. Pediatr Crit Care Med. 2009;10(1):1–11.
12. Jouvet PA, Payen V, Gauvin F, et al. Weaning children from mechanical ventilation with a computer-driven protocol: a pilot trial. Intensive Care Med. 2013; 39(5):919–25.
13. Deeter KH, Zimmerman JJ. Developing and implementing pull systems in the intensive care unit. In: Wellman J, Hagan P, Jeffries H, editors. Leading the lean healthcare journey. New York: CRC Press; 2011. p. 93–108.
14. Jouvet P, Hernert P, Wysocki M. Development and implementation of explicit computerized protocols for mechanical ventilation in children. Ann Intens Care. 2011;1:51.
15. Lellouche F, Mancebo J, Jolliet P, et al. A multicenter randomized trial of computer-driven protocolized weaning from mechanical ventilation. Am J Respir Crit Care Med. 2006;174(8):894–900.

16. Hermeto F, Bottino MN, Vaillancourt K, et al. Implementation of a respiratory therapist-driven protocol for neonatal ventilation: impact on the premature population. Pediatrics. 2009;123(5):e907–16.
17. Khemani RG, Sward K, Morris A, et al. Variability in usual care mechanical ventilation for pediatric acute lung injury: the potential benefit of a lung protective computer protocol. Intensive Care Med. 2011;37(11): 1840–8.
18. Burns KE, Meade MO, Lessard MR, et al. Wean earlier and automatically with new technology (the WEAN study). A multicenter, pilot randomized controlled trial. Am J Respir Crit Care Med. 2013;187(11):1203–11.
19. Liker JK. Principle 14: becoming a learning organization through relentless reflection *(Hansen)* and continuous improvement *(Kaizen)*. In: The Toyota way. New York: McGraw-Hill; 2004. p. 250–65.
20. Slutsky AS, Ranieri VM. Ventilator-induced lung injury. N Engl J Med. 2013;369(22):2126–36.
21. Jozwiak M, Teboul JL, Anguel N, et al. Beneficial hemodynamic effects of prone positioning in patients with acute respiratory distress syndrome. Am J Respir Crit Care Med. 2013;188(12):1428–33.
22. Gattinoni L, Taccone P, Carlesso E, et al. Prone position in acute respiratory distress syndrome. Rationale, indications, and limits. Am J Respir Crit Care Med. 2013;188(11):1286–93.
23. Venkatachalam V, Hendley JO, Willson DF. The diagnostic dilemma of ventilator-associated pneumonia in critically ill children. Pediatr Crit Care Med. 2011; 12(3):286–96.
24. Muszynski JA, Sartori J, Steele L, et al. Multidisciplinary quality improvement initiative to reduce ventilator-associated tracheobronchitis in the PICU. Pediatr Crit Care Med. 2013;14(5):533–8.
25. Sarter NB, Woods DD. Situation awareness: a critical but ill defined phenomenon. Int J Aviat Psychol. 1991; 1:45–7.
26. Baker D, Gustafson S, Beaubien J, Salas E, Barach P. Medical teamwork and patient safety: the evidence-based relation. AHRQ Publication No. 05–0053. 2005. Available at: http://www.ahrq.gov/qual/medteam/. Accessed 4 Apr 2014.
27. McGee DC, Gould MK. Preventing complications of central venous catheterization. N Engl J Med. 2003;348: 1123–33.
28. Merrer J, De Jonghe B, Golliot F, et al. Complications of femoral and subclavian venous catheterization in critically ill patients: a randomized controlled trial. JAMA. 2001;286:700–7.

Local Improvement Teams

21

Heather Freeman and Andrew Young Shin

Abstract

Improving how we safely and efficiently care for patients is a paramount issue for health care organizations. Yet, most institutions struggle with how to systematically achieve a continuously learning and improving program. Lack of organization, variability in clinical care, insufficient resources and competing agendas are common contributing factors to poor sustainability in quality improvement efforts.

Local Improvement Teams (LITs) are unit or patient population-based teams that apply structured problem solving methodologies to improve care processes toward achieving the Institute of Medicine's 6 aims: safe, timely, effective, efficient, equitable, and patient-centered care. LITs represent a fundamental aspect in creating an intelligent enterprise: the maturation of a frontline interface that connects the organization's core competency with the needs of the patient. Team structure, process, training and launch strategies are described in this chapter along with tactics to develop standard work, daily accountability process and standard work for leaders.

Keywords

Improvement Teams • Lean • Management System • Clinical Microsystems • A3 Thinking • 8-Step Problem Solving

H. Freeman, RN, MS, CNS, NNP-BC
Performance Improvement, Lucile Packard Children's Hospital at Stanford, 700 Welch Road, Ste. 125, Rm. 117, Palo Alto, CA 94304, USA
e-mail: hfreeman@lpch.org

A.Y. Shin, MD (✉)
Cardiovascular Intensive Care, Division of Pediatric Cardiology, Department of Pediatrics, Lucile Packard Children's Hospital, Stanford University Medical Center, 750 Welch Road, Suite 305, Palo Alto, CA 94304, USA
e-mail: drewshin@stanford.edu

P.R. Barach, J.P. Jacobs, S.E. Lipshultz, P.C. Laussen (eds.), *Pediatric and Congenital Cardiac Care: Volume 2: Quality Improvement and Patient Safety*, DOI 10.1007/978-1-4471-6566-8_21, © Springer-Verlag London 2015

Introduction

Since the publication of two landmark reports on the U.S. health care delivery by the Institute of Medicine (IOM), improving the quality of the health care system has become a national priority [1, 2]. In the report *Crossing the Quality Chasm: A New Health System for the 21st Century*, the committee builds a clear case for systematic improvement. The report openly states that health care today harms too frequently and routinely fails to deliver its potential benefit citing several publications that document significant quality shortcomings [1]. In a daunting report by the Institute of Healthcare Improvement (IHI), only 13 % of quality improvement initiatives are continued after 1 year providing perspective on the immense challenges in changing an organization's practice in a sustainable fashion. The IOM concludes that simply *trying harder will not work. Changing systems of care will.*

Local Improvement Teams (LIT's) represent a local milieu embedded within a larger organization in which providers, support staff, organizational leadership and patient representatives converge to analyze and implement systematic changes to improve the quality, efficiency and safety of health care. Like other clinical microsystems, LIT's are adaptive systems made up of front-line providers who are responsible for delivering most of the care to the patient. Because LIT's represent the most proximal constituent to the patient, they best understand the local subpopulation of patients and peers along with processes and patterns that make up their unit culture. LIT's represent a fundamental aspect in creating an intelligent enterprise: the maturation of a frontline interface that connects the organization's core competency with the needs of the individual customer – in this case, the patient.

The following chapter provides an overview of a unit-based local improvement team and its function in connecting larger organizational goals to frontline providers for measurable improvement in health care delivery. We will focus on the steps for successful implementation of a LIT within an institution describing organizational tools that promote consistency, efficacy and authority. Finally, a framework of the structure and support necessary for a creating a sustainable system with reliable processes and methodologies using case examples is described.

Local Improvement Team Overview

The LIT is based on the "Clinical Microsystems" improvement model originally developed at Dartmouth University [3]. The LIT is a permanent, multidisciplinary team that is specially trained in improvement methodologies with the goal of supporting the front line in producing highly reliable, safe, effective, timely care to our patients and families. The team's primary functions are to assess and prioritize complex problems, to develop and test countermeasures to address the problems, then create and continuously improve effective countermeasures (e.g., to create and manage standards). The LIT works in conjunction with strategic goal deployment (a.k.a. "hoshin kanri;" agreement and accountability at all levels) and daily management system (described below) [4].

Team Composition

The LIT's focus is not limited to one problem or project, but rather it is a permanent team structure formed to lead system improvement at the local level. The team is multidisciplinary, representing the roles within the local unit, including patient/family members, and are led in a dyad partnership by nurse-physician leaders [5–7] . The work of improving the system of care may be accomplished either within the LIT, or by training and guiding subgroups through an organized improvement process with LIT oversight. Improvement cannot be sustained within the small team—the team should continuously involve all other members (as applicable) of the local unit. The team also requires ancillary support from resources peripheral but integral to the local unit including, but not limited to analytics, clinical informatics, executive and administrative leadership. Ad hoc ancillary partners may also be included such as pharmacy, dietary, lab, respiratory therapy, and housekeeping.

Steps for Implementation

Defining the core team is an imperative first step in the implementation of a LIT [6]. The "core team" includes those interdisciplinary team members who will be actively involved in all improvement work. As outlined above, each team requires a nurse and physician lead to represent most of the perspectives of the local environment. One of the most necessary and essential resource for the core team is time. Committed time facilitates productivity, enables sustainability and establishes accountability. The allotment in dedicated time for the local leaders is a philosophical investment that has real gains measured by the economical implications in quality improvement work – specifically the optimization of clinical resource utilization and the reduction and elimination of preventable adverse events and hospital acquired conditions. The interdisciplinary core team should reflect and represent the important perspectives and components that define the interface between unit and patient. The development of a charter as an overarching guide should include short-term and long-term aims, membership expectations, meeting frequency, and a defined organizational decision-making process.

An important lesson for an initial team is to understand the culture of a local unit along with the specific challenges associated with institutional change. To understand the dynamics of change in a manageable way, it is important to start with a well-circumscribed, short-gain project so as to establish an efficacious and reliable process. Though the initial project should be small in scope, the process should still be rigorous and intentional. It begins with an assessment of the local unit using established methodologies for unit evaluation (*e.g.*, the 5 P's [Purpose, Patients, Professionals, Processes, and Patterns] or Assess, Diagnose, Treat Workbook) [5, 6]. The assessment includes documenting the steps of major processes, as experienced by the patients (also called "Value Stream Mapping") [8], and a review of clinical, service, and cost outcomes data [5].

Choosing a problem may invoke diverging opinions. Multiple perspectives from multiple stakeholders in a local environment pose challenges to the team to determine the direction in quality improvement work. The LIT should leverage available venues to include other unit members in the decision-making process. Concepts such as a Wall Chart of the top 5 or so processes to work on with a "polling" mechanism for each discipline that works in the unit to participate in problem selection [7] (see Table 21.1). It is important to remember that the scope of the initial problem should be fairly narrow with an estimated timeframe of 3–6 months. It should also be an important problem to work on at the time it is selected to ensure broad support; alignment with the institutional agenda is essential [9].

Table 21.1 Wall chart multi-voting example

Process	Never a problem	Sometimes a problem	A problem about ½ the time	A problem most of the time	Always a problem!	Patients and Families have concerns
Line Infection prevention	●● ●	●●				
Surgical site infection prevention			●	●●●●●● ●●	●●	
Pain management						
Hand-off from OR						
Discharge instruction						

Table 21.2 8-step problem solving [10]

Problem solving steps		Processes for each step
Plan	1. Clarify the problem	1. Identify the ultimate goal
		2. Identify the target condition (interim goal)
		3. Identify the gap between the target condition and current state
	2. Break down the problem	1. Break the problem down
		2. Select the specific problem to solve
		3. Specify the point of cause (go and see—who, when, where, why, how is it happening?)
	3. Set aim/target	1. Commit to solving the problem
		2. Set a measurable, concrete, challenging, time specific target/aim
	4. Root cause analysis	1. Without preconception, consider as many potential causes as possible
		2. Based on facts gathered by going and seeing, keep asking "why?"
		3. Specify the root cause
	5. Develop countermeasures	1. Develop as many as possible
		2. Narrow down to the most practical and effective
		3. Build consensus with others
		4. Create a clear and detailed action plan
Do	6. See countermeasures through	1. As a team, implement countermeasures (changes to test) quickly
		2. Share progress by following reporting, informing and consulting communication practices
		3. Never give up, and proceed to the next step quickly
Check	7. Monitor results and process	1. Evaluate the overall results and the processes used, share evaluation with involved team members
		2. Evaluate from three viewpoints: patient (customer), hospital, yours
		3. Understand factors behind success or failure (learn)
Adjust	8. Standardize successful processes	1. Structure successful process (standardize)
		2. Share new precedent through horizontal deployment
		3. Start next the round of incremental improvement

Training the Team

Team members likely have varying experience and knowledge of improvement techniques. To level-set and ensure team members are adequately prepared to do and lead improvement work, formal preparation should ideally be together. Training typically includes didactic lessons on education and improvement methodologies. More importantly and realistically, training should occur in "real time" and revolve around the problem selected. By receiving "in the moment" coaching with a relevant problem within the unit enhances success and promotes credibility of the LIT. There are many improvement methodologies including the Toyota's 8-Step Problem Solving [10] (Table 21.2) and A3-thinking [9] (Fig. 21.1). These improvement modalities are based on the Shewhart PDCA cycle [10]. Table 21.3 highlights an example to integrate improvement methods into a training program.

Designing Highly Reliable, Sustainable Processes

We in healthcare have had a pretty clear idea of *what* to do. There are innumerable reports that elaborate best practices. Yet, there continues to be important variation in care processes with significant variability between individuals, units, and centers. The reasons are likely multifactorial but in essence: (a) we do not agree on a standard way of doing our work and/or (b) we have not designed the process well. In order to build a highly reliable process, systems must be designed

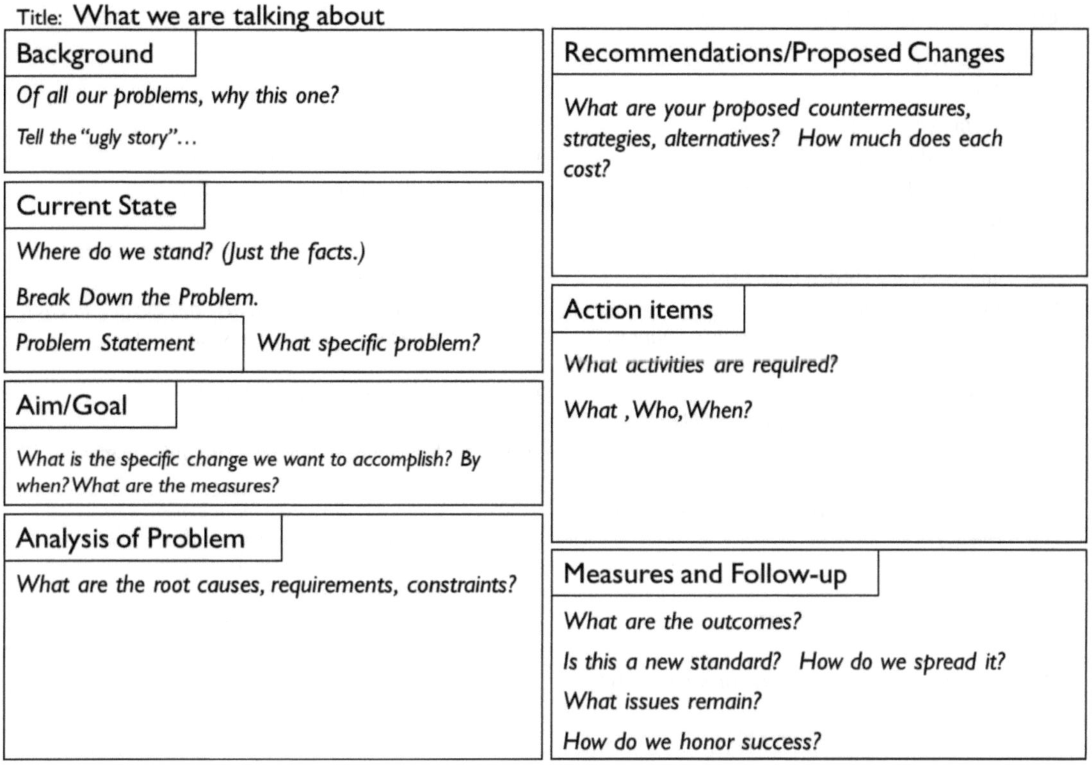

Fig. 21.1 A3 problem solving tool example [11]. Note: this tool has a method to its use. It is meant to be taken to the workplace, involve many other people, and be edited many times [8]

so that the right thing to do is either the only thing that can be done (error-proofed) or the easiest thing to do.

Designing Standard Processes

Each healthcare system has multiple standards in the form of policies and procedures. However, most institutional policies and procedures are overwhelmed with dense texts and numerous pages that defy utility. Not uncommonly, existing policies contradict one another or fall out of current practice, which contributes to confusion and threatens standard practice.

The most significant limitation lies when there are no existing standards. Taiichi Ohno famously said: "Without standards, there can be no improvement" [11]. Philosophically, it is not possible to have multiple "best ways" of doing something—especially when considering the patient's vantage point. Standardization of practice is a necessary process in order to improve practice. Stable and standard processes are the basis of system stability and provide the framework to improve the quality and safety of care.

Although evidence through scientific investigation is unavailable for most care processes, many different formats for developing standards exist. One of the better standard development methods comes from WWII training methods called "Training Within Industry" [18, 24]. Some basic questions should be answered by the standard, such as who should do the work, how it should be done, and why it is done this way. The job role (as applicable), steps, sequence, and timing points should be listed utilizing a format such as the Job Breakdown Sheet (Fig. 21.2 is an example of a job breakdown sheet).

Using a format such as a Job Breakdown Sheet will enhance the team's ability to teach the new standard. Though necessary, it is an insufficient

Table 21.3 Example LIT training program

Day 1		Day 2	
Time	Topic	Time	Topic
0:15	Team dynamics [12]	0:30	Data analysis and measurement [3]
0:10	System thinking [3, 13]	0:30	*Exercise*: *develop measures*
0:10	Clinical Microsystem overview [3, 5, 6]	0:20	Project management basics [5, 9, 14–16]
0:30	*Exercise*: *5 P's review* [5]	0:30	*Exercise*: *Plan your tests of change*
0:20	Clarifying and breaking down problems: understanding current state [9]	0:20	Change management/gaining agreement (A3 thinking) [9, 17]
1:30	*Exercise*: *go to the workplace and see* (*who, what, when, where, why does the problem happen*?). *Use timers, spaghetti diagrams, etc. as needed*	0:30	*Exercise*: *plan how to use A3 thinking to gain agreement, test changes, fill out A3*
1:00	*Exercise*: *debrief, draw current state map, record all data, give shape to problem*	0:15	Designing standards [18, 19]
0:10	Specifying the problem to solve: set target [9]	0:30	Managing standards: Daily management system overview [20]
0:30	*Exercise*: *set target* (*improve by how much, by when*?)	1:30	*Exercise*: *Go to see management system components*: *standards, audits, visual controls, leader standard work, daily accountability process*
0:15	Root cause analysis [9, 21]	0:45	*Exercise*: *Debrief, and plan/design management system*
0:45	*Exercise*: *analyze root cause* (*fishbone, 5 Whys*)	1:00	*Exercise*: *LIT planning*: *meeting times, communication, education, deliverables*
0:10	Selecting countermeasures [21]		
0:30	*Exercise*: *choose 1–2 countermeasures to try*		
0:20	Planning tests of change: PDCA [5, 10, 22, 23]		

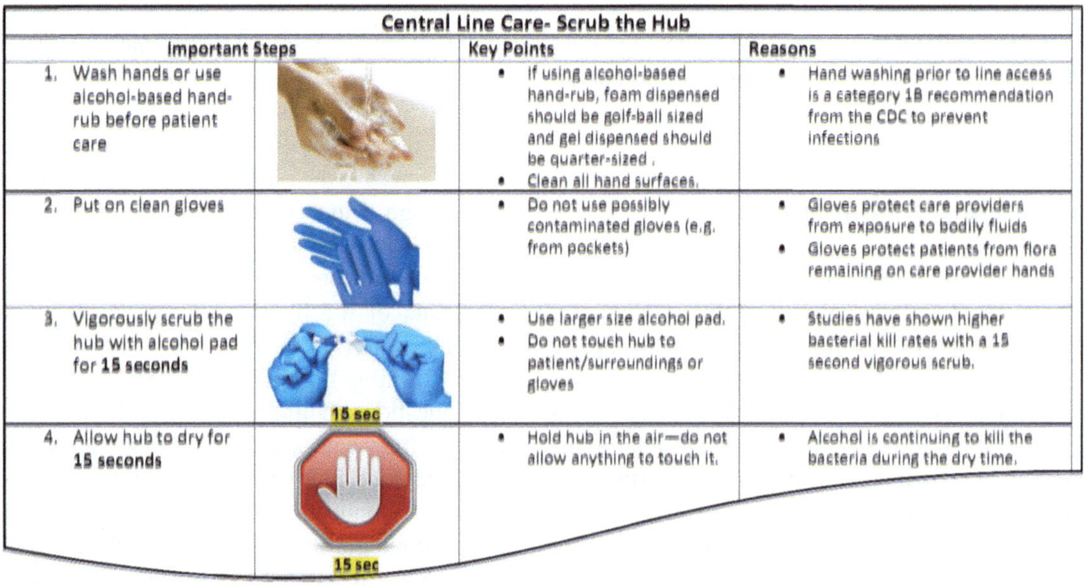

Central Line Care- Scrub the Hub

Important Steps	Key Points	Reasons
1. Wash hands or use alcohol-based hand-rub before patient care	• If using alcohol-based hand-rub, foam dispensed should be golf-ball sized and gel dispensed should be quarter-sized . • Clean all hand surfaces.	• Hand washing prior to line access is a category 1B recommendation from the CDC to prevent infections
2. Put on clean gloves	• Do not use possibly contaminated gloves (e.g. from pockets)	• Gloves protect care providers from exposure to bodily fluids • Gloves protect patients from flora remaining on care provider hands
3. Vigorously scrub the hub with alcohol pad for **15 seconds** (15 sec)	• Use larger size alcohol pad. • Do not touch hub to patient/surroundings or gloves	• Studies have shown higher bacterial kill rates with a 15 second vigorous scrub.
4. Allow hub to dry for **15 seconds** (15 sec)	• Hold hub in the air—do not allow anything to touch it.	• Alcohol is continuing to kill the bacteria during the dry time.

Fig. 21.2 Job breakdown sheet example

Table 21.4 Training within industry method

Steps	Key points
Step I: PREPARE the worker	Put him/her at ease
	State the job (process) and ask what he/she already knows about it
	Place learner in correct location/position
Step II: PRESENT the operation (process)	Tell, show, illustrate one important step at a time
	Stress each key point
Step III: TRY OUT performance	Have him/her do the job and correct errors
	Have him/her explain each key point as s/he does the job again
Step IV: FOLLOW UP	Allow him/her to perform independently. Designate who to go to with questions
	Check frequently, encourage questions
	Taper off coaching

component for sustainable and reliable practice. The standard process needs to be supported and well managed. Easily accessible supplies, equipment, and staffing must be available. The Central Line Care standard example above requires three components: a way to perform hand hygiene (gloves and alcohol wipes), clock, and a staff member (already apportioned). Inventory, accessibility, replenishment, and any other barriers to the standard practice are important items for daily management systems to investigate, audit and report back to ensure the reliability of the standard processes.

Training to the Standard

After developing the standard and ensuring that the right supplies, equipment, and staffing are in place, the people performing the standard need to be trained well enough to ensure they understand each step, how it is performed, and why it is important. Effecting change in behavior presents one of the most challenging aspects for improvement work and starts with transparency in goals and directed outcomes. Methodologies such as Training Within Industry [18, 24] have shown consistent results. The basic structure of this training is listed in Table 21.4 below [24]. This format for training, coupled with simulation is an ideal combination for training how to perform procedures or high-risk/low-volume processes [25].

Auditing the Standard

Standards that are not checked will inevitably breakdown and produce variable outcomes. Clinical or administrative circumstances change, new problems arise, new staff lacking in training arrive, missing supplies and equipment all contribute to challenges in sustainable processes. Standards need to be evaluated routinely for these and other problems—especially critical or time-sensitive standards. Audits are necessary tools to monitor for consistency and reliability and can be leveraged to understand ongoing challenges or blindspots to standard execution and reliable process.

The Management System: Managing and Improving Standards

Creating, training to, and auditing standards is not quite half the battle. This has been the typical method of improvement in healthcare, and although some positive changes have resulted, it has clearly not been enough to sustain the gains. Only 13 % of improvement efforts in healthcare are sustained after a year, but even more discouraging, after focused improvement efforts, the rate of harm has not dropped appreciably [26]. The system requires fundamental management and operational changes.

A "lean" management system is comprised of five main categories of elements: Stable and

Standard Processes (the section above describes this), Problem Identification (most notably via visual controls), the Daily Accountability Process, Problem Solving, and Standard Work for Leaders [20].

Problem Identification includes visual controls, immediate problem response, and audits. The purpose of visual controls is to highlight and make immediately apparent ongoing problems and to demonstrate actual compared to expected (or targeted) performance. There are many forms of visual controls, including process-based (such as results from audit or patient discharge processes), outcome-based (such as the CLABSI rate), work-focused (tasks of the day), and so forth. A good rule of thumb is that the visual display should be "understood from 5 ft away, within 5 s."

Immediate problem response (also termed "andon response") is an important systematic philosophy for getting help *in the moment* when a standard process cannot be followed as specified. Time-sensitive escalation to resolve small and large barriers to standard practice is an important factor to eliminate gaps in performance to ensure a highly reliable process.

As discussed above, audits are essential techniques to capture problems with specific standards. There are many ways of managing the audit process. An essential component to successful audit processes includes transparency. Visibility with the audit practice and the visibility with audit results help integrate this practice into the culture of the local environment. It is important to continuously link the results of the audit with the short-term and long-term aims of the LIT. Additionally, ensuring leadership are an integral part of the audit process establishes the standard and provides meaningful implications – both in audit process and further understanding best standard practice.

Placing data on a wall will not improve a process. Data needs to be checked frequently and acted upon. The daily accountability (or tiered huddle) process is crucial to maintaining the system and finding problems. Below is a list of suggested tiers [20]. The huddle meetings are brief, highlighting only abnormalities, ideally taking place at visibility boards. Adequate staff, supplies, equipment, and patient safety are among the common topics to review.

- Tier 1: Unit staff and team leader (e.g., charge nurse) meet at start of shift to review the activity of the day and known issues.
- Tier 2: Team leader and their immediate supervisors meet in tier 2 (manager/medical director or attending level) in the next huddle. Issues are discussed, problems assigned and escalated as needed.
- Tier 3: Manager/MD level meets with service line leader level. Same as above.
- Tier 4: Service Line Leaders meet with CNO/COO/Chief of Staff. Same as above.

Managing a system to support standard work must have active participation and investment from executive leadership. Standard work for LIT leaders is aimed at the express purpose of maintaining this subtle yet influential system of identifying and solving problems. Standard work for leaders should include routine reviews of visual boards to evaluate system status, conduct daily accountability meetings, identify real-time problems and facilitate real-time solutions [20].

An example of implementing daily management system to sustain and improve standards is below:

The Cardiovascular Intensive Care Unit Local Improvement Team aimed to reduce CLABSIs by 25 % in the next 6 months and 50 % in the next year.

The team constructed job aids (job breakdown sheets) for adequate hand washing utilizing alcohol-based hand-gel, proper sterilizing techniques for central venous catheter access, and standardized central line dressing changes.

Training was multi-modal utilizing existing venues such as staff meetings and daily huddles and unique venues such as simulation capitalizing on methods such as Training within Industry model (mentioned previously) [24, 25].

Audits were integrated into leader standard work. Process and outcome metrics were made visible on boards, and reviewed daily in huddles by frontline staff and executive leadership. Data from audits revealed several barriers to standard work such as inadequate supplies to which simple solutions were immediately implemented.

Leaders encouraged and specified a culture of immediate problem response. Each subsequent solution to a newly discovered barrier to "best practice" led to the maturation of a new standard work flow. With ongoing audits and removal of impediments to the standard process, the "best practice" was renovated into the easiest practice. Building a reliable and sustainable system contributed importantly to the unit's success in reducing the CLABSI rate by 30 % within 5 months.

Conclusions

A central element to bridge the gap between standard work and best practice is the ability for organizations and front line providers to reflect on their work and cultivate change at a system level. Pockets of excellence exist in our health care system but widespread inter-individual, unit and institutional variability contribute to inconsistent practices that undermine innovation and subvert reliable and sustainable processes.

A system of continuous quality improvement starts at the interface between the patient and the organization. Frontline healthcare providers are poised to be the most effective constituent of local change integrating both patient needs and institutional aims. Local improvement teams are discrete and proximal units that connect larger organizational goals to the patient. LITs can leverage deliberate improvement methodologies to understand and revise healthcare processes through organized efforts to reduce waste, complexity and redundancy. In the end, success in establishing a highly reliable management system is predictable and replicable when the investments from leadership are substantive, improvement teams reflect the frontline interface values and the methodologies are responsive and visibly organized.

References

1. Committee on Quality of Health Care in America, Institute of Medicine. Crossing the quality chasm: a new health system for the 21st century. Washington, DC: The National Academies Press; 2001.
2. Kohn LT, Corrigan JM, Donaldson MS, Committee on Quality of Health Care in America, Institute of Medicine, editors. To err is human: building a safer health system. Washington, DC: The National Academies Press; 2000.
3. Nelson EC, Batalden PB, Huber TP, Mohr JJ, Godfrey MM, Headrick LA, et al. Microsystems in health care: part 1. Learning from high-performing front-line clinical units. Jt Comm J Qual Improv. 2002;28(9):472–93.
4. Akao Y. Hoshin Kanri: policy deployment for successful TQM. Cambridge, MA: Productivity Press; 2004. 248 p.
5. Nelson EC, Batalden PB, Godfrey MM. Quality by design: a clinical microsystems approach. Lebanon/San Francisco: Center for the Evaluative Clinical Sciences at Dartmouth; Jossey-Bass/Wiley; 2007.
6. Godfrey MM, Nelson EC, Batalden PB. Assessing, diagnosing, and treating your inpatient unit [Internet]. Trustees of Dartmouth College; 2001. Available from: http://www.clinicalmicrosystem.org/materials/workbooks/.
7. Nelson EC. Value by design developing clinical microsystems to achieve organizational excellence [Internet]. 2011. [cited 2013 Jun 21]. Available from: http://proquest.safaribooksonline.com/?fpi=9780470385340.
8. Rother M, Shook J, Womack J, Jones D. Learning to see: value stream mapping to add value and eliminate MUDA. Version 1.4 Oct 2009 edition. Cambridge, MA: Lean Enterprise Institute; 1999.
9. Shook J. Managing to learn: using the A3 management process to solve problems, gain agreement, mentor and lead. Cambridge, MA: Lean Enterprise Institute; 2008.
10. Deming WE. Out of the crisis. Cambridge, MA: MIT Press; 2000.
11. Without standards there can be no kaizen [Internet]. The Lean Thinker. [cited 2013 Jul 6]. Available from: http://theleanthinker.com/2009/01/12/without-standards-there-can-be-no-kaizen/.
12. Tuckman BW. Developmental sequence in small groups. Psychol Bull. 1965;63(6):384–99.
13. Systems thinking [Internet]. Wikipedia Free Encycl. 2013 [cited 2013 Jul 5]. Available from: http://en.wikipedia.org/w/index.php?title=Systems_thinking&oldid=560631212.
14. Leach LP, Leach LP. Lean project management: eight principles for success. Boise: Advanced Projects, Inc.; 2005.
15. Project Management Institute. A guide to the project management body of knowledge (PMBOK Guide). Newtown Square: Project Management Institute; 2008.
16. Cohn M. Succeeding with agile: software development using Scrum. Upper Saddle River: Addison-Wesley; 2010.
17. Jellison JM. Managing the dynamics of change the fastest path to creating an engaged and productive workforce [Internet]. New York: McGraw-Hill; 2006. [cited 2013 Jul 6], Available from: http://site.ebrary.com/id/10150089.

18. Liker JK, Meier D. Toyota talent: developing your people the Toyota way. New York: McGraw-Hill; 2007.
19. Blancett SS, Flarey DL. Reengineering nursing and health care: the handbook for organizational transformation. Gaithersburg: Aspen Publishers; 1995.
20. Mann D. Creating a lean culture: tools to sustain lean conversions. New York: Productivity Press; 2010.
21. Marksberry P, Bustle J, Clevinger J. Problem solving for managers: a mathematical investigation of Toyota's 8-step process. J Manuf Technol Manag. 2011;22(7):837–52.
22. Institute for Healthcare Improvement: Science of Improvement: Testing Changes [Internet]. [cited 2013 Jun 21]. Available from: http://www.ihi.org/knowledge/Pages/HowtoImprove/ScienceofImprovementTestingChanges.aspx.
23. Liker JK, Franz JK. The Toyota way to continuous improvement: linking strategy and operational excellence to achieve superior performance. New York: McGraw-Hill; 2011.
24. Training USWMCB of. Job Instruction: Sessions Outline and Reference Material ... Training within Industry Service, Bureau of Training, War Manpower Commission; 1944. 76 p.
25. Halamek LP. Simulation-based training: opportunities for the acquisition of unique skills. Virtual Mentor. 2006;8(2):84–7.
26. Landrigan CP, Parry GJ, Bones CB, Hackbarth AD, Goldmann DA, Sharek PJ. Temporal trends in rates of patient harm resulting from medical care. N Engl J Med. 2010;363(22):2124–34.

Implementation Science—The Next Frontier

22

Brian S. Mittman

Abstract

The challenge of persisting gaps in the quality and outcomes of health care and public health continues to attract interest from the research, policy and practice communities. Public health programs can only deliver benefits if they are able to sustain activities over time. Implementation science is an emerging field of inquiry drawing from a diverse set of research traditions, methods and sources. This chapter reviews the origins and foundations of implementation science, discusses its strengths and weaknesses relative to closely-related bodies of activity in quality and safety improvement, and identifies opportunities for increased collaboration and mutually beneficial synergy across both fields. Implementation science and improvement science must enhance their attention to the significant levels of heterogeneity inherent in quality problems and their root causes, in the settings and contexts in which these problems occur, and in measuring the effects of strategies deployed to change clinical practices and improve patient outcomes. New research and practice strategies building upon the strengths and complementary perspectives of implementation and improvement sciences represent the "next frontier" in efforts to improve quality, value and outcomes in health. Such strategies offer considerable value if developed with a deep and balanced understanding of the magnitude and unique features of quality gaps, the need for multi-level,

B.S. Mittman, PhD
Department of Research and Evaluation, Kaiser Permanente Southern California, Pasadena, CA, USA

Implementation and Improvement Science Initiative, Clinical and Translational Science Institute, University of California Los Angeles, Los Angeles, CA, USA

VA Center for Implementation Practice and Research Support, US Department of Veterans Affairs Greater Los Angeles Healthcare System, 16111 Plummer Street, Sepulveda, CA 91343, USA
e-mail: brian.mittman@va.gov

P.R. Barach, J.P. Jacobs, S.E. Lipshultz, P.C. Laussen (eds.), *Pediatric and Congenital Cardiac Care: Volume 2: Quality Improvement and Patient Safety*, DOI 10.1007/978-1-4471-6566-8_22, © Springer-Verlag London 2015

multi-component, context-sensitive approaches, and the need for continuous monitoring, evaluation and refinement of improvement approaches.

Keywords
Healthcare delivery and organization • Healthcare delivery system science • Quality improvement • Performance improvement • Implementation science • Physicians' practice patterns • Complex interventions

Introduction

Nearly 15 years after publication of the landmark reports *To Err is Human* [1] and *Crossing the Quality Chasm* [2] in the United States and 25 years after the introduction of industrial quality improvement methods into the health care field [3, 4], interest in understanding and addressing deficiencies in the quality and outcomes of health care continues to grow. Recognition of substantial quality gaps in healthcare delivery and outcomes is widespread, documented in a diverse collection of publications quantifying and comparing these gaps in several countries throughout the world [5, 6]. Yet, despite widespread recognition of the problem and considerable investment in development of solutions, progress remains slow, and reliable strategies to improve the performance and quality of health care delivery remain scarce.

The challenge of improving health care performance has been the focus of an evolving mix of research approaches and fields, and a changing set of terms and labels describing these fields. Much of the early work (primarily in the 1970s and 1980s) was conducted under the heading "changing physician behavior" [7, 8], reflecting the prevailing view that health care quality is largely influenced by the decisions and actions of individual physicians and their diagnostic, management and treatment practices. Common strategies employed to influence these practices and enhance physician adherence to consensus-based clinical recommendations during this period included continuing medical education (CME), reminder systems [9, 10] and other narrowly focused strategies that were ultimately determined to have limited impact and value.

The introduction of industrial quality improvement concepts and approaches from outside the health domain began at the conclusion of the 1980s, led by Berwick and others, reflecting a shift of attention to the "system" rather than the individual physician [3, 4]. Accompanying this shift was an expanded interest in strategies to document, diagnose and correct flaws in healthcare system organizational policies and procedures. Research in this area, initially labeled "quality improvement" and "patient safety" research and, more recently, "improvement science," prioritized the development and evaluation of tools and approaches for identifying, documenting and diagnosing quality and safety gaps (via "root cause analyses") and related methods for treating these gaps via improvements in policies and procedures [11, 12]. This research activity expanded in parallel with rapid growth in the health industry's interest in quality improvement (QI), as evidenced (and stimulated) by organizations such as the Institute for Healthcare Improvement (IHI), Agency for Healthcare Research and Quality (AHRQ) and by the establishment and growth of new "quality and safety" journals such as *International Journal Quality in Health Care* [13], launched in 1989 as *Quality Assurance in Health Care*, and *BMJ Quality and Safety* [14], launched in 1992 as *Quality in Health Care*.

The label "implementation science" and the expansion of research activity and approaches under this label occurred during the mid-2000s [15] and continued into the current decade. This activity complemented and augmented existing interest in quality and safety improvement with interest in addressing the "translational

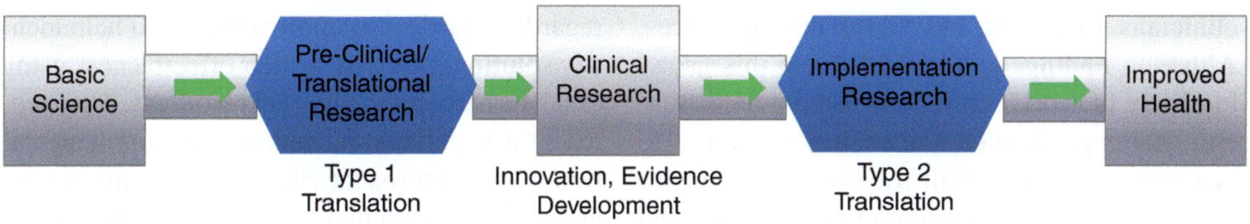

Fig. 22.1 Translational research phases

roadblocks" and implementation gaps identified by the Institute of Medicine's Clinical Research Roundtable [16, 17] and parallel entities in the UK and elsewhere. This work led to a widespread recognition and discussion of distinct categories of translational research, based on schemes that variously identify two, three, four or more translational research phases (i.e., T1, T2, T3, T4 phases) [18–20]. Despite different levels of sub-division of the two major phases described by the Institute of Medicine Clinical Research Roundtable and its counterparts internationally, each of these schemes directs attention to two broad categories of translational research activities (Fig. 22.1). The first, Type 1 translation (or T1), emphasizes the translation of basic science findings into effective clinical innovations via methods such as computational biology and the development and use of animal models of disease. Type 2 translation (or T2) and its sub-divisions, in contrast, works to facilitate appropriate, rapid adoption and implementation of effective clinical innovations and research findings into routine practice via their incorporation into clinical practice guidelines. Furthermore, this phase is devoted to the study of barriers and facilitators to implementation – and strategies to proactively accelerate practice change and implementation. Variously labeled knowledge translation research, research utilization, knowledge-to-action, and implementation science [21], research within the Type 2 translational phase examines barriers, facilitators, processes and strategies involved in achieving the benefits of research through its widespread implementation in community settings.

Although definitions and views about the scope of implementation science vary, a key feature is its approach to the problem of persisting quality gaps from the perspective of potential solutions, rather than problems. While quality and safety improvement generally proceeds from the starting point of suspected quality gaps that must be documented and diagnosed to guide the selection or identification of solutions, implementation science generally, and the commas and preceding and following it begins with the observation that effective, evidence-based practices (including practices for diagnosing, treating and managing disease) are under-utilized and require proactive efforts to facilitate broader implementation (or, alternatively, that ineffective practices are over-utilized and require efforts to achieve de-implementation) [22]. Consistent with this orientation and its close association with clinical research and the study designs and methods valued in clinical research, much of the effort within the field of implementation science has focused on experimental evaluation of specific implementation interventions or strategies, and the contextual factors—enablers and barriers to success—and other effect modifiers influencing their effectiveness in different circumstances.

Implementation Science and Improvement Science Contributions and Challenges

The emergence of the new discipline of implementation science has driven a rapid increase in studies of how new scientific discoveries are incorporated into new programs and policies and ultimately into routine practice by clinicians [23]. This ultimately is about engaging clinicians to accept and adopt new practices. Although findings and insights from this growing body of work continue to accumulate, several challenges remain and society continues to benefit from only a small fraction of its considerable investment in research in health care and public health.

The optimal application and the overall value of implementation science and improvement science in addressing quality and performance gaps in health care remain uncertain and are in flux. As policy and practice leaders have become increasingly aware of implementation science – and as they consider its potential to augment QI and improvement science approaches to accelerate progress – they quickly discover a lack of guidance or common vision in understanding the relationships and potential synergy between the two fields. This deficiency in published literature and the lack of useful guidance in combining the two closely-related but seemingly separate fields of inquiry reflect a degree of parochialism and an excessive inward-facing orientation by researchers and other experts in both domains. Simplistic characterizations of each field suggests that *improvement science* focuses too narrowly on the development of ad-hoc solutions to context-specific, unique problems – with insufficient attention to generalizable knowledge and broadly-applicable solutions and insights – whereas, *implementation science* is viewed as incorrectly assuming a level of homogeneity and stability in quality problems that rarely exists, and as seeking robust and very broadly applicable solutions that are similarly rare. While each of these views over-states the limitations of the improvement and implementation science fields, they both reflect underlying differences and similarities that offer potential value in developing future effective approaches to the problems of persistent quality gaps in health care.

Recognition of heterogeneity and complexity is inherent in improvement science, including rapid-cycle improvement methods, such as Plan-Do-Study-Act (PDSA) cycles that involve iterative cycles of planning, design, evaluation and refinement of improvement strategies [24]. These approaches generate context-specific evidence regarding barriers to improvement and help identify solutions and assess their effectiveness using quick turnaround in time and resources. They represent a significant advantage over implementation science approaches that assume homogeneity and resist incremental, real-time refinement and other threats to internal validity and external generalizability. An *improvement-science* approach recognizes the need for customized, site-specific and context-sensitive solutions based on careful study of current practices and local mental models, and careful surfacing and recognition of barriers to improvement. The *implementation-science* approach would contribute insights and guidance for addressing heterogeneity and guiding adaptation based on the all-important recognition of the context and contextual influences on the success and uptake of implementation processes and outcomes. Context is recognized as important within both fields (improvement and implementation sciences), and is the focus of a growing body of work within implementation science to identify and adapt social science theories and theoretical principles linking contextual factors to practice change process and outcome differences [25–27].

Improvement and implementation sciences offer complementary approaches in other respects as well. Implementation science aims to improve health care quality in part through the development of insights regarding variations in implementation success and the factors driving these variations. Implementation science theories and frameworks, such as the Promoting Action on Research Implementation in Health Services (PARIHS) framework [28] and the Consolidated Framework for Implementation Research (CFIR) [29], identify key factors driving variations such as features of evidence-based practices and innovations to be implemented, attributes of implementation settings and contexts, and the implementation and practice change strategies to be deployed to achieve improvement. Generalizable findings regarding the impacts of contextual factors (such as leadership, organizational culture, staffing sufficiency and stability, other resources and logistical arrangements) will enhance implementation approaches. Similarly, a sustained commitment to thoroughly assess quality gaps and their underlying causes will help improvement proponents increase the likelihood that a given practice change strategy will be compatible and effective in specific settings and for specific quality problems. This knowledge should also prove useful in reducing the number of improvement cycles required to achieve success. It will support a more nuanced, evidence-based approach to the development and evaluation of a series of potential solutions within a rapid-cycle, iterative approach [30].

Despite the potential for mutually beneficial contributions and synergy between the improvement and implementation science fields in their current forms, considerable development and enhancement are needed. Both fields are challenged by the need to better understand and achieve maintenance (sustainability) of improvements and to facilitate scale-up and spread of effective solutions across large multi-site systems and geographic regions. The implementation science field must balance its emphasis on experimental studies and rigor with increased study of naturally-occurring implementation processes to derive the insights they offer regarding factors influencing implementation success across diverse settings, quality problems and implementation strategies. And, both fields require additional development of tools and approaches for understanding the mediators, moderators and mechanisms of practice change.

Maintenance, Sustainability, Scale-up and Spread

An improvement program should ideally over time sustain various elements, including its activities, community-level partnerships, organizational practices, benefits to its clients, and the salience of the program's core issue. These are called "sustainability outcomes" by Scheirer and Dearing [31], and reflect the various ways that a program can continue to achieve its intended effects. However, this highlights the question of how a program can position itself to best ensure that these sustainability outcomes can be realized. It has been proposed that sustainability itself is the small set of organizational and contextual factors that build the capacity for maintaining a program over time. That is, sustainability is the ability to maintain programming and its benefits over time despite underlying factors that act to undermine and extinguish the effects of the intervention.

Despite its importance for outcomes, sustainability has received relatively little research attention. Findings and insights regarding improvement and implementation are generally documented and learned through reports of successful improvement projects as presented at conferences and seminars and via published articles in research, policy and practice journals. Because the majority of these present short-term impacts only, evidence regarding long-term maintenance of practice change and improvements is limited. Anecdotal evidence, however, suggests that long-term maintenance is rare and difficult to achieve and nearly impossible to document using traditional evaluation methods. The ultimate value of improvement and implementation science requires sustained, ongoing improvements (and measurements) rather than short-term benefits, and thus requires greater attention to the study of, and support for, institutionalization and maintenance of practice change. Recent publications in the implementation science literature advocate greater attention to sustainability and offer frameworks and guidance for studying and achieving sustainability, and represent important contributions to the growing recognition and need for sustainability research, practice and success [32, 33].

Closely related to sustainability challenges are questions of scale-up and spread. The heterogeneity of practice settings and quality problems limits the direct applicability and likely broad effectiveness of improvement and implementation strategies found to be useful in one or a small number of settings. Implementation researchers who recognize the rarity of spontaneous diffusion and widespread adoption of innovations in medical care and health care delivery often neglect to recognize that implementation strategies shown to be effective in one set of sites are unlikely to spontaneously diffuse to other sites, and that their suitability and likely effectiveness may be limited even if some natural spread occurs [34]. Research on scale-up and spread barriers, processes and strategies is limited in the same manner as research on maintenance and sustainability, and represents another "new frontier" for the fields of improvement and implementation sciences as they endeavor to better support more effective and evidence-driven public health policy and practice goals for quality improvement [35].

External Validity and Observational Research

Consistent with its foundations in clinical research and clinical research stakeholders' preference for rigorous, study designs prioritizing internal validity (e.g., randomized controlled trials), many implementation scientists similarly prefer experimental, interventional approaches to evaluate implementation strategies and understand implementation barriers and processes [36]. Although these maximize internal validity and meet standard scientific standards for rigor in study design, they entail considerable compromise in reduced external validity, policy and practice relevance [37, 38]. Investigator-initiated and directed implementation and improvement projects often require special arrangements and time-limited support and resources, including many that are not easily sustained nor replicated following the conclusion of the project. These additional resources and support preclude a valid conclusion that the specific practice change strategy under study is responsible for observed improvements in quality, rather than the special (and non-sustainable) support and resources provided. Observational studies of "natural experiments" and other naturally occurring implementation and improvement processes permit study of implementation and improvement processes and strategies without the complicating addition of artificial constraining circumstances and support. Increased interest in observational study designs that minimize threats to internal validity [39] will facilitate implementation research that balances internal and external validity and is better able to generate relevant and sustainable policy and practice insights.

Research on Mediators, Moderators and Mechanisms of Practice Change

The theories, tools and methods of implementation science prioritize implementation interventions and strategies and favor *summative evaluation* research designs and methods to evaluate their effectiveness and impacts. This focus on questions of *whether* improvement occurred emulates research approaches optimized to evaluate clinical interventions such as drugs and devices, but is less appropriate in situations characterized by high levels of heterogeneity and adaptability. These features of quality problems and solutions are implicitly recognized by improvement science methods and require a focus on the formative processes and mechanisms of improvement–*formative evaluation*–in addition to a focus on impacts and outcomes. Rapid-cycle improvement approaches are able to accommodate local variations in quality problems and causes, differences in contextual factors such as organizational resources and policies, and other factors that contribute to significant variations in improvement outcomes across sites and over time.

Quality improvement research has explicitly recognized the implications of heterogeneity and variation and their implications for research and evaluation methods [40, 41]. Increased use of process evaluation and approaches such as theory-based evaluation and realistic evaluation is needed to systematically and rigorously study the mediators and mechanisms of action of implementation and improvement strategies, to answer questions asking how, when, where and why these strategies operate, in addition to whether they are effective [42]. This approach assumes that the quality improvement challenge requires not just selection of an implementation strategy likely to be effective for a given quality gap and set of barriers in a given setting, but, will also require careful customization and adaptation over time, as well as an awareness of the importance of adaptation and management of the organization or setting. Research approaches that are able to generate useful insights and guide this expanded set of decisions and management actions are still under development and early use within the implementation and improvement science fields, but offer considerable potential.

Conclusions

Progress in improving the quality of health care across a wide range of clinical conditions and care delivery settings remains slow and inadequate. The field of implementation science, which has emerged and become well established only within the past 10 years, offers great value in complementing and augmenting approaches and insights from the fields of quality and safety improvement and improvement science.

Much of this potential remains untapped, however, and requires a range of efforts to enhance collaboration and communication across improvement and implementation science leaders and publication platforms. However, we have paid much less attention to what happens to programs once they have been implemented. Programs typically need time to reach a certain level of maturity and allow health benefits to accrue. If we as a society are to get the full benefit of the significant investment in public health research and subsequent program development, we need to better understand what factors can promote long-term program sustainability.

Increased attention to under-studied issues such as maintenance, sustainability, scale-up and spread, and research to better recognize the unique features of quality problems and settings, and implementation barriers, facilitators and strategies – and the implications of these unique features for research, policy and practice—are greatly needed.

Qualitative and mixed methods that assess potential influences on quality and outcomes across multiple levels are necessary to develop and refine hypotheses, to explain results of rigorous evaluations, and to understand the relationships between contextual factors, sustainability, maintenance outcomes, scale-up and spread. Growth in the "toolkit" of research approaches, designs and methods available to implementation and improvement researchers will help accelerate progress in developing valid and useful insights. These, in turn, will provide the needed guidance for policy and practice actions needed to close the quality gaps and to attain the full benefits from research and innovation in health care and public health.

References

1. Institute of Medicine. To err is human: building a safer health system. Washington, DC: National Academy Press; 2000.
2. Institute of Medicine. Crossing the quality chasm: a new health system for the 21st century. Washington, DC: National Academy Press; 2001.
3. Berwick DM. Continuous improvement as an ideal in health care. N Engl J Med. 1989;320(1):53–6.
4. Laffel G, Blumenthal D. The case for using industrial quality management science in health care organizations. JAMA. 1989;262(20):2869–73.
5. Hussey PS, Anderson GF, Osborn R, et al. How does the quality of care compare in five countries? Health Aff (Millwood). 2004;23(3):89–99.
6. Gauld R, Burgers J, Dobrow M, Minhas R, Wendt C, Cohen AB, Luxford K. Healthcare system performance improvement: a comparison of key policies in seven high-income countries. J Health Organ Manag. 2014;28(1):2–20.
7. Eisenberg JM. Doctors' decisions and the cost of medical care: the reasons for doctors' practice patterns and ways to change them. Ann Arbor: Health Administration Press; 1986.
8. Greco PJ, Eisenberg JM. Changing physicians' practices. N Engl J Med. 1993;329(17):1271–3.
9. McDonald CJ, Wilson GA, McCabe Jr GP. Physician response to computer reminders. JAMA. 1980;244(14):1579–81.
10. Davis DA, Thomson MA, Oxman AD, Haynes RB. Changing physician performance. A systematic review of the effect of continuing medical education strategies. JAMA. 1995;274(9):700–5.
11. Bagian JP, Gosbee J, Lee CZ, Williams L, McKnight SD, Mannos DM. The Veterans Affairs root cause analysis system in action. Jt Comm J Qual Improv. 2002;28(10):531–45.
12. Wu AW, Lipshutz AK, Pronovost PJ. Effectiveness and efficiency of root cause analysis in medicine. JAMA. 2008;299(6):685–7.
13. Jessee WF, Reerink E, Reizenstein P, Vuori HV. Quality assurance in health care editorial. Int J Qual Health Care. 1989;1(1):3.

14. Moss F. Quality in health care. Qual Saf Health Care. 1992;1:1–3.
15. Eccles MP, Mittman BS. Welcome to implementation science. Implement Sci. 2006;1:1.
16. Sung NS, Crowley Jr WF, Genel M, et al. Central challenges facing the national clinical research enterprise. JAMA. 2003;289(10):1278–87.
17. Crowley Jr WF, Sherwood L, Salber P, et al. Clinical research in the United States at a crossroads: proposal for a novel public-private partnership to establish a national clinical research enterprise. JAMA. 2004; 291(9):1120–6.
18. Rubenstein LV, Pugh J. Strategies for promoting organizational and practice change by advancing implementation research. J Gen Intern Med. 2006;21 Suppl 2:S58–64.
19. Khoury MJ, Gwinn M, Yoon PW, Dowling N, Moore CA, Bradley L. The continuum of translation research in genomic medicine: how can we accelerate the appropriate integration of human genome discoveries into health care and disease prevention? Genet Med. 2007;9(10):665–74.
20. Dougherty D, Conway PH. The "3T's" road map to transform US health care: the "how" of high-quality care. JAMA. 2008;299(19):2319–21.
21. McKibbon KA, Lokker C, Wilczynski NL, Ciliska D, Dobbins M, Davis DA, Haynes RB, Straus SE. A cross-sectional study of the number and frequency of terms used to refer to knowledge translation in a body of health literature in 2006: a Tower of Babel? Implement Sci. 2010;5:16.
22. Prasad V, Ioannidis JP. Evidence-based de-implementation for contradicted, unproven, and aspiring healthcare practices. Implement Sci. 2014;9:1.
23. Brownson RC, Colditz GA, Proctor EK, editors. Dissemination and implementation research in health: translating science to practice. Oxford/New York: Oxford University Press; 2012.
24. Berwick DM. A primer on leading the improvement of systems. BMJ. 1996;312(7031):619–22.
25. McCormack B, McCarthy G, Wright J, Slater P, Coffey A. Development and testing of the Context Assessment Index (CAI). Worldviews Evid Based Nurs. 2009;6(1):27–35.
26. Taylor SL, Dy S, Foy R, Hempel S, McDonald KM, Ovretveit J, Pronovost PJ, Rubenstein LV, Wachter RM, Shekelle PG. What context features might be important determinants of the effectiveness of patient safety practice interventions? BMJ Qual Saf. 2011; 20(7):611–7.
27. Kaplan HC, Provost LP, Froehle CM, Margolis PA. The Model for Understanding Success in Quality (MUSIQ): building a theory of context in healthcare quality improvement. BMJ Qual Saf. 2012;21(1):13–20.
28. Kitson AL, Rycroft-Malone J, Harvey G, McCormack B, Seers K, Titchen A. Evaluating the successful implementation of evidence into practice using the PARiHS framework: theoretical and practical challenges. Implement Sci. 2008;3:1.
29. Damschroder LJ, Aron DC, Keith RE, Kirsh SR, Alexander JA, Lowery JC. Fostering implementation of health services research findings into practice: a consolidated framework for advancing implementation science. Implement Sci. 2009;4:50.
30. Horbar JD, Rogowski J, Plsek PE, Delmore P, Edwards WH, Hocker J, Kantak AD, Lewallen P, Lewis W, Lewit E, McCarroll CJ, Mujsce D, Payne NR, Shiono P, Soll RF, Leahy K, Carpenter JH. Collaborative quality improvement for neonatal intensive care. NIC/Q Project Investigators of the Vermont Oxford Network. Pediatrics. 2001;107(1):14–22.
31. Scheirer MA, Dearing JW. An agenda for research on the sustainability of public health programs. Am J Public Health. 2011;101(11):2059–67.
32. Wiltsey Stirman S, Kimberly J, Cook N, Calloway A, Castro F, Charns M. The sustainability of new programs and innovations: a review of the empirical literature and recommendations for future research. Implement Sci. 2012;7:17.
33. Schell SF, Luke DA, Schooley MW, Elliott MB, Herbers SH, Mueller NB, Bunger AC. Public health program capacity for sustainability: a new framework. Implement Sci. 2013;8:15.
34. Fraser S. Undressing the elephant; why good practice doesn't spread in healthcare. This a self-published/vanity press book. The publisher is Lulu.com (an internet-based publisher). Lulu.com; 2008.
35. Norton WE, McCannon CJ, Schall MW, Mittman BS. A stakeholder-driven agenda for advancing the science and practice of scale-up and spread in health. Implement Sci. 2012;7:118.
36. Shojania KG, Grimshaw JM. Evidence-based quality improvement: the state of the science. Health Aff (Millwood). 2005;24(1):138–50.
37. Black N. Why we need observational studies to evaluate the effectiveness of health care. BMJ. 1996; 312(7040):1215–8.
38. Green LW, Glasgow RE. Evaluating the relevance, generalization, and applicability of research: issues in external validation and translation methodology. Eval Health Prof. 2006;29(1):126–53.
39. Concato J, Shah N, Horwitz RI. Randomized, controlled trials, observational studies, and the hierarchy of research designs. N Engl J Med. 2000;342(25):1887–92.
40. Walshe K, Freeman T. Effectiveness of quality improvement: learning from evaluations. Qual Saf Health Care. 2002;11(1):85–7.
41. Walshe K. Understanding what works—and why—in quality improvement: the need for theory-driven evaluation. Int J Qual Health Care. 2007;19(2):57–9.
42. Pawson R, Greenhalgh T, Harvey G, Walshe K. Realist review–a new method of systematic review designed for complex policy interventions. J Health Serv Res Policy. 2005;10 Suppl 1:21–34.

23 Leadership, Surgeon Well-Being, and Other Non-technical Aspects of Pediatric Cardiac Surgery

David S. Winlaw, Matthew M. Large, Jeffrey P. Jacobs, and Paul R. Barach

Abstract

The expectations of pediatric cardiac surgeons grow as the specialty evolves and yesterday's challenges become tomorrow's routine. The pioneering era of fast-paced major technical advances is behind us. Integration of surgery, cardiology, anesthesia, intensive care, and nursing is now the basis of incremental improvements in perioperative performance and long-term outcomes. Surgeons can be natural leaders of this process because their skills, roles, and experience are crucial in the preoperative, intra-operative, and postoperative care of the patient and their family. However, the personality traits that draw physicians to the specialty of surgery and contribute to the drive to become a successful technical surgeon may be at odds with the collaborative aspects of this microsystem, both inside and outside the operating room. The potential for disruptive behavior on the part of the surgeon to impede the functioning of a large multidisciplinary team providing care of the upmost complexity raises fundamental questions about how to design tools and checks to create reliable pediatric cardiac surgical teams.

D.S. Winlaw, MBBS (Hons), MD, FRACS (✉)
Paediatric Cardiac Surgery, Heart Centre for Children, The Children's Hospital at Westmead, Sydney, NSW, Australia

Sydney Medical School, University of Sydney, Sydney, NSW, Australia
e-mail: david.winlaw@health.nsw.gov.au

M.M. Large, BSc, MBBS, FRANZCP
Department of Mental Health Services, The Prince of Wales Hospitals, Randwick, NSW, Australia

University of New South Wales, Sydney, NSW, Australia
e-mail: mmbl@bigpond.com

J.P. Jacobs, MD, FACS, FACC, FCCP
Division of Cardiac Surgery, Department of Surgery, Johns Hopkins All Children's Heart Institute, All Children's Hospital and Florida Hospital for Children, Johns Hopkins University, Saint Petersburg, Tampa and Orlando, FL, USA

Division of Cardiac Surgery, Department of Surgery, Johns Hopkins University, Baltimore, MD, USA
e-mail: jeffjacobs@msn.com; jeffjacobs@jhmi.edu

P.R. Barach, BSc, MD, MPH
Department of Health Management and Health Economics, University of Oslo, Oslo, Norway
e-mail: pbarach@gmail.com

P.R. Barach, J.P. Jacobs, S.E. Lipshultz, P.C. Laussen (eds.),
Pediatric and Congenital Cardiac Care: Volume 2: Quality Improvement and Patient Safety,
DOI 10.1007/978-1-4471-6566-8_23, © Springer-Verlag London 2015

A new dynamic is needed to support members of the team, including the surgeon, in times of extreme stress, and to help members of the team avoid destructive, maladaptive responses. Focusing these efforts around the clinical microsystem requires a detailed analysis of the interactions of the team, the underlying culture and support, and the engagement of clinical staff. Building and nurturing a resilient system remains a constant challenge in a highly specialized environment where burnout, bullying, and loss of staff exist. Creating and nurturing an environment characterized by psychological safety for all team members requires development of trust to permit 'healthy conflict' and their successful resolution. Specific tools can be practiced to develop conscious competence in advanced methods of communication that facilitate trust. Patient safety and high value care depend on the development of trust within, between, and among team members.

For many, the questions are (i) how to build a sustainable model of quality improvement in a medium sized unit, (ii) how to create an enjoyable and rewarding working environment, and, (iii) how to build resilient systems that ensure excellent outcomes and protect against avoidable poor clinical outcomes.

Keywords
Pediatric cardiac surgery • Team dynamics • Quality • Psychological safety • Safety climate

Introduction

In just the past few decades, technical solutions for the majority of common congenital heart defects have been proposed and refined. A diagnosis of major structural cardiac disease remains a diagnosis for life, but a defined path and predictable outcome with relatively low mortality exist for the majority of lesions. This achievement and expectation now extend to 'standard risk' infants requiring complex reconstruction of a functionally univentricular heart (single ventricle) for hypoplastic left heart syndrome [1]. Nevertheless, many challenges remain to reduce morbidity, particularly of neonatal operations, and in addressing the life-long adult complications of repaired structural cardiac disease. In this chapter, we explore a range of non-technical aspects of the pediatric cardiac surgical practice, with reference to the literature and experiences common to pediatric cardiac surgical programs.

Risk, Complexity, and Cooperation in the Pediatric Cardiac Operating Room

One of the riskiest and most complex of all hospital environments is the pediatric cardiac surgery (PCS) operating suite. Pediatric cardiac surgical operations are among the most serious interventions in all of medicine, encompassing anatomic diversity, hemodynamic vulnerability, and the need of a highly skilled, multi-specialty team. Medical advances in the past three decades have resulted in increasing survival among children born with even the most complex cardiac defects [2]. In an analysis of 95,357 congenital and pediatric cardiac operations in the in the Society of Thoracic Surgeons (STS) Congenital Heart Surgery Database between 2007 and 2010, the mortality prior to hospital discharge was 3.5 % [3].

Although the overall mortality in pediatric cardiac surgery is below 4 %, in at least 20 % of cases where death occurs, it is postulated that preventable adverse events might occur and contribute to death. For neonates, a particularly low margin of error exists, accompanied by a very limited ability to rescue and retrieve from poor outcomes. In this neonatal age group, around 10 % of neonates undergoing complex pediatric cardiac surgery die within 30 days of surgery [4, 5]. As a result of the intensity of the work and the expectations of members of the team as well as those of the broader community, pediatric cardiac surgeons suffer a high rate of burnout, sometimes manifest as depression, and these challenges likely lead to a truncated working life [6, 7]. Although the affirming nature of successful pediatric cardiac surgical operations might be conceptualized as protecting the surgeon from depression, the impact of less successful outcomes and of other stressors can be significant and life lasting.

Pediatric cardiac surgery is a specialty with very low tolerance for error. Pediatric cardiac surgery encompasses many complex operations that are dependent upon a sophisticated organizational structure. Pediatric cardiac surgery requires the coordinated efforts of multiple individuals and has high demands on the cognitive skills and technical performance of the surgeon and team [8]. Factors that have been linked to poor outcomes in pediatric cardiac surgery include

- low institution and surgeon-specific volumes of surgical cases [9],
- complexity of cases [10], and
- systems failures [11, 12] such as miscommunications [13] and inadequate team planning.

Real opportunities exist to improve pediatric cardiac surgical outcomes, including in neonatal mortality and rates of complications, by addressing systems issues in the hyper-complex settings of pediatric cardiac surgery. Areas of consideration include

- striking the right balance between clinical responsibility and leadership versus an overly rigid hierarchy with consequent failure to identify and communicate errors in real time;
- pressures of time leading to suboptimal planning and briefing before operations and debriefing after operations; and,
- the tradeoffs between establishing safe and effective practices and the need for innovative change.

Good teamwork, in terms of both quality and quantity, is associated with shorter duration of operations, fewer adverse events, and lower postoperative morbidity [14]. Teamwork is a shorthand for a wide variety of processes that include good processes of communication and coordination that are required to bring together the individual knowledge, skills, and attitudes in the service of a common and valued goal of the team. Interventions focusing on teamwork have shown a positive relationship with improved teamwork and climate of safety. The 'working together' of a clinical microsystem is accomplished by a complex suite of 'nontechnical skills' [15, 16]. Teams that score low on independently observed non-technical skills make more technical errors, and in cases where teams infrequently display team behaviors, patients are more likely to experience death or major complications [17]. A significant correlation exists between subjective assessment of teamwork by members of the team themselves and postoperative morbidity. TeamSTEPPS is an evidence-based program for training surgical teams and requires ongoing assessment as to how best to implement and sustain the goals of the program [18].

Assessing team performance is key to understanding the methods to improve the performance of the team and increase the outcomes and safety of patients (see Table 23.1).

An ongoing tension in the literature exists regarding the relative importance of team *process* and *outcomes* [19]. Process is defined by the activities, strategies, responses, and behaviors employed by the team during the accomplishment of tasks, while outcomes are the clinical results of the patients cared for by the team. Process measures are important for training when the purpose of measurement of performance is to diagnose problems with performance and to provide feedback to trainees. Until recently, the medical community has focused more on outcomes than on measures of process. Medical educators have begun to appreciate the competencies that define effective processes of the team [20]. The key is to identify and measure processes that are directly related to outcomes of patients (e.g., successful resuscitation). Perhaps most

Table 23.1 Questions to ask when assessing the performance of the surgical team

Is the team the right ***size and composition***?
Are there adequate levels of ***complementary skills***?
Is there a shared ***goal*** for the team?
Does everyone ***understand the goals of the team***?
Has a set of ***goals of performance*** been agreed upon?
Do the members of the team hold one another ***accountable*** for the results of the group?
Are there shared ***protocols*** and ground rules of performance?
Is there mutual ***respect and trust*** between members of the team?
Does the ***leader of the team*** instill trust and mutual respect by the members of the team?
Do members of the team ***communicate*** and exhibit conflict resolution skills effectively?
Do members of the team know and appreciate each other's ***roles and responsibilities***?
When one member of the team is ***absent or not able to perform*** their assigned tasks, are other members of the team able to pitch in or help appropriately?

importantly, the results of the assessment must be translatable into specific feedback about technical or non-technical issues that can enhance the performance of the team in achieving a safer and more reliable outcome.

Non-technical Errors in the Pediatric Cardiac Operating Room

Research has shown that errors in the Operating Room (OR) occur both within and between clinical teams [21, 22]. Quite often, errors result from a breakdown in coordination and communication between the OR sub-teams [23]. For example, the scrub nurse and the surgeon failing to anticipate and synchronize their actions so that a particular instrument is not available at a critical moment, leading to excessive bleeding or hemodynamic instability; or, the anesthesiologist acting unilaterally because he does not understand the immediate priorities of the surgeon. Other things that are known to distract and aggravate the mindfulness of the team include [24, 25]:

- interruptions,
- traffic through the operating room (OR),
- uncertainty regarding availability of and access to beds in the pediatric intensive care (PICU),
- ambiguities about membership of the team, and
- communication.

The impact of errors committed by non-surgical members of the team, such as OR nurses, orderlies, and perfusionists, during open-heart surgery, is not well known, but is likely to be significant [26–28]. Instructions from the attending surgeon and anesthesiologist to their assistants (or vice versa) can also result in errors (e.g. failure to administer anticoagulants leading to a delay in being able to commence cardiopulmonary bypass). Faulty communication and effective handovers to the team in the intensive care unit have been identified as a particular problem [29]. Another major source of error is the handover of responsibility for a patient by one health professional to another.

In similar complex environments, referred also as complex socio-technical systems, research about human factors has been a major contributor to enhancement of safety and reliability [30]. The importance of research about human factors research about systems in improving outcomes of pediatric cardiac surgery was highlighted in the Bristol Royal Infirmary Report [31], the Report of the Manitoba Pediatric Cardiac Surgery Inquest [32], and ongoing multi-national professional groups [33]. A key lesson from the Bristol and the Mid Staffordshire inquiries [34] is that once a professional group normalizes a deviant organizational practice, it is no longer viewed as an aberrant act that elicits an exceptional response; instead, it becomes a routine activity that is commonly anticipated and frequently used [35]. This process is known as "normalized deviance". A permissive ethical climate and an inordinate emphasis on financial considerations in care can both contribute to managerial and clinician decisions to initiate deviance [36].

In pediatric cardiac surgery the expectations of families, administrators, and clinicians are uniformly high. Pediatric cardiac surgery has become a microcosm from which the wider medical community has sought to understand how to provide complex multidisciplinary care. Failures of units providing pediatric cardiac surgical care continue to occur with repeating themes including initial publication of apparent excess mortality from small units and the naming and shaming of surgeons involved [37]. Subsequent enquiries often highlight "system issues" including [37, 38]

- tenuous coverage at the admitting house officer level,
- excessive reliance on a small number of key individuals, and
- failures of effective communication between specialties.

Systems of clinical governance have generally focused on dealing with bad outcomes, and these suboptimal outcomes are generally not recognized in advance. Robust and widely adopted systems of risk stratification systems that allow cases to be classified on the basis of operative complexity and risk allow comparison of risk-adjusted outcomes between diverse pediatric cardiac units:

1. The Society of Thoracic Surgeons - European Association for Cardio-Thoracic Surgery Congenital Heart Surgery Mortality Categories (**STAT Mortality Categories**)
2. Aristotle Basic Complexity Levels (**ABC Levels**)
3. Risk Adjustment for Congenital Heart Surgery-1 Categories (**RACHS-1 Categories**).

It is generally accepted that open and transparent reporting of outcomes on a regular basis is ideal, as is commonly done in the UK [39, 40]. Real time analysis and reporting of outcomes for internal purposes, to identify early trends and under-performance of the system, is possible, but difficult to achieve in practice [41].

Improving Surgical Leadership of Teams

Most applicants for training in cardiac surgery are high achievers with high self-confidence. These applicants are goal oriented and have a strong sense in their ability to control their actions and environment. They are used to subjugating their personal needs to those of their career, although the balance considered acceptable is probably changing [42, 43]. 'Being' a cardiac surgeon also brings a degree of positional power within the institution and status within the medical and wider communities that may be attractive to some. Cardiac surgeons need to be able to marshal the resources in the operating room and initiate rapid changes in management, which require mature and adaptive skills in the command and control of others. There are also some surgeons, many of them undoubtedly talented, who blur the margins between forceful behavior and demonstration of narcissistic personality. Narcissistic traits, according to psychiatric nomenclature, include [44]:

- an exaggerated sense of self importance,
- unreasonable demands for special treatment or automatic compliance,
- a lack of consideration for the feelings of others, and
- arrogant and haughty conduct.

Other disruptive features include a tendency in some circumstances to externalize the reasons for failure where they exist, rather than taking responsibility or acknowledging the difficulty associated as a result of patient related factors. In extreme cases these behaviors might include throwing instruments, yelling, and diminishing members of the team.

These actions can be seen as intimidating and threatening to the psychological safety of other members of the team, hampering both the safety of patient care as well as the willingness of team members to speak up and to report failures of process and outcome [45]. Psychological safety is considered the cornerstone of enabling a culture of safety. Unchecked, such individuals tend to damage or destroy relationships within their working environment to the point where a serious breakdown–either personal or professional–is likely to occur. When recognized early, an understanding of the underlying complaints or frustrations needs to be addressed, in tandem with clear guidelines on what constitutes acceptable and unacceptable behavior. Often senior surgeons are involved, and the authority gradient makes those outside the operating environment reluctant to speak up and engage. These conflicts can only be resolved with meaningful commitment from such individuals and tackling the issues as a team problem. A calm analysis of episodes of unacceptable behavior might reveal genuine problems with training, competence, or cooperation on the part of team members. This candid discussion could improve the standard of care and lead to a reduction in the stress levels of the surgeon. Alternately, unacceptable behavior might give the surgeon and his or her colleagues an opportunity to reflect on their own levels of stress, be it due to occupational or personal circumstances.

The consequences of not acting are clear: a culture of blame and lack of psychological safety can lead to:

- real harm to patients,
- under reporting of incidents [46, 47],
- cover up strategies,
- justification of inadequate performance [48], and
- interpersonal situations where members of the pediatric cardiac surgical team refrain from speaking up about difficult issues or asking questions [49].

Expressions of frustration and real time verbalization of stress can have important functions such as communicating the urgency or seriousness of a situation, and some forms of disruptive behavior might even be tolerated by the team in the interests of doing the best for the patient. However, behavior that erodes the core concept of teamwork must be the concern of all members of the team, because ultimately it is the outcome of the patient that can clearly suffer [50].

Surgeons may overemphasize the contribution of a 'good operation' to successful organizational outcomes, and under-recognize the contribution of others, thus undermining trust within the team. It is easy to understand how this conclusion is reached, since a poor operation inevitably produces poor outcomes, but such logic is flawed. 'Teamwork' may be misunderstood as being simply a happy work environment where members do their best to help the surgeon gain a good outcome. This scenario, of course, can fail to deliver reliably good outcomes or a productive environment since leaders, including surgeons, are required to take collective responsibility for the known failings of 'teamwork', as articulated by Lencioni [51]. The 'five dysfunctions of teams' are well known to all in health care:

- absence of trust,
- fear of conflict,
- lack of commitment,
- avoidance of accountability, and
- inattention to results.

Teams that don't invest in measures to build trust have a harder time making sense (sense-making) of what others are doing. They are intimidated by debate that is necessary to generate 'healthy conflict', avoid clarity and closure, and then have a hard time holding each other accountable through confronting difficult issues while focusing on outcomes.

Improving Surgical Mentorship of Trainees

Surgeons commonly specialize in pediatric cardiac surgery after completing a general surgery residency and then a 1–4 years adult cardiac surgery fellowship that provides a solid theoretical and technical base. Training in pediatric cardiac surgery then requires them to step back from a reasonably high level of autonomy for a further 2–3 years whilst gaining experience before commencing in a consultant (attending) post. This period of mentorship brings its own challenges and opportunities.

The closeness of working relationships between pediatric cardiac surgeons and pediatric cardiologists is an attraction to some and a problem for others. This relationship requires intense communication and negotiation and intersects with the care and managing of the relationship with the family. Although much of the subsequent discussion deals with mentoring of surgeons by surgeons, some of the most expert mentoring of young surgeons is performed by pediatric cardiologists who are one step removed and are able to see the whole landscape.

Low volumes of pediatric cases make it more difficult to acquire a critical mass of experience and sustain the multiple competencies required for complex operations in a short fellowship when compared to adult practice. Younger pediatric cardiac surgeons need more experienced surgeons to mentor and direct them, inside and outside the operating room settings, and at least for the first

5 years of independent consultant (attending) practice [42, 43]. This formal mentorship requires a significant investment on behalf of the senior surgeon, and inevitably brings different stress, as junior colleagues are mentored through more complex cases. During this time, the senior surgeon is essentially taking responsibility for the conduct and outcomes of the operation. Learning is seen as a rational, linear, and developmental process involving the learning of new knowledge and skills around which improved service can be delivered. The act of learning can be portrayed as being free from bias and politically neutral, but a more realistic view is that questions of power, hierarchy, and control are interweaved with the processes of learning and mentorship [42, 43]. This relationship between mentee and mentor can be mutually satisfying [42, 43]; however, at times it can be tormenting. The relationship requires frequent renegotiation for which frameworks do not exist. It is not uncommon for these mentee-mentor relationships to become strained as the junior surgeon transitions to independent practice.

Identifying and retaining the 'joy' of operating is, for many, something that requires active awareness and attention [52]. Thoughtful mentorship is required throughout a surgical career, and consultant (attending) surgeons operating together on difficult or rare cases is more than simply 'sharing the load' or 'spreading the experience'. In some circumstances, consultant (attending) surgeons operating together is an uncontroversial way of

- staying in touch with colleagues,
- speaking a common language, and
- achieving a level of collegiality that powerfully models trust, respect, learning, and personal support within the operating environment.

Successful individuals usually cite strong mentors. As most pediatric cardiac surgeons are not ready to take on the full range of emergency and major elective operations at the time they finish formal training and become attending surgeons, mentorship is key to developing their talent, supporting their intellectual and technical growth and development, as well as actively addressing technical weaknesses [42, 43].

Low volumes of pediatric cardiac cases and financial incentives lead a significant proportion of practitioners into mixed adult and pediatric practice. This increased work can make it difficult to contribute to the non-operative elements of the pediatric cardiac surgical service, including mentoring and the development of the service and its personnel. It does bring advantages through cross-pollination with adult practice and participation in the innovations learned in the high volume settings of adult cardiac surgery. Diversity in the models of engagement (i.e. mixed adult practice vs. pediatric only practice) is a good strategy and assists in construction of a sustainable roster. Such individuals also bring with them the expectations of conduct in the operating room from the adult context that may be more hierarchical than the pediatric environment. It also, however, might lead to a lower overall number of pediatric cardiac surgical cases that must be factored into the overall competency in the early career of a surgeon.

We are well attuned to the need for management of challenges early in the career of a pediatric cardiac surgeon, but transitions at the other end of the career remain an important issue as well. In an ideal setting, older surgeons would be retained in the system to guide and coach younger colleagues to:

- support clinical decision-making,
- help in reflecting on process and outcomes,
- provide institutional memory, and
- develop their key strengths and contributions.

These older more senior surgeons would consciously create space to allow development of their younger colleagues; however, this strategy involves a level of clarity in planning and dialogue that is sometimes difficult to achieve. Since ending a career well is an important transition and many now have an expectation of working into their 70s, these considerations require close planning, attention, and candid conversations.

Recognizing Team Difficulties Before Bad Outcomes Occur

Pediatric cardiac surgery involves long and complex operations. All proceduralists will have observed that not all teams have equal capability. Some teams seem to be able to complete complex tasks with ease and in a good spirit whereas other teams show disharmony and conflict, sometimes with inferior clinical outcomes. Understanding what enables one team to perform more effectively and reliably than the other remains elusive and learning from 'mistakes' is difficult [53]. An obvious approach is for more harmonious and functional teams to work more closely with members of less functional teams in the hope of modeling better behavior of the team. Major operations that require additional hands present a natural opportunity for this cross fertilization. However, such cases in and of themselves are most likely to be stressful for all concerned and might not be ideal cases for illustrating good team dynamics.

Situations where known issues with individuals or combinations of individuals exist may create stress in anticipation because of the internal perception by many members of the team that they will need to rise above the usual input to achieve a good outcome. These expectations of 'compensating' for the other members of the team can be distracting and undermining. The challenges for the operating team are [54]:

- to learn how to improve their reliability, or consistent performance, at high levels of safety over long periods of time, and
- to differentiate between true underperformers and intrinsic failures of teamwork.

In instances where things go wrong, surgeons may become tense or angry, and fail to perform at their best. Collective responsibility would imply that that scrutiny of the conditions triggering these states, including an the individual performance of each member of the team, is important for every member of the team [55]. Systems theory suggests that the overall performance of the team is related to the individual performance of each member of the team; however, some surgeons can feel quite put out when poor outcomes are attributed to them when other members of them performed poorly [56].

Making Effective and Sustainable Teams

All members of staff experience the stress of 'doing' cardiac surgery. The surgeon carries with them the shared responsibility for the patient through the postoperative period and the lifetime of the patient. The unrelenting nature of the work, with very little 'down' time completely off call, and the need to routinely participate in care on the nights and weekends, generates ongoing occupational stress. A natural tension exists between:

- the need for individual learning and skills maintenance,
- practice building, and
- the need for a team that can allow for leave, research and learning opportunities.

This tension can be addressed by better sharing of work arrangements between surgeons. Yet, even when such arrangements exist, ***most pediatric cardiac surgeons report that they are never truly 'off call' unless they are out of the city and in some cases out of the country***. Vacations are interrupted by the demands of transplantation are common. With high levels of application to work, it is not surprising that surgeons report high levels of job satisfaction but also high rates of burnout [7], family discord, and the associated susceptibility to error and poorer outcomes [57]. High rates of self-reported de-personalization and emotional exhaustion are key findings. Difficulties in negotiating a home-work life balance [42, 43] and failure to look after one's own health are common manifestations of the burnout complex. Interestingly, in cardiac surgery, and particularly pediatric cardiac surgery, most of these aspects of the work are accepted as 'part of the job', but it is the apparently 'minor' factors that become incendiary, such as tardy members of the team, poor scheduling, and cancellation of cases because of constrained resources in the Pediatric Cardiac Intensive Care Unit (PCICU). These "incendiary factors" lead to flow-on implications of rescheduling patients and further upending the balance of their clinical and non-clinical priorities [58]. The cost of re-scheduling a case has far-reaching implications on the patient and the family of the patient, and often for the surgeon and the family of the surgeon.

The impact of an unpleasant and unsafe organizational and physical environment on younger surgeons can be particularly profound and is magnified by the importance of the master-apprentice relationship. This stressful setting with lack of safe and supportive mentorship was felt to have contributed directly to the isolation of the surgeon that greatly contributed to the poor outcomes of several children undergoing pediatric cardiac surgery in the Manitoba pediatric cardiac surgery inquiry [32, 33]. Although contemporary training programs emphasize the relationship between a trainee and the group as a whole, the senior surgeon is the gatekeeper to further operative experience, so there is an inevitable reluctance of the junior staff to disagree or express dissatisfaction with circumstances.

The inability to speak truth to power, even when patient care is at stake, can lead to patterns of withdrawal and assumption of a passive role [36]. These patterns can be a block to learning technical skills where self-confidence is an essential prerequisite. Younger trainees may have little life experience outside of medicine, or enter training after a period of high-achievement in another field such as medical research; regardless, these trainees need to learn new skills in an environment where simple mistakes have significant repercussions and a blame culture can be devastating for all involved.

In settings in which members of the pediatric cardiac surgical team feel unsafe to speak up, the ongoing threat can [59]:

- undermine safe practices,
- prevent tough conversations about the "undiscussable", and
- keep pediatric cardiac surgery from becoming more reliable.

The cognitive dissonance that providers and management feel when confronted by organizational secrecy is predictable and can lead to:

- a lack of sharing of information,
- a lack of learning, and ultimately,
- disruptive behaviors, frustration, burnout and high churn rates.

The need for consistent performance of pediatric cardiac surgical teams at high levels of safety over long periods of time is similar to other high-risk industries such as aviation and nuclear power [60]. In the face of health reform and increased competition in the market, moving to high reliability requires adopting and supporting a culture of mindfulness in understanding the relationship and synergy of a variety of organizational risk factors and their effect on producing harm and inefficiency [61]. This mindfulness goes beyond rearranging the vulnerabilities of the system and instead strives to understand how to manage best the technology and learning that are embedded in practice. This culture of mindfulness encourage norms and values of high reliability organizations [62]:

- preoccupation with failure,
- reluctance to simplify operations,
- commitment to resilience, and
- deference to sharp end, front line users.

Bigger Teams and Communities of Practice

Creating larger units with up to four full-time surgeons and greater depth of experience has been proposed in some countries such as the UK [37], and carried out successfully in others such as Norway and Sweden [38]. As an established path learned from other domains for increasing reliability [39], such larger units can gain superior outcomes through:

- internal sub-specialization,
- better efficiency, and
- opportunity for training, research and work-life balance.

Except where geography and distribution of population demand a local service, the days of small volume, single surgeon units seem numbered. Changing expectations of the workplace from younger surgeons is also driving this trend. It is now time to rethink the working environment including how best to create:

- the conditions for psychological safety needed to encourage staff members to speak up [45], and
- a more sustainable model of engagement of surgeons treating pediatric structural cardiac disease.

Despite the depth of expert opinion supporting centralization of highly specialized services, achieving this goal has been politically difficult in the UK [63], USA, and Australia. The organizational reflex to this reality involves establishment of networks designed to leverage the quality systems and experience of bigger centers in order to provide sustainable high quality care across two or more sites. The joining of teams with different values and ambitions presents a major exercise in management of change that requires a high level of engaged leadership to succeed. Fundamentals of success include articulating in an unambiguous way that the single most important driver for all change must be to provide:

- better care,
- safer outcomes, and
- value to the community.

Other shared principles include:

- robust transparency of data,
- delivery of equal standards of care and processes of triage of patients, irrespective of site,
- planned co-mingling of staff at all levels, and
- mandatory participation in network programs of quality assurance (QA).

Considerable evidence demonstrates several elements that are partially to blame for serious adverse events [23]:

- a lack of sharing of information,
- professional secrecy, and
- a failure to learn from mistakes.

Organizational vehicles such as 'learning collaboratives' and 'networks of communities' address such challenges and have emerged as a powerful tool in improving performance and safety in adult cardiac surgery. The Northern New England Cardiovascular Disease Study Group [64] has been able to dramatically improve outcomes across all members over a period of 20 years by

- sharing data,
- visiting each other's hospitals, and
- actively learning in practice how each cardiac team applies the knowledge of cardiac surgery in their own customized manner.

This community of practice is shaped less by managerially designed systems and more by activities of shared and reflective clinical practice and professional allegiance and honesty. Such informal networks are seen as providing a significant basis for learning [65]. The Pediatric Heart Network [66] and Congenital Heart Surgeons' Society (CHSS) [67] are two further examples.

The Joint Council on Congenital Heart Disease (JCCHD) National Pediatric Cardiology Quality Improvement Collaborative (NPC-QIC) (http://jcchdqi.org) is another example of a powerful tool to support pediatric cardiac programs and improve outcomes across the system. The JCCHD initiated the National Pediatric Cardiology Quality Improvement Collaborative (NPC-QIC) in 2006 with a vision to improve outcomes for patients with hypoplastic left heart syndrome [66]. The development of this collaborative is based on the Institute for Healthcare Improvement (IHI) Breakthrough Series Collaborative Model [68]. The relative rarity and heterogeneity of patients with hypoplastic left heart syndrome in most individual practices necessitates a multi-institutional approach to achieve sample sizes required for meaningful learning through measurements in process and outcome. The NPC-QIC has focused its initial efforts on the interstage period of patients with hypoplastic left heart syndrome. As outcomes after Norwood (Stage 1) palliation improve, interstage mortality and interstage "failure to thrive" have become increasingly important challenges. The NPC-QIC has addressed these challenges directly by stating that one of the desired outcomes is that "no infants experience growth failure during the interstage period".

These networks, or 'Communities of Practice', can help mentor and grow trust across geographic distances; these networks are often better suited for sharing of knowledge amongst clinicians by providing an informal, rapid, and service facing basis for problem solving and growth. These national and international collaborative efforts are similar to the regional effort of the Northern New England Cardiovascular Disease Study Group; however, because of the lower incidence of congenital heart disease and the large distance between many programs, regional pediatric cardiac collaboratives may be challenging to set up. These national or international quality improvement collaboratives may function as "virtual regional quality improvement collaboratives" and achieve the same objective as regional collaboratives such as the Northern New England Cardiovascular Disease Study Group. Evidence suggests that the quality of outcomes for complex neonates, as one example, is more dependent on the integration and orchestration of care than any single operative variable [69], highlighting the importance of this work.

Participation in an international registry of outcomes is a fundamental plank of a pediatric cardiac surgical quality system [70] and the first step in a feedback loop to modification of practice. Regional benchmarking may provide more valuable information than summary statistics based on unit comparisons that involve all database contributors. Analysis of regional outcomes through existing resources of data, such as disease-based registries or procedure-based registries, also shows great promise, as exemplified by the Australian and New Zealand Fontan Registry [71].

Conclusions and Recommendations

Pediatric cardiac surgery is a model of high complexity health care, where key determinants of outcomes of patients include technical performance, decision-making, and personal engagement. We have learnt from our well-publicized successes and failures, and are well placed to put these lessons into practice in our own institutions; however, we seek tools to implement these lessons. The development of the workforce of cardiac surgery will need to focus on technical as well as non-technical areas of practice.

Recommendations:

1. Individual surgeons and program directors regularly review their working environment and acknowledge the impact of ***safe climate and human factors*** on the quality of teamwork in their institution.
2. Assessment of the working environment includes the ***risk of burnout*** in individuals and the impact of ***related behaviors*** on other team members.
3. Particular attention should be given to ***mentorship*** of trainees during their graduated transition from trainee to accomplished providers; this process of mentorship should include a dedicated and committed overseeing surgeon who may need to be outside the place of employment. One trainee may have multiple mentors, with select a select mentor for different domains of practice.
4. Engage with like-minded institutions in ***'communities of practice'*** to support quality improvement in a collaborative, non-competitive manner.
5. Practitioners need to learn to take responsibility for outcomes of patients by ***discontinuing support arrangements known to be associated with poor outcomes***, including arrangements:
   - where outcomes are not widely disseminated,
   - where there is excessive reliance on key individuals, and
   - where volumes are insufficient to maintain a high quality and resilient team.

References

1. Ghanayem NS, Hoffman GM, Mussatto KA, Frommelt MA, Cava JR, Mitchell ME, et al. Perioperative monitoring in high-risk infants after stage 1 palliation of univentricular congenital heart disease. J Thorac Cardiovasc Surg. 2010;140(4):857–63.
2. Padley JR, Cole AD, Pye VE, Chard RB, Nicholson IA, Jacobe S, et al. Five-year analysis of operative mortality and neonatal outcomes in congenital heart disease. Heart Lung Circ. 2011;20(7):460–7.
3. Jacobs JP, Jacobs ML, Mavroudis C, Lacour-Gayet FG, Tchervenkov CI. Executive summary: the Society of Thoracic Surgeons Congenital Heart Surgery Database – Fourteenth Harvest – (January 1, 2007 – December 31, 2010). Durham: The Society of Thoracic Surgeons (STS) and Duke Clinical Research Institute (DCRI), Duke University Medical Center; 2010.
4. Jacobs JP, Mavroudis C, Jacobs ML, Maruszewski B, Tchervenkov CI, Lacour-Gayet FG, et al. What is operative mortality? Defining death in a surgical registry database: a report of the STS Congenital Database Taskforce and the Joint EACTS-STS Congenital Database Committee. Ann Thorac Surg. 2006;81(5):1937–41.
5. Odegard KC, DiNardo JA, Kussman BD, Shukla A, Harrington J, Casta A, et al. The frequency of anesthesia-related cardiac arrests in patients with congenital heart disease undergoing cardiac surgery. Anesth Analg. 2007;105(2):335–43.
6. Campbell DA, Sonnad SS, Eckhauser FE, Campbell KK, Greenfield LJ. Burnout among American surgeons. Surgery. 2001;130(4):696–702; discussion 702–5.
7. Shanafelt TD, Balch CM, Bechamps GJ, Russell T, Dyrbye L, Satele D, et al. Burnout and career satisfaction among American surgeons. Transactions of the meeting of the American Surgical Association. Ann Surg 2009; 250:107–115.

8. ElBardissi AW, Wiegmann DA, Dearani JA, Daly RC, Sundt TM. Application of the human factors analysis and classification system methodology to the cardiovascular surgery operating room. Ann Thorac Surg. 2007;83(4):1412–8; discussion 1418–9.
9. Hannan EL, Racz M, Kavey R, Quaegebeur JM, Williams R. Pediatric cardiac surgery: the effect of hospital and surgeon volume on in-hospital mortality. Pediatrics. 1998;101:963–9.
10. Wong DR, Vander Salm TJ, Agnihotri AK, Bohmer RM, Torchiana DF. Prospective assessment of intraoperative precursor events during cardiac surgery. Eur J Cardiothorac Surg. 2006;29:447–55.
11. Catchpole KR, Giddings AEB, Wilkinson M, Hirst G, Dale T, de Leval MR. Improving patient safety by identifying latent failures in successful operations. Surgery. 2007;142(1):102–10.
12. Catchpole KR, Giddings AEB, de Leval MR, Peek GJ, Godden PJ, Utley M, et al. Identification of systems failures in successful paediatric cardiac surgery. Ergonomics. 2006;49(5–6):567–88.
13. Arriaga AF, ElBardissi AW, Regenbogen SE, Greenberg CC, Berry WR, Lipsitz S, et al. A policy-based intervention for the reduction of communication breakdowns in inpatient surgical care. Ann Surg. 2011;253(5):849–54.
14. Carayon P, editor. Handbook of human factors and ergonomics in health care and patient safety. 2006. pp. 259–71. Available from: http://books.google.com/books?hl=en&lr=&id=7IJMP6UlHUIC&oi=fnd&pg=PP1&dq=Handbook+of+Human+Factors+and+Ergonomics+in+Health+Care+and+Patient+Safety+Second+Edition&ots=Cp37_ZbebQ&sig=yYTPJqXe5N6Kum78-2qeUaYb7EA.
15. Baker DP, Gustafson S, Beaubien J, Salas E, Barach P. Medical teamwork and patient safety: the evidence-based relation. Literature review. AHRQ publication no. 05–0053. Rockville: Agency for Healthcare Research and Quality; 2005.
16. Mohr J, Batalden P, Barach P. Integrating patient safety into the clinical microsystem. 2004. Available from: http://qualitysafety.bmj.com/content/13/suppl_2/ii34.short.
17. Sorbero ME, Farley DO, Mattke S, Lovejoy SL. Outcome measures for effective teamwork in inpatient care: final report. RAND Corporation, 2008.
18. Henriksen K, Battles JB, Keyes MA, Grady ML, King HB, Battles J, et al. TeamSTEPPS(™): team strategies and tools to enhance performance and patient safety. Rockville: Agency for Healthcare Research and Quality; 2008.
19. Cannon-Bowers JA, Salas E. A framework for developing team performance measures in training. Team performance assessment and measurement: Theory, methods, and applications. Series in applied psychology., (pp. 45-62). Mahwah, NJ, US: Lawrence Erlbaum Associates Publishers, xii, 370 pp. 1997.
20. Baker DP, Gustafson S, Beaubien JM, Salas E, Barach P. Advances in patient safety: from research to implementation. Medical Team Training Programs in Health Care. AHRQ Publication. 2005;(05–0021):4.
21. Keenan RL, Boyan CP. Cardiac arrest due to anesthesia. A study of incidence and causes. JAMA. 1985; 253(16):2373–7.
22. Eichhorn JH. Prevention of intraoperative anesthesia accidents and related severe injury through safety monitoring. Anesthesiology. 1989;70(4):572–7.
23. Helmreich RL. On error management: lessons from aviation. BMJ. 2000;320:781–5.
24. Henrickson Parker S, Yule S, Flin R, McKinley A. Towards a model of surgeons' leadership in the operating room. BMJ Qual Saf. 2011;20(7):570–9, BMJ Publishing Group Ltd.
25. Schraagen JM, Schouten T, Smit M, Haas F, van der Beek D, van de Ven J, et al. A prospective study of paediatric cardiac surgical microsystems: assessing the relationships between non-routine events, teamwork and patient outcomes. BMJ Qual Saf. 2011;20(7):599–603, BMJ Publishing Group Ltd.
26. Mejak BL, Stammers A, Rauch E, Vang S, Viessman T. A retrospective study on perfusion incidents and safety devices. Perfusion. 2000;15(1):51–61.
27. Jenkins OF, Morris R, Simpson JM. Australasian perfusion incident survey. Perfusion. 1997;12(5):279–88. SAGE Publications.
28. Ducat CM, Merry AF, Webster CS. Attitudes and practices of New Zealand anaesthetists with regard to emergency drugs. Anaesth Intensive Care. 2000;28(6): 692–7.
29. Donchin Y, Gopher D, Olin M, Badihi Y, Biesky M, Sprung CL, et al. A look into the nature and causes of human errors in the intensive care unit. Crit Care Med. 1995;23:692–7.
30. de Leval MR, Carthey J, Wright DJ, Farewell VT, Reason JT. Human factors and cardiac surgery: a multicenter study. J Thorac Cardiovasc Surg. 2000;119: 661–72.
31. Lim SS, Vos T, Flaxman AD, Danaei G, Shibuya K, Adair-Rohani H, et al. A comparative risk assessment of burden of disease and injury attributable to 67 risk factors and risk factor clusters in 21 regions, 1990–2010: a systematic analysis for the Global Burden of Disease Study 2010. Lancet. 2012;380(9859): 2224–60.
32. Associate Chief Judge Murray Sinclair. The report of the Manitoba pediatric cardiac surgery inquest [Internet]. Manitoba: Provincial Court of Manitoba; 1995 [cited 2011 Jul 3]. Available from: http://www.pediatriccardiacinquest.mb.ca/.
33. Jacobs JP, Jacobs ML, Mavroudis C, Backer CL, Lacour-Gayet FG, Tchervenkov CI, et al. Nomenclature and databases for the surgical treatment of congenital cardiac disease – an updated primer and an analysis of opportunities for improvement. CTY. 2008;18(S2):38.
34. Francis R. Report of the Mid Staffordshire NHS foundation trust public inquiry: executive summary. 2013.
35. Barach P, Phelps G. Clinical sensemaking: a systematic approach to reduce the impact of normalised

deviance in the medical profession. J R Soc Med. 2013;106(10):387–90.
36. Vaughan D. The dark side of organizations: Mistake, misconduct, and disaster. 1999. Available from: http://www.jstor.org/stable/223506.
37. South Central Strategic Health Authority. Review of paediatric cardiac services at the Oxford Radcliffe Hospitals NHS Trust. NHS South Central, UK. 2010.
38. The Bristol Royal Infirmary Inquiry. Learning from Bristol: the report of the public inquiry into children's heart surgery at the Bristol Royal Infirmary 1984–1995 [Internet]. 2001. Available from: http://www.bristol-inquiry.org.uk/index.htm.
39. The United Kingdom Central Cardiac Audit Database (UKCCAD). http://www.ccad.org.ukcongenital.
40. Jacobs JP. Introduction–Databases and the assessment of complications associated with the treatment of patients with congenital cardiac disease. CTY. 2008;18 Suppl 2:1–37, Cambridge University Press.
41. Grigg OA, Farewell VT, Spiegelhalter DJ. Use of risk-adjusted CUSUM and RSPRT charts for monitoring in medical contexts. 2003rd ed. 2003;12(2):147–70. Available from: http://www.ncbi.nlm.nih.gov/pubmed/12665208.
42. Cohen MS, Jacobs JP, Quintessenza JA, Chai PJ, Lindberg HL, Dickey J, et al. Mentorship, learning curves, and balance. CTY. 2007;17 Suppl 2:164–74.
43. Jacobs JP. Introduction to part III of the 2007 supplement to cardiology in the young: controversies and challenges facing paediatric cardiovascular practitioners and their patients. CTY. 2007;17(S4):133–7. Cambridge University Press.
44. American Psychiatric Association, American Psychiatric Association Task Force on DSM-IV. Diagnostic and statistical manual of mental disorders: DSM-IV-TR. 4th ed. Washington, DC: American Psychiatric Association; 2000. 944 p.
45. Edmonson A. Psychological safety and learning behavior in work teams [Internet]. Johnson: Cornell University; 1999. Available from: http://findarticles.com/p/articles/mi_m4035/is_2_44/ai_55306277/?tag=content;col1.
46. Waring JJ. Beyond blame: cultural barriers to medical incident reporting. Soc Sci Med. 2005;60(9):1927–35.
47. Barach P, Small SD. How the NHS can improve safety and learning. By learning free lessons from near misses. BMJ. 2000;320(7251):1683–4.
48. Weick KE, Sutcliffe KM. Managing the unexpected: assuring high performance in an age of complexity. San Francisco: Jossey-Bass; 2001.
49. Uhlig PN, Brown J, Nason AK, Camelio A, Kendall E. John M. Eisenberg Patient Safety Awards. System innovation: Concord Hospital. 2002nd ed. 2002; 28(12):666–72. Available from: http://www.ncbi.nlm.nih.gov/pubmed/12481601.
50. ElBardissi AW, Wiegmann DA, Henrickson S, Wadhera R, Sundt III TM. Identifying methods to improve heart surgery: an operative approach and strategy for implementation on an organizational level. Eur J Cardiothorac Surg. 2008;34(5):1027–33.
51. Lencioni PM. The trouble with teamwork. Leader to Leader. 2003;2003(29):35–40.
52. Endsley MR. Measurement of situation awareness in dynamic systems. Hum Factors. 1995;37(1):65–84.
53. Edmondson AC. Learning from failure in health care: frequent opportunities, pervasive barriers. Qual Saf Health Care. 2004;13 Suppl 2:ii3–9.
54. Amalberti R, Auroy Y, Berwick D. Five system barriers to achieving ultrasafe health care. 2005. Available from: http://annals.org/article.aspx?articleid=718374.
55. Cassin BR, Barach PR. Balancing clinical team perceptions of the workplace: applying "work domain analysis" to pediatric cardiac care. Prog Pediatr Cardiol. 2012;33(1):25–32.
56. Reason J. Human error: models and management. 2000 ed. 2000;320(7237):768–70. Available from: http://www.ncbi.nlm.nih.gov/pubmed/10720363.
57. Shanafelt TD, Balch CM, Bechamps G, Russell T, Dyrbye L, Satele D, et al. Burnout and medical errors among American surgeons. Ann Surg. 2010;251(6): 995–1000.
58. Wiegmann DA, ElBardissi AW, Dearani JA, Daly RC, Sundt III TM. Disruptions in surgical flow and their relationship to surgical errors: an exploratory investigation. Surgery. 2007;142(5):658–65.
59. Edmondson A. Psychological safety and learning behavior in work teams. Adm Sci Q. 1999;44(2):350–83, Sage Publications.
60. Weick KE, Sutcliffe KM, Obstfeld D. Organizing for high reliability: processes of collective mindfulness. Crisis Management. 2008. Chapter 34 in 'Volume III Part II Challenges in Crisis Management, pp31-66 Ed Arjen Boin, Sage Library in Business and Management. Sage Publications Ltd. London. ISBN: 978-1-84787-088-9.
61. Carroll JS. Organizational learning activities in high – hazard industries: the logics underlying self – analysis. J Manag Stud. 1998;35:699–717.
62. Sanchez JA, Barach PR. High reliability organizations and surgical microsystems: re-engineering surgical care. Surg Clin North Am. 2012;92(1):1–14.
63. Independent Reconfiguration Panel. Advice on safe and sustainable proposals for Children's Congenital Heart Services [Internet]. 2013. Available from: www.hsj.co.uk/Journals/2013/06/12/g/h/f/IRP-Report.pdf.
64. The Northern New England Cardiovascular Disease Study Group. [Internet]. [cited 2011 28/6/11]. Available from: http://www.nnecdsg.org/.
65. Lave J, Wenger E. Situated learning: legitimate peripheral participation. Cambridge: Cambridge University Press; 1991.
66. Ohye RG, Sleeper LA, Mahony L, Newburger JW, Pearson GD, Lu M, Goldberg CS, Tabbutt S, Frommelt PC, Ghanayem NS, Laussen PC, Rhodes JF, Lewis AB, Mital S, Ravishankar C, Williams IA, Dunbar-Masterson C, Atz AM, Colan S, Minich LL, Pizarro C, Kanter KR, Jaggers J, Jacobs JP, Krawczeski CD, Pike N, McCrindle BW, Virzi L, Gaynor JW; Pediatric Heart Network Investigators. Comparison of shunt types in the Norwood procedure for single-ventricle lesions. N Engl J Med. 2010;362(21):1980–92. PMID: 20505177.

67. Congenital Heart Surgeon's Society. [Internet]. [cited 2011]. Available from: http://www.chss.org/.
68. Kugler JD, Kugler JD, Beekman Iii RH, Beekman III RH, Rosenthal GL, Rosenthal GL, et al. Development of a pediatric cardiology quality improvement collaborative: from inception to implementation. From the Joint Council on Congenital Heart Disease Quality Improvement Task Force. Congenit Heart Dis. 2009; 4(5):318–28.
69. Karamlou T, Karamlou T, McCrindle BW, McCrindle BW, Blackstone EH, Blackstone EH, et al. Lesion-specific outcomes in neonates undergoing congenital heart surgery are related predominantly to patient and management factors rather than institution or surgeon experience: a Congenital Heart Surgeons Society Study. J Thorac Cardiovasc Surg. 2010;139(3):569–77.e1.
70. Jacobs JP, Jacobs ML, Austin EH, Mavroudis C, Pasquali SK, Lacour-Gayet FG, et al. Quality measures for congenital and pediatric cardiac surgery. World J Pediatr Congenit Heart Surg. 2012;3(1): 32–47.
71. Iyengar AJ, Winlaw DS, Galati JC, Gentles TL, Weintraub RG, Justo RN, et al. The Australia and New Zealand Fontan Registry: description and initial results from the first population-based Fontan registry. Intern Med J. 2013;44(2):148–55.

Part II

Safety Science and Systems

Quality and Safety in a Children's Hospital

24

Brigitta U. Mueller

Abstract

Patients and parents expect safe and high quality care when entering a children's hospital. However, pediatric care is confronted with unique challenges to safety, and errors are more common than we like to admit. Pediatric care is complicated by the differences in patient size and weight, requiring different medication doses, different sized devices with the potential for technical difficulties because of smaller sizes, such as insertion of intravenous catheter. Although great progress has been made to avoid errors in some institutions, there is still much more to be done. This chapter discusses some of the approaches and preliminary achievements in creating a patient safety program.

Keywords

Medication errors • High reliability • Culture of safety • Teamwork

Background

"Primum non nocere" or "first do no harm" is a fundamental tenet of medicine. However, several studies have demonstrated that errors, many of them leading to harm, can and do occur in every medical setting. In 1999, the Institute of Medicine (IOM) published its report *To Err is Human: Building a Safer Health Care System* and indicated that an estimated 44,000–98,000 deaths per year were caused by medical errors [1]. According to this report the majority of medical errors do not result from individual recklessness, but rather from basic flaws in the design of our health systems [1]. The IOM's initial definition of errors was subsequently expanded by the Quality Interagency Coordination task force (QuIC) and reads: "*An error is defined as the failure of a planned action to be completed as intended, or the use of a wrong plan to achieve an aim. Errors can include problems in practice, products, procedures, and systems*" [2]. Errors can occur at

B.U. Mueller, MD, MHCM
Pediatrics, All Children's Hospital,
Johns Hopkins University, 501 Sixth Avenue South,
St. Petersburg, FL 33701, USA
e-mail: bmuelle6@jhmi.edu

P.R. Barach, J.P. Jacobs, S.E. Lipshultz, P.C. Laussen (eds.),
Pediatric and Congenital Cardiac Care: Volume 2: Quality Improvement and Patient Safety,
DOI 10.1007/978-1-4471-6566-8_24, © Springer-Verlag London 2015

any time during an encounter with the healthcare system, and include errors in diagnosing, treating or preventing illness. Errors are due to many different factors, including lack of teamwork, incomplete communication, stress, workload, or equipment failures, but are rarely due to intentional and malicious acts [1, 3, 4]. An error represents an event that, once set into motion, passes through multiple systems defenses, each with a "hole" or error in it. The number of layers in the system and the size of the hole(s) in each one influence the probability of an error reaching the patient (as described in Reason's Swiss cheese model) [5]. In addition, all humans have lapses that can be promoted by such factors as fatigue, stress, and distractions [6]. Simplification and standardization decrease lapses, while poorly designed medical devices or processes can promote errors [6, 7].

The Joint Commission (TJC) investigates "sentinel events", i.e., events that signal the need for immediate investigation and response. Sentinel events are due to an unexpected occurrence involving death or serious physical or psychological injury (specifically loss of limb or function), or the risk thereof. The health care organization is required to share its root cause analysis when a reviewable sentinel event is reported to TJC. The events and their root causes are recorded in a de-identified database. Between 1993 and June 2013, twenty-six states and the District of Columbia had reported over 7,400 sentinel events, most of them (4,844) occurring in hospitals. The three most common categories were "unintended retention of a foreign body", "wrong-patient, wrong-site, wrong-procedure", and "delay in treatment". The most common reasons identified in root cause analyses include human factors, leadership issues and communication failures (http://www.jointcommission.org/sentinel_event.aspx). As of March 2014, 51 sentinel alerts have been issued. Sentinel Events are reported to TJC voluntarily by an accredited organization or reported via the complaint process.

Quality transformation is the conversion of a health care delivery system from its baseline service performance to one of reliably high quality care. The IOM defines health care quality as "*the degree to which health care services for individuals and populations increase the likelihood of desired health outcomes and are consistent with current professional knowledge*" [8]. High quality care is defined as care that is safe, effective, patient-centered, timely, efficient and equitable (Table 24.1) [8]. In its publication "Crossing the Quality Chasm" the IOM identifies five challenging goals: the reengineering of care processes; the effective use of information technologies; improved knowledge and skills management; the development of effective teams, and the coordination of care across patient-conditions, services, and sites of care over time [8].

Table 24.1 High quality care as defined by the Institute of Medicine [8]

Safe
Avoiding preventable injuries, reducing medical errors
Effective
Providing services based on scientific knowledge (clinical guidelines)
Patient centered
Care that is respectful and responsive to individuals
Efficient
Avoiding wasting time and other resources
Timely
Reducing wait times, improving the practice flow
Equitable
Consistent care regardless of patient characteristics and demographics

Quality improvement is not possible without measurements and transparent dissemination of the results. Standardized quality measurements are required by regulatory agencies, for example, the Joint Commission's ORYX measurements or the Healthcare Effectiveness Data and Information Set (HEDIS) of the Centers for Medicaid and Medicare Services (CMS). Although there are fewer validated pediatric measures (mainly related to childhood asthma and immunizations), an increase in their number can be expected in the next few years. Furthermore, the change from a volume-based model to value-based care has now reached the pediatric (Medicaid) population, connecting quality of care to financial reimbursement strategies. For example, preventable readmissions are targeted for both adults and children and, in the case of gastroenteritis and urinary tract infections, can result in 21–55 % of potential cost reductions, respectively [9]. The Joint Commission's *Top Performer on Key Quality Measures* program recognizes accredited hospitals that attain excellence in accountability measure performance. Recognition in the program is based on an aggregation of ORYX® accountability measure data reported to TJC during the previous calendar year. The data report on evidence-based interventions for heart attack, heart failure, pneumonia, surgical care, children's asthma care, inpatient psychiatric services, venous thromboembolism (VTE), stroke, and immunizations. Several children's hospitals received top performer recognition for asthma care in 2013 (http://www.jointcommission.org/accreditation/top_performers.aspx) Other quality indicators are Magnet® recognition by the American Nurses Credentialing Center (http://www.nursecredentialing.org/magnet.aspx), achieving high scores on the Leapfrog survey (http://www.leapfroggroup.org/), or becoming a winner of the Malcolm Baldrige National Quality Award (http://www.nist.gov/baldrige).

Status of Quality and Safety in Pediatrics

Patient safety and quality of care are the cornerstones of modern medicine and presumed to be practiced in all medical settings, and especially in a children's hospital. However, pediatric care is confronted with unique challenges to safety, and errors are not uncommon. Pediatric care is challenged by the differences in patient size and weight, requiring different medication doses, the use of different devices with the potential for technical difficulties because of size, such as the insertion of small gauge intravenous catheter. Children have unique susceptibility to certain infections at different stages of development, such as neonates and infants related to the immaturity of their immune system. Their metabolism is different at different ages, thus impacting the pharmacokinetics of medications. Children are unable to administer their own medications, identify potential mistakes, and be primary historians for reports of pain or illness, and thus are very much dependent on adults, including for their access to care. Some disease entities are unique to children, such as birth trauma, congenital heart disease or certain cancers, and many preventive interventions have the highest impact when initiated during childhood (smoking prevention, prevention of obesity, dental caries). In 2011, the Institute of Medicine (IOM) identified a significant gap due to the general absence of information about the content and quality of preventive services that are used by children and adolescents, and recommended a life-course approach to the measurement of health and health care quality [10].

Medication errors are the most common adverse event in children, in part due to the necessary weight and age adjustments for dosing. Diagnostic errors may occur because of the age of the child and the inability of the young child to verbalize complaints. Therapeutic errors can, like in adults, occur due to the failure to adhere to guidelines, staff fatigue, or interruptions during critical actions.

Diagnostic Errors

Diagnostic errors or a delay in diagnosis may be caused by a failure to employ indicated tests, the use of outmoded tests or therapy, or a failure to act on results of monitoring or testing. A study of 130 successful litigation claims against the National Health Service in England involving fatalities in children listed delayed or failed diagnosis in 47 % of the cases [11]. A study that surveyed academic, community, and trainee pediatricians showed that more than one-half (54 %) of respondents reported that they made a diagnostic error at least once or twice per month; this frequency was even higher (77 %) among trainees [12]. Almost one-half (45 %) of respondents reported diagnostic errors that harmed patients at least once or twice per year. The most-commonly reported breakdowns of processes included failure to gather information through history, physical examination, or chart review, and inadequate care coordination and teamwork were the most-commonly reported system factors. Not unexpectedly, viral illnesses being diagnosed as bacterial illnesses was the most-commonly reported diagnostic error, followed by misdiagnosis of medication side effects, psychiatric disorders, and appendicitis [12]. Participants listed several solutions to reduce diagnostic errors, including close follow-up of patients, improving teamwork, spending more time in clinical encounters, and empowering patients and families to be vigilant about the possibility of diagnostic errors. Access to electronic medical records that provide comprehensive clinical data was also ranked high, followed by availability of diagnostic decision-support tools [12]. Some areas, such as radiology, routinely audit their diagnostic accuracy through peer review. Comments made by peer reviewers were classified in one study as errors of observation (25.5 %), errors of interpretation (5.6 %), inadequate patient data gathering (3.7 %), and errors of communication (9.6 %). Inter-observer variability accounted for 21.3 % of the comments and the rest were either of informational nature, educational feedback or complimentary [13].

Errors in Care

Errors related to treatment include errors in the performance of an operation, procedure, or test; errors in administering the treatment; errors in the dose or method of using a drug (see below). However, it may also include avoidable delays in treatment or in responding to an abnormal test, or even inappropriate (not indicated) care. Furthermore, we now recognize that errors in prevention, such as failure to provide prophylactic treatment or the inadequate monitoring or follow-up of treatment, play an important role as well [8].

Healthcare-associated infections (HAIs) play an important role in causing morbity and mortality in children and adults. Many initiatives have successfully reduced the number of central line associated blood stream infections (CLABSIs), catheter-associated urinary tract infections (CAUTIs), ventilator-associated pneumonias (VAPs), and surgical site infections (SSIs). The incidence of CLABSIs in intensive care or pediatric oncology patients has successfully been reduced by using standardized "bundles" for insertion and maintenance of the catheters, as well as through the use of ancillary measures, such as daily baths with chlorhexidine [14–17]. The data on CAUTIs are not yet quite as robust, possibly due to the relative rarity of this event in pediatrics [18, 19], while VAPs, although rare in children overall and influenced by similar factors as in adults, are not uncommon in neonates, especially in the very low birth group [20–22]. Surgical site infections, their incidence and prevention have been most extensively studied in cardiac and orthopedic (especially spine) surgeries [23, 24]. In addition, preventable pressure ulcers may occur in critically ill children or patients with limited mobility. Especially vulnerable are neonatal patients, where the administration of oxygen via nasal prongs or masks can cause skin defects, sometimes with lasting cosmetic consequences [25, 26].

Medication Errors

Medication orders in pediatrics must not only be adjusted to the underlying disease but also to the age, weight, and height of the child. Most medications are formulated and packaged primarily for adults and the doses often need to be diluted or otherwise be altered to be practical for pediatric use. A study of hospitalized, non-newborn patients in the United States found a medication error rate of 1.81–2.96 per 100 discharges [27]. Teaching hospitals and settings where patients had more complex medical needs showed significantly higher error rates, while gender, payer and zip code did not significantly impact outcomes. Another report documented 55 medication errors per 100 inpatient admissions at a single, leading pediatric teaching hospital [28]. It is important to note that our reporting capabilities of medication errors that occur in the ambulatory or home setting are still limited [29, 30].

Many institutions rely on vigilance, either by self-checking or checking by others. This strategy tends to be ineffective for many reasons, including fatigue, distractions, and human imperfection. Flynn, et al studied the validity and cost-effectiveness of three methods for detecting medication errors in 36 hospitals and skilled-nursing facilities and concluded that direct observation was more efficient and accurate than reviewing charts and incident reports in detecting medication errors. Medication administration errors were studied using three methods: incident report review, chart review, and direct observation. Observers detected 300 of 457 pharmacist-confirmed errors made on 2,556 doses (11.7 % error rate) compared with 17 errors detected by chart reviewers (0.7 % error rate), and only 1 error detected by incident report review (0.04 % error rate). Thirty-five (8 %) of these errors were deemed potentially clinically significant and the majority of them (71 %) were detected by direct observation [31]. A pediatric-focused trigger tool may detect a much higher incidence of errors, as shown by Takata et al. [32] A review of 960 randomly selected charts from 12 children's hospitals revealed 2,388 triggers (2.49 per patient) and 107 unique adverse drug events. Almost a quarter (22 %) of all adverse drug events were deemed preventable, many could have been identified earlier (17.8 %), or could have been mitigated more effectively (16.8 %). Only 3.7 % of adverse drug events were identified in voluntary hospital-based incidence reports [32].

The Joint Commission issued a Sentinel Alert in 2008 regarding the prevention of pediatric medication errors and made several recommendations. These included, among others, the establishment of a pediatric formulary system, the availability of limited concentrations and dose strengths of high alert medications, and the use of oral (not intravenous) syringes for the administration of oral medications [33]. Another intervention that has been shown to be effective, is the presence of a unit-based pharmacist [34].

Quality Improvement and Patient Safety Initiatives

There are notable initiatives that have been established to improve the quality and safety of pediatric care. These include:

- The implementation of rapid response teams that can be activated by both staff and patients/parents [35] and the use of an early warning system [36] are among the most effective tools to increase patient safety and quality of care in a children's hospital.
- Several organizations are leading the quality improvement effort. One of the oldest national quality improvement networks is the Vermont Oxford Network (VON), an organization that has been tracking neonatal outcomes since 1988 and now encompasses more than 950 Neonatal Intensive Care Units around the world [37]. The Children's Hospital Association (CHA) Quality Transformation Network focuses on the prevention of central line associated blood stream infections (CLABSIs) both in the intensive care and oncology/bone marrow transplant setting. These efforts are beginning to show results: As of the first quarter of 2014 an estimated 5,015 infections and 603 deaths have been prevented and data on more than 1,000,000 central line days, >30,000 line insertion procedures, and >100,000 central line maintenance procedures have been accumulated [16, 38, 39]. Cincinnati Children's Hospital conducted a quality improvement initiative to implement cultural and system changes with the goal of reducing serious safety events (SSEs) . They were able to reduce SSEs per 10,000 adjusted patient-days from a mean of 0.9 at baseline to 0.3 ($P < .0001$) and to increase the number of days between SSEs from a mean of 19.4 at baseline to 55.2 ($P < .0001$) [40]. This initiative has now been expanded to a national network (Children's Hospitals' Solutions for Patient Safety®). Cardiology is another discipline that has a long-standing history of data collection and collaborative efforts to improve the quality of care (see Chap. 6) [41, 42].
- In 2005 a report entitled "Safe Medical Devices for Children" recommended that the Food and Drug Administration (FDA) should collaborate with industry, health care professionals and organizations, as well as parent and patient advocates to focus more attention on adverse device events, especially events involving children, and that it should establish a central point of responsibility for pediatric issues within the Center for Devices and Radiological Health to

evaluate the adequacy of the Center's use of pediatric expertise and its attention to pediatric issues in all aspects of its work [43].

- The American Board of Pediatrics (ABP) requires participation in a quality improvement project in part 4 of its Maintenance of Certification (MOC) process, and many organizations offer local opportunities to take an active role in quality improvement efforts [44, 45]. Most projects occur in the emergency room and the inpatient wards, fewer focus on the ambulatory environment [46–48].

Leadership/Governance

The Institute for Healthcare Improvement (IHI) has coined the term of the "triple aim" as a way to shift from a volume-based approach to value-based care: Improving the patient experience of care (including quality and satisfaction), improving the health of populations; and reducing the per capita cost of health care. Enhanced attention has been put on the role of leadership and governance in the quest to advance quality of care and assure safety for all patients [49–52]. Patient safety and quality of care has to be a priority for the executive leadership and the Board of an institution, but this requires providing training and education to the mainly lay members [52]. Board members and executive leaders should participate in regular patient safety rounds, hold the organization accountable for quality measures and be well informed regarding the organization's performance (see also Chap. 15) [53].

Culture (Accountability)

As important as education is the creation of a blame-free environment that is actively and visibly supported and nurtured by leadership. It has become clear that a major shift in culture from a punitive to a non-punitive environment is necessary to affect and maintain positive changes, especially when they emphasize teamwork instead of placing the blame on the end provider [54]. Organizations need to assess their culture of safety at regular intervals and share the results with front line providers, as well as develop action plans to address any deficiencies. Several instruments are available, including a well-validated tool from the Agency for Healthcare Research and Quality (AHRQ), available at http://www.ahrq.gov/professionals/quality-patient-safety/patientsafetyculture/index.html [55].

Patient and Family Involvement

An often under-utilized modality to prevent errors is the encouragement of patients and their families to become involved as guardians of safety and quality. Some institutions have given parents the option of activating a rapid response team, and a few make parents part of a root cause analysis [35, 56, 57]. However, many providers and staff still feel uncomfortable, feel criticized, or accused, if a patient or parent points out a mistake, or are hesitant to disclose an error themselves [58, 59]. Although disclosure to the patient and the family is encouraged and appropriate, this is often the most difficult part for the care providers involved [60]. A survey studied the opinions of members of a health plan and found that full disclosure of any errors or mistakes reduced the likelihood of changing physicians and increased patient satisfaction, trust and positive emotional response [61]. The overwhelming majority of responders (98.8 %) wanted to be told of an error.

Technology

The use of technology is widespread in medicine and most of it provides enhanced protection against human error. Electronic prescribing, and especially the use of order set templates developed for a specific aspect of care, can significantly reduce order errors by prompting the prescriber to provide necessary information in a standardized format [62]. However, although computerized physician order entry (CPOE) has been presented as the "solution" to prevent medication error, numerous studies have shown reduction but not elimination of errors [63].

CPOE systems have the potential to reduce errors in different ways, including forcing the entry of generic drug names, ensuring complete orders without missing data such as frequency, ensuring legibility of the order, and providing clear identification of the prescriber through the use of an electronic signature [63, 64]. CPOE can offer alerts and reminders designed to promote safer use of medication such as drug-allergy checking, drug-drug interaction checking, and medication guidelines, requiring deliberate overrides for doses or dosages that exceed predetermined maximums. As of 2009, CPOE for medications had been implemented in only 17 % of hospitals, but no pediatric-specific data are available [65]. As CPOE and other components of the electronic medical record are implemented in more pediatric institutions, specific pediatric challenges must be addressed, such as unique patient identifier for infants whose name changes; specific pediatric terminology for elements of the history or physical examination; age-based normal ranges; calculation of age in days or months when appropriate; prescribing of medications by weight or body surface area; and immunization support.

Bar-coding technology, prevalent in our daily lives, was first introduced into medical settings about 30 years ago for use in clinical laboratories and blood banks [66]. The use of bar codes to help match patients with their medication orders and administration is thought to be one of the most important mechanisms to decrease adverse medication events [67]. In 2004 the FDA proposed the introduction of rules requiring bar coding on medications, so that bar codes could be cross-matched with a patient's bar-coded wristband in an effort to reduce the number of errors. However, integration of the different electronic devices remains a challenge.

Computerized infusion devices (smart pumps) with built-in software that allows the pump to be programmed with institution-established dosage limits, are widely used and are especially helpful in pediatrics, since they can provide warnings to the clinicians when the dosage limits have been exceeded [68]. Ideally, they should be integrated with a bar-code system to facilitate the safe recognition of the patient about to receive the infusion, and their computer system can provide data regarding the proper adherence to safety parameters. However, human error can still occur and result in harm to the patient. In a study of errors related to Patient-controlled analgesia (PCA) pumps it was determined that 6.5 % of events were due to operator error, and most (81 %) of them involved pump misprogramming [69].

Teamwork and Communication

Care for many pediatric patients is based on a multi-disciplinary team approach, including social workers, nurses, physical therapists, physicians and other providers, as well as child life specialists, nutritionists, pharmacists and others. Hand-offs between different care providers are becoming ever more numerous and without a standardized approach that is regularly monitored for its quality will result in confusion, wasted time and resources, and in the end will lead to more errors that threaten our patients' safety. A study from a large children's hospital described the introduction of a resident handoff bundle, consisting of standardized communication and handoff training, a verbal mnemonic, and a new team handoff structure. Medical errors decreased from 33.8 per 100 admissions to 18.3 per 100 admissions, and preventable adverse events decreased from 3.3 per 100 admissions to 1.5 per 100 admissions [70].

Several tools are available to further improve team work. The Department of Defense and the Agency for Healthcare Research and Quality (AHRQ) have developed Team Strategies and Tools to Enhance Performance and Patient Safety (TeamSTEPPS™) as a systematic approach to integrate teamwork into practice. Other programs are modeled on the aviation industry's Crew Resource Management [71, 72] model, the Microsystems approach (http://www.clinicalmicrosystem.org/), or the Comprehensive Unit-based Safety Program (CUSP), developed initially to decrease catheter-associated blood stream infections (CLABSIs) in intensive care units (http://www.ahrq.gov/professionals/education/curriculum-tools/cusptoolkit/index.html).

High Reliability Organizations

Reliability is measured as the inverse of the system's failure rate. It is estimated that he US health system has a defect rate of 1 in 10 (i.e., we do it right only about 90 % of the time), thus performs at a level of 10^{-1}. A performance level of 10^{-1} relies on basic standardization, such as guidelines, standardized order templates, on memory aids, including checklists, and on feedback mechanisms regarding compliance with standards and awareness-raising, as well as training of new staff. To get to the next level (10^{-2}, or 95 % reliability) we need to implement real time identification of failures, introduce redundancy, such as double verification of chemotherapy orders, and create an environment that makes the right way the easy way to do it [73]. Level 3 (10^{-3} failures or fewer than 5 failures per 1,000) starts to get to the core principles of HRO (see below), but high reliability industries, such as the nuclear power industry or the airline industry function at or above the 10^{-6} level.

High reliability principles include [74]:

Preoccupation with failure: Real time awareness of failures, achieved by daily monitoring of processes, reporting of near misses, and an enhanced sensitivity to processes that could potentially fail <u>before</u> they actually do.

Reluctance to simplify: The first, obvious explanation for a failure may not be the right one, and it is rarely a single issue that leads to the error. Jim Conway, Executive Vice President and Chief Operating Officer at The Dana Farber Cancer Institute when a fatal chemotherapy error occurred, said: "Our systems are too complex to expect merely extraordinary people to perform perfectly 100 % of the time. We as leaders must put in place systems that support great practice by people who suffer from being human and thus will make mistakes."

Sensitivity to operations: Leaders and staff are constantly aware of how processes and systems affect the organization. Any process that does not work is highlighted and modified in real time. Transparency is a valuable tool to increase sensitivity to operations.

Commitment to resilience: Failures and especially near-miss situations are considered learning opportunities. High reliability organizations are constantly learning, improving, and testing new ways of operating. This takes skilled people that have the appropriate tools, as well as adequate time to evaluate, measure and implement. A commonly used tool is the Plan-Do-Study-Act (PDSA) cycle [75].

Deference to expertise: This includes taking advantage of the different levels and areas of expertise that team members contribute, and the recognition that the most senior person is often not the most knowledgeable. Just like we use multi-disciplinary teams to discuss patient care, we may use the same approach to discuss any real or potential failures.

We already know that such high performance levels are possible to achieve: the safety of blood transfusions or general anesthesia approach a low failure rate of 10^{-5}, similar to the airline industry [76]. In the new reimbursement system hospitals that experience safety events will be at risk, not just because of potential litigation, but also because insurance companies will no longer reimburse for events they consider preventable, such as ventilator-associated pneumonias, catheter-associated blood stream infections, or pressure ulcers. Without doubt, an investment will be necessary, not just in dollars, but also in people and time, but a study from Cincinnati Children's Hospital was able to demonstrate measurable savings for the organization after implementing HRO principles. Over a 2-year period estimated harm-related hospital costs decreased by 22 % due to a decrease in serious safety events (from 1.15 events to 0.19 events per 10,000 adjusted hospital-days), and a decrease in preventable harm events by 53 % [77]. The pediatric community can greatly benefit from collaborative efforts such as through the Children's Hospital Association (CHA) or the Solution for Patient Safety®.

References

1. Kohn LT, Corrigan JM, Donaldson MS, Committee on Quality of Health Care in America IoM, editors. To err is human: building a safer health care system. Washington, DC: National Academic Press; 2000. 1–29 p.
2. Eisenberg JM. Continuing education meets the learning organization: the challenge of a systems approach

to patient safety. J Contin Educ Health Prof. 2000; 20(4):197–207.
3. Brennan TA, Localio AR, Leape LL, Laird NM, Peterson L, Hiatt HH, et al. Identification of adverse events occurring during hospitalization. A cross-sectional study of litigation, quality assurance, and medical records at two teaching hospitals. Ann Intern Med. 1990;112(3):221–6.
4. Leape LL, Brennan TA, Laird N, Lawthers AG, Localio AR, Barnes BA, et al. The nature of adverse events in hospitalized patients. Results of the Harvard Medical Practice Study II. N Engl J Med. 1991;324(6):377–84.
5. Reason J. Human error: models and management. BMJ. 2000;320(7237):768–70.
6. Weinger MB, Ancoli-Israel S. Sleep deprivation and clinical performance. JAMA. 2002;287(8):955–7.
7. Rozich JD, Howard RJ, Justeson JM, Macken PD, Lindsay ME, Resar RK. Standardization as a mechanism to improve safety in health care. Jt Comm J Qual Saf. 2004;30(1):5–14.
8. Institute of Medicine. Crossing the quality chasm: a new health system for the 21st century. Washington, DC: National Academy Press; 2001.
9. Torio CM, Elixhauser A, Andrews RM. Trends in potentially preventable hospital admissions among adults and children, 2005–2010. Agency for Healthcare Research and Quality (AHRQ), Mar 2013. Report No.
10. Institute of Medicine. Child and adolescent health and health care quality. Measuring what matters. Washington, DC: National Research Council of the National Academies; 2011.
11. Sen G, Keene J, Raine J. An analysis of successful litigation claims in childhood fatalities in England. Eur J Pediatr. 2012;171(11):1657–60.
12. Singh H, Thomas EJ, Wilson L, Kelly PA, Pietz K, Elkeeb D, et al. Errors of diagnosis in pediatric practice: a multisite survey. Pediatrics. 2010;126(1):70–9.
13. Iyer RS, Swanson JO, Otto RK, Weinberger E. Peer review comments augment diagnostic error characterization and departmental quality assurance: 1-year experience from a children's hospital. AJR Am J Roentgenol. 2013;200(1):132–7.
14. Klieger SB, Potter-Bynoe G, Quach C, Sandora TJ, Coffin SE. Beyond the bundle: a survey of central line-associated bloodstream infection prevention practices used in US and Canadian pediatric hospitals. Infect Control Hosp Epidemiol. 2013;34(11):1208–10.
15. Quach C, Milstone AM, Perpete C, Bonenfant M, Moore DL, Perreault T. Chlorhexidine bathing in a tertiary care neonatal intensive care unit: impact on central line-associated bloodstream infections. Infect Control Hosp Epidemiol. 2014;35(2):158–63.
16. Rinke ML, Chen AR, Bundy DG, Colantuoni E, Fratino L, Drucis KM, et al. Implementation of a central line maintenance care bundle in hospitalized pediatric oncology patients. Pediatrics. 2012;130(4): e996–1004.
17. Ting JY, Goh VS, Osiovich H. Reduction of central line-associated bloodstream infection rates in a neonatal intensive care unit after implementation of a multidisciplinary evidence-based quality improvement collaborative: a four-year surveillance. Can J Infect Dis Med Microbiol. 2013;24(4):185–90.
18. Bi XC, Zhang B, Ye YK, He HC, Han ZD, Dai QS, et al. Pathogen incidence and antibiotic resistance patterns of catheter-associated urinary tract infection in children. J Chemother. 2009;21(6):661–5.
19. He W, Wang D, Ye Z, Qian W, Tao Y, Shi X, et al. Application of a nanotechnology antimicrobial spray to prevent lower urinary tract infection: a multicenter urology trial. J Transl Med. 2012;10 Suppl 1:S14.
20. Gautam A, Ganu SS, Tegg OJ, Andresen DN, Wilkins BH, Schell DN. Ventilator-associated pneumonia in a tertiary paediatric intensive care unit: a 1-year prospective observational study. Crit Care Resusc. 2012;14(4):283–9.
21. Simpson VS, Bailey A, Higgerson RA, Christie LM. Ventilator-associated tracheobronchitis in a mixed medical/surgical pediatric ICU. Chest. 2013; 144(1):32–8.
22. Hocevar SN, Edwards JR, Horan TC, Morrell GC, Iwamoto M, Lessa FC. Device-associated infections among neonatal intensive care unit patients: incidence and associated pathogens reported to the National Healthcare Safety Network, 2006–2008. Infect Control Hosp Epidemiol. 2012;33(12):1200–6.
23. Atchley KD, Pappas JM, Kennedy AT, Coffin SE, Gerber JS, Fuller SM, et al. Use of administrative data for surgical site infection surveillance after congenital cardiac surgery results in inaccurate reporting of surgical site infection rates. Ann Thorac Surg. 2014; 97(2):651–8.
24. Glotzbecker MP, Riedel MD, Vitale MG, Matsumoto H, Roye DP, Erickson M, et al. What's the evidence? Systematic literature review of risk factors and preventive strategies for surgical site infection following pediatric spine surgery. J Pediatr Orthop. 2013;33(5): 479–87.
25. Schindler CA, Mikhailov TA, Cashin SE, Malin S, Christensen M, Winters JM. Under pressure: preventing pressure ulcers in critically ill infants. J Spec Pediatr Nurs. 2013;18(4):329–41.
26. Schluer AB, Schols JM, Halfens RJ. Risk and associated factors of pressure ulcers in hospitalized children over 1 year of age. J Spec Pediatr Nurs. 2014;19(1):80–9.
27. Slonim AD, LaFleur BJ, Ahmed W, Joseph JG. Hospital-reported medical errors in children. Pediatrics. 2003;111(3):617–21.
28. Kaushal R, Bates DW, Landrigan C, McKenna KJ, Clapp MD, Federico F, et al. Medication errors and adverse drug events in pediatric inpatients. JAMA. 2001;285(16):2114–20.
29. Neuspiel DR, Stubbs EH, Liggin L. Improving reporting of outpatient pediatric medical errors. Pediatrics. 2011;128(6):e1608–13.
30. Walsh KE, Roblin DW, Weingart SN, Houlahan KE, Degar B, Billett A, et al. Medication errors in the home: a multisite study of children with cancer. Pediatrics. 2013;131(5):e1405–14.

31. Flynn EA, Barker KN, Pepper GA, Bates DW, Mikeal RL. Comparison of methods for detecting medication errors in 36 hospitals and skilled-nursing facilities. Am J Health Syst Pharm. 2002;59(5):436–46.
32. Takata GS, Mason W, Taketomo C, Logsdon T, Sharek PJ. Development, testing, and findings of a pediatric-focused trigger tool to identify medication-related harm in US children's hospitals. Pediatrics. 2008;121(4):e927–35.
33. The Joint Commission. Preventing pediatric medication errors. Sentinel Event Alert. 2008;(39):1–4.
34. Kaushal R, Bates DW, Abramson EL, Soukup JR, Goldmann DA. Unit-based clinical pharmacists' prevention of serious medication errors in pediatric inpatients. Am J Health Syst Pharm. 2008;65(13):1254–60.
35. Van Voorhis KT, Willis TS. Implementing a pediatric rapid response system to improve quality and patient safety. Pediatr Clin North Am. 2009;56(4):919–33.
36. Duncan KD, McMullan C, Mills BM. Early warning systems: the next level of rapid response. Nursing. 2012;42(2):38–44; quiz 5.
37. Horbar JD. The Vermont-Oxford Neonatal Network: integrating research and clinical practice to improve the quality of medical care. Semin Perinatol. 1995; 19(2):124–31.
38. Rinke ML, Bundy DG, Chen AR, Milstone AM, Colantuoni E, Pehar M, et al. Central line maintenance bundles and CLABSIs in ambulatory oncology patients. Pediatrics. 2013;132(5):e1403–12.
39. Billett AL, Colletti RB, Mandel KE, Miller M, Muething SE, Sharek PJ, et al. Exemplar pediatric collaborative improvement networks: achieving results. Pediatrics. 2013;131 Suppl 4:S196–203.
40. Muething SE, Goudie A, Schoettker PJ, Donnelly LF, Goodfriend MA, Bracke TM, et al. Quality improvement initiative to reduce serious safety events and improve patient safety culture. Pediatrics. 2012;130(2):e423–31.
41. Burstein DS, Rossi AF, Jacobs JP, Checchia PA, Wernovsky G, Li JS, et al. Variation in models of care delivery for children undergoing congenital heart surgery in the United States. World J Pediatr Congenit Heart Surg. 2010;1(1):8–14.
42. Jacobs JP. Introduction–databases and the assessment of complications associated with the treatment of patients with congenital cardiac disease. Cardiol Young. 2008;18 Suppl 2:1–37.
43. National Research Council. Safe medical devices for children. Washington, DC: The National Academies Press; 2005.
44. Lannon CM, Peterson LE. Pediatric collaborative networks for quality improvement and research. Acad Pediatr. 2013;13(6 Suppl):S69–74.
45. Miles PV, Moyer VA. Quality improvement and maintenance of certification. Acad Pediatr. 2013;13 (6 Suppl):S14–5.
46. Fortescue EB, Kaushal R, Landrigan CP, McKenna KJ, Clapp MD, Federico F, et al. Prioritizing strategies for preventing medication errors and adverse drug events in pediatric inpatients. Pediatrics. 2003; 111(4 Pt 1):722–9.
47. Guttmann A, Razzaq A, Lindsay P, Zagorski B, Anderson GM. Development of measures of the quality of emergency department care for children using a structured panel process. Pediatrics. 2006;118(1):114–23.
48. Neuspiel DR, Hyman D, Lane M. Quality improvement and patient safety in the pediatric ambulatory setting: current knowledge and implications for residency training. Pediatr Clin North Am. 2009;56(4):935–51.
49. Jiang HJ, Lockee C, Bass K, Fraser I. Board oversight of quality: any differences in process of care and mortality? J Healthc Manag. 2009;54(1):15–29; discussion 29–30.
50. Gandhi TK, Graydon-Baker E, Barnes JN, Neppl C, Stapinski C, Silverman J, et al. Creating an integrated patient safety team. Jt Comm J Qual Saf. 2003;29(8):383–90.
51. The Joint Commission. Leadership in healthcare organizations. San Diego: The Governance Institute; 2009.
52. Conway J. Getting boards on board: engaging governing boards in quality and safety. Jt Comm J Qual Patient Saf. 2008;34(4):214–20.
53. Swensen S, Pugh M, McMullan C, Kabcenell A. High-impact leadership: improve care, improve the health of populations, and reduce costs. Cambridge, MA: Institute for Healthcare Improvement; 2013.
54. Stump LS. Re-engineering the medication error-reporting process: removing the blame and improving the system. Am J Health Syst Pharm. 2000;57 Suppl 4:S10–7.
55. Sorra JS, Dyer N. Multilevel psychometric properties of the AHRQ hospital survey on patient safety culture. BMC Health Serv Res. 2010;10:199.
56. Shepherd HL, Barratt A, Trevena LJ, McGeechan K, Carey K, Epstein RM, et al. Three questions that patients can ask to improve the quality of information physicians give about treatment options: a cross-over trial. Patient Educ Couns. 2011;84(3):379–85.
57. Frey B, Ersch J, Bernet V, Baenziger O, Enderli L, Doell C. Involvement of parents in critical incidents in a neonatal-paediatric intensive care unit. Qual Saf Health Care. 2009;18(6):446–9.
58. Matlow AG, Moody L, Laxer R, Stevens P, Goia C, Friedman JN. Disclosure of medical error to parents and paediatric patients: assessment of parents' attitudes and influencing factors. Arch Dis Child. 2010; 95(4):286–90.
59. Loren DJ, Klein EJ, Garbutt J, Krauss MJ, Fraser V, Dunagan WC, et al. Medical error disclosure among pediatricians: choosing carefully what we might say to parents. Arch Pediatr Adolesc Med. 2008;162(10):922–7.
60. Liang BA. A system of medical error disclosure. Qual Saf Health Care. 2002;11(1):64–8.
61. Mazor KM, Simon SR, Yood RA, Martinson BC, Gunter MJ, Reed GW, et al. Health plan members' views about disclosure of medical errors. Ann Intern Med. 2004;140(6):409–18.
62. Wasserfallen JB, Butschi AJ, Muff P, Biollaz J, Schaller MD, Pannatier A, et al. Format of medical order sheet improves security of antibiotics prescription: the experience of an intensive care unit. Crit Care Med. 2004;32(3):655–9.

63. Meisenberg BR, Wright RR, Brady-Copertino CJ. Reduction in chemotherapy order errors with computerized physician order entry. J Oncol Pract. 2014;10(1):e5–9.
64. Bates DW, Evans RS, Murff H, Stetson PD, Pizziferri L, Hripcsak G. Detecting adverse events using information technology. J Am Med Inform Assoc. 2003;10(2):115–28.
65. Jha AK, DesRoches CM, Campbell EG, Donelan K, Rao SR, Ferris TG, et al. Use of electronic health records in U.S. hospitals. N Engl J Med. 2009;360(16):1628–38.
66. Murphy MF, Kay JD. Barcode identification for transfusion safety. Curr Opin Hematol. 2004;11(5):334–8.
67. Bates DW, Cohen M, Leape LL, Overhage JM, Shabot MM, Sheridan T. Reducing the frequency of errors in medicine using information technology. J Am Med Inform Assoc. 2001;8(4):299–308.
68. KLAS. Smart pumps: in an area where decimal-point medication errors can be fatal, smart infusion pumps are adding a line of defense. Healthc Inform. 2008;25(12):20.
69. Schein JR, Hicks RW, Nelson WW, Sikirica V, Doyle DJ. Patient-controlled analgesia-related medication errors in the postoperative period: causes and prevention. Drug Saf. 2009;32(7):549–59.
70. Starmer AJ, Sectish TC, Simon DW, Keohane C, McSweeney ME, Chung EY, et al. Rates of medical errors and preventable adverse events among hospitalized children following implementation of a resident handoff bundle. JAMA. 2013;310(21):2262–70.
71. Buljac-Samardzic M, Dekker-van Doorn CM, van Wijngaarden JD, van Wijk KP. Interventions to improve team effectiveness: a systematic review. Health Policy. 2010;94(3):183–95.
72. Buljac-Samardzic M, van Woerkom M, Paauwe J. Team safety and innovation by learning from errors in long-term care settings. Health Care Manage Rev. 2012;37(3):280–91.
73. Chassin MR, Loeb JM. The ongoing quality improvement journey: next stop, high reliability. Health Aff (Millwood). 2011;30(4):559–68.
74. The Joint Commission aims for high-reliability health care, unveils framework to move hospitals toward zero harm. ED Manag. 2013;25(12):suppl 3–4, 139.
75. Gillam S, Steel N. The quality and outcomes framework–where next? BMJ. 2013;346:f659.
76. Amalberti R, Auroy Y, Berwick D, Barach P. Five system barriers to achieving ultrasafe health care. Ann Intern Med. 2005;142(9):756–64.
77. Brilli RJ, McClead Jr RE, Crandall WV, Stoverock L, Berry JC, Wheeler TA, et al. A comprehensive patient safety program can significantly reduce preventable harm, associated costs, and hospital mortality. J Pediatr. 2013;163(6):1638–45.

The Children's Hospital of Michigan Quality and Safety Journey: Making Safety First and Making It Last

25

Rudolph P. Valentini

Abstract

Quality improvement, while commonplace in manufacturing for decades, is a newer concept in health over the past 10–15 years. Accountability and transparency of patient care quality and safety metrics are becoming expectations of hospitals today. There is an increasing emphasis on the provision of quality care in the most cost effective manner, thereby yielding the highest value to our consumers (patients and families). The delivery of value is also highly desired by third party payers.

To increase the safety of patient care delivery at our pediatric hospital, our journey to transform our safety culture took place 2 years ago, and was led by our hospital board and our executive leadership team. The collective passion for driving safety permeated through to the frontline staff of the hospital. Points of emphasis were daily safety huddles, increased event reporting, and intensive investigation of hospital safety events through root cause analysis and peer review. Positive reinforcement for near miss or "great catch" reporting is a regular occurrence, and has contributed to earlier identification of problems. Our 2-year journey has resulted in a marked increase in event reporting and reduction in serious safety events. Further, improved safety outcomes including reduction in central line associated blood stream infections and catheter associated urinary tract infections have led to our hospital achieving national recognition in 2013.

Keywords

Safety huddle • Serious safety events • Hand hygiene compliance • CLABSI • CAUTI

R.P. Valentini, MD
Pediatric Nephrology, Children's Hospital of Michigan, Wayne State University School of Medicine, 3901 Beaubien Blvd, Detroit, MI 48201-2119, USA
e-mail: rvalenti@dmc.org

P.R. Barach, J.P. Jacobs, S.E. Lipshultz, P.C. Laussen (eds.),
Pediatric and Congenital Cardiac Care: Volume 2: Quality Improvement and Patient Safety,
DOI 10.1007/978-1-4471-6566-8_25, © Springer-Verlag London 2015

Introduction

Quality improvement is a concept that has existed in manufacturing for decades, but it has only been a part of health care for the past 10–15 years—a topic introduced by the 1999 Institute of Medicine's report, *To Err is Human*. This report highlighted the fact that deaths attributable to medical errors exceed those from motor vehicle accidents, breast cancer and AIDS. In addition to drawing attention to this matter, this article emphasized that most errors are not due to individual errors from reckless practice; rather, the healthcare industry is ripe for these type of errors due to the fragmented nature of our practices with caregivers in one setting often lacking the full clinical picture. System based errors were the focus, with the authors noting that individuals must still need to be accountable. This landmark report called for: a national focus on patient safety, mandatory nationwide public reporting of errors leading to deaths or serious injury and voluntary reporting of potential serious events. Further, committed organizational and regulatory expectations for improved patient safety were needed, and finally, health care organizations were called to create a safety culture, and implement systems that improve safety which do not rely upon the memory of practitioners [1].

In the era of increasing accountability and transparency, it is no longer acceptable for hospitals to improve at their own pace; they must do so quickly because improvement is certain to have financial impacts on their long-term well being, both in terms of treating patients more cost-effectively and in competing in a challenging health care marketplace. Insurance companies now can choose to pay for procedures or treatment provided only in centers meeting their criteria, which may include performance thresholds or treatment costs. For instance, an insurer can mandate that an approved kidney transplant be performed at a "center of excellence," where excellence is measured by several means, such as the number of transplants in the past year, 1-year allograft survival rates, median hospital length of stay, hospital readmission rates following renal transplantation or overall cost of the transplant. As their health care budgets continue to tighten, insurers are now linking reimbursement more closely to quality of hospital care. One such example is the Centers for Medicare and Medicaid Services (CMS), which introduced hospital value-based purchasing as a program to reward acute care hospitals for achieving quality outcomes for Medicare patients [2].

Terms such as "hospital value-based purchasing" have entered the lexicon of hospital leaders who want to deliver the most value for the health care dollar spent. Value in the health care setting is classically defined as quality divided by cost [3]:

$$\text{value} = \text{quality} / \text{cost}$$

This equation is critical because the focus has to be primarily on delivering *high-quality* care. If high-quality care can be delivered, the next focus is to provide it at the lowest possible *cost*. Hence, delivering quality care at a responsible cost provides excellent *value*, and high value is what patients, families, and third-party payers, such as CMS, are seeking. Hospital-acquired conditions (HAC's), such as blood stream infections and urinary tract infections associated with medical devices such as indwelling catheters, are now carefully monitored; and they are no longer part-and-parcel of hospitalization in an intensive care setting. Hospitals now must be accountable for their outcomes, although research results linking reimbursement to outcomes in a pay-for-performance model have been mixed [4, 5].

Evolution of a Safety Culture

Hospitals have begun learning how to improve safety and quality from industries such as aviation and nuclear power operations [6]. These complex organizations are mindful of failures, as well as of successes; and they focus on system solutions and standardization of processes as a means to improve safety. Preoccupation with failure and the relentless pursuit of improvement are ways that high-reliability organizations produce fewer than the expected number of problem events for a given high-risk situation [7, 8]. For hospitals to take on a likeness of a high reliability organization, they must focus on detecting errors and improving faulty processes with the goal of reducing the risk of recurring errors [9]. The mindset needed to drive change toward institutional improvement starts by a better understanding of how errors are committed. The epidemiology of errors in pediatric hospital care has been recently reviewed [8].

The Children's Hospital of Michigan Safety Story

The commitment to patient safety needs to permeate throughout the hospital. This commitment must begin at the highest levels of the organization, including the Board of Trustees and the executive leadership team. Those at the patient-care level must also hold this same commitment-, including nursing, physicians, pharmacists, radiology technicians, transportation services, and environmental services.

Children's Hospital of Michigan (CHM) is a 228-bed, freestanding pediatric hospital founded more than 125 years ago. This urban hospital is staffed by pediatric medical and surgical specialists who serve children in the local community, in addition to children across the region and state. The Hospital is the lone pediatric center in a larger, seven-hospital medical system. Like most pediatric hospitals, CHM offers comprehensive and specialized care, including programs for solid organ and bone marrow transplantation and burn and trauma care.

The hospital strives to be the best, but achieving quality requires establishing appropriate metrics, such rates of central-line associated bloodstream infections, and showing that data pertaining to these metrics have improved over baseline and benchmarked values.

When we decided we could do more to improve safety, we formed workgroups, such as our hospital safety event team (HSET), and implemented our daily "safety huddle" to begin changing our institutional culture. Importantly, we also engaged our board of trustees early on. These steps set the stage for several initiatives, especially in training our staff on error prevention techniques and on the importance of event reporting. Firmly engaging staff in this way has been critical to achieving and sustaining our success in quality and safety initiatives.

Staff Training in Safety Initiatives

Both our medical staff and other hospital personnel were trained in error-prevention techniques. Mandatory workshops and on line tutorials were instituted to increase the skills and engagement of physicians, nurses, and support staff. Safety coaches were identified among hospital leaders in an effort to reinforce safety principles and to disseminate updates on new safety initiatives. This training in error recognition and prevention strategies created the necessary building blocks to drive event reporting, which is so critical to our improvement efforts. A key message to staff was that patient safety is everyone's responsibility. A second key message was that anyone who witnesses an unsafe situation has the duty to speak up and change the situation in the interest of patient safety.

Reporting Safety Events

As earlier discussed, high reliability organizations have a high sensitivity to operations-the systems and processes that influence patient care, and are preoccupied with failure-looking at near misses as opportunities to improve these systems and processes to safeguard against recurrence [10]. The need to report errors is paramount to becoming a high reliability organization. Categorizing error reports by event type and responsible service allows us to develop or improve strategies to prevent recurrence. Creating a culture of expectation around event reporting is essential; event reporting must be seen by every employee as a responsibility needed to improve hospital safety.

Identifying barriers to reporting is also important because an arduous, time-consuming process discourages consistent reporting. An anonymous reporting process can reassure employees that reporting is safe if they fear retaliation for "whistle blowing". These fears should subside as the safety culture becomes further embedded in the institution.

Creating a culture of increased reporting is necessary for success of a patient safety program. The result of an aggressive reporting environment, is a large number of reports that must be sorted through and organized in a meaningful way. Our quality team, which is comprised of the Director of Quality, the Chief Medical Officer, and other members of HSET, has developed a systematic way to organize these event reports, to direct them to the appropriate service for investigation, and to allow close out of these reports with action plans to enable improvements. Further review of high frequency events, (medication errors, for example), might trigger the development of a work group to focus on common underlying causes of these events. Thus, event reporting is essential to starting the process, but it is the analysis of the events by the quality team that allows a deeper understanding of the opportunities for improvement.

Classifying Safety Events

The Healthcare Performance Improvement system classifies an event as a near miss, a precursor event, or a serious safety event [11]. Near miss events do not reach the patient. Precursor events reach the patient but result in no or only minor, temporary harm, such as a wrong dose of medication that has no adverse effect. A serious safety event reaches the patient and causes moderate to severe temporary harm, permanent harm, or death. An example of a serious safety event would be a wrong dose of medication that leads to acute kidney injury requiring hemodialysis and placement of a hemodialysis catheter. Although this error caused only temporary harm, the need to subject the patient to additional procedures and their associated risks makes this error a serious safety event. This classification system allows us to report our near miss-to-safety-event percentage: the number of near-miss events divided by the total number of safety events. This percentage is reported on our hospital safety dashboard to increase the visibility of events and to reinforce the importance of protecting our patients against harm.

Celebrating and Rewarding Success

We acknowledge successes in error prevention. A medication error caught by a pharmacist or nurse can turn a potential serious safety event into a near miss error instead. These "Great Catches" occur throughout the institution: a transporter recognizes that two patients with the same last name are to be taken to radiology and takes the time to determine which patient is which, or a housekeeper calls attention to an unusual odor in a cleaning closet before a chemical spill worsens. We publicly celebrate and recognize these Great Catches in hospital town hall meetings-large employee forums led quarterly by the hospital president, which focuses on new activities and accomplishments of the hospital. We also acknowledge the individuals privately with a thank you note and a copy of the Great Catch announcement to the responsible individual(s). In general, the staff response to this approach has been to embrace our safety culture, which is paramount, because the staff will make or break the overall success of a quality improvement program.

Investigating Safety Events

Converting reported error events into quality improvement changes requires effort. We can inform leaders of safety concerns in several ways. We first describe these ways before describing our investigations.

Notification Mechanisms for Safety Concerns

The Safety Huddle

At CHM, we begin each weekday morning with a "safety huddle." This 30-min meeting is attended by the hospital president, chief nursing officer, and chief operating officer, and is led by the chief medical officer. Other attendees include nurse leaders from various acute care units, including neonatal and pediatric intensive care, and clinical service areas, such as the emergency department, operating room, radiology, and pharmacy. Other attendees come from quality, risk management, transportation, facilities, environmental services, social work, and care management.

Each meeting is begun with the discussion of Great Catches in the past 24 h, followed by the reporting of serious safety events. The former sets the tone of the meeting by celebrating success and helping others feel empowered to share their successes and encourage their front-line staff to participate. The latter helps hospital leadership quickly identify problems. At huddle, we may learn of critical supply shortages with equipment, pharmacy, or staff. We may learn of a new safety event that occurred a few hours before huddle, which has not yet made it through our event-reporting pathway. Whenever safety events are discussed, those reporting are asked to be certain that an event report is also filed to assist with our follow-up investigation and accounting of event occurrences.

Daily Summary Reports and Hospital Safety Event Team

Our quality department sorts the event reports from the prior 24 h by location of occurrence and severity (near miss, precursor, or serious safety events) and records them in a spreadsheet. This daily report is circulated to quality and safety leaders 2 h before safety huddle. This spreadsheet helps bridge the gap between safety huddle meetings. The daily report includes relatively minor events (e.g., infiltrated intravenous catheters) as well as any major events that occurred after the previous day's safety huddle, thereby giving leaders a preview of a safety huddle discussion for that morning.

The HSET consists of the directors of quality, risk management, and pharmacy; the chief and associate chief medical officers; and the chief nursing officer. At weekly meetings, the Team looks for trends in precursor events and identifies those that require more detailed investigation. Team members review non-physician event reports and the corresponding responses from the supervisors overseeing the front line staff involved. Hospital leaders are reminded to complete the investigation of events in a reasonable time and receive feedback about the event and its associated response. Providing feedback to hospital staff is important because it emphasizes that time spent entering event reports is valued by hospital leadership. Further, highlighting changes made in response to an event report helps validate the difference that event reporting can make in improving patient safety.

The HSET focuses primarily on precursor and serious safety events. Events deemed worthy of a deeper level of investigation might be subjected to a Root Cause Analysis or a Peer Review Root Cause Analysis (see below). Minor, physician-related events are sent for traditional peer review.

Root Cause Analysis

One way we review errors is with a retrospective, systems-based process called root cause analysis (RCA). The events selected for RCA include serious safety events, and precursor or near miss events with potential for severe harm. We cannot depend on good fortune when a potential serious event occurs; the focus has to be on understanding why it occurred.

The HSET determines who should be invited to the RCA, and attendance is expected; a conference call is also arranged to encourage maximal participation. Invitees include any front-line staff relevant to the event. The standing membership is essentially the HSET team, thereby allowing consistency in the meeting format. The meeting is led by our quality director, and tension is quickly diffused by introductions and establishing the ground rules of a non-blame environment. We seek to understand the problem so we can identify system solutions and realize long-term improvement. The team utilizes "fish bone" diagrams to identify cause-and-effect relationships among factors that may have led to or contributed to the event. Everyone is invited to share his or her understanding of the situation. The meeting is concluded with a thank you to all participants, and an action item list is disseminated 1–2 days later with assignments to individuals responsible for driving change.

Peer Review and Peer Review RCA

Peer review is the methodology we use to evaluate physicians. Our team includes our pediatrician-in-chief and our surgeon-in-chief. The process begins with the quality department reassigning the event report to the division chief overseeing the involved physician; the division chief's response is then sent back to the quality department.

The peer review committee reviews both the event and the chief's response without knowing the name of the physician involved. The event, not the individual, is reviewed, and a ruling of not preventable, possibly preventable, or preventable is rendered, and whether or not harm has occurred. After the event is scored, the physician name is revealed so that the pediatrician-in-chief or surgeon-in-chief can note that information. A letter is then sent to the involved physician informing him or her of the committee's decision. Descriptions of preventable and possibly preventable events are placed in the physician's file, which is available to the chief when privileges are up for renewal.

Serious events that involve physician judgment or behaviors are investigated in a peer-review RCA; attendees at this meeting that are involved in the analysis include: our peer review committee, directors of quality and risk management, and the involved physician(s). This format allows a more expedient response to serious matters and allows the discussion to be documented. The event is also classified regarding its preventability and associated harm.

Involvement of the Hospital Board

Sustaining the highest safety and quality standards requires that they be a core value throughout the organization [12]. Safety and quality must be topics of conversation at every huddle and at every conference so that they are always seen as priorities. At Children's Hospital of Michigan, we are blessed with a highly engaged board of trustees comprised of community leaders, many of whom have a personal connection to our hospital. It is a volunteer board, but one whose members are passionate about making our hospital safer and better.

Our hospital board has members from the private sector, hospital executive leadership, and physician leaders and meets quarterly. Because a major focus of our board is quality and safety, we are fortunate to have a quality committee within the board, which meets bimonthly. This committee is co-chaired by the vice chair of our board, who has an engineering background and extensive experience in quality and safety management in the automotive industry. Other members of the committee come from the manufacturing, healthcare services, automotive, and retail sectors. Our meetings focus on discussing quality results. A healthy dialogue from our non-hospital board members challenges us to think differently.

One outcome of our quality committee was our Quality-Safety Education Day, which took place in May 2012, for hospital managers and supervisors. The workshop was hosted by our chief medical officer and led by our quality committee members who invited colleagues with expertise in process improvement. The morning featured didactic sessions on process-improvement techniques and problem-solving strategies used in the automotive and healthcare manufacturing industries. Key concepts from these sessions included the importance of identifying an "Interim Containment Action" plan, or "tourniquet" whenever a problem is identified [13]. These sessions emphasized the need to immediately stop the problem from happening elsewhere as soon as the circumstances leading to it are identified. Developing a perfect solution to a problem can take several months, but the problem must not be allowed to recur in the meantime.

Specific safety concerns were the focus of the afternoon session. Two workgroups were formed, and attention was directed at two areas of need: reducing central-line associated bloodstream infections and improving the early recognition of sepsis in children. After a case presentation highlighting the problem, attendees, including our guests with expertise in Six Sigma process improvement techniques, suggested alternative approaches to these important clinical problems. At the end of the day, both work groups reconvened and reported their recommendations.

The workshop was well received by participants, who saw it as evidence that our hospital board and executive leadership were committed to improving quality and safety. The workshop definitely helped jump-start our quality and safety journey. It emphasized to the doctors and nurses struggling with these issues that central-line associated bloodstream infections and delayed recognition of pediatric sepsis were hospital-wide problems that were taken seriously by the entire hospital, not simply by those in the pediatric intensive care units and emergency departments.

Outcomes

The impact of our safety culture can be measured in several ways. Qualitatively, the staff may speak the language of safety, but have our efforts really translated into meaningful results and, if so, what are they?

Increased Event Reporting

As noted earlier, to reduce serious safety events, the hospital needs to increase the number of events reported to capture more near miss events. A hospital whose culture encourages event reporting often sees a sharp increase in the number of reported safety events early on [11]. The goal of event reporting, however, is to first increase the number reported so that all events are known and then to shift the percentages away from serious events toward near miss and precursor events.

We track reports every month (Table 25.1). Event reporting increased by 12 % from 2011 to 2012 and by another 28 % from 2012 levels in 2013. These trends indicate that the staff is making safety a high priority.

Table 25.1 Event Reports for the Children's Hospital of Michigan, 2011–2013

Fiscal year	Average number of event reports per month	Reporting rate per 10,000 adjusted patient days	Percent change from prior year	Percent change from 2011 baseline rate
2011	187	…	…	…
2012	211	483	+12.2	+12.2
2013	270	644	+28.0	+43.6

Other Safety Metrics

Hand Hygiene Adherence

Hand hygiene was a metric that challenged us for some time. We measured adherence with "secret shopper" observations in various hospital settings, such as the acute care units, emergency department, operating room, and ambulatory clinics. Adherence was 86.5 % from July 2010 through April 2011. Until then, a non-blame, accountability culture predominated. Although this tradition is in keeping with our general approach to quality and safety, it is difficult to not assign some level of personal accountability for washing one's hands [14, 15]. As such, we placed a new emphasis on hand hygiene scores as a first step in reducing hospital-associated infections.

Our hand-hygiene compliance officers were re-educated about reporting. No longer was the epidemiology department content with generic designations such as "nurse," "resident," "medical student," or "transporter"; we now expected the compliance officers to report specifics such as, "resident John Smith was observed not washing his hands before entering a room on hospital ward X at 2 PM on June 8, 2011." Reports with this degree of specificity were gathered over a month and shared with the hospital chief medical officer, who drafted an e-mail to the leader overseeing the responsible individual. The baseline period lasted from May 2011 through June 2011. One year later, the hand hygiene adherence rate had increased to 98.7 %. Our methodology changed slightly in July 2012 when we allowed parents to assess hand hygiene adherence with a questionnaire in select outpatient clinics. The result for fiscal 2013 was 96 %. Increased awareness and monitoring with feedback markedly improved and sustained hand hygiene.

Hospital Acquired Infections

The rates of central-line associated bloodstream infections and catheter-associated urinary tract infections should be reduced by improved hand hygiene. Both causes of infections have been tracked hospital-wide for some time. We hypothesized that both rates would decrease by the increased emphasis on infection prevention, such as improving hand hygiene. Of course, we use an insertion-bundle checklist for central-line placement; the importance of this approach has been well described [16, 17]. Indeed, both infection rates declined significantly. These favorable trends reflect an institutional commitment to safety and quality beginning with hand hygiene, reduction of catheter usage, and timely removal of indwelling devices whenever possible. The improvement in these important hospital safety metrics has many implications: first and foremost, patient safety is improved; second, hospitalization costs and patient length of stay are decreased.

As a testament to our improved safety scores, The Leapfrog Group recognized CHM as 1 of 13 Top Children's Hospitals in 2013; our last receipt of this designation was in 2008. The criteria used for award qualification included best safety practices to reduce medication errors (computerized physician order entry-a Leapfrog recommended practice), adequacy of intensive care unit (ICU) physician staffing, low frequency of never events, and low rates of hospital acquired conditions such as infections [18].

Lessons Learned

As we have continued our safety journey, we have tried to use the results of our root cause analysis as "take away lessons." One issue consistently identified during our patient safety event investigations has been communication breakdowns, in which nurses and residents are reluctant to escalate safety concerns to their supervising nurses and/or attendings, respectively. Too often, for example, a nurse had repeatedly contacted the resident on call, despite the fact that this individual's response was suboptimal. One outcome from our quality

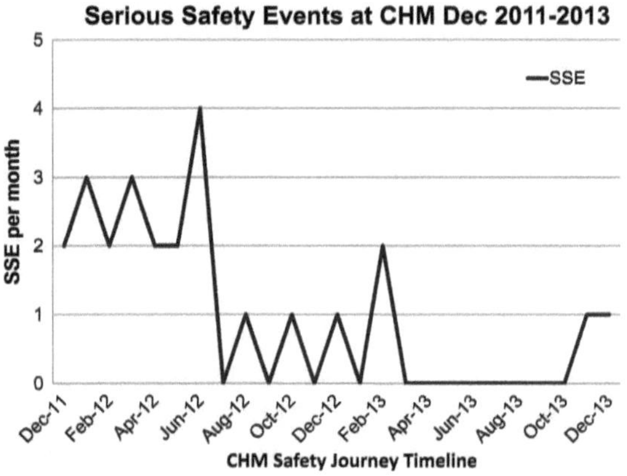

Fig. 25.1 The frequency of serious safety events at Children's Hospital of Michigan, 2012 and 2013. A serious safety event reaches the patient and causes moderate to severe temporary harm, permanent harm, or death

department was our "escalation communication algorithm." This tool empowers nurses to pursue the issue with supervisors above a resident if they are concerned. For stable patients, the nurse is asked to wait no more than 20 min for an appropriate response and to shorten the wait to 10 min if the patient's clinical status is concerning. Of course, if the patient is unstable, a rapid response or code blue can be called at any time. The escalation pathway moves from the senior resident, to the fellow (if applicable), to the responsible attending, to the Division Chief overseeing the responsible attending, to the Specialist-in-Chief (either the Pediatrician-in-Chief or the Surgeon-in-Chief) to the Chief Medical Officer, to the hospital president. This tool, in conjunction with our aggressive event reporting and our relentless commitment to safety, has reduced the frequency of serious safety events over the past 25 months from 2.6 events/month for the first 7 months to 0.6 events/month for the next 8 months, followed by 0.2 events/month for the most recent 10 months (Fig. 25.1).

An example of an action item from a hospital safety event included the development of white "time out" boards, which have traditionally been used in operating rooms (Fig. 25.2). The time-out board used in our cardiac catheterization lab has checklist items on patient demographics, important laboratory values, and safety items, such as confirmation that two forms of identification were used to confirm the patient's identify, the

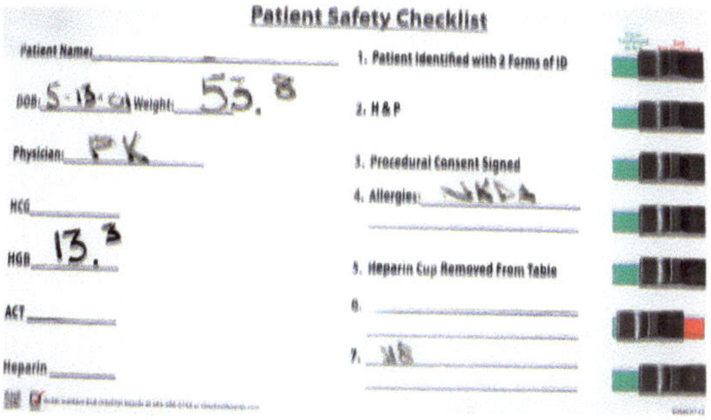

Fig. 25.2 A Patient Safety Checklist on a white board in a cardiac catheterization lab at the Children's Hospital of Michigan. The checklist has helped the Hospital reduce the likelihood of safety events occurring during cardiac catheterizations

consent form was signed, allergies were confirmed, and that the heparin cup had been removed from the procedure table. This checklist has increased the likelihood of performing cardiac catheterizations without incident.

Conclusions

The safety journey at our hospital is well underway, but more work is needed. We need to continue to learn from our quality and safety investigations and to translate these lessons into better value. This chapter described our efforts to improve hand hygiene and to lower the rates of hospital-acquired infections and serious safety events. Our future efforts need to further and sustain these improvements at lower costs. The Detroit Children's hospital will continue to be a model of leadership for driving quality improvement at lower costs for pediatric healthcare.

References

1. Medicine Io. To Err is human: building a safer health system. Washington, DC: National Academies Press; 1999.
2. CMS.gov. Hospital value-based purchasing. Centers for Medicare & Medicaid Services [Website]. 2014. Accessed 2nd Jan 2014.
3. Porter ME. What is value in health care? N Engl J Med. 2010;363(26):2477–81.
4. Calikoglu S, Murray R, Feeney D. Hospital pay-for-performance programs in Maryland produced strong results, including reduced hospital-acquired conditions. Health Aff (Project Hope). 2012;31(12):2649–58.
5. Lee GM, Kleinman K, Soumerai SB, et al. Effect of nonpayment for preventable infections in U.S. hospitals. N Engl J Med. 2012;367(15):1428–37.
6. Nance JJ. Why hospitals should fly: the ultimate flight plan to patient safety and quality care. Bozeman: Second River Healthcare Press; 2008.
7. Weick KE, Sutcliffe KM. Managing the unexpected: assuring high performance in an age of complexity. San Francisco: Jossey-Bass; 2001.
8. Steering Committee on Quality Improvement and Management and Committee on Hospital Care. Policy statement–principles of pediatric patient safety: reducing harm due to medical care. Pediatrics. 2011;127(6):1199–210.
9. Leonard MS. Patient safety and quality improvement: medical errors and adverse events. Pediatr Rev. 2010;31(4):151–8.
10. Hines S, Luna K, Lofthus J, et al. Becoming a high reliability organization: operational advice for hospital leaders. Rockville: Agency for Healthcare Research Quality Publication; 2008; No. 08–0022.
11. Throop C, Stockmeier C. The HPI SEC & SSER Patient Safety Measurement System for Healthcare. HPI white paper series. 2009.
12. Millar R, Mannion R, Freeman T, Davies HT. Hospital board oversight of quality and patient safety: a narrative review and synthesis of recent empirical research. Milbank Q. 2013;91(4):738–70.
13. Stamatis DH. Six sigma and beyond: problem solving and basic mathematics. Boca Raton: St. Lucie Press (CRC Press); 2002.
14. Goldmann D. System failure versus personal accountability–the case for clean hands. N Engl J Med. 2006;355(2):121–3.
15. Wachter RM, Pronovost PJ. Balancing "no blame" with accountability in patient safety. N Engl J Med. 2009;361(14):1401–6.
16. Pronovost P, Needham D, Berenholtz S, et al. An intervention to decrease catheter-related bloodstream infections in the ICU. N Engl J Med. 2006;355(26):2725–32.
17. Gawande A. The checklist manifesto: how to get things right. New York: Metropolitan Books; Henry Holt and Company; 2009.
18. Group TL. The Leapfrog Group 2013 Top Hospital Methodology and Description. 2014. http://www.leapfroggroup.org/media/file/2013TopHospitalMethodology.pdf. Accessed 2nd Sept 2014.

Resilience and Systems Engineering

26

Karen Harrington and Peter C. Laussen

Abstract

Pediatric cardiac surgery is a complex, high-risk field characterized by a vulnerable patient population, technically demanding surgery, and technological and team challenges. Human factor studies have identified the importance of teamwork, communication, and standardization of some processes of care to improve outcomes. With demonstrable improvement in safety still lacking, continued reflection is warranted on the fundamental concepts which underlie safety efforts. Most studies have adapted a linear accident model with emphasis on error commission and recovery, adverse events, and latent conditions. More recent approaches to safety based on systems and resilience engineering are more applicable to complex systems of care, such as cardiac surgery. Systems engineering seeks to minimize risk through redesign. Resilience engineering explores how individuals and organizations negotiate complexity to *create* safety.

Keywords

Pediatric cardiac surgery • Patient safety • Accident model • Complexity • Systems engineering • Resilience

K. Harrington MDCM, MSc (✉)
Departments of Pediatrics and Critical Care,
CHU Ste Justine, 3175 Côte Ste Catherine,
Montreal, QC H3T 1C5, Canada
e-mail: karen.harrington.hsj@ssss.gouv.qc.ca

P.C. Laussen, MBBS, FCICM
Department of Critical Care Medicine,
The Hospital for Sick Children, Toronto, ON, Canada

Department of Anaesthesia, University
of Toronto, 555 University Avenue,
Toronto, ON M5G 1X8, Canada
e-mail: peter.laussen@sickkids.ca

Introduction

It has been over a decade since the Institute of Medicine Report (IOM), To Err is Human [1] with alarming estimates of preventable medical harm. The report demanded a new approach to safety, highlighted systemic issues, and called for a 50 % reduction in medical errors by 2004. This was not achieved, despite dedicated efforts at local, regional and national levels, as well as

P.R. Barach, J.P. Jacobs, S.E. Lipshultz, P.C. Laussen (eds.),
Pediatric and Congenital Cardiac Care: Volume 2: Quality Improvement and Patient Safety,
DOI 10.1007/978-1-4471-6566-8_26, © Springer-Verlag London 2015

turning to other high-risk industries and organizational safety models for instruction.

Initiatives to improve patient safety have continued to gain momentum over recent years, yet it is worthwhile to remember that significant efforts to improve safety and outcomes had already started within pediatric cardiac surgery prior to the IOM report being published. Marc de Leval introduced the concept of human factors to the field [2] and adapted an organizational accident model to study the role of human factors in surgical outcomes [3]. Two high profile inquiries into pediatric cardiac surgery deaths in the United Kingdom [4] and in Canada [5] highlighted the presence of system-wide problems, which echoed the call for a systemic approach to safety in the treatment of children with congenital heart disease.

More than a decade after the first IOM report, and despite significant effort and financial investment, it is unclear in fact if patient safety has improved [6–9]. While efforts have gone into refining error counting and data collection, continued reflection is warranted not only on how to reliably measure safety [8], but also on the fundamental concepts of safety that guide our safety improvement efforts.

All efforts to improve safety are based on an underlying understanding, and conceptual model, of safety and risk. As in many industries, traditional emphasis in healthcare has been on the frontline practitioner, and more recently a linear accident model has been applied to explore all contributing factors. Complex linear accident models portray adverse events as the results of a chain of events and failures, which may be active or latent [10]. Linear models are appealing for their clarity and ease of understanding, and they offer conceptually straightforward solutions: eliminate root causes, strengthen defences, and/or introduce barriers between the hazard and the patient. The very simplicity that makes them appealing, however, limits their applicability to complex systems. By artificially simplifying complex interactions into linear causal chains, the adaptive function that a "failure" in one chain of events may have in another system function is not recognized. Opportunities to explore *why* people acted as they did are limited, and solutions (for example, punishing/banning certain actions or introducing barriers) may inadvertently introduce more complexity and risk into the system.

While fault-based and linear accident models may remain useful in simple systems, in which processes are linear and there is one best way of doing things, they are insufficient to adequately describe risks in complex systems. With the development of increasingly complex systems scientific thinking about safety has increasingly moved towards a "systemic view", in which outcomes are seen to emerge from the complex functioning of the system as a whole [11], It is not sufficient to understand and improve the function of one system component; interdependencies and relationships must be recognized, explored, and optimized.

Safety research in pediatric cardiac surgery has developed in a parallel course to safety theory in general, concentrating first on the performance of the individual surgeon [2], with more recent studies highlighting team and organizational factors [3, 12, 13]. Methods and measures have predominantly been adapted from a linear accident model (Swiss Cheese analogy [10], with an emphasis on error commission and recovery, adverse events, and latent conditions. The existing research has identified the importance of teamwork, communication, and standardization of some processes of care.

Pediatric cardiac surgical care delivery *is* a complex system. It is characterized by a highly vulnerable patient population, technically demanding surgery, complex monitoring and life support technology, and the coming together of individuals from several disciplines to form a team at each stage of patient care. Advances in diagnosis, surgical technique, perfusion and ICU management have allowed younger, patients with more complex lesions to be treated, and survival has increased significantly. Paradoxically, these same advances have also increased system complexity and introduced new sources of risk that cannot adequately be studied and addressed using a linear accident model.

This chapter will briefly review the contributions and limitations of the linear accident model to our understanding of safety in pediatric cardiac surgery. It will then discuss two systems approaches to safety in complex systems, systems engineering and resilience engineering. The approaches are complementary when studying a complex socio-technical system. Systems engineering emphasizes design and process and seeks to minimize risk through system redesign, and resilience engineering has a stronger focus on the human dimension, exploring how individuals and organizations create safety by managing complexity.

Traditional View of Safety: The "Person Model"

> I will prescribe regimens for the good of my patients according to my ability and my judgment and never do harm to anyone -Hippocratic Oath, 4th Century BC

The traditional understanding of safety, in healthcare as in other industries, emphasizes the frontline individual's contribution to an outcome. The underlying belief is that competent individuals will produce a desired, "safe" outcome. Undesired outcomes are the result of error, and error is caused by incompetence or complacency. In this view, sometimes called the "bad apple theory", the system is inherently safe, but is threatened by incompetent or complacent individuals (bad apples). Once offending individuals are identified, removed, or rehabilitated ("naming, shaming, blaming, retraining") [14], system safety is restored.

Belief in the bad apple/person model of safety remains strong in healthcare. The medical culture is rooted in a deep sense of personal responsibility, accountability and patient ownership [15]. Healthcare, and especially surgery, is often delivered in a one-to-one or few-to-one manner [16], and patients as well as healthcare professionals believe that safety "lies foremost in the hands through which care ultimately flows to the patient" [17]. As such, poor surgical outcome is still often ultimately concluded to be the "fault" of an individual surgeon. A failed intubation attempt or line insertion is due to the lack of skill, error or complacency of the anesthetist. A medication error is caused by the incompetence or carelessness of the doctor prescribing, or the nurse administering the drug.

While individual competence remains essential, and while a high degree of personal accountability is laudable, as Dekker asks: *are individual virtue, competence, and strength of character the only things, the main things, we want to rely on"* [17] to optimize patient safety? Is the system so frail that the difference between a good outcome and catastrophe is one person?

The deeply held belief that competence equals perfection, that error equals incompetence, and that good doctors do not make mistakes has fostered a culture of secrecy, shame, and blame that has not only limited opportunities for safety learning, but offers few strategies for safety growth beyond insisting that people be better and try harder. Far from producing demonstrable improvement in safety, this is the approach that is alleged to cause upwards of 100,000 deaths each year in the United States alone. The first IOM report [1], the Bristol inquiry [4] and the Winnipeg inquiry [5] all demanded a new approach to patient safety, moving beyond the traditional person-based model to examine systemic factors.

Early "Systems" Approach: The Linear Accident Model

> Rather than being the main instigators of an accident, operators tend to be the inheritors of system defects. Their part is that of adding the final garnish to a lethal brew that has been long in the cooking." Reason [18]

At the time that safety research in pediatric cardiac surgery began, James Reason's Swiss cheese analogy [10] had recently emerged. It has provided the framework for most of the safety research in this field.

The Swiss cheese analogy is a linear accident model. An accident is seen as the result of a number of contributing factors, some active and some latent, that come together at a particular place and time. Reason's metaphor describes layers of defenses, barriers and safeguards between a hazard and its potential victim. The Swiss cheese imagery refers to the weaknesses ("holes") that exist in each defensive layer. Weaknesses are the result of "active failures' by people- slips, lapses, fumbles, mistakes and procedural violations- and of "latent conditions" within the system itself, for example, understaffing or chronic worker fatigue resulting from managerial decisions. An accident occurs when the holes in many layers line up, allowing the hazard through. In this model, risk can be managed proactively by tracing back and eliminating the root cause, by identifying and remedying latent conditions in the system and/or by introducing barriers into the hazard trajectory.

The Swiss cheese metaphor has been widely adopted in healthcare and in safety research in pediatric cardiac surgery [3, 12, 13, 19]. In this analogy, if the "hazard" is improper transfer of a coronary artery during the arterial switch operation, layers "upstream" from the surgeon might include pre-operative diagnosis and decision-making and latent conditions in the cardiac surgery department, hospital management, and healthcare organization [20] causing distraction and suboptimal surgical performance. A layer "downstream" might be diagnostic techniques to detect the coronary problem before separation from cardiopulmonary bypass, allowing immediate revision. A "hole" in this layer of defense could be failure by the cardiologist to identify an incorrect coronary attachment on the postoperative echocardiogram. A "hole" in the anesthesia layer of defense might be *"cognitive tunnel vision on insertion of lines to the neglect of monitoring the ECG screen* [3], which could delay the identification of patient instability and reevaluation of coronary blood flow.

Contributions and Limitations of the Linear Accident Model

> One of the greatest obstacles to progress on safety is, paradoxically, the attraction of neat solutions
> -Charles Vincent [21]

There is no doubt that the widespread adoption of the linear accident model has added to our understanding of adverse events in healthcare. It has helped to deflect blame from frontline workers and to increase our awareness of upstream factors. Safety studies in pediatric cardiac surgery have used a linear accident model to highlight the importance of teamwork, clear communication, and standardization of some processes. But is a linear accident model such as the Swiss cheese metaphor *sufficient* to understand safety? Does it accurately and fully describe how things go wrong, and more importantly for future learning, does it explain *why* they did?

Paradoxically, the very simplicity that has given the linear accident model such appeal and resulted in its widespread use may hinder further progress on safety by artificially reducing the complexity of real work. The model reduces complex interactions into artificially simple linear sequences, and hindsight provides a seemingly predictable view of the path to failure. The inherent outcome bias of an accident model further limits progress on safety by labeling behavior and actions as errors and failures, rather than considering alternative explanations for why people behaved as they did with the information available to them at the time.

Using a linear accident model approach, a multi-center study of human factors in the arterial switch operation [3] classified similar events as "minor" or "major" according to outcome. For example, *"cognitive tunnel vision on insertion of lines to the neglect of monitoring the ECG screen (where no major event results)"* is classified as a minor event, while *"delayed diagnosis of a major deterioration in the patient's condition"* [3] is listed as a major event. In this case, who determines that tunnel vision and neglect of monitoring occurs? If line insertion was difficult, was the attentiveness of the anesthetist to the task of inserting the lines "tunnel vision", and was it inappropriate? The same behavior "event" can therefore be classified as either minor or major *according to the outcome.*

The linear accident model has increased our understanding of upstream contributions to accidents by identifying vulnerabilities throughout the system, rather than implicating only the frontline worker. However, over reliance on the linear accident model may hinder further progress in safety by artificially representing complex processes as linear sequences, and by concluding the investigation at the identification of fault or error rather than considering how observed actions made sense to clinicians at the time. Beyond sequencing observable events and listing problems, a different mental model and tools are required to develop meaningful understanding of complex work [22].

Systems Approach to Safety

Faced with increasingly complex systems that stretched the limits of traditional industrial accident models and safety engineering techniques [11], scientific thinking about safety has evolved towards a "systems view", in which outcomes are seen to emerge from the complex functioning of the system as a whole.

The International Council of Systems Engineering (INCOSE) [23] defines a system as:

> A system is a construct or collection of different elements that together produce results not obtainable by the elements alone. The elements, or parts, can include people, hardware, software, facilities, policies, and documents; that is, all things required to produce systems-level results. The results include system level qualities, properties, characteristics, functions, behaviour, and performance. The value added by the system as a whole, beyond that contributed independently by the parts, is primarily created by the relationship among the parts; that is, how they are interconnected.

Reductionist approaches to improve safety by optimizing individual system components are simply not sufficient in complex systems; relationships and interdependencies between different parts of a system must be understood (systems analysis) in order to identify areas of vulnerability that can be improved through design (systems engineering).

Karsh and Alper [24] describes the main steps shared by several systems analysis methodologies:

1. Determine what system will be the subject of analysis
2. Produce a preliminary work system map.
3. Using the preliminary work system map, identify stakeholders in the system under analysis.
4. Stakeholders conduct an initial scan of the system by gauging the accuracy of the preliminary work system map and by "scanning the horizon" for upcoming internal or external factors that could impact the system.
5. Set boundaries on the system, realizing that setting them too narrow may miss important variables and setting boundaries wide will increase analysis time.
6. Determine specific, measurable performance goals for each step in the system.
7. Begin formal data collection to revise and update the work system map, gauge current performance, and determine baseline measures that will be used to evaluate the effectiveness of system redesign.
8. Analyse data in order to identify weaknesses and prioritize areas for redesign.
9. Develop control strategies for identified hazards.
10. Conduct a system analysis on the redesign hazard-control ideas prior to implementation.

This framework can be applied at a regional or national healthcare level to describe the current structure of healthcare delivery and identify targets for change [25]. It can also be applied at an institutional and clinical microsystem level [26–29] to provide a meaningful blueprint of local work systems by which events can be analysed and processes understood and redesigned.

Barach and Johnson [26] used systems analysis to develop a process map of pediatric cardiac surgical care. Note that each step in the larger system process map can represent a process map of its own; boundaries may be set large initially and then narrowed depending on the focus of analysis and complexity of clinical steps involved (see Fig. 3.3).

The authors suggest the following questions when developing and analysing the process map:

- What is the goal of the process?
- Does the process work as it should?
- Are there obvious redundancies or complexities?
- How different is the current process from the ideal process?
- What are the various factions within the larger group, and how does this division support/hinder more effective processing of patient care?
- What are the work-arounds to the proscribed process?

A key concept is that a work process is mapped *as it is* rather than as *it is desired* in order to identify areas of vulnerability. This is a fundamental difference from the widespread accident model approach, in which events associated with an undesired outcome are judged against an imagined ideal process. For example, consider the event (failure): "cognitive tunnel vision on insertion of lines to the neglect of monitoring the ECG screen" [3] against the backdrop of the process map. What is the usual process for line insertion, and under what circumstances- how does it interact with other elements of the surgical process map? What are the constraints (eg time pressure from surgical team?) and competing demands (eg insert line while also responsible to watch the monitor). Are there redundancies and/or safeguards (eg audible alarm on monitor? Second person assigned to watch monitor and respond while anesthetist is occupied with line insertion task?). By moving beyond identifying that a behaviour or process was not ideal to explore *why* (beyond calling it an error or failure), valuable information is obtained about the competing pressures and inter-dependent elements that make up normal work, which can then inform system redesign.

The systems approach and systems engineering offer tremendous opportunities for safety learning and improvement in healthcare. Engaging engineering partnerships at the sharp end of healthcare delivery will be essential at local as well as the national level to develop a systems approach.

Resilience Engineering

The systems approach introduced the idea of safety emerging from interactions among system parts. Systems engineering seeks to minimize risk by optimizing design, with an emphasis on structure and processes.

Resilience engineering adds the dimension that while certain risks may be decreased through redesign, *risk cannot be eliminated*, and that in complex systems, risks are ever changing. Safety, then, is not something that a system *has* by design and *maintains* by following procedure. Rather, safety is something that people and organizations *create*, by recognizing and negotiating constantly changing conditions, pressures and competing demands [30]. In this view, "failure" is not caused by deviations in standard procedure, as deviations and workarounds are recognized as adaptations developed to handle complexity. Failure is the (temporary) inability to cope with complexity. As such, risk is not "managed" by limiting performance variation and adding barriers and constraints (which, paradoxically, increase system complexity). Rather, risk is understood as emerging from competing demands and limited resources that make tradeoffs, workarounds and performance variation necessary. Safety is not defined solely as the *absence* of adverse events, but is explored as the *presence* of resilience: "the ability of an organization to continue operations during and after a major mishap or in the presence of continued significant stresses" [31].

Resilience engineering does not abandon the study of accidents, rather it *adds* the dimension of studying normal work in order to identify conflicting goal pressures, safety boundaries, and leadership and teamwork characteristics that may both create success and become vulnerabilities at times of stress.

The focus of accident analysis is thus shifted:

> Rather than looking for causes we should look for concurrences, and rather than seeing concurrences as exceptions we should see them as normal and therefore also as inevitable. This may at times lead to the conclusion that even though an accident happened nothing really went wrong, in the sense that nothing happened that was out of the ordinary. Instead it is the occurrence of a number of events, just on the border of the ordinary, that constitutes an explanation of the accident or event [31].

Studies of complex socio-technical systems reveal that there are often mismatches between actual work and written guidelines, and that this is not unique to adverse outcomes [17]. As systems grow in complexity, policies and procedures tend to become less relevant because conditions change too quickly for written guidelines to keep up, and because written guidance cannot capture all the complex adaptations and permutations necessary to maintain production in the face of ever changing resources and conditions. Clinicians work around the rules rather than carelessly disregarding regulations, but they are usually adapting their performance where regulations are underwritten, and are making necessary tradeoffs among competing demands to get things done. Simon called this *satisficing*: a combination of satisfying and sufficing [17]. Hollnagel calls it efficiency-thoroughness tradeoffs (ETTO): *"in their daily activities, at work or at leisure, people routinely make a choice between being effective and being thorough, since it is rarely possible to be both at the same time"* [32]. Production pressures and limited resources demand that people be effective. In hindsight after an accident, it seems clear exactly where they should have been thorough.

Accident analysis will always be subject to hindsight and outcome biases. Investigators must make a concerted effort when reconstructing events to follow the **local rationality principle** [33]: that people behave in a way that is reasonable to them, that makes sense to them given *the way the world looked to them at the time*. People are not deliberately erring, violating and deviating from correct procedure; they are balancing pressures to try to get things done right. What data was available to people at the time? What did the situation look like to them each step of the way? What other pressures existed? Where was their attention focused? Why did they behave the way they did? As Dekker urges: "Be relentless: press on their behavior until it makes sense to you" [33].

Example

Recall the example of an anesthetist's "*cognitive tunnel vision on insertion of lines to the neglect of monitoring the ECG screen*" [3]. The anesthetist is performing at least two simultaneous tasks: that of inserting a line, and that of monitoring the ECG screen. In hindsight after the delayed identification of a problem on the monitor, we assume that the anesthetist had full knowledge of the undesired outcome, and therefore *chose* wrongly to concentrate on the line insertion rather than on the screen. In reality, the anesthetist was attending to and negotiating two (at least) goals and risks: the goal of monitoring, with the risk of not succeeding at line insertion from focusing on the ECG screen and the goal of line insertion, with the risk of missing an important change in vital signs on the monitor. If the "failure" in this case had been an unsuccessful line insertion, the anesthetist could just have easily have been faulted for not paying enough attention to the line and too much attention to the ECG screen. The risk here is not the "erring" anesthetist, but the competing demands. Rather than insisting the anesthetist, in hindsight, choose better, a systems engineering approach would redesign workflow so as to minimize competing demands. Risk cannot be completely eliminated, and so individual and team resilience needs to be increased by explicitly calling attention to sometimes unavoidable competing demands in order to facilitate urgent communication, backup, and teamwork when the undesired situation arise.

Schraagen et al. [34] move away from error-based descriptions in a prospective study of pediatric cardiac surgical microsystems. Using a pre-operative questionnaire to explore team preparedness and intraoperative observations, the authors avoid "error" and "failure" based definitions, and instead introduce the term "non routine event"(NRE), defined as "any event that is perceived by care providers or skilled observers to be unusual, out-of-the-ordinary or atypical". In keeping with previous studies of Human Factors in the operating room [3, 12], more procedural NREs were associated with a more complicated post-operative course. In contrast to previous studies, good teamwork was associated with poorer patient outcomes. The authors believe this may reflect a flaw in previous studies, which rated teamwork mostly in hindsight, with knowledge of the outcome. They suggest that teamwork processes are adaptive mechanisms, emerging primarily when operations become more difficult. They hypothesize that during difficulty, poor teams will display ineffective teamwork while excellent teams such as the one they observed will display good teamwork, even if the outcome is ultimately adverse.

A resilience engineering approach to accidents challenges the strong outcome bias that has dominated traditional accident investigations.

If we accept that a system is complex, and that performance variation is *necessary*, then we must also be prepared to discover that an adverse outcome emerged from the same work processes that usually produce the desired outcome, and that "even though an accident happened, nothing really went wrong, in the sense that nothing happened that was out of the ordinary" [31]. By acknowledging the imperfection of *normal* work, we take the first steps towards a genuine understanding of risk and safety in a complex socio-technical system.

Resilience engineering [31] seeks to expand on the traditional definition safety as the *absence* of an accident or adverse event and explore safety as the *presence* of something: what is it that people do to make things go right? Safety is reframed as the *presence* of resilience. To fully understand safety, we must not only seek to understand accidents, but also to understand how people create success.

Dekker describes four characteristics [30] of resilient organizations:

1. They do not take past success as a guarantee of future safety
2. They keep a discussion of risk alive even when conditions appear safe
3. They are open to new perspectives, invite minority opinions and doubt, and remain curious and sensitized to risk
4. They promote a culture of refusing to trade safety for production concerns.

Is resilience engineering relevant to healthcare systems? There has been a strong held premise in the patient safety movement that all errors are discoverable, and preventable, and that the goal of patient safety should be achieving zero error and zero harm [22]. Yet more than a decade on from the first IOM report, we are no closer to that ambitious goal.

Dekker makes the important distinction between *complicated* and *complex* systems. A *complicated* system may be difficult and intricate, but is "ultimately knowable" [17], can be described, and can be controlled by discovering the one best way to operate. In a complicated system, accidents result from deviation from the one best way of operating. Systems engineering can be used to redesign processes in order to decrease hazards in even very complicated systems. A *complex* system, however, is never fully knowable. Boundaries are blurred; relationships are non-linear and interdependent, in ways that *cannot* be fully appreciated or understood. Success is not guaranteed by designing and following the one-best-way of doing things; there is no one-best way to balance forever changing and competing demands. Success is achieved by constantly adapting to changing conditions and pressures. Failure is not deviation from the one-best-way, but is the inability to adapt to complexity. In order to make meaningful progress in patient safety, we must decide whether healthcare is complicated, or truly complex; the answer is that it shares both properties.

What about pediatric cardiac surgery? It is a high-risk field characterized by a vulnerable patient population, technically demanding surgery, invasive life-support technology, highly technical monitoring systems, and multidisciplinary care teams. Few would argue that the system is complex. Some *elements* of the system are complicated; these are the most readily studied, and it is these elements that have already adopted some degree of standardization. For example, the surgical act of coronary transfer is arguably complicated rather than complex. The physical transfer of a patient, and the structure of a handover, may be complicated rather than complex. The system in which these complicated processes take place though, is complex, characterized by multiple interactions and interdependencies of social and technological actors and components, and at its center, the complexity of a critically ill patient with a limited tolerance of physiological variations, be they the result of error or not. Safety initiatives based on the principle that this system is fully knowable will always come up short.

How Do We Measure Resilience?

One of the greatest challenges facing safety theorists and practitioners is the struggle to demonstrate measurable improvements in safety. The accident-based view of safety is appealing because accidents are visible, and countable. A "measure" of safety based on tallies of preventable adverse events will always be limited, however, by the influences of hindsight and of outcome, which make the determination of preventability very subjective. The resulting numbers may not mean very much at all. Safety as resilience is even more difficult to measure; as visible as accidents are, safety often goes by unnoticed, a "dynamic non-event" [35]. As Galvan stated: "*Despite the results reported in this study*" (which associated negative events with outcome), "***positive** events existed. They were too numerous to record...and they were hard to separate from normal procedures*" [12].

As Carthey states: "the only realistic goal of safety management is to achieve, not zero adverse events, but the maximum degree of intrinsic resistance *consistent with the organization's reason for existence*" [20]. Resilience engineering is a new and emerging field, and robust methods by which to assess organizational resilience have yet to be developed. Until specific methods emerge from resilience engineering theory, organizations individuals and organizations can gauge their resilience, and strive for resilience, by gauging their characteristics and abilities to those described above.

Summary

Pediatric surgery is a complex, high-risk field characterized by a highly vulnerable patient population, technically demanding surgery, technological and team complexity and low error tolerance. The role of human factors has long been acknowledged, and a number of studies have now explored the application of a linear accident model surgical outcomes. While instrumental in directing blame away from frontline workers and introducing the concept of blunt end contributions, the linear accident model is limited in its application to complex systems.

Scientific thinking about safety has evolved towards a systems view, in which outcomes, including safety, are emergent properties. Systems cannot be analysed or understood as the sum of individual parts, but must be considered as a whole. Systems analysis is essential to describe work as it is, rather than as it is ideally imagined.

Systems engineering seeks to minimize risk through systems redesign. Resilience engineering explores how individuals and organizations negotiate complexity to *create* safety. Both fields represent a new way of looking at safety in our field, and have tremendous potential for future application.

Acknowledgements The authors offer their sincere thanks to Sidney Dekker and Nancy Poirier for their review of this chapter and for their helpful comments.

Portions of this chapter are reprinted from Harrington K. Patient safety in pediatric cardiac surgery [MSc thesis]. Lund, Sweden: Lund University, Sweden; 2011.

References

1. Kohn LT, Corrigan J, Donaldson MS. To err is human: building a safer health system. Washington, DC: National Academy Press; 2000, xxi, 287 p.
2. de Leval MR. Analysis of a cluster of surgical failures: application to a series of neonatal arterial switch operations. J Thorac Cardiovasc Surg. 1994;107(3): 914–24.
3. de Leval MR, Carthey J, Wright DJ, Farewell VT, Reason JT. Human factors and cardiac surgery: a multicenter study. J Thorac Cardiovasc Surg. 2000;119 (4 Pt 1):661–72.
4. Kennedy I. Learning from Bristol: the report of the Public Inquiry into Children's Heart Surgery at the Bristol Royal Infirmary 1984–1995. HMSO. 2001.
5. Sinclair CM. The report of the Manitoba Peadiatric Cardiac Surgery Inquest: an Inquiry into Twelve Deaths at the Winnipeg Health Sciences Center in 1994. Winnipeg Provincial Court of Manitoba. 2000.
6. Martinez EA, Thompson DA, Errett NA, Kim GR, Bauer L, Lubomski LH, et al. Review article: high stakes and high risk: a focused qualitative review of hazards during cardiac surgery. Anesth Analg. 2011;112(5):1061–74.
7. Stelfox HT, Palmisani S, Scurlock C, Orav EJ, Bates DW. The "to err is human" report and the patient safety literature. Qual Safe Health Care. 2006;15(3):174–8.
8. Pronovost P, Holzmueller CG, Needham DM, Sexton JB, Miller M, Berenholtz S, et al. How will we know patients are safer? An organization-wide approach to measuring and improving safety. Crit Care Med. 2006;34(7):1988–95.
9. Wachter RM. Patient safety at ten: unmistakable progress, troubling gaps. Health Aff. 2010;29(1):165–73.

10. Reason JT. Managing the risks of organizational accidents. Aldershot/Hants/England/Brookfield: Ashgate; 1997, xvii, 252 p.
11. Leveson N. System safety engineering: back to the future. http://sunnyday.mit.edu/book2.pdf2002.
12. Galvan C, Mohr J, Barach P. A human factors approach to understanding patient safety during pediatric cardiac surgery. Prog Pediatr Cardiol. 2005;20(1):13–20.
13. Catchpole KR, de Leval MR, McEwan A, Pigott N, Elliott MJ, McQuillan A, et al. Patient handover from surgery to intensive care: using Formula 1 pit-stop and aviation models to improve safety and quality. Paediatr Anaesth. 2007;17(5):470–8.
14. Reason J. Human error: models and management. BMJ. 2000;320(7237):768–70.
15. Van Eaton EG, Horvath KD, Pellegrini CA. Professionalism and the shift mentality: how to reconcile patient ownership with limited work hours. Arch Surg. 2005;140(3):230–5.
16. Reason J. Beyond the organisational accident: the need for "error wisdom" on the frontline. Qual Safe Health Care. 2004;13 Suppl 2:ii28–33.
17. Dekker S. Patient safety: a human factors approach. Boca Raton: CRC Press; 2011, xii, 249 p.
18. Reason JT. Human error. Cambridge England/New York: Cambridge University Press; 1990, xv, 302 p.
19. Catchpole A, Giddings KR, de Leval MR, Peek GJ, Godden PJ, Utley M, Gallivan S, Dale T. Identification of systems failures in successful pediatric cardiac surgery. Ergonomics. 2006;15(5-6):567–88.
20. Carthey J, de Leval MR, Reason JT. Institutional resilience in healthcare systems. Qual Health Care. 2001; 10(1):29–32.
21. Vincent C. Patient safety. Edinburgh: Churchill Livingstone; 2006.
22. Cassin BR, Barach PR. Making sense of root cause analysis investigations of surgery-related adverse events. Surg Clin North Am. 2012;92(1):101–15.
23. Engineering ICoS. What is system engineering: a consensus of the INCOSE fellows 2006 [cited 2014 March]. Available from: http://www.incose.org/practice/fellowsconsensus.aspx.
24. Karsh BT, Alper SJ. Work system analysis: the key to understanding health care systems. 2005. In: Advances in patient safety: from research to implementation [internet]. http://www.ncbi.nlm.nih.gov/books/NBK20518/. Agency for Healthcare Research and Quality.
25. Reid PP, Compton WD, Grossman JH, Fanjiang G, National Academy of Engineering, Institute of Medicine (U.S.), et al. Building a better delivery system: a new engineering/health care partnership. Washington, DC: National Academies Press; 2005, xiv, 262 p.
26. Barach P, Johnson JK. Understanding the complexity of redesigning care around the clinical microsystem. Qual Safe Health Care. 2006;15 Suppl 1:i10–6.
27. Carayon P. Sociotechnical systems approach to healthcare quality and patient safety. Work. 2012;41 Suppl 1:3850–4.
28. Kopach-Konrad R, Lawley M, Criswell M, Hasan I, Chakraborty S, Pekny J, et al. Applying systems engineering principles in improving health care delivery. J Gen Intern Med. 2007;22 Suppl 3:431–7.
29. Ravitz ADSA, Pham JC, Doyle PA. Systems approach and systems engineering applied to health care: improving patient safety and health care delivery. John Hopkins APL Tech Dig. 2013;31(4):354–65.
30. Hollnagel E, Nemeth CP, Dekker S. Resilience engineering perspectives. Aldershot/Hants/England/Burlington: Ashgate; 2008.
31. Hollnagel E, Woods DD, Leveson N. Resilience engineering: concepts and precepts. Aldershot/England/Burlington: Ashgate; 2006, xii, 397 p.
32. Hollnagel E. The ETTO principle: efficiency-thoroughness trade-off: why things that go right sometimes go wrong. Burlington: Ashgate; 2009, vii, 150 p.
33. Dekker S. The field guide to human error investigations. Aldershot/Hants/England/Burlington: Ashgate; 2002, ix, 160 p.
34. Schraagen JM, Schouten T, Smit M, Haas F, van der Beek D, van de Ven J, et al. A prospective study of paediatric cardiac surgical microsystems: assessing the relationships between non-routine events, teamwork and patient outcomes. BMJ Qual Safe. 2011; 20(7):599–603.
35. Weick K. Organizational culture as a source of high reliability. Calif Manage Rev. 1991;29:112–27.

Measuring and Assessing Adverse Medical Events

27

René Amalberti

Abstract
The measurement of safety in healthcare is challenging, yet the simple actions of identifying and measuring adverse events, accessible to all professionals, has the potential to be highly beneficial. The chapter provides an overall view of pragmatic concepts, methods and key points that may serve this objective.

Keywords
Patient safety • Adverse events • Human errors • Complications • Measurement

Since the 1990s, the deployment of Quality and Patient safety initiatives has been tremendous, sustained by an impressive series of policies, regulations, monitoring mechanisms (namely certification and accreditation), and organizational changes imposing new standards of care. The identification and measure of adverse events has been a pivotal action for all of these initiatives since no risk management strategy makes sense in the absence of knowledge on the nature of risks, their frequency and severity.

Probably the most valuable lesson that industry has learned is that safety management is more than buying and applying a set of tools and techniques: without the proper changes in culture, perspective, and attitude toward errors, failures and their causes, introducing tools with the hope of a "quick fix" will largely miss the point. Safety must be recognised as a systems problem instead of "blaming and shaming" of individuals working at the sharp end. The focus of incident investigations must therefore be on the latent factors and not just on the immediate precursors and local triggers [1].

Definitions of Harm

Identifying problems and measuring safety are more complex in healthcare than in many other industries. The primary reasons relate to variation in the natural history of disease and variable

R. Amalberti, MD, PhD
HAS, 2 avenue du Stade de France,
Saint-Denis La Plaine 93218, France
e-mail: rene.amalberti@wanadoo.fr

P.R. Barach, J.P. Jacobs, S.E. Lipshultz, P.C. Laussen (eds.),
Pediatric and Congenital Cardiac Care: Volume 2: Quality Improvement and Patient Safety,
DOI 10.1007/978-1-4471-6566-8_27,

responses to management within patient populations, as well as practice variability among clinicians. Even when the error is obvious, the severity of consequences often depends on the patient's underlying condition. Whether all harms and complications should be viewed as safety-related events, especially when the underlying disease is fast-evolving and no single obvious error is evidenced, is subject to discussion.

Healthcare has adopted the definitions of adverse events (AEs), human error (HE), and negligence as used in industry. In addition, because of the evolution of disease and response to management, the terminology of Preventable Adverse Event (PAE) is used in healthcare to identify safety events that were not associated with the underlying disease.

- Adverse events (AEs) are defined as harm caused by medical management–rather than by the underlying disease–which prolongs hospitalization, produces a disability at the time of discharge, or both [2]. Charles Vincent adds a dynamic dimension to the definition: The avoidance, prevention and amelioration of adverse outcomes or injuries stemming from the process of healthcare [3]. Preventable adverse events are all AEs that can be avoided by an appropriate error mitigation and management strategy and by avoiding negligence (care that fell below the standard expected of physicians in their community).
- Human errors (HEs) are defined as circumstances in which planned actions fail to achieve the desired outcome [4].

Despite the definition PAEs may be subject to varying interpretations, yet it is essential to not exclude complication and events for *a priori* reasons without considering the preventability of these events.

The Complex Relationship Between Errors, Adverse Events, and Categories of Adverse Events

There are several traps in the process of risk measurement, especially in healthcare.

Human Error and Preventable Adverse Events

Not all adverse events are preventable, nor are they always the result of medical errors. Not all medical errors lead to adverse events, and when medical errors do lead to adverse events, in many circumstances they are minor with minimal or no patient harm.

Errors are common in human behaviour. James Reason has stated that errors and intelligence are the two sides of the same coin [3], and that relatively few events impact safety because of the capacity and resilience of humans and organizations to recover from errors. The error frequency in tightly coupled systems can be high. In aviation, as an example, numerous studies show that the minimum rate of error for professional pilots is around one per hour, whatever its outcome and the quality of the workplace design [5, 6]. Detection performance is the true marker of expertise, while error production is not. The rate of self-detection is very high, above 70 %, and is integrated in the natural cognitive resources that individuals have to manage. Routine errors are better detected than mistakes. Detection and recovery are sensitive to high workload, task interruptions, and system time management [7].

This essential distinction between error production and error recovery applies to the systems view in healthcare. The safest hospitals are not those where no HEs, AEs and complications occur, but those that detect and recover from these errors and complications.

Identifying Preventable Adverse Events

The identification of Preventable Adverse Events (PAEs) relies on four different tools.

The first tool relies on voluntary or mandatory reporting. Under reporting of events is common [8, 9]. Moreover, most provider-reported events are made by nurses or other non-physician staff and often relate to events considered to be nursing issues (e.g. wrong medication administered, patient falls or skin breakdown from inadequate attention to pressure care) [10]. While reporting tools are necessary for enhancing a safety culture (engaging workers to adopt a culture of transparency), they are limited and inaccurate for capturing medical adverse events.

The second tool relies on medical file analysis. The most widely known method of medical file analysis is the Institute for Healthcare Improvement's Global Trigger Tool (GTT). Trigger tools [11] are sentinel words, precursors, or conditions found in a relatively quick review of the medical record to detect the possibility of the occurrence of an adverse event. The presence of one of these conditions 'triggers' a more extensive record review by multiple reviewers, including a physician, to assess the cause of the condition. The method can be easily captured within an electronic patient record. The Global Trigger Tool found at least ten times more confirmed serious events than captured by other methods [12]. Trigger tools are a good and productive method for detecting Adverse Drug Events (ADE), but limited as the method detects only what is searched.

The third tool relies on automatic surveillance of the system through patient safety indicators (PSIs) that have 'reasonable face and construct validity, specificity and potential for fostering quality improvement'. Each indicator is defined by selected ICD-9-CM diagnosis or procedure codes on a specific type of case (e.g. surgery, obstetrics or all inpatients) that suggests the occurrence of an adverse event. For example, a surgical patient with a secondary diagnosis of streptococcal septicemia (ICD-9 diagnosis code 038.0) would be considered as having postoperative sepsis (PSI 13). Many PSI indicators have specific exclusions to reduce the likelihood of false positive cases. With this tool, detection of complications can be achieved directly, whatever the causes (preventable or not).

The fourth tool relies on the detection of medical complications. The method relies on internal and external registries or administrative databases in which data of the patient journey is collected systematically. The occurrence of a complication does not mean that it was a preventable, but should feed into a systematic analysis, such as a Mortality-Morbidity review, to determine deficiencies in care delivery. This is possibly the most comprehensive mode in monitoring risk for clinicians, and it is recommended out of the four tools when commencing a safety review.

Categories of AEs

The perception of safety for patients needs to consider within the framework of two different categories of adverse events [13].

The first category of AEs relates to any suspected medical complication. With the advance of medicine, many complications may not reflect poor quality of care (non-quality AE) or problems arising from deviances to recommended protocols of care. Nevertheless, compliance with even well accepted safety recommendations remains low. For example, only 55 % of surgical patients receive antimicrobial prophylaxis and only 58 % of those at risk of venous thromboembolism receive the recommended preventive treatment [14–16]. It is also true that non-compliances does not necessarily lead to complications, and at times may be considered as an appropriate exception to quality measures [17] because of the variability among patients and the need for a case-by-case analysis. This category of AEs is well appreciated by medical professionals, such AEs are frequent enough that they can be benchmarked among hospitals, and their detection automated with GTT methods. For those AEs related to medical complications or non-quality AEs, specific recommendations can be generated to reduce their risk of occurrence, and it is therefore easy to measure drifts and trends, and change behaviors accordingly to improve.

The second category of AEs corresponds to unusual and often isolated problems. Examples include a post-operative patient stuck in an elevator, a junior physician alone on duty at the emergency hospital without back up, or a surgery on a wrong patient. There are many "out-of-thinking" low frequency events that may unfortunately occur in the journey of patients and fall into this category. Such uncommon problems are not possible to measure or even predict, (most have a frequency below 10^{-4} [18], although the sum makes a significant contribution to overall patient safety events (about a quarter of the overall AEs). Measuring the frequency of these events is problematic in that neither the numerator nor denominator of these events can be reliably assessed. Runciman [19] makes a strong argument for large scale reporting systems by pointing out that many of the rare events reported would not be identified and would be dismissed as isolated incidents at a local level.

While this category of events is difficult to measure because of the low frequency, they often have a high impact and profile, compared to the more frequent complications and non-quality AEs. Such events may also not be related to specific technical issues (as in Non Quality AE), but more so to organizational issues and an audit of the entire governance structure is required, with a specific emphasis on the (poor) safety culture. It is important to not concentrate on local solutions alone when a low frequency event occurs, as the event may be a symptom of a global disorganization and poor management of the hospital that could lead to other unsuspected and incredible events.

The problem for ensuring safety is to precisely understand the barriers contributing to and associated with a poor culture; organizational audits usually point to the weakness of the middle and top managers which may not be appreciated as clearly as local solutions for non-quality AEs. It is also important to acknowledge that this category of incredible and unanticipated AEs is very sensitive to the growth in complexity and changes in systems of care provided by organisations, and as such may well increase rather than decrease in the near future.

Measurement of Adverse Events

It is important to acknowledge that safety does not just mean avoiding emotional and insurance-driven responses to AEs that have occurred during acute care in hospitals, and that have often drawn high media attention. Most national patient safety programmes have given high priority to these AEs (e.g. wrong side surgery, infections), with immediate sanctions being imposed. However, these publicized AEs, also termed "never events", relate to relatively few patients, and give an incorrect impression that prevention strategies are the only acceptable safety strategies for healthcare, whereas recovery strategies are much more adaptable and needed for most adverse events.

There is strong evidence that differences in mortality between hospitals is not associated with large differences in complication rates. Instead, these differences seem to be associated with the ability of a hospital to effectively rescue patients from complications [20, 21].

It is also as important for a safe and successful patient journey to reengineer hospital discharge programs, rehabilitation care, and home care to decrease readmission. This priority given to patient's journey is even more important in pediatric cardiac surgery, since the success of any care is necessarily a mix of technique and social factors, with mid or long term rehabilitation phases [22, 23].

Advances in patient safety are hampered by the narrow timeframe used in AE detection and analysis. We recommend considering three different timeframes to detect and analyze AEs, and to better define the perimeter of patient safety [24]. The shortest timeframe covers simple problems relating to the direct coupling between wrong action and the immediate consequence to the patient (e.g. treatment to the wrong patient). A somewhat longer timeframe covers potential medical complications (that may be attributed to care or the lack of care), which alters the course of the disease during an entire acute episode of care from initial worsening to in-hospital admission, discharge and rehabilitation. The longest timeframe covers the entire patient journey and the integrated consequences of avoidable hospital admissions, preventable morbidity and mortality.

Accidents and Near-Misses

A continuum or cascade of effects exists from apparently trivial incidents to near misses to actual adverse events. The identical patterns of causes for failure and their relationships precede both adverse events and near misses. Only the presence or absence of recovery mechanisms determines the actual outcome [25]. The analysis of near misses is therefore crucial for drawing up new guidelines, building defences, and enhancing quality and safety. Reporting near-misses rather than AEs has many advantages: greater frequency, fewer barriers to data collection, limited liability, and recovery patterns that can be captured, studied, and used for improvement.

However, near misses should not be confused with AEs. There is a ratio factor of about 1,000 between the raw number of errors made by humans at work and those consequential for safety [7]. Most of the errors are recovered by different mechanisms before causing an AE, and may be captured by any reporting or measurement mechanism. For example, consider these cases: rewriting some drug prescriptions every day because of interruptions (but finally without harming the patient); prescriptions sent to the nurse with a dose missing (but finally without harming the patient due to recovery process); doctors on duty in the operating theatre, unable to leave, passing information via the telephone to the nurses for adjusting doses and drugs in the wards, and confirm only later when they can come and visit the patient (not a recommended practice); a patient recognizes that the pills given by the nurse were not the usual pills taken over preceding days. All of these stories are near misses, stopped at different temporal distance from harm. As the 'time distance to harm' is not specified the inclusion/exclusion of these stories and near-misses varies considerably from one professional to another, therefore making the actual measurement of risk for an AE subjective rather than objective.

Many risk managers mistakenly consider the near-miss from 'non-compliance with checking procedures' on a par with an AE such as 'wrong patient', yet only the AE and not the near-miss has an immediate impact on the patient. Including near misses with AEs unnecessarily inflates risk statistics and makes health professionals believe that the cause of an AE is the same thing as the AE itself. The cause of an AE is rarely a single factor, although there can be circumstances in which an incident may have been avoided if an isolated causal factor had not occurred [26]. Multiple factors and root causes usually contribute to a given AE and threat to the safety system. Each contributory factor may be necessary for the AE to occur, but is insufficient on its own. In addition, the context of the AE may contribute indirectly to the incident by providing the conditions in which the AE took place. It may thus also be possible to establish that certain factors are NOT significant in the events leading to failure [19].

Reporting, identifying and analysing near misses is useful for identifying precursors of AEs and working on recovery strategies. Conversely, because of their intrinsic unstable and interpretative nature, near misses should not be confused with AEs, nor lead to any calculation of their raw numbers for the purpose of safety measurement.

Are We Getting Safer?

After 15 years of continuous quality and safety efforts, whether or not there has been progress in patient safety is still debated [27].

Well conducted adverse event studies published over the past decade [28, 29] have demonstrated little improvement in the frequency of events. The methodology used for quality and safety studies is important to understand, and should be consistent with evaluations of the rate of AEs conducted using cross sectional (data gathered in 1 day), prospective (data gathered during hospital stay), or retrospective methods (review of medical records), but excluding methods based on voluntary or mandatory reporting [30].

On the positive side, a number of disease-specific epidemiological studies conducted over the last decade (such as for cancer, stroke, myocardial infarction, diabetes, AIDS) show a significant and continuous improvement in the prognosis and a lower complication rate, a longer life, and a greater health expectation. In part, these successes are related to specific, improved and standardized quality and safety efforts in these fields.

There are at least three explanations for the intriguing data on patient safety and seeming lack of improvement.

First, the innovation rate is much higher in healthcare compared to the rest of industry (5.5 years for half-life of knowledge [31, 32] compared to 13 years in Aviation, and 17 years in the Nuclear industry). This higher rate of innovation makes our list of errors unstable. We continuously change and add new protocols, modify recommended strategies, and alter paradigms and management practices. At least 10 % of recommended practices of the mid 2000s are considered as errors in the early 2010s, and even more in a few innovative specialties like oncology. As medicine continually advances the standard of acceptable care continually changes, and consequently also the standard of unacceptable care. The concept of what constitutes an error therefore moves over time, and the count of AEs over time therefore loses relevance.

Second, we have multiplied by 4 (at least) the number of process driven quality and safety protocols within a period of 10 years, and changed several times the tools for measuring AE (Manual chart review in the 90s, voluntary reporting in the early 2000, Global Trigger tools in the mid 2000, and now PSIs). These evolutions have moved the standards of acceptability (protocols), and the detection of many more adverse events. The more we generate process driven protocols and change guidelines, the more we automatically increase the visibility of noncompliance and deviance, and the measurement of more errors [16].

Third, the desire to continuously improve the standards and of quality care is at the core of medicine. It gives the hope for improved outcomes, longer life expectancy and quality of life. As such, quality initiatives fundamentally convey a positive vision, process driven, giving priority to preventive strategies as much as possible, and avoidance of noncompliance with the ideal scope of care. On the other hand, setting the quality bar at maximum is demanding for healthcare workers. Anytime this standard is not attained, and the disease not controlled, the patient may consider that there is a causal relationship between the prognosis and the noncompliance to the standard. For example, until a few years ago, strokes were regarded as untreatable. Brain cells were thought to die within minutes after a stroke began, so acute stroke treatment was believed unhelpful. The only onsite medical treatment was stabilization and "wait and see." It is now understood that treatment following a stroke, *especially if begun within 3 h of onset*, can help preserve brain tissue[1]. Before the last decade, there were few AE occurring with strokes, because the standards of quality were poor and limited. Nowadays, avoidable adverse events occur because patients cannot access care within the 3 h window due to organizational failures of the healthcare system; nevertheless, these AEs are often considered as harm due to the noncompliance with new standards.

The measures of safety are subject to biases. The report of Charles Vincent and colleagues published by the Health Foundation on the measurement of safety [27] gives a perfect view on the complexity and the size of challenges and leads to a fundamental question "Is the goal of healthcare intending to improve care… or to improve safety… or both as if the two ideas are similar?"

The ultimate level of safety observed in a socio-technical system is always the result of a systemic vision, with a four-step construction process [33].

The first step is always to identify the risks and establish an ideal model of defence. This is the classical field of risk mapping, decision-making matrices and safety measurement, extended to include human reliability. This step leads to the definition of lines of defence (barriers) to reduce the occurrence of the accidents that are of concern. The second step is to set this ideal model alongside the real situation. In many circumstances, operators do not use this model and suffer no particular penalty, at least for a period of time; many divergences occur for many different reasons, and it is useful to understand these. It is therefore necessary to establish a feedback loop to adjust the ideal model. The third step is systemic in nature. No-one imagines that a complex system can be made completely safe simply by relying on putting procedures and recommendations in place. A further step needs to be taken to strengthen the "system", based on a strategy of "safe governance" of this system, and balancing the tradeoffs between efficiency, economy, profitability, and safety. The fourth step concerns the ultimate resilience of the resulting model.

Conclusion

In this chapter we focused on important steps towards patient safety, starting with definitions of error, adverse event and negligence, then trying to capture what are the priorities and traps existing with the measurement of safety in healthcare, and finally providing some avenues for pragmatic improvements.

The measurement of safety in healthcare is anything but obvious. The simple action of identifying and measuring AEs, visible and accessible to all clinicians, is highly beneficial. It is important to avoid being more or less blinded by complicated calculations that detract from the larger picture. Clinicians are busy, time-constrained and care-focused, often with minimal time or opportunities to engage and attend meetings and debriefings using complex methodologies for the purpose of populating and analyzing incident/accident date bases. This certainly does not mean clinicians are ignorant of, or unconcerned with, the prevention of harm, but pragmatic solutions, easy-to-learn, easy-to-do, with clear benefit to alter practices are required.

References

1. Van der Shaaf T. Medical applications of Industrial Safety science. Qual Saf Health Care. 2002;11:205–6.
2. Brennan T, Leape L, Laird N, Localio A, Lawthers A, Newhouse J, et al. Incidence of adverse events and negligence in hospitalized patients: results of the Harvard medical practice survey study I. N Engl J Med. 1991;324:370–6.
3. Vincent C. Patient safety. 2nd ed. Chichester: Wiley; 2010. Institute of Medicine. To err is human: building a safer health system. National Academy of Sciences; 2000.
4. Reason J. Human error. Cambridge: Cambridge University Press; 1990.
5. Helmreich R. On error management: lessons from aviation. BMJ. 2000;320:721–85.
6. Amalberti R. The paradoxes of almost totally safe transportation systems. Safety Science. 2001;37:109–26.
7. Amalberti R, Hourlier S. Human error reduction strategies. In: Carayon P, editor. Handbook of human factors and ergonomics in healthcare and patient safety. 2nd edn. Hillsdale; 2011, chapter 24, 562-385-98, New Jersey: LEA; 2010.
8. Cullen D, Bates D, Small S, Cooper J, Nemeskal A, Leape L. The incident reporting system does not detect adverse drug events: a problem for quality improvement. Jt Comm J Qual Improv. 1995;21(10):541–8.
9. Aylin P, Tanna S, Bottle A, Jarman B. How often are adverse events reported in hospital statistics? BMJ. 2004;329:369–70.
10. Lawton R, Parker D. Barriers to incident reporting in a healthcare system. Qual Saf Health Care. 2002;11:15–8.
11. Resar R, Rozich J, Classen D. Methodology and rationale for the measurement of harm with trigger tools. Qual Safe Health Care. 2003;12:39–45.
12. Classen D, Resar R, Griffin F, Federico F, Frankel T, Kimmel N, Whittington J, Frankel A, Seger A, James B. 'Global trigger tool' shows that adverse events in Hospitals may be ten times greater than previously measured. Health Aff. 2011;30(4):581–8.
13. Amalberti R, Benhamou D, Auroy Y, Degos L. Adverse events in medicine: easy to count, complicated to understand, and complex to prevent. J Biomed Inform. 2011;44(3):390–4.
14. Bratzler D, Houck P, Richards C, Steele L, Dellinger P, Fry D, et al. Use of antimicrobial prophylaxis for major surgery. Arch Surg. 2005;140:174–82.
15. Cohen A, Tapson V, Bergmann J-F, Goldhaber S, Kakkar A, Deslandes B, et al. Venous thromboembolism risk and prophylaxis in the acute hospital care setting (ENDORSE study): a multinational cross-sectional study. Lancet. 2008;371:387–94.
16. Carthey J, Deelchand V, Vincent C, Griffiths W. Breaking the rules: understanding non-compliance with policies and guidelines. BMJ. 2011;343:d5283.
17. Persell S, Dolan N, Friesema E, Thompson J, Kaiser D, Baker D. Frequency of inappropriate Medical exceptions to Quality Measures. Annals Intern Med. 2010;152:225–31.
18. Clarke J, Johnston J, Finley E. Getting surgery right. Ann Surg. 2007;246(3):395–405.
19. Runciman WB. Lessons from the Australian Patient Safety Foundation: setting up a national patient safety surveillance system–is this the right model? Qual Saf Health Care. 2002;11(3):246–51.
20. Ghaferi A, Birkmeyer J, Dimick J. Hospital volume and failure to rescue with high risk surgery. Med Care. 2011;49(12):1076–81.
21. Ghaferi A, Birkmeyer J, Dimick J. Variation in Hospital Mortality Associated with inpatient surgery. N Engl J Med. 2009;361:1368–75.

22. Shepperd S, Doll H, Angus R, Clake M, Iliffe S, Ricauda N, TIbaldi V, Wilson A. Avoiding hospital admission through provision of hospital care at home: a systematic review and meta-analysis of individual patient data. CMAJ. 2009;180(2):175–82.
23. Jack B, Chetty V, Anthony D, Greenwald J, et al. A reengineered hospital discharge program to decrease rehospitalization. Ann Int Med. 2009;150:178–87.
24. Amalberti R, Benhamou D, Auroy Y, Degos L. Adverse events in medicine: easy to count, complicated to understand, complex to prevent. J Biomed Inform. 2011;44(3):390–4.
25. Barach P, Small S. Reporting and preventing medical mishaps: lessons from non-medical near miss reporting systems. BMJ. 2000;320:759–63.
26. Johnson C. Failure in safety-critical systems: a handbook of accident and incident reporting. Glasgow: University of Glasgow Press; 2003.
27. Vincent C, Burnett S, Carthey J. The measurement and monitoring of safety, report 2013. Health Foundation.
28. Vincent C, Aylin P, Francklin BD, Holmes A, Iskander S, Jacklin A, Moorthy K. Is health care getting safer? BMJ. 2008;337:a2426.
29. Landrigan C, Jarry G, Bones C, Hackbarth A, Goldmann D, Sharek P. Temporal trends in rates of patient harm resulting from medical care. N Eng J Med. 2010;363:2124–34.
30. Michel P, Quenon JL, de Sarasqueta AM, Scemama O. Comparison of three methods for estimating rates of adverse events and rates of preventable adverse events in acute care hospitals. BMJ. 2004;328:1–5.
31. Sjohania K, Sampson M, Ansari M, Ji J, Douvette S, Moher D. How quickly do systematic reviews go out of date? A survival analysis. Ann Int Med. 2007;147:224–33.
32. Dixon Woods M, Amalberti R, Goodman S, Bergman B, Glaziou P. Problems and promises of innovation: why healthcare needs to rethink its love/hate relationship with the new. BMJ Qual Saf. 2011;20:i47–51.
33. Amalberti R. Navigating safety, necessary compromises and trade-offs – theory and practice. Berlin: Springer; 2013.

28 The Role of Communication and Patient Handovers in Pediatric Cardiac Care Centers

Brian F. Joy and Timothy F. Feltes

Abstract

Optimal care of patients with complex congenital heart disease requires multidisciplinary collaboration and clear communication amongst team members on all levels and between all disciplines. Multidisciplinary case conferences, daily rounding communication, and the cardiac care center leadership structure are all opportunities to maintain communication. Accurate and efficient handovers are also essential to preserving this communication and collaboration. The handovers from the operating room to the cardiac intensive care and from the nursing unit to hospital discharge are two especially important transitions of care in pediatric cardiac care centers.

Keywords

Handover • Communication • Cardiac intensive care • Multidisciplinary • Collaboration

The heart center model (or the pediatric cardiac care center) that centralizes the leadership and administrative structure of the pediatric cardiology and cardiac surgery programs has been successful in several institutions. This model combines the disciplines of pediatric cardiology, interventional cardiology, cardiac critical care, cardiothoracic surgery, and cardiac anesthesia, in addition to nursing and support personnel, under a single organizational and leadership umbrella. The goal of this centralization is to improve the efficiency and quality of care for the complex population of children with heart disease. Central to the success and maintenance of a heart center is effective communication across all disciplines throughout the duration of treatment.

Multidisciplinary case conferences are an essential part of caring for pediatric cardiac patients. These conferences should present all relevant clinical data, including a detailed patient history, non-invasive imaging, exercise stress tests, electrophysiology procedures,

B.F. Joy, MD (✉) • T.F. Feltes, MD
Department of Pediatrics, Nationwide Children's Hospital, The Ohio State University, Second Floor Tower T2278 700 Children's Drive, Columbus, OH 43205, USA
e-mail: brian.joy@nationwidechildrens.org; timothy.feltes@nationwidechildrens.org

P.R. Barach, J.P. Jacobs, S.E. Lipshultz, P.C. Laussen (eds.),
Pediatric and Congenital Cardiac Care: Volume 2: Quality Improvement and Patient Safety,
DOI 10.1007/978-1-4471-6566-8_28, © Springer-Verlag London 2015

cardiac catheterizations, and surgical procedures. They are a formal venue in which to review and discuss the anticipated and ongoing medical and surgical management of patients. All members of the cardiac care team are expected to attend, and the conferences are scheduled regularly and at least weekly.

Handovers in the Pediatric Cardiac Care Center

Many handovers take place in caring for patients with congenital heart disease. Some of the main handovers are: within each discipline (nurse to nurse, physician to physician) at change of shift or transition of service responsibilities; multidisciplinary handovers, such as the transition from the operating room to the cardiac intensive care unit (CICU); and the discharge handover from the nursing unit to the parents and outpatient care providers after hospitalization. In pediatric cardiology, several studies have investigated the multidisciplinary postoperative handoff [1–6], fewer studies have looked at the discharge of patients [7–9], and even fewer studies have evaluated the shift-to-shift handover [10].

The Handover from the Operating Room to Cardiac Intensive Care

The handover from the operating room to the CICU after cardiac surgery is one of the most complex and crucial handovers in pediatrics. This handover involves the transfer of equipment and technology, the verbal handover of a detailed patient history and surgical information, and the transfer of responsibility for the care of the patient. All these transfers occur during a time of substantial hemodynamic and physiologic vulnerability for the patient [11].

Several studies have attempted to standardize and improve this handover, and many of techniques and strategies have been taken from high reliability organizations. These organizations function in a hazardous environment and have a commitment to resilience and excellence, as well as a preoccupation with failure that allows for reducing and mitigating errors to maintain safety [12]. Examples of high reliability organizations are found in the aviation industry, car racing, nuclear power plants, and NASA. Handover strategies used by these organizations include a face-to-face verbal update with interactive questioning, limiting interruptions, clear delineation of handover responsibilities, discussion of the outgoing team's stance toward changes to plans, and an unambiguous transfer of responsibility and delay of such transfer when the status of the process becomes a concern [13, 14].

A standardized protocol for the operating-room-to-CICU handover can improve teamwork [1, 3], reduce technical errors [1, 3], reduce information omissions [1–4], and reduce interruptions during the verbal handover [2, 3]. Given the variability among hospitals, a handover protocol should be tailored and adjusted to fit the particular hospital and unit of its intended use. A multidisciplinary team of key stakeholders should create the protocol to promote buy-in and ownership. Before widespread implementation, the protocol should be tested and revised with several plan-do-study-act (PDSA) cycles.

The operating-room-to-CICU handover can be divided into four parts: the pre-handover preparation, the physical transfer of the patient's equipment and technology, the verbal handover of patient information, and the transfer of responsibility for the care of the patient.

Preparations to be completed by CICU providers before the patient arrives in the CICU include setting up all monitors and equipment, obtaining the necessary intravenous fluids or medications, and reviewing the patient's history. The operative team updates the CICU team on the surgical progress and alerts the CICU providers so they are ready when the patient arrives.

When the patient arrives in the CICU, the individual in charge of coordinating the handover leads and interacts with the team, as would a code team leader. The urgent tasks required for the physical transfer of the patient and equipment are completed before the verbal information is transferred. The time that the patient is unmonitored and off the ventilator should be minimized during this part of the handover.

OR to CICU Sign Out Present (OR Team): Surgeon __ Anesthesiology __ Perfusionist __
Present (CICU): Attending__ APN__ Nurse__ RT__
***Sign out Time out:** Are we ready for sign out: OR team ___ ICU med team ___ ICU Nursing team___ Room Silence ____

Patient Name______________________ **MR#**_______________ **Age**____ **Weight**______kg **Date**_______________
Diagnosis/Problems____
Surgical Repair____

Pertinent Past History
PMHx__________________________ **Pre-op Medications**________________________ **Allergies**______________

Airway/Respiratory
Endotracheal Tube size_____ **depth** ____cm **Laryngoscope** Miller / Mac ___ **Airway** Easy / Difficult
Ventilator Setting PIP___ **PEEP**___ **Rate**___ **FiO2**___ **NO** ___ppm
Baseline SpO2 ____ **Most Recent SpO2**___ **Most Recent ABG pH**____**/pCO2**____**/pO2**____**/HCO3**____
Precautions/Plan: ____

Cardiovascular
Access: PIV__________ **Arterial Catheter** ___________ **Central Venous Catheters**____________ **Thoracic Catheters**__________
Times: CPB______mins **Aortic XClamp**_______mins **DHCA**______mins **MUF** yes / no
ECG Rhythms: Pre-CPB NSR / _____________ **Post-CPB** NSR / ____________
Inotropic Support: None / Milrinone Load___mcg/kg / Milrinone gtt ___mcg/kg/min / Epinephrine ___mcg/kg/min / ______________
Most Recent HR_____ **Most Recent BP**_____ **CVP/RAP**____ **PAP**_____ **LAP**_____
Precautions/Plan: ____

Neurologic
Pain Meds Given __________________________________ **Last Dose**________________________
Precautions/Plan: ____

Renal
Urine Output _____ml **Most Recent Chemistries Na**_____ **K**_____ **Glucose**_____
Precautions/Plan: ____

Hematologic
Most Recent Hgb _____ **Hct** _____
Blood Products Given RBC / FFP / PLTS / CRYO / Cell Saver / Autologous **Available** RBC / FFP / PLTS / CRYO / Cell Saver / Autologous
Precautions/Plan: ____

ID
Last dose of Antibiotic Ancef____mg at ___:___ / Other _______________

Additional Surgical Concerns: **Additional Anesthesia Concerns:**

Fig. 28.1 Handover template for the operating-room-to-cardiac critical care unit handover

The verbal handover proceeds after the physical transfer of the patient and once all relevant members of the surgical and receiving teams are ready. The participants of the information handover, at a minimum, should include the anesthesiologist, operating room nurse, perfusionist, cardiac surgeon, bedside nurse, and CICU physician. Only one care provider speaks at a time, and interruptions, disruptions, and distractions should be minimized. Throughout the handover, a "sterile cockpit" environment should be maintained. This term, adapted from the aviation industry, means that during critical periods (take-off and landing in aviation or handovers and code situations in healthcare) only patient-specific conversations should occur.

A structured handover template (a form or reference card) can guide communication and ensure that all information is transferred. Their use is strongly encouraged, particularly in the learning phase of handovers but it should be pointed out that they are not universally in use (Fig. 28.1). If used it should be stressed that making an effort to measure compliance with completion is advocated. The verbal handover consists of detailed information about the patient's history and condition, anesthetic course and complications, surgical course and complications, current condition, predicted patient trajectory, and care plan. Questions, clarifications, and concerns can be voiced after the information handover. The completion of the handover is confirmed when the receiving team accepts responsibility for the care of the patient with a formal statement such as "The CICU team has received a handover from the OR team." as a means to document (and measure) handover compliance.

Discharge Handover

The discharge handover is also critical, particularly in the care of neonates with complex congenital heart disease. The National Pediatric Cardiology Quality Improvement Collaborative (NPC-QIC) evaluated the handover that takes place after the Norwood operation between the discharging institution and the outpatient cardiologist and primary care provider. A complete handover was defined as providing the outpatient providers a written list of medications, a nutrition plan, and a list of "red flag" events. The NPC-QIC study found that only 45 % of outpatient cardiologists and 26 % of primary care providers received all three components of the complete handover [8].

The handover from the nursing unit to the parents and primary caregivers is another important component of the discharge process. The parents and caregivers need to learn how to assume the medical care of their child, including administering, for example, multiple medications, complex high-calorie formula feeding regimens, gastric and nasogastric tube feedings, and oxygen. Rooming-in before discharge is one strategy used by many centers to facilitate this handover for complex neonates, especially shunt-dependent and single-ventricle neonates. Parents stay overnight in the hospital for 24 h before their child is discharged. During this time, they are responsible for performing all of the care and therapies, as well as administering all medications themselves.

Home monitoring programs for high-risk and interstage single-ventricle patients are becoming more common, especially after the Children's Hospital of Wisconsin (Milwaukee, WI) heart center group reported a decrease in the interstage mortality rate after implementing a home monitoring program [7]. These programs consist of several components. Patients need to meet certain minimum nutritional and weight requirements before discharge. Parents are trained before discharge to monitor daily oxygen saturations, patient weight, and volume of enteral intake. They are educated on breeches, such as decreased saturations, poor weight gain, or "red flag" events that require notifying the monitoring team. The team communicates regularly with the family by phone, and all breeches must be evaluated by a member of the team. More recently, the Milwaukee group has reported that their home monitoring program has resulted in normal infant weight gain in their interstage single-ventricle patients [15].

Videoconferencing with parents after discharge decreases parental anxiety more than do phone calls alone [16]. Clinicians participating in the videoconference report feeling more confident in making medical decisions than they do after telephone conferencing [17].

Daily Rounding Communication

Communication during daily rounds is crucial for maintaining quality of care. Daily rounds involve a multidisciplinary team, are performed at the patient's bedside, and involve the patient's family, if possible. The optimal make-up of the multidisciplinary team includes the bedside nurse, CICU physician, possibly a cardiology consult physician, pharmacist, dietician, respiratory therapist, patient's family, and front-line providers (fellows, residents, advance practice nurses, medical students).

Daily goal sheets are increasingly being used in the CICU (Fig. 28.2). The daily goals sheet outlines the tasks to be completed and the care plan for the day. Daily goal sheets have improved physician-nurse communication in pediatric intensive care units and increased the team's agreement on daily goals [18, 19]. In adult intensive care units, daily goals sheet have reduced ICU length of stay [20, 21]. Modifications to the goal sheet can target areas of team weakness, such as the need to ask, "if the parents wish to join rounds," or "has the referring physician been updated?" Goal sheets should also require "read backs" on new medications or modifications to medications that include dose, route of administration, and frequency of administration.

Additional strategies to improve the quality of care and reduce errors during daily rounds include limiting interruptions during patient presentations, keeping all members of the team on

CTICU DAILY GOAL SHEET

RN 7A-7P: ____________ APN: ____________ Date: ________

RN 7P-7A: ____________ Attending Physician: ____________

Patient Label

Respiratory Plan Vent wean Y N N/A Non invasive wean Y N N/A Extubate Y N N/A Other Pulmonary Therapies needed? **Goal Met? 7a-7p Y/N 7p-7a Y/N**	**Sedation/Analgesia Plan** Sedation/Analgesia: □ Increase □ Decrease □ Δ Drug □ Δ to PO □ No Δ □ NA Neuromuscular Blockade: □Continue □D/C □Holiday □ NA Restraints: □Continue □D/C □ NA □Active Order? **Goal Met? 7a-7p Y/N 7p-7a Y/N**
Cardiovascular Plan Cerebral Saturation Monitor: □ START □ CONT □ D/C □ N/A Vasoactive Titration: Y N N/A Vasoactive Wean: Y N N/A Pacemaker Battery Change: Y N N/A **Goal Met? 7a-7p Y/N 7p-7a Y/N**	**Infection Surveillance** Lines/Hardware Present: □CVL □PICC □A-line □UAC □UVC □RA □CT □Wires □ Foley Lines/Hardware to be removed: □CVL □PICC □A-line □UAC □UVC □RA □CT □Wires □ Foley Lab draws/meds that can be consolidated________ Can meds be switched to enteral? Yes No **Goal Met? 7a-7p Y/N 7p-7A Y/N**
FEN/GI Plan Dosing Wt______ Current Wt_______ □ NPO □MIVF □TPN □Enteral Feeds □ Regular Diet Calories Receiving_______ Needed_______ Fluid Balance: □ No Δ □More Negative □Less Negative Diuretic Regimen: □Increase □ Decrease □No Δ Electrolyte Adjustment Y N Dosing Weight Adjustment Y N **Goal Met? 7a-7p Y/N 7p-7a Y/N**	**Skin Care Issues** Wound Consult needed? Y N Surgical dressing change needed? Y N **Goal Met? 7a-7p Y/N 7p-7a Y/N**
ID Plan Antibiotics: □ START □ CONT □ D/C □ N/A Drug (s)/Day #____________ Rule Out/ Prophylaxis / Treatment Course **Goal Met? 7a-7p Y/N 7p-7a Y/N**	**Tests/Procedures:** | **MEDS:** Are there any Meds Scheduled To end today? | **Therapy:** □ OT □ PT □ Speech □ Massage □ Lactation □ Child Life □ N/A □ Other

Fig. 28.2 Cardiac critical care unit daily rounding goal sheet

task, and providing ordered read back of information before moving onto the next patient. Nurse presentations on daily rounds increase the bedside nurse's engagement on rounds and improve family and staff satisfaction [22, 23]. For example, the bedside nurse presents a brief patient history, notable events over the previous 24 h, current patient status, fluid balance, vital sign trends, review of systems, and recent laboratory and radiologic exam results. The assessment and plan can then be completed by a front-line provider on the CICU team.

Summary

The increasing complexity of congenital heart disease patients and the expanding teams required to care for these patients requires effective communication on all levels. This chapter focused on two of the most complex and challenging handovers (from the OR to the CICU and from the nursing unit to hospital discharge) along with strategies to improve daily rounds. These examples highlight the importance of multidisciplinary collaboration and the value of structured protocols and handover templates. These tools and techniques can be used to improve communication and handover in all aspects of the care of patients with congenital heart disease.

References

1. Catchpole KR, de Leval MR, McEwan A, Pigott N, Elliott MJ, McQuillan A, et al. Patient handover from surgery to intensive care: using Formula 1 pit-stop and aviation models to improve safety and quality. Paediatr Anaesth. 2007;17(5):470–8.

2. Craig R, Moxey L, Young D, Spenceley NS, Davidson MG. Strengthening handover communication in pediatric cardiac intensive care. Paediatr Anaesth. 2011;22(4):393–9.
3. Joy BF, Elliott E, Hardy C, Sullivan C, Backer CL, Kane JM. Standardized multidisciplinary protocol improves handover of cardiac surgery patients to the intensive care unit*. Pediatr Crit Care Med [Internet]. 2011;12(3):304–8. Available from: http://eutils.ncbi.nlm.nih.gov/entrez/eutils/elink.fcgi?dbfrom=pubmed&id=21057370&retmode=ref&cmd=prlinks.
4. Agarwal HS, Saville BR, Slayton JM, Donahue BS, Daves S, Christian KG, et al. Standardized postoperative handover process improves outcomes in the intensive care unit. Crit Care Med. 2012;40(7):2109–15.
5. Chen JG, Wright MC, Smith PB, Jaggers J, Mistry KP. Adaptation of a postoperative handoff communication process for children with heart disease: a quantitative study. Am J Med Qual. 2011;26(5):380–6.
6. Henriksen K, Battles JB, Keyes MA, Grady ML, Mistry KP, Jaggers J, et al. Using Six Sigma(®) methodology to improve handoff communication in high-risk patients. Rockville: Agency for Healthcare Research and Quality (US); 2008.
7. Ghanayem NS, Hoffman GM, Mussatto KA, Cava JR, Frommelt PC, Rudd NA, et al. Home surveillance program prevents interstage mortality after the Norwood procedure. J Thorac Cardiovasc Surg. 2003;126(5):1367–75.
8. Schidlow DN, Anderson JB, Klitzner TS, Beekman RH, Jenkins KJ, Kugler JD, et al. Variation in interstage outpatient care after the Norwood procedure: a report from the Joint Council on Congenital Heart Disease National Quality Improvement Collaborative. Congenit Heart Dis. 2011;6(2):98–107.
9. Hansen JH, Furck AK, Petko C, Buchholz-Berdau R, Voges I, Scheewe J, et al. Use of surveillance criteria reduces interstage mortality after the Norwood operation for hypoplastic left heart syndrome. Eur J Cardiothorac Surg. 2012;41(5):1013–8.
10. Sharit J, McCane L, Thevenin DM, Barach P. Examining links between sign-out reporting during shift changeovers and patient management risks. Risk Anal. 2008;28(4):983–1001.
11. Tweddell JS, Hoffman GM. Postoperative management in patients with complex congenital heart disease. Semin Thorac Cardiovasc Surg Pediatr Card Surg Annu. 2002;5:187–205.
12. Wilson KA. Promoting health care safety through training high reliability teams. Qual Safe Health Care. 2005;14(4):303–9.
13. Patterson ES. Handoff strategies in settings with high consequences for failure: lessons for health care operations. International J Qual Health Care. 2004;16(2):125–32.
14. Catchpole K, Sellers R, Goldman A, McCulloch P, Hignett S. Patient handovers within the hospital: translating knowledge from motor racing to healthcare. Qual Safe Health Care. 2010;19(4):318–22.
15. Hehir DA, Rudd N, Slicker J, Mussatto KA, Simpson P, Li S-H, et al. Normal interstage growth after the Norwood operation associated with interstage home monitoring. Pediatr Cardiol. 2012;33(8):1315–22.
16. Morgan GJ, Craig B, Grant B, Sands A, Doherty N, Casey F. Home videoconferencing for patients with severe congential heart disease following discharge. Congenit Heart Dis. 2008;3(5):317–24.
17. McCrossan B, Morgan G, Grant B, Sands AJ, Craig BG, Doherty NN, et al. A randomised trial of a remote home support programme for infants with major congenital heart disease. Heart. 2012;98(20):1523–8.
18. Agarwal S, Frankel L, Tourner S, McMillan A, Sharek PJ. Improving communication in a pediatric intensive care unit using daily patient goal sheets. J Crit Care. 2008;23(2):227–35.
19. Rehder KJ, Uhl TL, Meliones JN, Turner DA, Smith PB, Mistry KP. Targeted interventions improve shared agreement of daily goals in the pediatric intensive care unit. Pediatr Crit Care Med. 2012;13(1):6–10.
20. Pronovost P, Berenholtz S, Dorman T, Lipsett PA, Simmonds T, Haraden C. Improving communication in the ICU using daily goals. J Crit Care. 2003;18(2):71–5.
21. Narasimhan M, Eisen LA, Mahoney CD, Acerra FL, Rosen MJ. Improving nurse-physician communication and satisfaction in the intensive care unit with a daily goals worksheet. Am J Crit Care. 2006;15(2):217–22.
22. Ellis M, Clark K, Coyle J, Dobbelhoff D, Dennis D, Tzanetos DT, et al. Nurses take center stage: nurse driven bedside rounds [abstract]. World J Pediatric Congenit Heart Surg. 2012;3(2):NP29.
23. Goebel BL, Buckley C, Plant J, Parrish M. Patient data presentation by bedside nurse at PCICU multidisciplinary rounds [abstract]. World J Pediatr Congenit Heart Surg. 2012;3(2):NP44.

The Role of Technology and Medical Devices in Enhancing Pediatric Cardiac Critical Care Outcomes

29

Amanda L. King, Orkun Baloglu, and Matthew C. Scanlon

Abstract

Medical technologies of all types are ubiquitous in pediatric cardiac critical care. Despite the widespread use of technology in the PICU there is a paucity of evidence directly linking these technologies to improved outcomes. This chapter first places technology in the larger context of healthcare systems. It further explores the evidence for technologies ranging from electrocardiograms to mechanical support and electronic health records. Additional attention is given to special topics of the impact of alarms and alerts, as well as the role of technology in human cognition.

Keywords

Technology • Systems • Cognition • Outcomes • Alarms

A significant factor in the advancement of outcomes among critically ill children with cardiac disease is the explosion of medical devices and technology in the intensive care unit (ICU). Arguably many of the children alive today would not be without these life-sustaining tools. However, all of these tools have the potential for harm as well as benefit. Further, each of these tools comes with an economic cost that may or may not be justified. Thus any consideration of the role of these devices and technologies in enhancing outcomes of pediatric cardiac critical care (PCCC) must be made from a broad perspective. With this context in mind, this chapter first frames tools and technologies in the context of systems. Then categories of tools and technology are explored in more depth.

A.L. King, MSN, RN
M.C. Scanlon, MD, CPPS (✉)
Department of Pediatric Critical Care Medicine, Medical College of Wisconsin, 9000 West Wisconsin Ave. Mail Station 681, 1997, Milwaukee, WI 53226, USA
e-mail: aking@mcw.edu; mscanlon@mcw.edu

O. Baloglu, MD
Department of Pediatric Critical Care Medicine, Children's Hospital of Wisconsin/Medical College of Wisconsin, 9000 West Wisconsin Ave. Mail Station 681, 1997, Milwaukee, WI 53226, USA
e-mail: obaloglu@mcw.edu

P.R. Barach, J.P. Jacobs, S.E. Lipshultz, P.C. Laussen (eds.),
Pediatric and Congenital Cardiac Care: Volume 2: Quality Improvement and Patient Safety,
DOI 10.1007/978-1-4471-6566-8_29,

Systems, Tools, and Outcomes

Medical devices and technologies are merely tools to be used for any number of purposes. Just as it is short sighted, if not dangerous, to view the function of a patient's heart without an understanding of its interactions with other organs, so it is a mistake to view these tools without placing them in the context of a system. For the purpose of illustration, we will consider one model of systems thinking. The Systems Engineering Initiative for Patient Safety [1] model states that, **people** use **tools** to perform **tasks** in a specific **environment** within the context of an **organization** (Fig. 29.1). Safety (or harm) is an emergent property of the interactions of these five systems elements. People include providers (surgeons, intensivists, nurses, etc.). Tools range from a marker pen and a white board to an electronic health record (EHR). Tasks may include gathering data for rounds or placing a patient on extracorporeal membrane oxygenation (ECMO). Environments range from a cardiology clinic to the operating room (OR) to the ICU. Finally, organizations include the rules, financial decisions, staffing, and culture.

There are two important implications of this model. First, safe or unsafe outcomes are an emergent property resulting from the interaction of these five elements. However, none of the elements alone can guarantee good outcomes. Second, changes to any of the elements affect all the other elements *and the ultimate outcomes.* For instance, a team may be adept at emergently cannulating a patient with low cardiac output

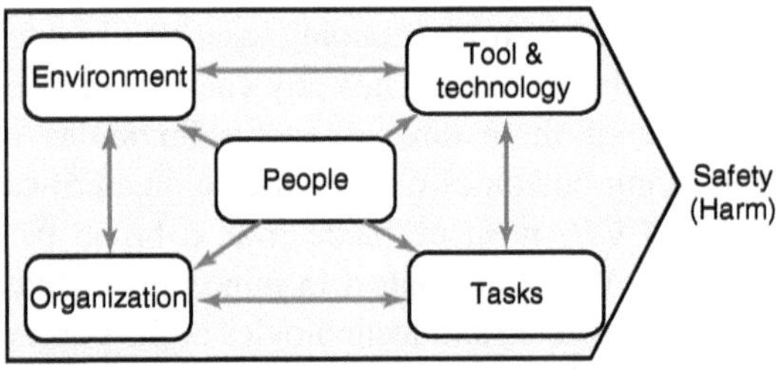

Fig. 29.1 SEIPS Model of Systems in Healthcare: safety and harm are emergent properties of systems (Redrawn with permission from Carayon Qual Saf Health Care 2006)

with good outcomes. However, simply changing the environment from the ICU to the parking structure will have dramatic influence on the outcomes, regardless of keeping the other elements the same. Similarly, a team that is skilled at performing emergent cardiac bypass on adults is not necessarily qualified to perform a palliative procedure on a child with hypoplastic left heart syndrome. Thus, whether any tool used to enhance PCCC outcomes is beneficial or not is contingent on the how well the tool fits in the larger system. As with another common tool, your mileage may vary. With this in mind, the following sections illustrate several categories of tools and technologies: monitoring, mechanical assist devices and medication and care delivery.

Monitoring Technologies and Tools

Arguably, the perioperative and postoperative care of children with cardiac disease has been enhanced through the development of both invasive and non-invasive monitoring tools. However, like any tool, monitoring can be used correctly or incorrectly. And, applying the Systems Engineering Initiative for Patient Safety (SEIPS) model, a monitoring tool without the skilled people to interpret the data and an environment conducive to using the tool is essentially useless or may even create a false sense of security thus increasing risk to patients. Further, as the "people" component of the SEIPS model includes patients, safe and effective use of monitoring technologies requires that appropriate alarm ranges and "normal" values be used. This requirement creates a major challenge for the pediatric cardiac population. The range of normal heart rates differs widely based on age range and the presence or absence of dysthymias. Similarly, normal values of oxygenation depend significantly on whether a patient has pathophysiology that leads to mixing of deoxygenated blood or not. Thus "one size fits all" is a potentially dangerous approach to the use of monitors that can produce false alarms (and thus desensitization to alerts) as well as failure to detect true hazards.

The **clinical electrocardiogram** (ECG) is considered one of the most valuable and widely used diagnostic tools in modern medicine and is considered the standard of care in the postoperative pediatric cardiac critical care population [2, 3]. Guidelines have been published for ECG monitoring in both adults and children by the American Heart Association, which states that all children after cardiac surgery have an indication for ECG monitoring, given they can be prone to arrthythmias, ischemia, conduction defects, and low cardiac output [3, 4]. Common pediatric postoperative arrhythmias following surgical repair include atrial flutter, junctional ectopic tachycardia, and ventricular tachycardia, all of which can be diagnosed with ECG monitoring and if diagnosed and treated early, can minimize adverse outcomes [5]. There have been numerous adult clinical trials demonstrating that an aggressive approach to treatment of myocardial ischemia, evidenced by ST elevation, improves patient outcomes by decreasing incidence of infarction and cardiac arrest [5]. This finding has not been clearly demonstrated in the pediatric studies, but similar assumptions can be extrapolated. Despite several advantages and benefits of ECG monitoring, it isn't without its downsides. Human oversight is essential for interpretation of the data to filter out erroneous alarms, which can be frequent and distracting. Cardiac monitor algorithms are purposely designed to have a high sensitivity for the value being measured, but at the expense of specificity, thus leading to numerous false alarms [5]. It is essential that well-trained individuals interpret the data prior to initiating any interventions to avoid overtreatment, particularly when that treatment is invasive with associated risks. Waveform artifact can contribute to false alarms, which can arise from muscle activity such as shivering, seizures, or fasiculations, thus leading to inaccurate heart rate displays [3]. Though there are no pediatric studies evaluating the frequency of false readings, it could lead to inaccurate interpretations of patient condition and possibly unnecessary or missed interventions. A potential risk associated with ECG monitoring is sustaining burns at the electrode sites, which have been reported in adult studies, one such situation resulted in second to third degree burns for a patient who underwent magnetic resonance imaging (MRI) with supposedly "MRI-safe" ECG leads in place [6]. There is also potential for skin breakdown at the lead placement sites, thus necessitating routine changes by the nursing staff, and could lead to venues for infection if breakdown occurs [2]. Finally, there are reports of electrocution when the leads are inadvertently connected to line power (120 volts alternating current) [7]. While none of the real or potential harm from ECG monitoring would justify abandoning wide scale monitoring of cardiac (and even non cardiac) patients, this technology nicely illustrates the importance of understanding both benefits and risks of tools in healthcare.

Invasive hemodynamic monitoring encompasses intraarterial lines, central venous lines, pulmonary artery catheters and intra-cardiac lines. When used to measure pressures as an indication of volume status or cardiac function, these intravascular catheters are attached to a transducer, which converts the pressure waves obtained by the catheter into electrical signals to be analyzed and converted to value, e.g., central venous pressure (CVP), or left atrial pressure (LAP). The potential value of these tools comes from providing real time data on filling pressures which may assist in monitoring and decision making of a patient's status. Theoretically, a range of clinical conditions that manifest through changes in intravascular pressures could be detected early allowing timely intervention.

However, like ECG monitoring, invasive hemodynamic monitoring requires providers who can interpret the data provided by the monitor and place this information in the larger context of the patient condition. A high CVP associated with high PCO_2 in an agitated and hypoxic patient with known pulmonary hypertension requires different interventions than a patient with high CVP and signs of low cardiac output due to a disconnect in a epinephrine infusion. When multiple pieces of information are available, providers may be faced with selecting which data to include or discard in their decision-making. This, coupled with theoretic limits of information processing [8, 9] may result in incorrect interpretations of large numbers of variables.

Beyond the issues of misinterpretation of monitoring data, invasive lines, whether venous or arterial, have been associated with a range of other complications including ischemia distal to insertion site, vascular trauma, arterial and venous thrombosis, thromboembolism, pneumothorax, hemothorax, dysrhythmias, bleeding and local and blood stream infections [10, 11]. Applying a concept of hazard reduction, while multiple steps can be taken to try and minimize these complications, the most effective interventions to improve outcomes include never placing lines unless truly indicated, and then removing the line as soon as no longer needed.

Capnography involves measuring carbon dioxide concentration. End tidal and transcutaneous carbon dioxide (CO_2) can be measured episodically or continuously, the latter graphically displayed over time. The use of capnography is well accepted in the context of delivering anesthetics, and can aid in assessing alveolar ventilation, confirmation of endotracheal tube placement and determining the effectiveness of cardiopulmonary resuscitation [4]. Further, the slope of the displayed waveform can provide information about airway resistance. At the same time, concerns have been expressed about the added dead space an inline sensor can add. Despite this, numerous societies have stated support for use of capnography on mechanically ventilated patients [12, 13]. Though there may not be randomized controlled trials proving the value of capnography, these authors agree with publications calling for the routine use of capnography in ICUs barring a contraindication [4, 14].

Pulse oximetry has been used widely in ICUs for decades despite the lack of robust clinical trial. Clinical experience has demonstrated this technology has important component of assuring safe care, leading to expert consensus advocating the routine use of pulse oximetry in ICU settings [4].

A more controversial tool is that of **near-infrared spectroscopy** (NIRS) monitoring devices for non-invasive continuous regional tissue oxygenation (rSO_2) monitoring at the bed side. NIRS devices utilize the principle that oxygenated hemoglobin and deoxygenated hemoglobin molecules have different absorption of light at different wavelengths. The calculated absorption of near-infrared light by hemoglobin molecule in tissues reflects the oxygenation of venous weighed capillary blood in NIRS monitoring. Unlike pulse oximetry, NIRS devices do not analyze for an arterial pulsatile signal, but for the average or nonpulsatile optical component, which is highly related to capillary–venous hemoglobin saturation [15]. This venous-weighted measurement provides an estimation of the regional oxygen supply– demand relationship.

Cerebral NIRS monitoring is most commonly used in intraoperative monitoring of infants and children who undergo congenital cardiac surgery. Interventions based on intraoperative neurophysiologic monitoring including cerebral NIRS appear to decrease the incidence of postoperative neurologic sequelae and reduce the length of stay [16]. In a series of 79 infants who underwent stage 1 palliation, somatic NIRS measurements less than 60 %, and a progressive somatic ischemia indicated by a somatic– cerebral NIRS value difference approaching zero predicted biochemical shock, complications, and longer intensive care unit length of stay [17].

Concerns about this technology include cost, accuracy and thus utility in an ICU setting [18]. Additionally, it is unclear what threshold or level of reading translates into harm to organs [15]. Despite these concerns, a 2011 evaluation made a recommendation for selected use of NIRS based on Class II, level B evidence [15].

The **bispectral index** (with the dyslexic acronym BIS) **monitor** is a processed electroencephalographic parameter that integrates time domain, frequency domain, and higher-order spectral analysis of electroencephalogram (EEG) signals (obtained from two electrodes placed over the frontal cortex), which creates a univariate descriptor of the patient's level of sedation, represented as a numerical value from zero (isoelectric) to 100 (awake with eyes open) [19, 20]. The BIS monitor was initially developed with data from the adult population, but now has widespread use intraoperatively in the pediatric population with a goal to assess conscious level and avoid prolonged periods of cerebral hypoperfusion during the procedure [20]. More recently, the BIS monitor has been utilized in other venues in pediatrics including the emergency room as well as the intensive care unit (ICU) to more objectively titrate sedation to desired effect prior to encountering any adverse sequelae from the medications. A BIS index of less than 40 denotes a deep hypnotic state; 40–60 is general anesthesia, which has been verified in several intraoperative studies; and 70–90 is light to moderate sedation [19, 21]. There is some debate amongst intensivists whether or not this modality of monitoring aids in sedation management decisions for critically ill children given it has some inherent limitations and costs.

The notion that BIS monitoring can improve patient outcomes, decrease medication costs, and reduce the incidence of withdrawal is enticing, though this has not been clearly demonstrated in literature. BIS monitoring provides a way to objectively assess a patient's sedation level in the face of altered heart rate, blood pressure, and physical examination to avoid possible over- or under-sedation, which may be associated with increased morbidity and costs [22]. There have been a limited amount of studies evaluating BIS monitoring in the pediatric ICU, which had similar results emphasizing that BIS scores can be an adjunct to already established methods of assessing level of sedation, but may be beneficial when physiologic parameters are altered by other medications (sedation, inotropes) or with neuromuscular blockade [20, 22].

There are some limitations to BIS monitoring which need to be considered to justify its use. Erroneous measurements have been widely reported, particularly with facial movements and eternal stimuli, which can be difficult to control at times in a busy and noisy ICU [21]. In a pediatric ICU case series, the sedation agent chosen impacted the utility of the BIS scores showing that patients receiving certain sedating medications showed a less accurate correlation with BIS scores to sedation scores [20]. Another question is whether or not BIS monitoring is sensitive enough to differentiate between the different levels of sedation, which would be it's main utility in the pediatric intensive care environment. In a pediatric prospective study, BIS scores reliably differentiated between inadequate and adequate sedation, but was relatively insensitive for differentiating between adequate and over-sedation [22]. It should also be noted that BIS monitoring was developed using adult EEG data and was not designed to incorporate the developmental changes of the pediatric EEG. There have been no documented injuries associated with BIS monitoring, but given the electrodes in place for potentially prolonged periods of time, the risk for skin breakdown must always be a concern for the provider. The are a limited amount of cost-benefit analyses of BIS monitoring in cardiac and non-cardiac surgical patients, which find the costs of the technology trivial when weighed against the potential benefits of more precise sedation, shorter intubation times, and less hemodynamic sequelae as a results of over-sedation [23].

Studies incorporating the use of BIS monitoring for critically ill children are promising given the possibility of improving patient outcomes, reducing costs, and being able to objectively titrate sedation, though further evaluation is needed to justify its use in the ICU environment.

Mechanical Support Technologies

Mechanical circulatory support, the mainstay being **extracorporeal membrane oxygenation** (ECMO) and the **ventricular assist device** (VAD), may be used in children as a bridge to recovery or a bridge to cardiac transplantation [24].

ECMO has been demonstrated to improve outcomes in select pediatric populations (acute respiratory failure, neonatal respiratory failure) though data on ECMO in the post operative cardiac population shows survival ranging from 33 to 64 % [25, 26]. A study of neurologic outcomes in a mixed pediatric population who underwent extracorporeal membrane oxygenation during cardiopulmonary resuscitation (E-CPR) showed favorable outcome in 95 % of patients [27]. Mahle et al. 2005 analysis of cost-utility of salvage ECMO in 32 children (84 % of whom had cardiac disease) demonstrated justifiable cost-utility [28]. Of note, of the technologies discussed so far in this chapter, ECMO is the one with such an analysis.

However, ECMO is not free of risk. Complications include bleeding, thromboembolic events including strokes, infection, and death [29–32]. While some of these complications are beyond the control of providers, when ECMO is considered from the standpoint of systems thinking, many of these risks are potentially manageable. Because of the interdisciplinary nature of ECMO (involving surgeons, intensivists, nurses, perfusionists, anesthesiologists, pharmacists and more), effective team performance is imperative [33]. Not surprisingly, safety tools such as failure modes and effects analysis (FMEA) have been successfully applied to the domain of ECMO with a reduction in risk [34]. Such applications may be appropriate for the other technologies considered.

VADs have been widely used in the adult population for years with very good outcomes, but the use of these devices in children has historically been limited, though the use has expanded in recent years, particularly in the congenital heart disease population. There are two main types of VADs used in children: centrifugal pump (the Bio-Pump) and pulsatile (Heartmate, Thoratec, Berlin Heart, ABIOMED BVS 5000, and MEDOS HIA). Indications for placement of a VAD are similar to that of ECMO including failure to separate from cardiopulmonary bypass (CPB) following surgical repair, or right, left, or biventricular failure, but the patient but still be able to adequately maintain oxygenation through their lungs [35]. There are pediatric studies reporting good outcomes with the use of VADs, particularly as a bridge to transplant. A study of the Pediatric Heart Transplant Study database found a survival to transplantation rate of 77 % using VADs from 1993 to 2003 with even better survival in the later years from 2000 to 2003 of 86 % [24]. But it is important to note that the success rate with VAD usage is significantly lower in patients with congenital heart disease and in the smaller, younger patients, which is where they are often utilized [24]. And there are numerous inherent risks and adverse outcomes associated with VADs in addition to their associated costs that must be considered when determining how beneficial they are to the pediatric cardiac surgical population.

There are limited studies with VAD use in pediatrics, but some have reported excellent outcomes of their use both with postoperative recovery or as a bridge to transplant [36]. There are studies with Thoratec usage in children, some reporting nearly 70 % survival to hospital discharge, though the best outcomes were seen with patients diagnosed with cardiomyopathy or myocarditis with only minimal survival and significant neurologic complications in patients with congential heart disease [37, 38]. The Berlin Heart VAD system is widely used and comes in five sizes as is suitable for patients of all ages ranging from neonates (>2.5 kg) to adolescents [24]. Survival to discharge with the Berlin Heart has been better in the older pediatric patients aged 6–16 years with a 52 % survival rate [35]. There are few long-term follow-up studies of children supported with VADs, but one was done at Children's Hospital of Boston over a decade, which reported that 37 children supported with mechanical circulatory support (11 of them with VADs), the overall survival rate was 95 % with one reported death [39]. Of these survivors, they reported 80 % of them were in good to excellent health with 90 % having normal ventricular function on echocardiogram at follow up years later [39]. A major advantage of utilizing a VAD versus ECMO for a pediatric patient is the lower rates of neurologic complications associated with VADs, likely due to the decreased anticoagulation need for this modality of support resulting in fewer intracranial hemorrhages. However, often times ECMO is indicated over VADs due to the degree of complexity of illness in the child and if they need respiratory support as well as cardiac support due to pulmonary hypertension or hypoxemia.

In addition to sharing many of the same risks associated with ECMO, there are some reported adverse outcomes with the usage of VADs in the literature. Left ventricular assist devices (LVADs) may contribute to right ventricular failure, and thereby significant morbidity and mortality for pediatric patients [40]. It has been speculated that the acute unloading of the left ventricle after placement of an LVAD leads to shifting shift of the ventricular septum, thus altering the right ventricle shape and size, which inturn alters its contractility [41]. Alternatively, intrinsic right ventricular impairment may be more evident once an LVAD is placed and there is an increase in the right heart preload [42]. Regardless of the etiology for the predisposition to right heart failure following LVAD placement, it is evident how important it is to identify risk factors in selecting patients for the appropriate VAD type, whether it be single ventricle or biventricular support. Placement of biventricular support (BiVAD) in patients at high risk for developing right heart failure, as opposed to waiting for it to occur after LVAD placement, may lead to better patient outcomes [43]. In this circumstance, the RFAV maintain prelad to the LVAD and therefore preserved systemic perfusion [41]. There are also conflicting studies which report improved right ventricle function following LVAD placement, which may occur as a result of decreased right heart afterload leading to better preload for the LVAD and the right ventricular workload [40].

Another major adverse outcome reported with VAD implantation is the development of antibodies, which has been widely reported in adult literature but with some reports in the pediatric cardiac population as well. A review of pediatric literature shows that sensitization seems most pronounced following implantation of the Heartmate I and Thoratec VADs, though it has been reported with other devices as well [44, 45]. Some studies have proposed that VADs can induce B-cell hyperreactivity due to the textured internal surface of the VAD (which is porcine tissue), thus producing HLA antibodies [45]. There have been conflicting reports as to whether or not the development of antibodies has adverse outcomes in the pediatric cardiac surgical population. One study showed that sensitized pediatric cardiac transplant candidates had longer waiting times and an increased likelihood of death awaiting transplantation, while other studies showed that sensitization had no effects on survival pre or post-transplantation [44, 46].

Mechanical circulatory support will continue to play an increasing role in the pediatric cardiac population with the advances in congenital heart surgery and management of heart failure or bridge to transplantation. ECMO will continue to play an acute recovery role, but the use of VADs is likely to increase for longer-term support with less sequelae compared to ECMO. With the increasing adolescent single-ventricle population who may well require cardiac transplantation, VADs can be used as a bridge to transplant, or in some cases as destination therapy. Further research is needed regarding cost benefit analysis of this modality of circulatory support in the pediatric population.

Medication and Care Delivery Technologies and Tools

A final group of tools used extensively in the aim of improving the outcomes of the pediatric cardiac patient population include computer provider order entry (CPOE), EHR, bar coding medication administration (BCMA) and "smart" infusion pumps. An exhaustive discussion of each of these tools merits chapters or books of their own. Thus, this section provides an overview of the tools while noting some provocative comparisons. CPOE (with or without clinical decision support (CDS)) is intended to aid in assuring safe prescribing of medications by eliminating illegible handwriting and human calculations while potentially guiding optimal decisions on choice of medication and dose [47]. EHR refers to any of a range of tools including computerized patient notes, digital imaging, CPOE, computerized lab results in any possible combination. "Smart" infusion pumps and BCMA are tools intended to improve the safety of medication administration. In the case of the former, drug libraries are leveraged to provide patient-specific dosing limits in an attempt to mitigate overdoses of infused parenteral medications [48]. In contrast, BCMA is intended to assure that any administered medication matches what is prescribed for a given patient [49].

These tools share several things in common. First, each represents an expensive solution targeted at improving the safety of patients, primarily through reducing medication errors. Second, each of these tools represents a complex technology that is added to an already complex system of care in the ICU. Third, while many have been linked to a reduction in errors, there remains no evidence that any of these costly solutions actually improves outcomes. This point seems at odds with the reduction of errors, yet the errors prevented seem to be not the same failures leading to preventable harm [50, 51]. Finally, each of these solutions has the potential to cause harm, in large part through failure to understand how introducing complex technologies into a complex system can worsen safety.

The reason for the lack of clear benefit from these much-lauded technologies is multifactorial [51]. Karsh et al. [52] explore many in their 2010 exploration of fallacies about healthcare information technology. Additional explanations include lack of maturity of the devices (relative to their promise), inadequate consideration of existing models of technology adoption, lack of attention to known success factors in implementing technologies, and an absence of user centered design, a cornerstone of human factors engineering [53–57]. While these issues may seem beyond the scope of those providing care to the pediatric cardiac population, each of these technologies represent significant system changes which will ultimately affect outcome. Whether this is for the better or not remains unanswered.

Alarm and Alert "Fatigue"

Two of the well intended but poorly considered byproducts of many of the technologies in the ICU setting are alarms and alerts. In the case of the former, alarms are meant to indicate physiologic distress or potential hazards associated with a device, e.g., infusion pump or ventilator alarm. Similarly, alerts are typically associated with technologies like CPOE and are intended to warn an end-user that their action may have been in error or simply ill advised.

Both alarms and alerts are associated with the phenomenon of fatigue or desensitizing end-users. Drawing from Pavlov's work on classical conditioning, Wolpe later showed that exposure to an anxiety provoking stimulus followed by a period of relaxation (as in a false alarm) leads to counter conditioning [58]. This *systematic desensitization* has been demonstrated with both alarms and alerts, and has reached the point of national attention because of the associated harm. The Joint Commission cited 80 deaths attributable to alarm fatigue in their 2013 Sentinel Event Alert, while other sources cite alarm-associated deaths in the range of 216–566 patients [59, 60]. While the harm related to alerts in computer systems in not well characterized, literature has estimated that up to 96 % of all alerts are overridden [61].

There are a number of factors that have been linked to causing desensitization. For alarms, these causes include alarm configuration and thresholds, alarm algorithms, and the resultant low signal-to-noise ratio [62]. Additional considerations in the child with congenital heart disease include the range of age- and pathology-related norms for heart rate, respiratory rate and oxygen saturation, as well as motion artifact in infants and small children. For alerts, causes include signaling known interactions or concerns, clinically irrelevant alerts, and where the perceived benefit of therapy outweighs the alerted hazard [63]. Additionally, the concept of alerting as clinical decision support is arguably backwards; rather than assisting providers in ordering context appropriate care, the device allows them to err and only then alerts the end-user.

What is perhaps most disturbing about the topics of alert and alarm desensitization is that there is no literature on recovery from desensitization. Thus, as one considers introducing new technologies that depend on alarms and alerts to assure safety, there is reason to think carefully before implementing any alerts that have a low signal-to–noise ratio do to real or perceived false positives. Until designers of technologies rethink the fundamental concept of alerts and alarms, prevention of desensitization appears to be the only hope.

Technology and Cognition

Cognition can be described as the "process of coordinating, mediating, and redistributing knowledge representations that are internal… and external…" [64]. This is important because, while safety as often been described as an emergent property of symptoms, it has also been framed as "the product of how well health care providers (HCPs) perform cognitive work processes" [65]. This second consideration is critical to understanding the role of technology in care delivery because technology can *improve or hamper human cognition.* A thorough discussion of all the ways technology can influence human cognition would require a textbook, not a paragraph in a chapter. Interested readers should start with works by Lawler and Holden [65, 66]. Not surprisingly, the issue of alerts and alarms are potentially disruptive to cognition and thus the delivery of safe care. Despite an extensive body of literature, more work remains on how to optimize technologies to optimize cognition. Until the issue of technology-cognition interactions are fully understood and addressed, it is likely we will continue to see technologies having a negative impact (direct or indirect) on PCCC outcomes.

Tools, Technologies and Outcomes

While outcomes can simply be framed in terms of "dead or alive" at the end of a clinical encounter, most would argue that functional outcomes are of far greater importance. What is striking in reviewing the literature associated with these technologies is just how few can be linked to meaningful improvement in either survival or functional outcome. Similarly, with a few notable identified exceptions, few of these technologies have undergone formal cost-benefit analysis. This leaves providers faced with both a void of useful information guiding which technologies truly matter to patient centered outcomes. This void also offers an opportunity for ongoing research into what aspects of our care actually matter.

Despite the lack of outcomes data, it is safe to conclude that the introduction of tools and technologies to the care of pediatric cardiac patients is not a neutral endeavor. Assuredly, such introductions will bring about fundamental changes to care delivery as well as to outcomes. Paraphrasing a public service announcement, simply knowing that technologies will create changes to systems and outcomes is half the battle [67].

References

1. Carayon P, Hundt AS, Karsh B-T, Gurses AP, Alvarado CJ, Smith M, Brennan PF. Work system design for patient safety: the SEIPS model. Qual Saf Health Care. 2006;15(Suppl I):i50–8.
2. Jevon P. An introduction to electrocardiogram monitoring. Nurs Crit Care. 2010;15(1):34–8.
3. Halley GC, Tibby S. Hemodynamic monitoring. In: Nichols DG, Rogers MC, editors. Rogers' textbook of pediatric intensive care. 4th ed. Philadelphia: Lippincott Williams & Wilkins; 2008. p. 1039–63.
4. Sivajaran VB, Bohn D. Monitoring of standard hemodynamic parameters: heart rate, systemic blood pressure, atrial pressure, pulse oximetry, and end-tidal CO2. Pediatr Crit Care Med. 2011;12(4):S2–11.
5. Drew BJ. Practice standards for electrocardiographic monitoring in hospital settings: an American Heart Association scientific statement from the councils on cardiovascular nursing, clinical cardiology, and cardiovascular disease in the young. Circulation. 2004; 110(17):2721–46.
6. Kugel H, Bremer C, Puschel M, Rischbach R, Lenzen H, Tombach B, et al. Hazardous situation in the MR bore: induction in ECG leads causes fire. Eur Radiol. 2003;13:690–4.
7. ECRI Institute. Risk of electric shock from patient monitoring cables and electrode wire leads. Hazard Health Devices. 1993;22(5–6):301–2. Available at: http://www.mdsr.ecri.org/summary/detail.aspx?doc_id=8161. Accessed 2 Aug 2013.
8. Miller GA. The magical number seven, plus or minus two: some limits on our capacity for processing information. Psychol Rev. 1956;63:81–97.
9. Florance V, Marchionini G. Information processing in the context of medical care. SIGIR '95 Proceedings of the 18th annual international ACM SIGIR conference on Research and development in information retrieval. New York: Springer; 1995. p. 158–63.
10. Costello JM, Clapper TC, Wypij D. Minimizing complications associated with percutaneous central venous catheter placement in children: recent advances. Pediatr Crit Care Med. 2013;14(3):273–83.
11. Karapinar B, Cura A. Complications of central venous catheterization in critically ill children. Pediatr Int. 2007;49(5):593–9.
12. Walsh BK, Crotwell DN, Restrepo RD. Capnography/capnometry during mechanical ventilation: 2011. Respir Care. 2011;56(4):503–9.
13. Oridion Medical. Standards mandating capnography monitoring. 2011. p. 1–16. Available at: www.multileadmedics.com/www.multileadmedics.com/Capnography_files/capnogrpahy%20standards-final.pdf. Accessed 15 July 2013.
14. Whitaker DK. Time for capnography everywhere. Anaesthesia. 2011;66:539–49.
15. Ghanayem NS, Wernovsky G, Hoffman GM. Near-infrared spectroscopy as a hemodynamic monitor in critical illness. Pediatr Crit Care Med. 2011;12 (4 Suppl):S27–32.

16. Austin 3rd EH, Edmonds Jr HL, Auden SM, Seremet V, Niznik G, Sehic A, Sowell MK, Cheppo CD, Corlett KM. Benefit of neurophysiologic monitoring for pediatric cardiac surgery. J Thorac Cardiovasc Surg. 1997;114(5):707–15.
17. Hoffman GM, Ghanayem NS, Mussatto KS, Berens RJ, Tweddell JS. Postoperative two-site NIRS predicts complications and mortality after stage 1 palliation of HLHS. Anesthesiology. 2007:A234. Available at: http://www.asaabstracts.com/strands/asaabstracts/abstract.htm;jsessionid=CCBCF7BE71A4FCAFBE686CC53266F3F5?year=2007&index=16&absnum=1585. Accessed 1 Aug 2013.
18. Drayna PC, Abramo TJ, Estrada C. Near-infrared spectroscopy in the critical setting. Pediatr Emerg Care. 2011;27(5):432–9.
19. Bell MJ, Chang T. Central nervous system monitoring. In: Wheeler DS, Wong HR, Shanley TP, editors. Pediatric critical care medicine: basic science and clinical evidence. London: Springer; 2007. p. 865–71.
20. Grindstaff RJ, Tobias JD. Applications of bispectral index monitoring in the pediatric intensive care unit. J Intensive Care Med. 2004;19(2):111–6.
21. Levine DA, Platt SL. Novel monitoring techniques for use with procedural sedation. Curr Opin Pediatr. 2005;17(3):351–4.
22. Berkenbosch JW, Fichter CR, Tobias JD. The correlation of the bispectral index monitor with clinical sedation scores during mechanical ventilation in the pediatric intensive care unit. Anesth Analg. 2002;94(3):506–11.
23. Klopman MA, Sebel PS. Cost-effectiveness of bispectral index monitoring. Curr Opin Anaesthesiol. 2011;24(2):177–81.
24. Bronicki R, Chang A. Management of the postoperative pediatric cardiac surgical patient. Crit Care Med. 2011;39(8):1974–84.
25. Kulik TJ, Moler FW, Palmisano JM, Custer JR, Mosca RS, Bove EL, Bartlett RH. Outcome-associated factors in pediatric patients treated with extracorporeal membrane oxygenator after surgery. Circulation. 1996;94(9 Suppl):II63–8.
26. Duncan BW, Ibrahim AE, Hraska V, et al. Use of rapid deployment extracorporeal membrane oxygenation for the resuscitation of pediatric patients with heart disease after cardiac arrest. J Thorac Cardiovasc Surg. 1998;116(2):305–11.
27. Raymond TT, Cunnyngham CB, Thompson MT, Thomas JA, Dalton HJ, Nadkarni VM. Outcomes among neonates, infants, and children after extracorporeal cardiopulmonary resuscitation for refractory in hospital pediatric cardiac arrest: a report from the national registry of cardiopulmonary resuscitation. Pediatr Crit Care Med. 2010;11(3):362–71.
28. Mahle WT, Forbess JM, Kirshbom PM, Cuadrado AR, Jimsic JM, Kantner KR. Cost-utility analysis of salvage cardiac extracorporeal membrane oxygenation in children. J Thorac Cardiovasc Surg. 2005;129(5):1084–90.
29. DeBerry BB, Lynch J, Chung DH, Zwischenberger JN. Emergencies during ECLS and their management. In: Van Meurs K, Lally KP, Peek G, Zwischenberger JN, editors. ECMO: extracorporeal cardiopulmonary support in critical care. 3rd ed. Ann Arbor: Extracorporeal Life Support Organization; 2005. p. 133–56.
30. O'Neill J, Schutze G, Heulitt M, et al. Nosocomial infections during extracorporeal membrane oxygenation. Intensive Care Med. 2001;27:1247–53.
31. Thiagarajan RR, Laussen PC, Rycus PT, Bartlett RH, Bratton SL. Extracorporeal membrane oxygenation to aid cardiopulmonary resuscitation in infants and children. Circulation. 2007;116:1693–700.
32. Thiagarajan RR, Barrett CS. ECMO-indications and outcomes. Society of Critical Care Medicine Critical Connections. 2011. Available at: http://www.sccm.org/Communications/Critical-Connections/Archives/Pages/ECMO---Indications-and-Outcomes.aspx. Accessed 5 Aug 2013.
33. Guerguerian AM, Ogino MT, Dalton H, SHekerdemian LS. Setup and maintenance of extracorporeal life support programs. Pediatr Crit Care Med. 2013;14(5 Suppl):S84–93.
34. Meyer MT, Braby J, Scanlon MC. Using failure mode and effects analysis to design a mobile extracorporeal membrane oxygenation team. Air Med J. 2011;30(4):201–7.
35. Graciano AL, Meliones JN, Kocis KC. Treatment of heart failure in infants and children: mechanical support. In: Nichols DG, Rogers MC, editors. Rogers' textbook of pediatric intensive care. 4th ed. Philadelphia: Lippincott Williams & Wilkins; 2008. p. 1109–16.
36. Kamdar F, John R, Eckman P, Colvin-Adams M, Shumway S, Liao K. Postcardiac transplant survival in the current era in patients receiving continuous-flow left ventricular assist devices. Cardiothorac Transplant. 2013;145(2):575–81.
37. Reinhartz O, Keith F, El-Banayosy A. Multicenter experience with the thoratec ventricular assist device in children and adolescents. J Heart Lung Transplant. 2001;20(4):439–48.
38. Reinhartz O, Hill J, Al-Khaldi A. Thoratec ventricular assist devices in pediatric cardiac patients: update on clinical results. ASAIO J. 2005;51(5):501–3.
39. Ibrahim A, Duncan B, Blume E. Long-term follow-up of pediatric cardiac patients requiring mechanical circulatory support. Ann Thorac Surg. 2000;69:186–92.
40. John R, Lee S, Eckman P, Liao K. Right ventricular failure – a continuing problem in patients with left ventricular assist device support. J Cardiovasc Transl Res. 2010;3:604–11.
41. Kormos R, Moazami N, Milano C, Massey T, Miller L, John R, et al. Right ventricular failure in patients with the HeartMate II continuous-flow left ventricular assist device: incidence, risk factors, and effect on outcomes. J Thorac Cardiovasc Surg. 2010;139(5):1316–24.
42. Farrar D. Ventricular interactions during mechanical circulatory support. Semin Thorac Cardiovasc Surg. 1994;6:163–8.

43. Fitzpatrick J, Howell E, O'Hara M, Laporte C, Kozin E, McCormick R, et al. Early planned institution of biventricular mechanical circulatory support results in improved outcomes compared with delayed conversion of a left ventricular assist device to a biventricular assist device. J Thorac Cardiovasc Surg. 2009;137(4):971–7.
44. O'Connor M, Ravishankar C, Kaufman B, Paridon S, Hanna B, Gaynor J, et al. Ventricular assist device-associated anti-human leukocyte antigen antibody sensitization in pediatric patients bridged to heart transplantation. J Heart Lung Transplant. 2010;29(1):109–16.
45. Grutter G, Amodeo A, Brancaccio G, Parisi F. Panel reactive antibody monitoring in pediatric patients undergoing ventricle assist device as bridge to heart transplantation. Artif Organs. 2013;37(5):435–8.
46. Feingold B, Bowman P, Zeevi A, Girnita A, Quivers E, Miller S, et al. Survival in allosensitized children after listing for cardiac transplantation. J Heart Lung Transplant. 2007;26(6):565–71.
47. Abramson EL, Kaushal R. Computerized provider order entry and patient safety. Pediatr Clin North Am. 2012;59:1247–55.
48. Scanlon MC. The role of "smart" infusion pumps in patient safety. Pediatr Clin North Am. 2012;59(6):1257–67.
49. Karsh BT, Wetterneck TB, Holden RJ, Rivera-Rodriguez J, Faye H, Scanlon MC, Carayon P, Alper SJ. Bar coding in medication administration. In: Yih Y, editor. Handbook of healthcare delivery systems. Boca Raton: CRC Press; 2010.
50. Kaushal R, Shojania KG, Bates DW. Effects of computerized physician order entry and clinical decision support systems on medication safety- a systematic review. Arch Intern Med. 2003;163:1409–16.
51. Leapfrog Group. Factsheet: computerized physician order entry. 2012. Available at: https://leapfroghospitalsurvey.org/web/wp–content/uploads/FScpoe.pdf. Accessed 27 Aug 2013.
52. Karsh BT, Weinger MB, Abbott PA, Wearls RL. Health information technology: fallacies and sober realities. J Am Med Inform Assoc. 2010;17:617–23.
53. Holden RJ, Karsh B. The technology acceptance model: its past and its future in health care. J Biomed Inform. 2010;43(1):159–72.
54. Holden RJ, Brown RL, Scanlon MC, Karsh BT. Modeling nurses' acceptance of bar coded medication administration technology at a pediatric hospital. J Am Med Inform Assoc. 2012;19(6):1050–8. doi: 10.1136/amiajnl-2011-000754. Epub 2012 Jun 3. PMID:22661559.
55. Karsh BT. Beyond usability: designing effective technology implementation systems to promote patient safety. Qual Saf Health Care. 2004;13:388–94.
56. Scanlon MC, Karsh BT. The value of human factors to medication and patient safety in the ICU. Crit Care Med. 2010;38(6 Suppl):S90–6.
57. Russ AL, Fairbanks RJ, Karsh BT, Miletello LG, Saleem JJ, Wears RL. The science of human factors: separating fact from fiction. Qual Saf Health Care. 2013;00:1–7.
58. Wolpe J. Psychotherapy by reciprocal inhibition. Stanford: Stanford University Press; 1958.
59. The Joint Commission. Medical device alarm safety in hospitals. Jt Comm Sentinel Event Alert. 2013;(50):1–2. Availble at http://www.jointcommission.org/assets/1/18/sea_50_alarms_4_5_13_final1.pdf.
60. Kowalczyk L. Groups target alarm fatigue at hospitals. Boston Globe, 18 Apr 2011.
61. Van der Sijs H, Aarts J, Vulto A, et al. Overriding of drug safety alerts in computerized order entry. J Am Med Inform Assoc. 2006;13:138–47.
62. Solet JM, Barach PR. Managing alarm fatigue in cardiac care. Prog Pediatr Cardiol. 2012;33:85–90.
63. Taylor L, Tamblyn R. Reasons for physician non-adherence to electronic drug alerts. Stud Health Technol Inform. 2004;107:1101–5.
64. Horsky J, Zhang J, Patel VL. To err is not entirely human: complex technology and user cognition. J Biomed Inform. 2005;38:264–6.
65. Karsh B, Holden RJ, Alper SJ, Or CKL. A human factors engineering paradigm for patient safety-designing to support the performance of the health care professional. Qual Saf Health Care. 2006;15:i59–65.
66. Lawler EK, Hedge A, Pavlovic-Veselinovic S. Cognitive ergonomics, soci-technical systems, and the impact of healthcare information technologies. Int J Ind Ergon. 2011;41:336–44.
67. Hasbro Games. GI Joe public service announcements. Available at: http://www.gametrailers.com/videos/s7x099/all-gi-joe-psas. Accessed 15 Aug 2013.

Human Factors and Outcomes in Pediatric Cardiac Surgery

30

Ken Catchpole

Abstract

Medical accidents are estimated to be the sixth leading cause of death in the US and may cost up to $980 billion per year. To determine their causes, these accidents need to be understood in terms of the systems model of accidents and of human factors, or the study of the relationship between individuals and work systems. Healthcare systems create errors through a complex mix of factors that shape human performance, including cost and throughput demands, poor technology design, interruptions, tolerance of violations, team tensions and miscommunication, and a limited understanding and application of human factors expertise.

Pediatric cardiac surgery outcomes are particularly susceptible to such problems, because children are already seriously at risk. Checklists, teamwork training, patient and parental involvement, and other improvements have all been beneficial, but all need to be considered carefully in terms of the mechanisms of their effects, their broader impact on work systems of work, their diffusion, and their sustainability. Small problems can escalate to create serious adverse outcomes, but good teamwork can help avoid these problems, avoid escalating them to more serious problems, and help recover from these problems without leading to adverse outcomes.

Keywords

Human Factors • Error • Safety • Performance • Systems • Accidents • Checklists • Teamwork

Pediatric cardiac surgery has particular task demands that make highly specialized teamwork training potentially extremely valuable, yet the understanding and training of these skills is poor, especially in the context of the complex and high-risk surgical environment.

K. Catchpole, BSc, PhD
Department of Surgery,
Cedars-Sinai Medical Center,
8700 Beverly Blvd., Los Angeles,
CA 90048, USA
e-mail: ken.catchpole@cshs.org

P.R. Barach, J.P. Jacobs, S.E. Lipshultz, P.C. Laussen (eds.),
Pediatric and Congenital Cardiac Care: Volume 2: Quality Improvement and Patient Safety,
DOI 10.1007/978-1-4471-6566-8_30, © Springer-Verlag London 2015

Prospective safety measures introduced from the bottom up are likely to be far more effective than reactive, top-down measures, and focusing only on behavioral solutions does not acknowledge that at all accidents are ultimately management issues. Truly high-risk, low-error surgery can be accomplished with a carefully designed structure of safety data, training, communication systems, teamwork, information technology, simulation, user-centered design, and continuous prospective data monitoring.

Patient Safety

The incidence of errors that harm hospitalized patients is 5–15 % [1–5]. Patients receive only about 55 % of their recommended care [6]. Every year, 45,000–98,000 Americans die as a result of preventable medical errors in US hospitals, and up to one million more experience some type of preventable harm [7]. Risky events or near misses may be even more frequent, occurring in perhaps one-third of patients [8, 9]. Direct costs are estimated to be $19.5 billion per year but may range as high as $980 billion [10].

Studies routinely attribute a large proportion of healthcare accidents—possibly up to 80 %—to communication failures [7, 11, 12], in part because a huge proportion of clinical work is communication. However, more sophisticated understanding of the causes of accidents in several high-risk industries and many high-profile catastrophes, indicates that blaming individuals (the "individual defect" model) or single causes predisposes to repeat incidents rather than solutions [13–16]. Instead, these tragic events need to be understood in terms of the systems model [17, 18]. In fact, humans have created safety in several work systems characterized by complexity, unreliability, unpredictability, and intolerant of variations inhuman performance. It is the mismatches between these challenges in work demands (defined by the design of the system) and human abilities (defined through evolution) that lead to errors and accidents.

Human factors (HF) is the study of the relationship between individuals and the systems in which they work. The field grew from the combination of management science and applied psychological research in aviation [19, 20]. It has since become a key component of safety and performance improvement in other high-risk industries, including road and rail transport [21], aviation [22–24], shipping [25], nuclear power [26], and military technologies and operations [27, 28]. One of the principles derived from studying accidents across industries is that human beings create safety, efficiency, and high levels of performance, whereas work systems are insufficient, unreliable, and unsafe and thus predispose workers to make errors. That is, human errors are a symptom of deeper system problems. Learning about these deeper problems can help to make healthcare systems more resilient to failure, before patients are harmed. Although this principle is well recognized and taught as part of a culture of safety in most high-risk industries, this human-centered approach is considerably less prevalent in healthcare.

Successful surgery requires coordinating many complex and independent components. It requires a skilled team of surgeons, anesthesiologists, nurses and other specialists, a patient who has undergone an appropriate diagnostic process, a set of well rehearsed procedures matched closely to the requirements of the patient, and a range of equipment, drugs, and blood products that must be appropriately organized in a supporting workspace. It also requires an institutional organization and culture that sustains the progress of the patient through treatment and the activities of the teams.

Pediatric cardiac surgery outcomes are particularly susceptible to systems problems because the patients are already seriously at risk and anatomically unique, often with multi-factorial comorbidities, so each requires a specifically tailored intervention. The surgery is complex, extremely invasive, requires substantial and rapid adaptation, and uses many different technologies, skills, people, drugs, and treatments, yet the outcomes still largely depend on a large, highly specialized team of experts. In such complex treatment, the capacity for failure is huge.

A recent summary article on behalf of the American Heart Association emphasizes the importance of human factors in cardiac surgery. Although the benefits of teamwork and generic training are acknowledged, understanding how optimal communication models and the wider system's effects impact teamwork and processes is incomplete [29]. Learning about these interactions, why they occur, and what can be done about them is fundamental for improving patient safety.

The Systems Model of Human Performance

Healthcare systems create errors through a complex mix of factors that affect human performance. The managerial and administrative "blunt end" of care creates opportunities for harm by organizational pressures, such as cost and throughput demands [30]; unreliable reporting of incidents [31–33]; failure to learn from previous events [34, 35]; hindsight bias in analysis [36, 37]; limited prospective hazard prediction [38, 39]; continued emphasis on behavioral solutions and training [20]; limited teaching of systems thinking in medical education [40]; poorly developed rules and interventions [41]; implementation that ignores clinical complexity or expertise [42]; drift in organizational standards and processes [43, 44]; poor ergonomics [29, 45]; and poor implementation of technology [46]. These factors affect the ability of healthcare providers at the "sharp end" of care to cope with unusual or unexpected features of the patient [47, 48]; risk, uncertainty and variation in surgical tasks [49]; equipment failures and poor design [45, 48]; diagnostic deficiencies [1, 14, 50]; lack of resources to support surgery [51]; interruptions, absences [52–55], and a culture tolerant of safety violations [43, 56, 57]. These factors are exacerbated by non-technical or teamwork performance deficiencies [58–60]; team hierarchies that rely on the most senior team member not to fail [61, 62]; tensions between professional groups [63]; lack of feedback and learning mechanisms that encourage recurrent problems and alternative solutions [47, 64]. The problems are perpetuated by ethical and cultural barriers to improving safety and by limited knowledge about human error among clinicians and hospital administrators [65, 66].

In the years since the publication of To Err is Human [7, 67], extensive efforts have been made to improve safety. New elements of work, such as checklists [68–70], briefings [71, 72], care pathways [73], protocols [74], and technological developments [75] can improve teamwork, shared knowledge, and workflow. The greatest successes are achieved by involving clinicians in the process [76, 77] and by designing systems around their needs [78].

Involving patients is also vital for improving safety and diagnosis [79, 80]. Involving parents of children with congenital heart problems is particularly important [81], not only for communication during care [82] but also for the eventual return home [83, 84]. However, although many studies initially found improved processes and some improved outcomes [47], most involved supposedly simple one-dimensional solutions, poorly identified causal mechanisms [14], did not address the complexity of healthcare systems or human behavior, and relied on behavioral change, training, or extra documentation [15]. This reliance has resulted in problems with implementation, the diffusion of interventions, rule violations and drift in standards and processes [9]. The danger is that too many procedures and rules make it impossible not to violate at least some of them and that they create a complex, brittle system with little resilience [5]. Furthermore, these changes do not remove the professional and administrative silos within the healthcare system or the circumstances in which teams form, develop, coordinate, complete, and dissipate. As a result, sustained change has been a challenge, especially for teamwork and communication training.

The Systems Engineering Initiative for Patient Safety (SEIPS) model is useful for framing HF in healthcare [85]. The model recognizes that task, technology, environment, and organization affect human performance and that these components can have complex interactions.

Acknowledging that these interactions exist also benefits interventions by providing a broader range of solutions to particular problems, as well as by reinforcing the view that reliable solutions need to be multi-dimensional to provide "defence in depth" [18]. The HF approach can optimize healthcare delivery by designing care around the abilities and behaviors of those delivering care and by acknowledging the important effects that work demands, equipment, environment, and organization have on those behaviors.

Task, Team and Technology Interactions

In 2000, inquiries into surgical deaths in Winnipeg, Canada [86], and Bristol, UK [87], were among the first to highlight the complex range of systemic influences on surgical performance. These inquiries revealed a huge range of organizational systems problems. Subsequent prospective direct observations in cardiac [51, 88–90], orthopedic [51], laparoscopic, vascular [49, 60], and other surgeries found a range of small recurrent and frequent process problems that, on their own, seemed innocuous but that in certain situations contributed to errors [60, 91]. These observations led to searches for a mechanism by which minor problems might lead to harm. Critical errors, even rare technical errors, occur in close proximity to usually innocuous failures, frequently described as "flow disruptions" [92]. This accumulation of small problems can cause adverse events. A sequence of small failures can build to create something more dangerous or exacerbate (fail to recover from) a single, more serious mistake [47].

Both accumulation and exacerbation processes an occur together, so the propagation of error from minor isolated disruptions to major failure sequences is likely to be a combination of the cumulative effect of flow disruptions. When this combination coincides with some critical stage or process in the operation, otherwise minor communication errors can lead to devastating outcomes [29]. This effect is more pronounced in higher-risk or more complex operations, both because they are more difficult and naturally have more problems and because they have more critical stages, so the likelihood of a disruption occurring at the time of a critical event is increased [47, 48]. Crucially, deLeval and Carthey [93–95] found that minor problems could affect outcomes in pediatric cardiac surgery and that the team's failure or success in meeting a challenging situation is what made the difference. Indeed, good teamwork helps to avoid minor problems, helps avoid the escalation of these problems to more serious ones, and helps to recover from these situations without leading to adverse outcomes.

The ability of operating room teams to avoid failures or capture them before they can accumulate to influence outcome, may be critical [7] because the cascade of disruptions to a major failure may also be prevented by effective teamwork [82–85]. Teamwork, critical team absences, communication problems, poor coordination, and equipment failures can all exacerbate an already difficult and uncertain case and are related to intraoperative performance [89, 96–98] and outcome [95, 99]. These factors involve skills that are, at present, not formally included in training curricula. Surgical teams can be extremely ill-prepared for some of the unexpected systems problems they encounter. This problem is particularly critical in the management of perfusion, which is shared between surgeon, anesthesiologist, and perfusionist. Management requires close coordination between the team members, their equipment, and the procedures that need to be carried out to ensure the successful recovery of the patient. Management can also become unstable in periods of high workload and close interaction, such as immediately after weaning from cardiopulmonary bypass. These issues make perfusion fundamentally more complex and higher risk than many other tasks in the operating room (OR). The anesthesiologist and surgeon may give the perfusionist conflicting commands, and miscommunication can lead to task deviations, equipment misuse, and near-miss exsanguination [47]. Simply training in teamwork or technical skills would miss the subtleties of the tightly coupled relationship in cardiac surgery [100]. Thus, we argue that the effectiveness of generic teamwork training models and checklist is limited. Rather, it is this complex mix of task, team, technology, and environment that creates the opportunities for desirable or undesirable outcomes.

Case Study

A 6-month old boy underwent a Norwood Stage 2 procedure for hypoplastic left heart syndrome. As the attending anesthesiologist prepared for the operation, he realized only 2 units of blood had been ordered and left the anesthetic resident in the OR while he went to arrange for more. During the initial sternotomy, performed by the experienced assistant surgeon, the heart and great arteries were found to have adhered to the sternum, and an unusual bleeding site was noted. Placing pressure on the bleed, the assistant surgeon asked for the attending anesthesiologist and surgeon to be called, since neither were present in the OR. Both arrived within 2 min, but in that time, bleeding had become severe. The assistant surgeon asked for heparin to be given to the patient, which would allow rapid initiation of cardio-pulmonary bypass and re-use of the blood being lost. The attending surgeon said no to heparin, and went to scrub up. By this time, heart rate, arterial pressure, CVP, oxygen saturation and ETCO2 had all fallen markedly. Seeing the bleeding get worse, the assistant surgeon again asked the attending anesthesiologist for the heparin, and the anesthesiologist agreed. Looking up from scrubbing, the attending surgeon stated angrily that he had specifically said no heparin. However, on viewing the anesthetic monitor and the surgical field, he realized the seriousness of the situation.

The aortic homograft from the previous surgery had been ruptured during the sternotomy. Vigorous cardiac massage was given, and an aortic cannula was placed with considerable difficulty. Adrenaline and blood volume were given, but 20 min after the bleeding was identified, defibrillation was required. Fortunately, sinus rhythm was regained, and 6 min later, the heart rate began to rise again. The patient was placed on cardio-pulmonary bypass 34 min after the initial bleeding, by which time the heart had been bradycardic for 22 min, the blood had a pH of 6.9, and haematocrit was at 19.

Several other difficulties were encountered in re-configuring the hastily initiated bypass, but the surgery was successful, and the patient was moved to ICU after a 279-min operation. A post-operative neurological examination found no adverse effects from the incident.

Commentary

The absence of attendings, the awareness failure by the attending surgeon, and the lack of blood products all delayed the response to the initial discovery of the problem. Although clearly the rupture of the homograft was the triggering event, contributing to the event were the patient, who was predisposed to the rupture by having particularly adherent arteries, and the procedure, for which rupture a known complication. The decision by the assistant surgeon and the senior anesthesiologist, to overrule the wishes of the attending surgeon was critical to the eventual successful outcome, but the sequence of further problems in configuring bypass made this an extremely challenging situation. Fortunately, the team then worked exceptionally well together, appropriately managing the resources available and prioritizing their responses to the situation. With better preparation, the response would have been faster and more effective and would not have risked the life of the patient (Adapted from Catchpole et al. [47]).

In 2007, we published an influential handoff protocol that has now been adopted in many units around the world (including Saudi Arabia and Brazil) [101]. To improve our flawed process, we sought to learn from aviation and motor racing. We found in both industries a no-blame culture that was led from the highest level of management; a detailed database for recording errors or faulty equipment, allowing access to information at several levels and performance tracking of every element in the system; clear procedures and extensive use of checklists; well rehearsed contingency plans for time-critical events and strategic change; extensive auditable briefings at a variety of levels to plan for future events and to learn from experiences; quiet and calm leadership, with an ability to step back from proceedings to assess the situation and the ability to learn from other teams, particularly when major accidents occurred. At the operational level, we implemented checklists, process re-design (allocation and sequence), and specific teamwork processes (a structured briefing, discussion, and agreed plan). These changes substantially improved our handoff process, which has since provided a framework for a number of other studies [102–105], and reinforced the view that learning from other industries, combined with human factors expertise and a multidimensional approach to interventions, can have transformative effects.

Challenges

Despite successes and large numbers of interventions, healthcare-associated accidents have been reduced only slightly. Intraoperative events are rarely recorded, so there is little feedback for process improvement. Often, there is no further attention paid to "near miss" events, no postoperative debriefing, and no assessment of why events happened. Consequently, nothing is learned about how these clear deficiencies might be improved. Attention to minor failures could have a considerable impact on mortality and morbidity, particularly in high-risk operations. Few studies track flow disruptions, an activity that can provide detailed quantitative and qualitative data on the threats to safe and efficient systems' function. Although each case is unique, the underlying problems are common, and the resulting failures can be major and common. This circumstance provides a huge learning opportunity that is lost unless tracked. Instead, something goes wrong, which leads to an extra check or a new checklist, which frequently does not address the underlying problem. Prospective, ground-up solutions are likely to be far more effective than reactive, top-down interventions [42].

Resilience—the ability to sustain work effectively under long-term, systems-related stress—is even less frequently described. We need to solutions that are effective and sustainable by identifying the mechanisms of failure and success at both at the sharp end of care delivery, and at the blunt end of management. This dual approach is particularly important given that, in complex human systems, the source of a problem may be spatially and temporally separated from the manifestation of that problem. For example, communication problems may be underpinned by a lack of sufficient time, space, and medium to communicate rather than by a lack of ability or willingness to communicate. Alternatively, the ability to adapt to unexpected situations can be reduced by over-standardization, which has resulted in problems with implementation [106], spread [107, 108], rule and process violations, and drift [57]. As stated above, the danger of too many procedures and rules is that at least some are likely to violated and that they also make a system brittle and unresponsive to changing stresses or needs [30, 109].

Summary

Medical error is among the top ten causes of death, carries with it great personal tragedy and huge costs, and remains persistent [8], despite huge efforts and some progress [67, 110]. Improving healthcare safety is an extraordinarily complex task, yet is usually approached with little knowledge of human-system interactions [20]. By employing a carefully designed structure of safety, training, communication, teamwork, and clinical systems, it is possible to perform truly high-risk, low-error surgery. This safety structure should include checklists, simulations, user-centered design, continuous performance monitoring and improvement, data dashboards, information technology, and equipment integration. The structure should be based on detailed process data; better use of that data based on the development of systems models; the specific modeling of teamwork and communication before, during and after surgery; patient and parent involvement in care and in the development of measures and models; and multi-dimensional interventions with known mechanisms of affect.

The systems view [17] ultimately challenges many concepts held by clinicians, such as the idea that Randomized Controlled Trials are always the best evidence [111], the fallacy that good outcomes indicate good processes [34], and the fallacy of self-determinism, especially the view that errors can be avoided through force of will or more training. Good outcomes are shaped by the equipment, tasks, environment, and organization, as well as by people. The core message of systems safety is that good outcomes are not so much about individual heroes—though clearly some key individuals can be extremely influential upon outcomes—but about establishing a team that can deliver every day, reliable, predictable, individualized care that treats the patient in the safest and most efficient way.

References

1. Leape LL, Brennan TA, Laird N, et al. The nature of adverse events in hospitalized patients. Results of the Harvard Medical Practice Study II. N Engl J Med. 1991;324(6):377–84.
2. Gawande AA, Thomas EJ, Zinner MJ, Brennan TA. The incidence and nature of surgical adverse events in Colorado and Utah in 1992. Surgery. 1999;126(1):66–75.
3. Thomas EJ, Studdert DM, Runciman WB, et al. A comparison of iatrogenic injury studies in Australia and the USA. I: context, methods, casemix, population, patient and hospital characteristics. Int J Qual Health Care. 2000;12(5):371–8.
4. Vincent C, Neale G, Woloshynowych M. Adverse events in British hospitals: preliminary retrospective record review. Br Med J. 2001;322:517–9.
5. Department of Health. An organisation with a memory: report of an expert group on learning from adverse events in the NHS. London: HMSO; 2000.
6. McGlynn EA, Asch SM, Adams J, et al. The quality of health care delivered to adults in the United States. N Engl J Med. 2003;348(26):2635–45.
7. Kohn LT, Corrigan JM, Donaldson MS. To err is human: building a safer health system. Washington, DC: National Academy Press; 2000.
8. Classen DC, Resar R, Griffin F, et al. 'Global trigger tool' shows that adverse events in hospitals may be ten times greater than previously measured. Health Aff (Millwood). 2011;30(4):581–9.
9. Kreckler S, Catchpole KR, New SJ, Handa A, McCulloch PG. Quality and safety on an acute surgical ward an exploratory cohort study of process and outcome. Ann Surg. 2009;250(6):1035–40.
10. Andel C, Davidow SL, Hollander M, Moreno DA. The economics of health care quality and medical errors. J Health Care Finance. 2012;39(1): 39–50.
11. Neale G, Woloshynowych M, Vincent C. Exploring the causes of adverse events in NHS hospital practice. J R Soc Med. 2001;94(7):322–30.
12. Gawande AA, Zinner MJ, Studdert DM, Brennan TA. Analysis of errors reported by surgeons at three teaching hospitals. Surgery. 2003;133(6): 614–21.
13. Davidson TM. Anatomy of a medical accident. West J Med. 2000;172(4):267–70.
14. Hofer TP, Hayward RA. Are bad outcomes from questionable clinical decisions preventable medical errors? A case of cascade iatrogenesis. Ann Intern Med. 2002;137(5):327–33.
15. Woolf SH, Kuzel AJ, Dovey SM, Phillips RL. A string of mistakes: the importance of cascade analysis in describing, counting, and preventing medical errors. Ann Fam Med. 2004;2:317–26.
16. Reason J. Human error: models and management. Br Med J. 2000;320(7237):768–70.
17. Reason JT. Human error. Cambridge: University Press; 1990.
18. Reason J. Managing the risks of organisational accidents. Aldershot: Ashgate; 1997.
19. Gurses AP, Ozok AA, Pronovost PJ. Time to accelerate integration of human factors and ergonomics in patient safety. BMJ Qual Saf. 2012;21(4):347–51.
20. Russ AL, Fairbanks RJ, Karsh BT, Militello LG, Saleem JJ, Wears RL. The science of human factors: separating fact from fiction. BMJ Qual Saf. 2013; 22(10):802–8.
21. Lawton R, Ward NJ. A systems analysis of the Ladbroke Grove rail crash. Accid Anal Prev. 2005;37(2):235–44.
22. Helmreich RL, Foushee HC. Why crew resource management? Empirical and theoretical bases of human factors training in aviation. In: Cockpit resource management. San Diego: Academic; 1993. p. 3–45.

23. Helmreich RL. Anatomy of a system accident: the crash of Avianca Flight 052. Int J Aviat Psychol. 1994;4(3):265–84.
24. Helmreich RL, Merritt AC. Culture at work in aviation and medicine. Aldershot: Ashgate; 1998.
25. Hetherington C, Flin R, Mearns K. Safety in shipping: the human element. J Safety Res. 2006;37(4): 401–11.
26. Carvalho PV, Dos S, Vidal MC. Safety implications of cultural and cognitive issues in nuclear power plant operation. Appl Ergon. 2006;37(2):211–23.
27. Burke CS, Salas E, Wilson-Donnelly K, Priest H. How to turn a team of experts into an expert medical team: guidance from the aviation and military communities. Qual Saf Health Care. 2004;13 Suppl 1(1475–3898 (Print)):i96–104.
28. Klein G. Naturalistic decision making. Hum Factors. 2008;50(3):456–60.
29. Wahr JA, Prager RL, Abernathy JH, et al. Patient safety in the cardiac operating room: human factors and teamwork: a scientific statement from the American Heart Association. Circulation. 2013; 128(10):1139–69.
30. Cook R. "Going solid": a model of system dynamics and consequences for patient safety. Qual Saf Health Care. 2005;14(2):130–4.
31. Stanhope N, Crowley-Murphy M, Vincent C, O'Connor AM, Taylor-Adams SE. An evaluation of adverse incident reporting. J Eval Clin Pract. 1999; 5(1):5–12.
32. Evans SM, Berry JG, Smith BJ, et al. Attitudes and barriers to incident reporting: a collaborative hospital study. Qual Saf Health Care. 2006;15(1):39–43.
33. Kreckler S, Catchpole K, McCulloch P, Handa A. Factors influencing incident reporting in surgical care. Qual Saf Health Care. 2009;18(2):116–20.
34. Dekker SW. The field guide to human error investigations, vol. 1. Aldershot: Ashgate; 2002.
35. Dekker SW. Accidents are normal and human error does not exist: a new look at the creation of occupational safety. Int J Occup Saf Ergon. 2003;9(2): 211–8.
36. Wood G. The I-knew-it-all-along effect. J Exp Psychol Hum Percept Perform. 1978;4:345–53.
37. Berlin L. Hindsight bias. Am J Roentgenol. 2000; 175(3):597–601.
38. Sujan MA, Harrison MD, Steven A, Pearson PH, Vernon SJ. Demonstration of safety in healthcare organisations. In: Gorski J, editor. Computer safety, reliability, and security, proceedings, vol 4166. 2006. p. 219–32.
39. Sujan MA, Koornneef F, Chozos N, Pozzi S, Kelly T. Safety cases for medical devices and health information technology: involving health-care organisations in the assurance of safety. Health Informatics J. 2013;19(3):165–82.
40. Gordon M, Catchpole K, Baker P. Human factors perspective on the prescribing behavior of recent medical graduates: implications for educators. Adv Med Educ Pract. 2013;4:1–9.
41. Gagliardi AR, Brouwers MC, Palda VA, Lemieux-Charles L, Grimshaw JM. How can we improve guideline use? A conceptual framework of implementability. Implement Sci. 2011;6:26.
42. Dixon-Woods M, McNicol S, Martin G. Ten challenges in improving quality in healthcare: lessons from the Health Foundation's programme evaluations and relevant literature. BMJ Qual Saf. 2012;21(10):876–84.
43. de Saint MG, Auroy Y, Vincent C, Amalberti R. The natural lifespan of a safety policy: violations and system migration in anaesthesia. Qual Saf Health Care. 2010;19(4):327–31.
44. Catchpole K. Toward the modelling of safety violations in healthcare systems. BMJ Qual Saf. 2013; 22(9):705–9.
45. Gurses AP, Kim G, Martinez EA, et al. Identifying and categorising patient safety hazards in cardiovascular operating rooms using an interdisciplinary approach: a multisite study. BMJ Qual Saf. 2012; 21(10):810–8.
46. Staggers N, Clark L, Blaz JW, Kapsandoy S. Why patient summaries in electronic health records do not provide the cognitive support necessary for nurses' handoffs on medical and surgical units: insights from interviews and observations. Health Informatics J. 2011;17(3):209–23.
47. Catchpole K, Godden PJ, Giddings AEB, et al. Identifying and reducing errors in the operating theatre. Patient Safety Research Programme. 2005:PS012. Available at: http://pcpoh.bham.ac.uk/publichealth/psrp/publications.htm.
48. Catchpole KR, Giddings AE, de Leval MR, et al. Identification of systems failures in successful paediatric cardiac surgery. Ergonomics. 2006;49(5–6): 567–88.
49. Catchpole K, Mishra A, Handa A, McCulloch P. Teamwork and error in the operating room: analysis of skills and roles. Ann Surg. 2008;247(4): 699–706.
50. Thammasitboon S, Singhal G. System-related factors contributing to diagnostic errors. Curr Probl Pediatr Adolesc Health Care. 2013;43(9):242–7.
51. Catchpole KR, Giddings AE, Wilkinson M, Hirst G, Dale T, de Leval MR. Improving patient safety by identifying latent failures in successful operations. Surgery. 2007;142(1):102–10.
52. Alvarez G, Coiera E. Interruptive communication patterns in the intensive care unit ward round. Int J Med Inform. 2005;74(10):791–6.
53. Brixey JJ, Tang ZH, Robinson DJ, et al. Interruptions in a level one trauma center: a case study. Int J Med Inform. 2008;77(4):235–41.
54. Kreckler S, Catchpole K, Bottomley M, Handa A, McCulloch P. Interruptions during drug rounds: an observational study. Br J Nurs. 2008;17(21): 1326–30.
55. Grundgeiger T, Sanderson P. Interruptions in healthcare: theoretical views. Int J Med Inform. 2009;78(5): 293–307.

56. Alper SJ, Holden RJ, Scanlon MC, et al. Self-reported violations during medication administration in two paediatric hospitals. BMJ Qual Saf. 2012;21(5):408–15.
57. Amalberti R, Vincent C, Auroy Y, de Saint MG. Violations and migrations in health care: a framework for understanding and management. Qual Saf Health Care. 2006;15 Suppl 1:i66–71.
58. Flin R, Patey R. Improving patient safety through training in non-technical skills. BMJ. 2009; 339(1468–5833 (Electronic)):b3595.
59. Undre S, Sevdalis N, Healey AN, Darzi SA, Vincent CA. Teamwork in the operating theatre: cohesion or confusion? J Eval Clin Pract. 2006;12(2):182–9.
60. Mishra A, Catchpole K, Dale T, McCulloch P. The influence of non-technical performance on technical outcome in laparoscopic cholecystectomy. Surg Endosc. 2008;22(1):68–73.
61. McFerran S, Nunes J, Pucci D, Zuniga A. Perinatal patient safety project: a multicenter approach to improve performance reliability at Kaiser Permanente. J Perinat Neonatal Nurs. 2005;19(1):37–45.
62. Leonard M, Graham S, Bonacum D. The human factor: the critical importance of effective teamwork and communication in providing safe care. Qual Saf Health Care. 2004;13 Suppl 1(1475–3898 (Print)):i85–i90.
63. Sexton JB, Thomas EJ, Helmreich RL. Error, stress and teamwork in medicine and aviation: cross sectional surveys. Br Med J. 2000;320:745–9.
64. Catchpole K. Who do we blame when it all goes wrong? Qual Saf Health Care. 2009;18(1):3–4.
65. Hignett S, Carayon P, Buckle P, Catchpole K. State of science: human factors and ergonomics in healthcare. Ergonomics. 2013;56(10):1491–503.
66. Catchpole K. Spreading human factors expertise in healthcare: untangling the knots in people and systems. BMJ Qual Saf. 2013;22(10):793–7.
67. Leape LL, Berwick DM. Five years after to err is human: what have we learned? JAMA. 2005;293(19): 2384–90.
68. Lingard L, Regehr G, Orser B, et al. Evaluation of a preoperative checklist and team briefing among surgeons, nurses, and anesthesiologists to reduce failures in communication. Arch Surg. 2008;143(1):12–7.
69. Haynes AB, Weiser TG, Berry WR, et al. A surgical safety checklist to reduce morbidity and mortality in a global population. N Engl J Med. 2009;360(5):491–9.
70. Verdaasdonk EG, Stassen LP, Widhiasmara PP, Dankelman J. Requirements for the design and implementation of checklists for surgical processes. Surg Endosc. 2009;23(4):715–26.
71. Makary MA, Mukherjee A, Sexton JB, et al. Operating room briefings and wrong-site surgery. J Am Coll Surg. 2007;204(2):236–43.
72. Berenholtz SM, Schumacher K, Hayanga AJ, et al. Implementing standardized operating room briefings and debriefings at a large regional medical center. Jt Comm J Qual Patient Saf. 2009;35(8):391–7.
73. de Vries EN, Hollmann MW, Smorenburg SM, Gouma DJ, Boermeester MA. Development and validation of the SURgical PAtient Safety System (SURPASS) checklist. Qual Saf Health Care. 2009;18(2):121–6.
74. Arora V, Johnson J. A model for building a standardized hand-off protocol. Jt Comm J Qual Patient Saf. 2006;32(11):646–55.
75. Dobson I, Doan Q, Hung G. A systematic review of patient tracking systems for use in the pediatric emergency department. J Emerg Med. 2013;44:242–8.
76. Dickson EW, Singh S, Cheung DS, Wyatt CC, Nugent AS. Application of lean manufacturing techniques in the Emergency Department. J Emerg Med. 2009;37(2):177–82.
77. McCulloch P, Kreckler S, New S, Sheena Y, Handa A, Catchpole K. Effect of a "Lean" intervention to improve safety processes and outcomes on a surgical emergency unit. BMJ. 2010;341(0959-535X (Linking)):c5469.
78. Berguer R. Surgery and ergonomics. Arch Surg. 1999;134(9):1011–6.
79. McDonald KM, Bryce CL, Graber ML. The patient is in: patient involvement strategies for diagnostic error mitigation. BMJ Qual Saf. 2013;22 Suppl 2:ii33–9.
80. Nathan AT, Hoehn KS, Ittenbach RF, et al. Assessment of parental decision-making in neonatal cardiac research: a pilot study. J Med Ethics. 2010; 36(2):106–10.
81. Torowicz D, Lisanti AJ, Rim JS, Medoff-Cooper B. A developmental care framework for a cardiac intensive care unit: a paradigm shift. Adv Neonatal Care. 2012;12 Suppl 5:S28–32.
82. Nascimento LC, Strabelli BS, de Almeida FC, Rossato LM, Leite AM, de Lima RA. Mothers' view on late postoperative pain management by the nursing team in children after cardiac surgery. Rev Lat Am Enfermagem. 2010;18(4):709–15.
83. Hartman DM, Medoff-Cooper B. Transition to home after neonatal surgery for congenital heart disease. MCN Am J Matern Child Nurs. 2012;37(2):95–100.
84. Wray J, Sensky T. Psychological functioning in parents of children undergoing elective cardiac surgery. Cardiol Young. 2004;14(2):131–9.
85. Carayon P, Schoofs HA, Karsh BT, et al. Work system design for patient safety: the SEIPS model. Qual Saf Health Care. 2006;15 Suppl 1(1475–3898 (Linking)):i50–i58.
86. Davies JM. Painful inquiries: lessons from Winnipeg. CMAJ. 2001;165(11):1503–4.
87. Kennedy I. Learning from Bristol: the report of the public inquiry into children's heart surgery at the Bristol Royal Infirmary 1984–1995. 2001. Command Paper: CM 5207.
88. Wiegmann DA, Eggman AA, Elbardissi AW, Parker SH, Sundt TM. Improving cardiac surgical care: a work systems approach. Appl Ergon. 2010;41(5): 701–12.
89. Barach P, Johnson JK, Ahmad A, et al. A prospective observational study of human factors, adverse events, and patient outcomes in surgery for pediatric cardiac disease. J Thorac Cardiovasc Surg. 2008; 136(6):1422–8.

90. Elbardissi AW, Wiegmann DA, Dearani JA, Daly RC, Sundt TM. Application of the human factors analysis and classification system methodology to the cardiovascular surgery operating room. Ann Thorac Surg. 2007;83(4):1412–8.
91. Wiegmann DA, Elbardissi AW, Dearani JA, Daly RC, Sundt TM. Disruptions in surgical flow and their relationship to surgical errors: an exploratory investigation. Surgery. 2007;142(5):658–65.
92. Parker SE, Laviana AA, Wadhera RK, Wiegmann DA, Sundt TM. Development and evaluation of an observational tool for assessing surgical flow disruptions and their impact on surgical performance. World J Surg. 2010;34(2):353–61.
93. Carthey J, de Leval MR, Wright DJ, Farewell VJ, Reason JT. Behavioural markers of surgical excellence. Saf Sci. 2003;41:409–25.
94. Carthey J, de Leval MR, Reason JT. The human factor in cardiac surgery: errors and near misses in a high technology medical domain. Ann Thorac Surg. 2001;72(1):300–5.
95. de Leval MR, Carthey J, Wright DJ, Reason JT. Human factors and cardiac surgery: a multicenter study. J Thorac Cardiovasc Surg. 2000;119(4):661–72.
96. Bognar A, Barach P, Johnson JK, et al. Errors and the burden of errors: attitudes, perceptions, and the culture of safety in pediatric cardiac surgical teams. Ann Thorac Surg. 2008;85(4):1374–81.
97. Schraagen JM, Schouten T, Smit M, et al. Assessing and improving teamwork in cardiac surgery. Qual Saf Health Care. 2010;19(6):1–6.
98. Schraagen JM, Schouten T, Smit M, et al. A prospective study of paediatric cardiac surgical microsystems: assessing the relationships between non-routine events, teamwork and patient outcomes. BMJ Qual Saf. 2011;20(7):599–603.
99. Young-Xu Y, Neily J, Mills PD, et al. Association between implementation of a medical team training program and surgical morbidity. Arch Surg (Chicago, Ill: 1960). 2011;146(12):1368–73.
100. Catchpole KR. Task, team and technology integration in the paediatric cardiac operating room. Prog Pediatr Cardiol. 2011;32:85–8.
101. Catchpole KR, de Leval MR, McEwan A, et al. Patient handover from surgery to intensive care: using Formula 1 pit-stop and aviation models to improve safety and quality. Paediatr Anaesth. 2007;17(5):470–8.
102. Nagpal K, Abboudi M, Fischler L, et al. Evaluation of postoperative handover using a tool to assess information transfer and teamwork. Ann Surg. 2011;253(4):831–7.
103. Zavalkoff SR, Razack SI, Lavoie J, Dancea AB. Handover after pediatric heart surgery: a simple tool improves information exchange. Pediatr Crit Care Med. 2011;12(3):309–13.
104. Catchpole K, Sellers R, Goldman A, McCulloch P, Hignett S. Patient handovers within the hospital: translating knowledge from motor racing to healthcare. Qual Saf Health Care. 2010;19(4):318–22.
105. Catchpole KR, Gangi A, Blocker RC, et al. Flow disruptions in trauma care handoffs. J Surg Res. 2013; 184(1):586–91.
106. Pickering SP, Robertson ER, Griffin D, et al. Compliance and use of the World Health Organization checklist in UK operating theatres. Br J Surg. 2013;100(12):1664–70.
107. Bion J, Comm W, Richardson A, et al. 'Matching Michigan': a 2-year stepped interventional programme to minimise central venous catheter-blood stream infections in intensive care units in England. BMJ Qual Saf. 2013;22(2):110–23.
108. Dixon-Woods M, Leslie M, Tarrant C, Bion J. Explaining Matching Michigan: an ethnographic study of a patient safety program. Implement Sci. 2013;8:13.
109. Nemeth C, Wears RL, Patel S, Rosen G, Cook R. Resilience is not control: healthcare, crisis management, and ICT. Cogn Technol Work. 2011;13(3): 189–202.
110. Wachter RM. Patient safety at ten: unmistakable progress, troubling gaps. Health Affairs (Project Hope). 2010;29(1):165–73.
111. Smith GCS, Pell JP. Parachute use to prevent death and major trauma related to gravitational challenge: systematic review of randomised controlled trials. Br Med J. 2003;327(7429):1459–61.

Information Management and Hospital Enterprise Information Systems

31

Melvin C. Almodovar

Abstract

Effective information management in knowledge-based industries, such as healthcare, is crucial to their success in achieving desired outcomes and product goals. Advances in computer and information technology, along with the evolution of the field of biomedical informatics, have contributed to the maturation of healthcare electronic information systems whose purposes are to support patient care and sustain hospital operations. Access to data across application systems through better integration of system components has become a preferred model for information system architecture and, as a result, institutions often choose to adopt enterprise-wide systems architecture formats using single-vendor application packages. Whether the information system architecture is comprised of multiple, variably, or non-integrated core components or is an integrated enterprise-wide system, this chapter emphasizes how data access, even using a hybrid information system structure, can be used to drive and, hopefully, advance the delivery of care.

Keywords

Health information technology • Enterprise information systems • Enterprise-wide clinical information systems • Biomedical informatics • Application system integration • Healthcare quality

Introduction

Complex business organizations, or "enterprises," rely heavily on information technology (IT) for their viability and competitiveness. This reliance is true for large and small businesses across all industries, particularly those that are *knowledge-based*, in which workers manage

M.C. Almodovar, MD
Division of Cardiac Intensive Care,
Department of Cardiology,
Boston Children's Hospital,
300 Longwood Avenue, Bader 600,
Boston, MA 02115, USA
e-mail: mel.almodovar@cardio.chboston.org

P.R. Barach, J.P. Jacobs, S.E. Lipshultz, P.C. Laussen (eds.),
Pediatric and Congenital Cardiac Care: Volume 2: Quality Improvement and Patient Safety,
DOI 10.1007/978-1-4471-6566-8_31,

information, either through its production or receipt or its use or distribution [1].

Since the early 1990s, enterprise resource planning information management software applications have been employed to integrate departments and their functions within a company. The concept, now commonly referred to as "enterprise information system integration," employs integrated enterprise information system (IEIS) software to maximize efficiency while reducing costs across the company. The benefits, challenges, and controversies associated with IEIS implementation have been popular subjects in the business literature and, increasingly, in the healthcare management literature [2, 3]. It is evident that advances in computer and information technology, beginning with the task-specific use of software applications and extending to the broader IEIS approach, have benefited industry, particularly on business process efficiency and performance, especially when combined with other resources (ie, a strategy in which the application of IT is complimented with the company's human and business resources) [4].

Simultaneously, expectations around the use (and now reliance) of IT have spread to all aspects of society, including healthcare services, training, and research. However, the adoption of IT uniformly across healthcare enterprises or hospitals has lagged substantially behind that of non-healthcare industries and, in the United States, has lagged even behind that of similarly developed peer countries [5]. Reasons for this lag include cost, concerns about privacy and information security, and the fact that healthcare information is highly complex. Despite the lag, there are benefits common to both healthcare and non-healthcare industries:

- Real-time access to important and relevant information
- Efficient and secure internal and external communications
- Enhanced productivity and precision in the performance of certain work-related tasks and decision support
- Performance tracking of business processes (including financial accounting and product outcomes)
- Training and monitoring worker's performance
- Compliance with evolving regulatory requirements

With the evolution and the increased penetration of healthcare IT that is partly driven by governmental and societal mandates [6–9], the science of medical information management, or *biomedical informatics*, has greatly influenced how information and knowledge are applied in medical care delivery.

This chapter will review the data hierarchy concept and briefly introduce the field of biomedical informatics before describing existing hospital information systems structure. It concludes with a discussion of how current information management systems and approaches may be used to provide and evaluate medical care.

The Data Hierarchy

Advances in technology that support data collection, presentation, and distribution, have become more plentiful (sometimes overwhelmingly so), and are readily available to frontline healthcare providers. Because healthcare workers must effectively manage large amounts of data and information to provide medical care, perform research, or even make business decisions, a short review of the data-to-knowledge hierarchy is in order.

The terms *data* and *information* are often used interchangeably, but they are not synonymous. Data are raw observations and facts that, when processed, become information. Information is, thus, data that has been processed to any degree. The threshold beyond which data becomes information is not always easily determined, but the boundary may be irrelevant because information itself, like data, is further processed in our minds to become *knowledge*. At the top of the data hierarchy, knowledge is the product of information processing or analysis as influenced by the experience of the individual or system, the assessment of relationships among information elements, and the application of rules to the information. Important applications of knowledge are the formulation of opinions and decisions that become manifest through actions in everyday life or professional activities. Hence, in the process of information management, it is vital to have reliable data to generate high quality information and knowledge on which decisions and actions can be optimized.

Biomedical Informatics

The practice of medicine requires clinicians to gather, process, and communicate information about individuals or groups of patients. Data and information must also be managed to identify and understand medical problems and to evaluate the appropriateness and effectiveness of diagnostic and treatment strategies. The interdisciplinary field of biomedical informatics (or health informatics) can be defined as the discipline of information management and processing for the purposes of providing medical care, supporting education, and enabling research activities [10–14]. Knowledge creation and information processing are the key fundamental elements; hence the overlay between medicine, cognitive and information science, and computer technology [15, 16].

The four major applications traditionally thought to comprise the field of biomedical informatics are (1) bioinformatics, (2) imaging informatics, (3) clinical informatics (health informatics), and (4) population health informatics. *Bioinformatics* relates to data associated with the basic sciences, such as that involved in the study of genes and proteins. *Imaging informatics*, or radiology informatics, is concerned with digital image acquisition, processing, and applications associated the visual study of organs and organ systems. *Clinical informatics* relates to the acquisition, storage, retrieval, and application of patient information. Health or clinical information systems and their components, such as the electronic medical record, laboratory results reporting tools, and pharmacy systems, all fall under this category. Finally, *public health informatics* is concerned with population-level data and analytic methodologies that pertain to groups of patients. Benchmarking across populations as a means comparing performance between similar groups or against an acceptable standard is contained within this domain.

Collectively, all four of the biomedical informatics subtypes described here encompass rigorous data management techniques along a continuum, beginning with molecular biology and basic science, moving to sophisticated organ system image information processing, then to the comprehensive medical care of individuals, and ending with population-focused data assessment, capture, and analysis.

Health Care Information Systems

An information system is defined as a collection of data, processes, people, and information technology that interact to acquire, process, store, and transmit an output (data or information) to meet an organization's goals [17]. In health care organizations, information systems are classified according to the data management needs for the following: (a) administrative functions or non-clinical operations, and (b) clinical operations [18]. *Administrative systems* deal with information-associated hospital business processes (i.e., patient registration, scheduling, billing, care utilization, etc.), hospital finance accounting, personnel management accounting, and equipment and supplies management. In health care, the use of information technology to support non-clinical activities has progressed faster than its use in support of patient care. *Clinical information systems (CIS)* address the information management needs for all aspects of clinical care and may be organized in several ways (Fig. 31.1). Integration and communication between CIS components, both internally and with external systems, are active areas of focus when considering the overall ability of the system as a whole. Individual hospital departments or ancillary services, such as radiology, pharmacy, or laboratory medicine, typically have their own separate CISs to support internal workflow needs. Traditionally, they have been robust enough to exist independently of other systems because of their unique processes and requirements. They were among the first CISs implemented in hospitals, yet integrating them with other CIS systems has required substantial effort, especially as the overall CIS infrastructure changes.

Clinical activities or specialty areas may need to customize systems to perform specific

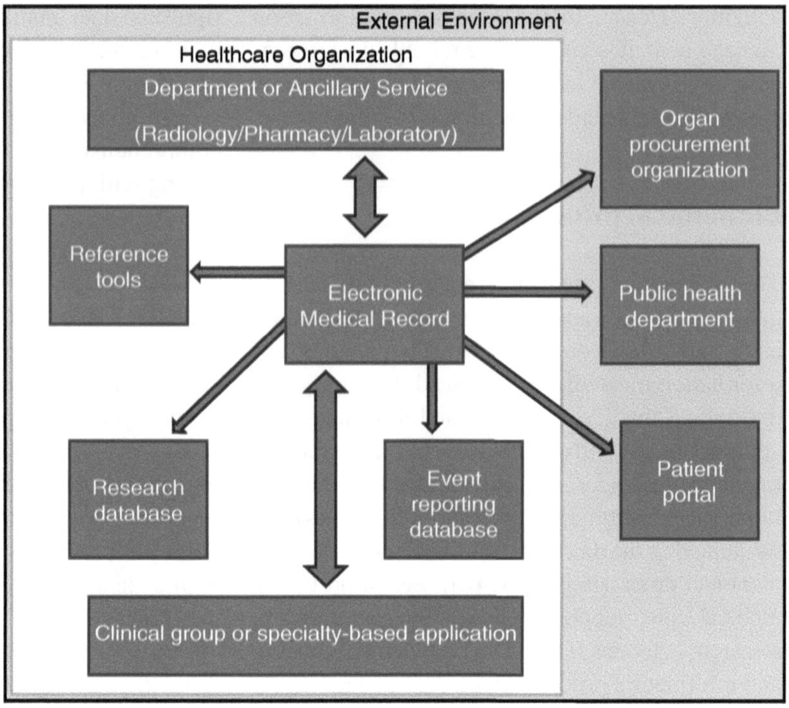

Fig. 31.1 Components of a clinical information system with the electronic medical record as the core component that communicates with internal and external systems

functions not attainable within the broader system architecture. Specialty notes documentation, disease-specific tracking and management, order entry, and medication processing may be supported in this way. Health organizations that have been early adopters of CISs have typically done so using department or group-specific information systems, many of which were locally created. Computerized order entry and decision-support systems are such examples [19].

Knowledge-based reference systems, such as medication formularies and other online reference tools, are readily accessed through the Internet and have become strongly embedded in the day-to-day care of patients across all clinical settings. The electronic medical record (EMR) and the electronic health record (EHR) represent, perhaps, the most inclusive of the CIS types. The designation "EMR" generally refers to the collection of medical information related to a specific event or encounter in a single organization and usually sits at the center of the CIS structure in a healthcare organization (Fig. 31.1). The EHR refers to the repository of patient information collected over time and across organizations. Both hold the same health information contained in the paper-based medical record and are the product of the push for universal conversion to useful health information solutions.

Some of the forces driving this transition towards greater health IT adoption include advances in computer and information technology, a desire to reduce costs while enhancing efficiency, government and societal policy initiatives [6, 7], and the growing focus on patient safety, quality of care, and public health. The Institute of Medicine has stipulated, in its report from the Committee on Data Standards for Patient Safety, that the EMR and EHR should include the following core functions: collection of health information and data (data repository), results management, medication order entry, clinical decision support, communication capability among care providers and with the patient, administrative process support, patient support, and population health management and reporting [20]. Traditionally paper-based medical record systems, which are often highly fragmented both within and across hospital departments, continue to evolve into more accessible and integrated electronic clinical and administrative information systems [21].

Information Systems Architecture

An institution's information systems architecture is guided by its values, IT goals, and requirements for the system. The architecture will, in turn, reflect the capabilities and features of the system, which are enabled by the specific core technologies, applications software, and desired workflow characteristics built into it. Several factors influence the construction and implementation of a system, including (1) the potential return on investment; (2) the financial, personnel, expertise, and existing IT infrastructure resources needed to acquire, implement, and develop the system; (3) the extent of customization efforts; and (4) the desired or expected workflows. The impact on workflow most directly affects the end users or clinical staff who expect that the system will enhance their ability to perform their duties, not hinder it, especially in the era of increased regulatory oversight and focus on care quality and safety outcomes.

The most common hospital IS approaches specifically related to the use of IT for clinical care across an institution are the integrated enterprise-wide system approach (using a single-vendor application software package); the multiple, non-integrated applications system approach, and a hybrid strategy (Figs. 31.2 and 31.3).

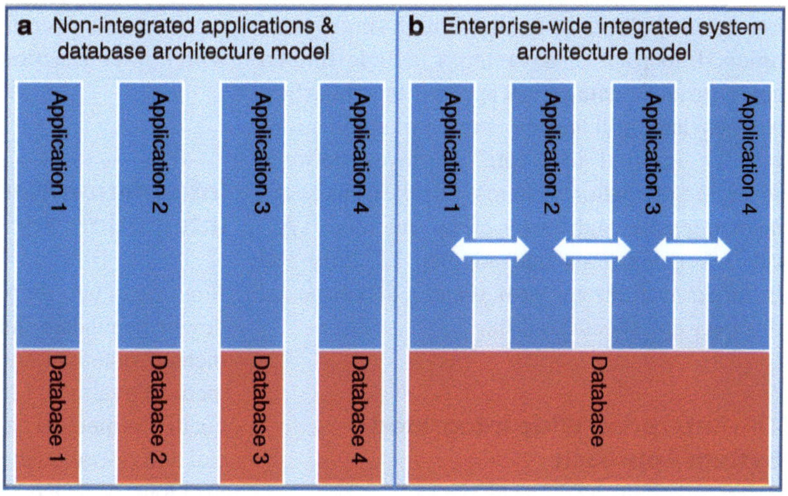

Fig. 31.2 Clinical information system architecture models. (**a**) The non-integrated model consists of separate applications and databases that are not integrated. (**b**) The integrated enterprise-wide model in which applications are integrated and rest on a common database

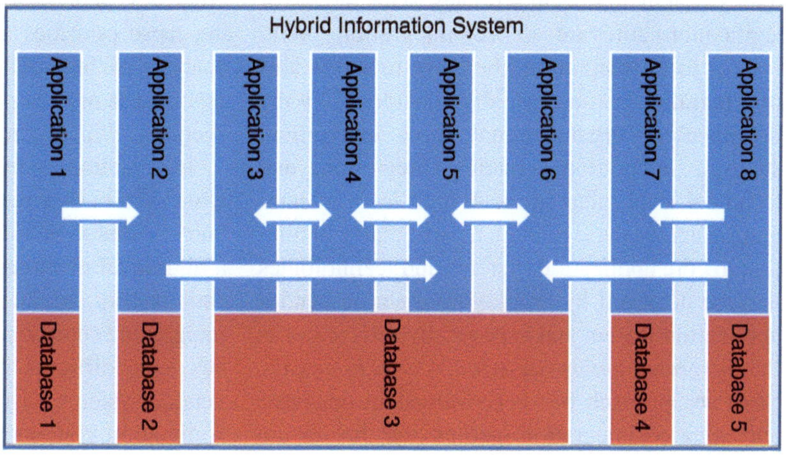

Fig. 31.3 A hybrid information system architecture model. Applications 3 through 6 and Database 3 are fully integrated. The other applications and their respective databases are separate except for variable, unidirectional integration at the application level

The Multiple, Non-integrated Applications Approach

An organization seeking to achieve multiple IS goals through the use of specialized, industry-established, customizable application system components may create what has been traditionally referred to as a *best-of-breed* system. Best-of-breed systems are comprised of core components, thought to be the best in the industry, that support departmental or group-specific workflow and software needs. They are also referred to as "stovepipe" systems, a term reflecting the parallel, non-integrated nature of their component systems in many circumstances (Fig. 31.2). Important advantages are that departments or specialty groups can select the best, usually most mature and customizable components, to achieve multiple IS goals within a single institution. Important disadvantages include limited ability to share data across applications. Interface engines and middleware software applications may be inserted to create interfaces between separate application systems, but these fixes are labor-intensive and costly. They are more typical in organizations that adopted IT early and in larger institutions with greater departmental diversity and specialization.

The Enterprise-Wide Integrated System Approach

Another organizational perspective that determines system architecture relates to the degree of application software or IS integration. With respect to IS integration, there are four domains of integration that are usually considered by the organization: organizational level integration, strategic integration, systems integration, and technical level integration. A high level of integration across these domains, particularly in relation to core application systems and technologies may be achieved by employing a single vendor application system and is generally referred to as the *integrated enterprise-wide system approach.* Such an approach has been valued in business, and greater integration across the healthcare enterprise has become a highly desired feature of contemporary healthcare information systems as indicated by studies of health IT management strategy [22–24].

Selected characteristics of the best-of-breed and integrated enterprise-wide system approaches, including key benefits and advantages related to implementation and usability are displayed in Table 31.1 [25]. Hybrid system architecture represents a third approach and will be discussed later in the chapter. Yet another method of achieving integration, though at the application level, involves the creation of a common user interface (using a separate, web-based application) to provide front-end access to multiple, otherwise separate applications. This is referred to as *visual integration,* which can be achieved, relatively superficially, with little disruption to the overall system infrastructure, albeit with limited functional characteristics.

Information Management, Systems Integration, and Care Delivery

Biomedical informatics supports several key priorities of healthcare delivery. Given the well documented potential for harm to patients receiving medical treatment [26], maximizing the safety and quality of medical care is a top priority. The financial and operational challenges to healthcare organizations have led to the need to refine hospital processes toward better resource use, operational efficiency, and cost containment. Crucial to meeting these priorities are the effective capture and analysis of high-quality data, in addition to the optimal use of IT in personnel and operations management, clinical care, and research activities.

Information management in the enterprise-wide system is enhanced by two important attributes: a shared or common database structure and a high level of integration across multiple applications (Fig. 31.2). However, achieving a truly integrated enterprise-wide information system has been difficult, even though several single-vendor systems have integrated many important application systems ranging from event schedul-

Table 31.1 Selected characteristics of multiple, non-integrated applications and integrated enterprise-wide electronic information systems

	Multiple, non-integrated applications system		Integrated enterprise-wide system	
Functionality	Multiple software applications	+	Single vendor applications	+
	Specialty-focused	+	Organization-focused	–
	Applications more mature	+	Limited application maturity	–
			Some now have clinical area/ specialty focused modules	+
Design	Highly customizable	+	Limited customization	–
	Variable or no integration	–	Highly integrated	+
	Less standardization	–	Highly standardized	+
	Interfaces required for integration	–	Decreased need for interfaces	+
	More rapid design as impact limited to fewer or small areas	+	Design impacts more broadly; need buy in; time consuming	–
Implementation and maintenance	Shorter timeline for implementation	+	Longer timeline for entire system life cycle development	–
	Complicated maintenance requirements	–	Maintenance less complicated, but changes may impact across applications	+
End users	Need to learn multiple systems	–	Need to learn one system	+
	Redundant data entry may be necessary	–	Decreased need for redundant data entry	+
Data sharing	Difficult without substantial interfaces	–	Common database- better reporting capabilities	+
	Multiple places to find data	–	Easier to view data across multiple care areas and encounters	+

Benefits and disadvantages are indicated by a + or – sign, respectively

ing, to imaging viewing and archiving, pharmacy management, laboratory results reporting, and patient care documentation.

Currently, many single-vendor systems have several components that cannot replace or are not superior to other, already on-the-market solutions [25]. Hence, the more realistic scenario involves a CIS architecture comprised of a primary system (possibly a single-vendor system) that integrates certain components while other department or specialty-focused systems are employed alongside. The primary system typically comprises the EMR, whereas the separate, non-integrated component systems may support clinical care directly or be used for other purposes, such as quality-of-care tracking for real-time benchmarking, clinical research activities, and as a reference tool to guide decision making. Such a hybrid system lies somewhere between the completely integrated system architecture and the multiple non-integrated application system construct (Fig. 31.3).

Example of a CIS Profile and Information Management Opportunities

To illustrate how information systems can be employed within a health enterprise, selected examples from the author's institution are summarized in this section. The institutional information system architecture is effectively a hybrid system, although the organizational strategy since 2004 has been to establish an integrated enterprise-wide system. The organization has nevertheless attained the Healthcare Information and Management Systems Society's (HIMSS) highest level (Level 7) for the adoption of the complete EMR [27]. This feat reflects the ability to share data across all capabilities of the EMR, which is remarkable because fewer than 2 % of centers at any stage of EMR conversion have achieved this level as of early 2013.

At the author's institution, EMR conversion is being achieved by implementing a single-vendor enterprise application system encompassing the medical record and several fully integrated department-specific systems. Separately, and for the support of information management and patient care within the hospital's cardiovascular program, are multiple application systems that are integrated to some degree with the EMR and to each other. Admission, discharge, and transfer data are shared across most applications, which is the most consistent example of data sharing. The following are systems or applications that support patient care, quality improvement, research, and tracking of resource utilization.

- *Cardiology clinical database/longitudinal health record.* Using cardiology and congenital heart disease-specific diagnostic coding, separate applications are used to access patient diagnoses, hospital and clinic encounters, surgical and catheter procedures, and primary caregivers. Reports and queries by patient and diagnostic or procedural codes can quickly be performed. Reports from imaging studies and catheter procedures interface with the EMR from the original source application.
- *Hospital serious event reporting system.* A hospital-wide, self-reporting, web-based application captures and classifies patient care or system variances for review and quality tracking. The application is customizable, and events are classified according to type, category, severity, and preventability. Regular review by care area teams and local administrators and by hospital quality coordinators allows real time surveillance of safety and quality metrics with opportunities to benchmark and intervene as necessary.
- *Hospital acquired infection surveillance database.* Initially focused in the critical care units, nosocomial infections (catheter-associated bloodstream infection, urinary catheter-associated infection, ventilator-associated pneumonia, and surgical site infections) are tracked and classified for regular unit-based and hospital-wide review. Data for each infection type are benchmarked against that for similar, pooled patient populations. Rapid review cycles and a ready-to-intervene approach have resulted in beneficial practice and process changes.
- *Standardized care pathway database.* To reduce unnecessary practice variation and optimize care outcomes while improving resource utilization, the institution created formal evidence-based, hypothesis-driven standardized care plans for selected patient populations. Deviations from suggested care practices are identified, and plausible outcomes of the pathways are reviewed for efficacy on an iterative basis, usually in 6-to-9-month cycles. On the basis of this review, practices are modified and new plausible outcomes are generated, if appropriate.
- *Patient tracking, trajectory, and trigger tool.* For critically ill patients, an application was developed to capture, display, and store physiologic information from the continuous bedside monitoring system and some biomedical devices. Physiologic data can be viewed continuously over the entire intensive care unit stay, and trends can be discerned before and after events, which can be annotated in the system. The user interface provides a robust, customizable view of trends, allowing a patient's trajectory to be assessed. Stored physiologic data is integrated with clinical data collected from the EMR and is being used to develop predictive models and algorithms to aid in real-time decision support.
- *Cost stratification by patient type.* From hospital and cardiovascular program financial databases, cardiac procedure costs are matched to patient clinical characteristics. Analysis of patients undergoing catheter and surgical procedures resulted in a cost-stratification model that predicted resource use by diagnosis and procedure type. Predicting resource intensity from financial and clinical data may guide resource planning for patients, third-party payers, and the healthcare organization.

Summary

In this chapter, a parallel has been drawn between healthcare and business enterprises with respect to the application of information technology and evolution towards integrated enterprise-wide information systems to improve information management. Although such systems have become a highly sought means by healthcare organizations as they transition to the complete EMR, success is variable, as is the degree to which complete integration has been achieved. Good data are crucial, and there are many ways to achieve a high level of integration within the IS architecture of an organization. Clearly, as we gain experience in the science of data and information management, and as IT capabilities and applications continue to evolve, better integration of systems will enable safer and higher quality healthcare, research, and efficiency in the medical care delivery process.

References

1. Olson DL, Kesharwani S. Analysis and framework to EIS. In: Enterprise information systems: contemporary trends and issues. Singapore: World Scientific; 2010. p. 1–28.
2. Sumner M. Critical success factors in enterprise wide information management systems projects. In Proceedings of the 1999 ACM SIGCPR conference on Computer personnel research (SIGCPR '99). 1999; 297–303.
3. Davenport TH. Putting the enterprise in the enterprise system. Harv Bus Rev. 1998;76(4):121–31.
4. Powell TC, Dent-Micallef A. Information technology as competitive advantage: the role of human, business, and technology resources. Strateg Manage J. 1997;15(5): 375–405.
5. Jha AK, Doolan D, Grandt D, Scott T, Bates DW. The use of health information technology in seven nations. Int J Med Inform. 2008;77(12):848–54.
6. Bush GW. Executive Order 13335- Incentives for the Use of Health Information Technology and Establishing the Position of the National Health Information Technology Coordinator. Federal Register. April 30, 2004; 69(84): 24059–61.
7. H.R. 1–111th Congress: American Recovery and Reinvestment Act of 2009. (2009).http://www.govtrack.us/congress/bills/111/hr1.
8. California Senate Bill 1875. www.leginfo.ca.gov/.../bill/.../sb.../sb_1875_bill_20000928_chaptered.pdf.
9. Kohn LT, Corrigan JM, Donaldson MS. To err is human: building a safer health system. Washington, DC: The National Academies Press; 2000.
10. Johnson KB, Kim GR. Informatics in pediatric health care. In: Lehmann CU, Kim GR, Johnson KB, editors. Pediatric informatics: computer applications in child health. New York: Springer; 2009. p. 5–18.
11. Greenes RA, Shortliffe EH. Medical informatics: an emerging academic discipline and institutional priority. JAMA. 1990;263(8):1114–20.
12. Hersh WR. A stimulus to define informatics and health information technology. BMC Med Inform Decis Mak. 2009;9:24. doi 10.1186/1472-6947-9-24.
13. Imhoff M, Webb A. Goldschmidt on behalf of the ESICM A. Health Informatics Intensive Care Med. 2001;27(1):179–86.
14. Greenes RA, Siegel ER. Characterization of an emerging field: approaches to defining the literature and disciplinary boundaries of medical informatics. IEEE Computer Society Press; Washington, DC. 1987. p. 411–5.
15. Patel VL, Kaufman DR. Medical informatics and the science of cognition. J Am Med Inform Assoc. 1998; 5(6):493–502.
16. Shortliffe EH, Blois MS. The computer meets medicine and biology: emergence of a discipline. In: Shortliffe E, Cimino J, editors. Biomedical informatics. New York: Springer; 2006. p. 3–45.
17. Whitten J, Bentley L. Systems analysis and design methods. 7th ed. New York: McGraw-Hill/Irwin; 2005.
18. Wager KA, Lee FW, Glaser JP. Health care information systems: a practical approach for health care management. San Francisco: Jossey-Bass; 2009.
19. Campbell E, Guappone K, Sittig D, Dykstra R, Ash J. Computerized provider order entry adoption: implications for clinical workflow. J Gen Intern Med. 2009; 24(1):21–6.
20. Institute of Medicine, Committee on Data Standards for Patient Safety. Key capabilities of an electronic health record system. Washington, DC: Institute of Medicine; 2003.
21. Blumenthal D, Glaser JP. Information technology comes to medicine. N Engl J Med. 2007;356(24): 2527–34.
22. Burke D, Yu F, Au D, Menachemi N. Best of breed strategies–hospital characteristics associated with organizational HIT strategy. J Healthc Inf Manag. 2009;23(2):46–51.
23. Cruz-Correia R, Vieira-Marques P, Ferreira A, Oliveira-Palhares E, Costa P, Costa-Pereira A. Monitoring the integration of hospital information systems: how it may ensure and improve the quality of data. Stud Health Technol Inform. 2006; 121:176–82.
24. Cruz-Correia R, Vieira-Marques P, Ferreira A, Almeida F, Wyatt J, Costa-Pereira A. Reviewing the integration of patient data: how systems are evolving in practice to meet patient needs. BMC Med Inform Decis Mak. 2007;7(1):14.
25. Altavilla S, Thornton JM, Almodovar MC. Assessing the introduction of enterprise-wide clinical information systems in pediatric medical center. Prog Pediatr Cardiol. 2011;32(2):141–5.
26. Institute of Medicine (US). Crossing the quality chasm: a new health system for the 21st century. Washington, DC: National Academies Press; 2001.
27. Health Information and Management Systems Society. HIMSS analytics EMR adoption model. HIMMS Analytics web site. 2013 [cited 2013 Jun 9]. Available from: http://www.himssanalytics.org/emram/emram.aspx.

Towards Effective Data Utilization in Congenital Cardiac Critical Care

32

Dimitar Baronov, Jesse Lock, Sam Phillips, Melvin C. Almodovar, Peter C. Laussen, and Evan Butler

Abstract

Critical care is among the most data intensive fields in health care, with multiple sources of physiologic measurements that are tracked both continuously and intermittently for the purpose of guiding ongoing treatment. Clinicians have a limited capacity to convert this data into actionable information, and thus there is an ongoing effort to develop sophisticated analytic support systems. The immediate technical issues of aggregating this data for analysis are significant but manageable. Analytical models may be generally categorized based on their abstraction of underlying physical principles. Models may be derived from experimental data through statistical processing (black box), from first physiologic principles (white box), or some combination of the two (grey box). Ultimately, successful analytic technologies will *distill* and *reduce* data and present the resultant information in a *centralized*, *intuitive*, and *efficient* manner.

Keywords

Data • Analysis • ICU • Information • computing • Model physiology

D. Baronov, PhD (✉) • J. Lock, MD, PhD
E. Butler, MS
Etiometry LLC, 119 Braintree Street,
Suite 210, Allston, MA 02134, USA
e-mail: baronov@etiometry.com;
jlock@etiometry.com; evan@etiometry.com

S. Phillips, MEng
Arcadia Solutions, Burlington, MA, USA
e-mail: sam.phillips@arcadiasolutions.com

M.C. Almodovar, MD
Division of Cardiac Intensive Care, Department of Cardiology, Boston Children's Hospital,
300 Longwood Avenue, Bader 600,
Boston, MA 02115, USA
e-mail: mel.almodovar@cardio.chboston.org

P.C. Laussen, MBBS, FCICM
Department of Critical Care Medicine,
The Hospital for Sick Children,
Toronto, ON, Canada

Department of Anaesthesia,
University of Toronto,
555 University Avenue,
Toronto, ON M5G 1X8, Canada
e-mail: peter.laussen@sickkids.ca

P.R. Barach, J.P. Jacobs, S.E. Lipshultz, P.C. Laussen (eds.),
Pediatric and Congenital Cardiac Care: Volume 2: Quality Improvement and Patient Safety,
DOI 10.1007/978-1-4471-6566-8_32, © Springer-Verlag London 2015

Introduction

The critical care management of newborns, infants and children with cardiac disease is among the most data intensive fields in health care, with dozens of asynchronous physiologic measurements that are tracked for the purpose of informing ongoing treatment. Despite the raw computational power of the ubiquitous medical devices, clinicians are the principal analytical entity charged with evaluating data and extracting the appropriate actionable information. Humans are inherently limited in their capacity to evaluate multiple complex interrelated information streams, sometimes leading to suboptimal care [1, 2]. Clearly, there is a role for technology that can extract meaningful attributes of the patient state and deliver them to clinical decision-makers.

A useful abstract hierarchy of idea development within the human mind defined by Ackoff [3] follows a progression through *data*, *information*, *knowledge*, and ultimately *wisdom*.

Data is the raw primitive source, which must be processed and structured to create information. Knowledge provides a framework for connecting this information to decision making. Wisdom is the process by which knowledge can be extrapolated from one domain to another. Thus useful formulation of wisdom derives from the creative processing, analysis, and extrapolation of data.

Within the context of the intensive care, it is apparent that there is a huge amount of raw data for clinicians to interpret, from continuous physiologic monitoring through to periodic laboratory and pharmacy data. However, only a small fraction of this data is integrated, captured, stored and translated into meaningful information to assist with knowledge acquisition and decision making. The development of knowledge is a challenging task, and therefore there is inherent value in encapsulating knowledge in a way that makes it transferable and sharable through universal standards of care. However, clinical protocols only provide treatment solutions when the available data is translatable into actionable information. Thus it is an appropriate goal to use advanced analytical technology to improve the proportion of data that is converted into information.

The sections of this chapter provide a framework for analyzing the challenges of data overload in critical care, and the methodologies that can be used to overcome this burden by extracting actionable clinical information.

Data Overload: Causes and Consequences

The critical care environment is an extraordinarily data-rich environment where the volume and variety of signals produced by a patient are highly correlated to acuity. Standard care of a critically ill patient includes the monitoring of many continuously measured physiologic variables (i.e., ECG, SpO_2, invasive blood pressures, etc.), along with intermittently measured laboratory data and biomarkers (lactic acid, hemoglobin, etc.). While the vendor-specific monitors and electronic healthcare records are designed to capture, parse, and deliver intermittent data, the clinicians are required to do the overwhelming majority of the processing and analysis. Despite extensive training and cultivated skills, individual physicians cannot always contend with and assimilate the entirety of these signals [4].

The term "Big Data" refers to systems in which the data volume is too great to be processed by traditional database tools [5], and beyond the capabilities for immediate human integration and interpretation. In a 2001 technical report, Laney [6] describes three distinct components of Big Data: velocity, volume, and variety. *Velocity* is the speed at which data is captured and delivered, *variety* is the number and diversity of data sources, and *volume* is the amount of stored data that requires processing to yield meaningful information. In the following sections we discuss each of these and the challenges they present to physicians when interpreting ICU data.

Velocity

Signals from monitoring in critical care transmit at a variety of rates over many orders of magnitude, from ECG waveforms (>1 kHz), to photoplethysmography (120 Hz) to intermittent

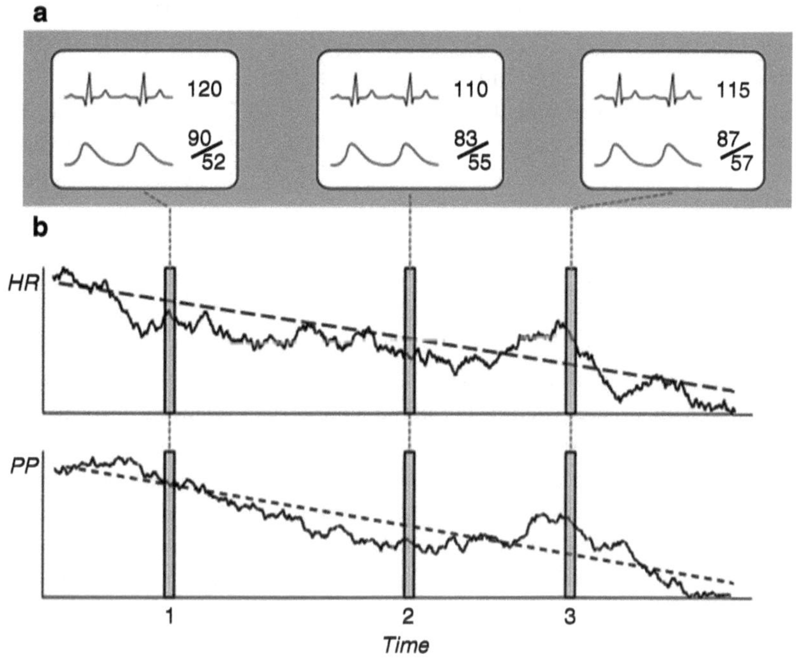

Fig. 32.1 Schematic of evolving patient data. Data that is observed only intermittently (**a**) may not reveal critical underlying clinical trends (**b**).

laboratory data. To contend with these disparate rates, patient data is most often presented as a snap-shot view, usually over a limited time frame and with limited information regarding the history and evolution of that data. This limits the bandwidth with which the clinician can utilize the data, effectively hiding important trends that can indicate critical developments of the patient clinical trajectory. Figure 32.1 shows a schematic of patient data showing a progressively decreasing heart rate (HR) and narrowing pulse pressure (PP). As shown, the inherent variability in these signals can obscure the dominant trend and impending physiologic failure.

Variety

Data in critical care comes from multiple interrelated sources that can serve to illuminate or cloud the relevant underlying clinical state. As an example, consider the evaluation and monitoring of adequate oxygen supply/demand balance. Estimating this factor for a critically ill patient is arguably the most important aspect of pediatric critical care [7]. While the balance between oxygen demand and delivery can be estimated and calculated with intermittent data points, it is difficult to measure continuously. Moreover, there is no way to measure the effective utilization of oxygen for oxidative phosphorylation at the mitochondrial level. Instead, clinicians use a variety of signals that serve, to some degree, as indirect measurements. These proxy measurements include general hemodynamic parameters (e.g. heart rate, perfusion pressure), end-organ perfusion parameters (urine output and biochemical indices of function), metabolic byproducts (lactic acid, and mixed venous O_2 level), and other hematologic parameters (hemoglobin). Although none of these individual proxies provide sufficient information to properly assess adequate oxygen delivery, taken as a group they can theoretically provide a more accurate physiologic picture.

In practice, clinicians have a limited capacity to interpret multiple dissimilar data sources [1, 8]. In a study by Tibby et al. [9] clinicians were asked to stratify the cardiac output of ventilated children (high, normal, low) when provided with all available hemodynamic, laboratory, and physical examination findings. When their responses were compared to the current gold-standard measurement derived from femoral artery thermodilution, researchers found low correlation (r = 0.24) independent of the level of training of the clinician, thus demonstrating the inherent challenge of complex clinical assessment.

Volume

The frequent and standardized repetition of specific circumscribed care will improve a clinician's technical skills. This is much more difficult for complex and varying clinical situations in critical care, such as the management of multi-organ failure or postoperative cardiac surgical care. For a clinician treating such a patient, it is difficult to abstract the enormous volume of data into meaningful information at the moment of care, let alone to derive important and new clinical knowledge that will be relevant to the next patient.

Despite years of experience with ostensibly similar patients, clinicians often reach markedly divergent conclusions about patient care. In an unpublished study, the authors conducted a survey of attending-level physicians to assess the perceived critical bounds of physiologic variables for post-operative management of single-ventricle infants after stage 1 palliation. Physicians were asked to specify three regions for each variable: (1) Physiologically optimal (Green), (2) Physiologically non-optimal (Yellow), and (3) Imminent physiologic failure (Red). The bounds assigned by the clinicians were then compared with the actual physiologic histograms from 39 patients.

Figure 32.2 shows frequency data for Heart Rate (HR), Oxygen Saturation (SpO_2) and Mean Arterial Pressure (ABPm) for this cohort, and demonstrates considerable inconsistencies between individual practitioners in the perceived bounds. Specifically, some practitioners set bounds implying imminent clinical failure more than 40 % of the time, and others assigned values that were >3 standard deviations from the mean as normal. Thus despite years of training and experience, it is challenging to integrate patient data into consistent and accurate clinical guidelines.

Components of Effective Data Utilization

Technologies that seek to overcome the problems caused by data overload in critical care will inevitably need to address several common components of data analysis and utilization. First, data must be captured from multiple heterogeneous sources, formatted universally, and aggregated into a single cluster. Next, the data must be analyzed to extract information relevant to a specific patient's state and trajectory. Finally, the resulting information must be presented to clinicians so as to effectively assist the care process. The following sections present an overview of the specific challenges presented by each of these components, and some technological solutions to these challenges.

Data Capture

Sources of patient information include those directly attached to patients, such as external sensors/devices, and external software systems, such as the electronic health records. Each of these may be locally self-contained, networked back to a local hub within a patient room, or networked centrally within the hospital.

Data may exist in one of many standardized formats, and exchanged using protocols that span multiple conceptual levels. The process of information exchange is often described as the connection between "stacks" of protocols, where each protocol acts on a higher conceptual level than the one preceding it. The conceptual levels can be summarized generically, in increasing conceptual level, as (a) the method of delivery, (b) the structure of the message, (c) the content of the message, and (d) the expected behavior of the recipient. Only when these rules are defined and understood by stakeholders will the exchange proceed in an efficient and expected manner. In order to successfully collect and collate data from multiple healthcare data sources it is imperative that the exchange mechanisms are compatible at each level of the protocol. The mechanisms of interoperation are beyond the scope of this document, but one could imagine that the challenges of information exchange depend largely on which protocols need to be adapted.

A deceptively challenging task is to associate data with its originating patient. While some devices can do this locally by collecting and displaying data only within a patient room, networked data requires a system to associate the correct source of data with other levels of information, such as from the admission, discharge, transfer and patient demographic systems, to ensure there is system-wide agreement. This type of challenge, known as the "multi-master problem" arises whenever two systems assert the same piece of information and a third system has to adjudicate to determine which it should accept. For example, if a monitor in room 123 is associated with Patient A, but the EMR associates room 123 with Patient B, a third system which integrates information from both systems has the option to either (a) assume that the monitor is correct, (b) assume that the EMR is correct, or (c) assume neither and disregard messages until the discrepancy is resolved. The correct resolution

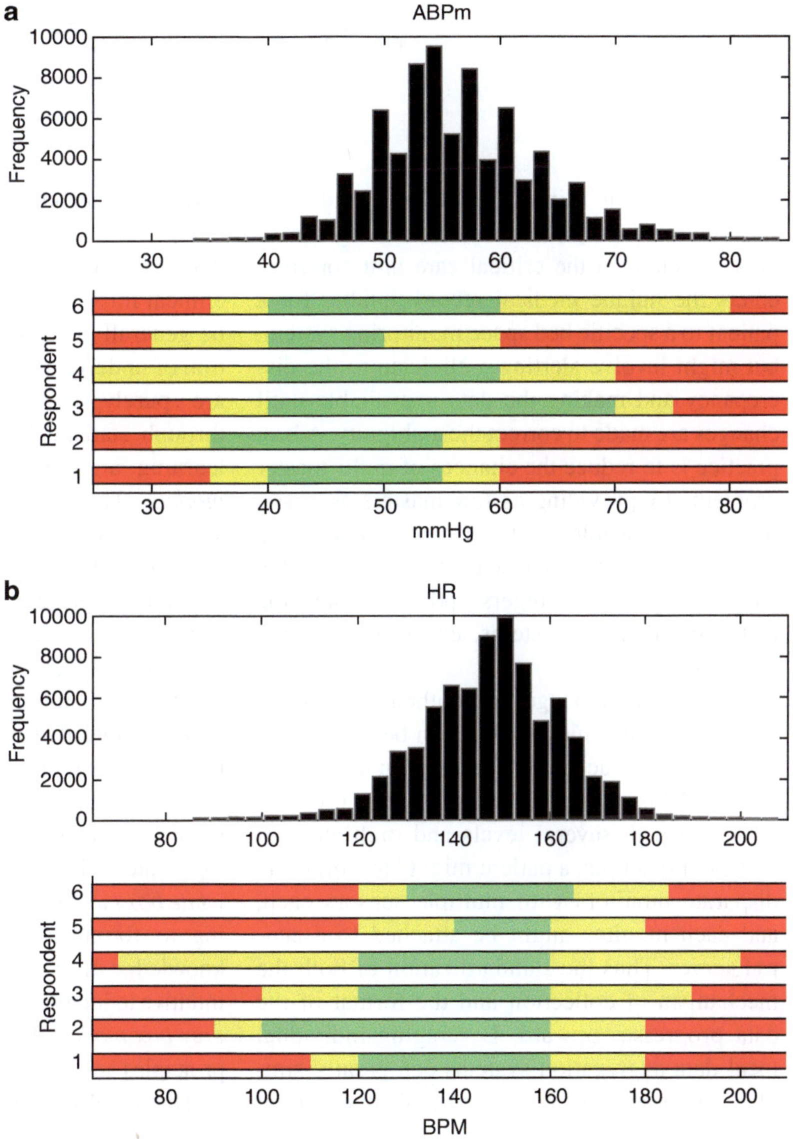

Fig. 32.2 Histograms of patient data frequency vs. clinician's assignment of physiologically optimal (*Green*), physiologically non-optimal (*Yellow*), and imminent physiologic failure (*Red*) for Mean Arterial Blood Pressure (**a**), Heart Rate (**b**), and Oxygen Saturation (**c**).

Fig. 32.2 (continued)

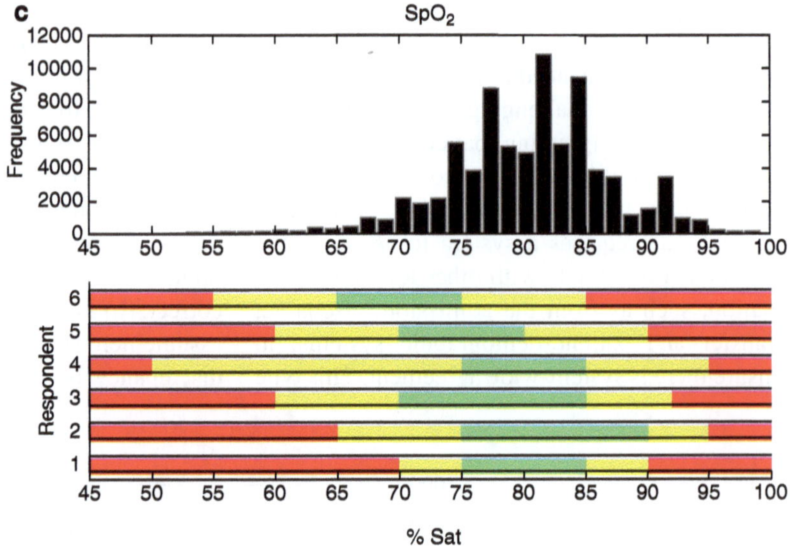

will depend on clinical workflows and site-specific requirements, such as ensuring that a nurse or clerk in the critical care unit correctly enters the unique medical record number for a patient to a specific bed space monitoring system, but might involve alerting a clinician to the discrepancy and making the data unavailable until changes are made to correct the ambiguity. A best practice is to reduce the chances of multi-master problems by providing as few masters as possible. When feasible, systems can be connected such that one upstream change (e.g. during the admission process) triggers updates to both the EMR and monitor systems, ensuring they stay synchronized.

Once data exchange and authenticity protocols have been achieved, data can be aggregated into a centrally accessible location in a common format. This aggregation can occur progressively through several levels and multiple systems. For example, a patient might have multiple disparate monitors with multiple sensors each, and each monitor might be attached to a central server. Thus the standardization of both the mechanism of collection and the format of the data progresses upward. Leveraging individual local data aggregation systems can greatly simplify the process of collecting real-time patient health information.

Modeling and Analysis

Analytical models are used to extract relevant clinical information from patient data. These can be generally categorized based on their abstraction of underlying physical principles. Those that are purely derived from experimental data through statistical processing, such as machine learning algorithms, are known as *black box models*. These types of models are generally straightforward to implement, but have a number of drawbacks in that they (a) disregard known physiologic principles, and (b) are challenging to correlate with larger clinical context. As an example, a black box algorithm that purports to identify impending cardiovascular collapse is less valuable if it cannot concomitantly express the underlying physiological reasoning.

Models that are derived from first physiologic principles by abstracting well understood physiologic interactions and dependencies are known as *white box models*. These models are more challenging to formulate because they require a priori knowledge of the underlying system, but are more intuitive to interpret. Additionally, there exist hybrid *grey box models* that embed both clear underlying principles and data derived dependencies.

Historically, the first models to be utilized for analyzing critical care data were static black box models used to assess severity of illness. These include indices such as the APACHE, SAPS, ASCOT, and PRISM scores. The general format for each of these scores is to use weighted combinations of easily obtainable variables (e.g. age, responsiveness, physiologic signs) to assign a relation to a particular level of acuity or likely outcome (e.g. length of stay, mortality). Despite their simplicity, few of these models are commonly used prospectively to make medical decisions due to limited immediate clinical value or technical requirements. More recently, a number of dynamic indices, such as the Pediatric Early Warning System (PEWS) [10] and the Stability Index [11] have been developed to monitor *changes* in variables to capture evolving physiologic trends.

Grey box models used in critical care generally seek to interpret data in the context of maintaining physiologic homeostasis (e.g. matching oxygen supply and demand). The most well-known examples of grey box models are those that measure the variability of vital signs (such as Heart Rate) to assess autonomic system function. These models start from the rationale that homeostasis is maintained through interactions of multiple decentralized systemic components [12]. For example, oxygen delivery is governed both globally through chemoreceptors and locally within tissue through active and reactive hyperemia. This results in a networked system whose stability emerges as a natural result of its interactions, and loss of variability is a sign of the system failing. Algorithms based on variability analysis have had some success identifying impaired oxygen delivery in patients with single ventricles [13], hemorrhagic shock [14], and sepsis [15].

White box models attempt to illuminate homeostasis by interpreting data using first-principle physiologic models. The general structure of a cardiovascular white box model can be divided into two components: a *dynamic model* and an *observational model*. The dynamic model abstracts physiologic auto-regulation and the respective regulated variables such as oxygen delivery or mean arterial pressure. The observational model relates the regulated variables to available data streams. An example of this model architecture using hemodynamics of a single ventricle congenital heart population is provided by McManus et al. [16]. One critical feature of this model is that it is stochastic, which enables it to capture the inherent uncertainties of both the measurements and the physiology model itself. As a result, the model provides probability density functions for estimated variables, as opposed to specific estimations with unknown precision and accuracy. As shown Fig. 32.3, readily available data may be processed through a dynamic physiology model to obtain probabilistic estimates of relevant underlying hidden variables.

Information Delivery

Once information has been created from data it must be delivered effectively to clinicians. In an environment already at risk for sensory and data overload, the delivery of new information must conform to the medical workflow without overwhelming clinicians. A report by Osheroff et al. [17] outlines a national roadmap for successful implementation of clinical decision support systems, that starts with optimized technology. Within critical care, optimized analytic technology will *distill* and *reduce* data as opposed to adding another monitor or index to the mix, allowing clinicians to focus on the most relevant material. Second, it will present information in a *centralized, intuitive*, and *efficient* manner. Third, it will be integrated into the clinical workflow and permit the clinician to provide feedback to encourage engagement and provide continuous clinical and analytic improvement. Technologies that have fallen short on these criteria in the past have suffered from poor adoption and usage. The development of individual medical knowledge is derived over many years of experience, making clinicians skeptical of significant or rapid changes in medical guidelines. For analytical models to be broadly accepted they must definitively demonstrate return on investment and they must improve the clinical workflow. While return on investment is certainly an important factor, the challenges to achieving this milestone will be specific to each individual technology.

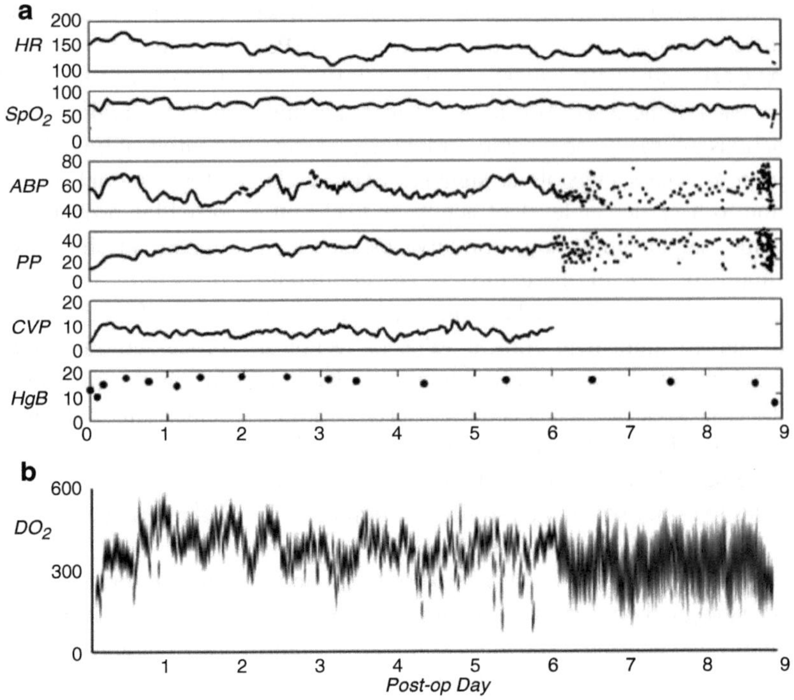

Fig. 32.3 Patient data showing (**a**) Continuous and intermittent measurement employed by the risk-based monitoring system use to infer: (**b**) Probabilities of inadequate oxygen delivery. Each time slice of (**b**) represents a probability density function, and this function widens notably after the removal of the continuous indwelling monitor on day 6

Conclusion

Data overload in critical care is a pressing concern that will likely worsen in the near term as signals from new devices and tests come to market. The immediate technical issues of aggregating this data are significant but manageable. A greater challenge is the development of successful analytic methods. While black-box analytic methods may yield quick results, the use of white-box models are strongly preferred to provide a more thorough understanding of the underlying physiology. Ultimately, successful analytic technologies will provide an intuitive funnel from raw data into actionable information.

References

1. Soleymani S, Borzage M, Noori S, Seri I. Neonatal hemodynamics: monitoring, data acquisition and analysis. Expert Rev Med Devices. 2012;9(5):501–11.
2. Blount M, Ebling MR, Eklund JM, James AG, McGregor C, Percival N, Smith KP, Sow D. Development and deployment of the artemis analytic system. IEEE Eng Med Biol Mag. 2010;29(2):110–118.
3. Ackoff R. From data to wisdom. J Appl Syst Anal. 1989;16:3–9.
4. Scanlon MC, Karsh B-T. Value of human factors to medication and patient safety in the intensive care unit. Crit Care Med. 2010;38(6 Suppl):S90–6.
5. Manyika J, Chui M, Brown B, Bughin J, Dobbs R, Roxburgh C, Byers AH. Big data: the next frontier for innovation, competition, and productivity. Washington, DC: McKinsey Global Institute; 2011.
6. Laney D. 3D data management: controlling data volume, velocity, and variety. META Group Research Note, 6, 2001.
7. Checchia P, Laussen P. The cardiac intensive unit perspective on hemodynamic monitoring of oxygen transport balance. Pediatr Crit Care Med. 2011;12(4):S69–71.
8. Bohn D. Objective assessment of cardiac output in infants after cardiac surgery. Semin Thorac Cardiovasc Surg Pediatr Card Surg Annu. 2011;14(1):19–23.
9. Tibby S, Hatherill M, Marsh M. Clinicians' abilities to estimate cardiac index in ventilated children and infants. Arch Dis Child. 1997;77(6):516–8.
10. Parshuram CS, Hutchison J, Middaugh K. Development and initial validation of the Bedside Paediatric Early Warning System score. Crit Care. 2009;13(4):R135.
11. Baronov D, Butler EJ, Lock J, Mcmanus M, Laussen PC. Stability index retrospective validation in post-operative patients with single ventricle palliation. 2013.
12. Buchman TG. The community of the self. Nature. 2002;420(6912):246–51.
13. Kaltman JR, Hanna BD, Gallagher PR, Gaynor JW, Godinez RI, Tanel RE, Shah MJ, Vetter VL, Rhodes LA.

Heart rate variability following neonatal heart surgery for complex congenital heart disease. Pacing Clin Electrophysiol. 2006;29(5):471–8.

14. Cooke WH, Convertino VA. Heart rate variability and spontaneous baroreflex sequences: implications for autonomic monitoring during hemorrhage. J Trauma Inj Infect Crit Care. 2005;58(4):798–805.
15. Moorman JR, Carlo WA, Kattwinkel J, Schelonka RL, Porcelli PJ, Navarrete CT, Bancalari E, Aschner JL, Whit Walker M, Perez JA, Palmer C, Stukenborg GJ, Lake DE, Michael O'Shea T. Mortality reduction by heart rate characteristic monitoring in very low birth weight neonates: a randomized trial. J Pediatr. 2011;159(6):900–6.e1.
16. McManus M, Baronov D, Almodovar M, Laussen P, Butler E. Novel risk-based monitoring solution to the data overload in intensive care medicine. In: 52nd conference on decision and control. Firenze: Italy; 2013. p. 1009–16.
17. Osheroff JA, Teich JM, Middleton B, Steen EB, Wright A, Detmer DE. A roadmap for national action on clinical decision support. J Am Med Inform Assoc. 2007;14(2):141–5.

Clinical Decision Making

33

Pat Croskerry

Abstract

In every domain of medicine, decisions are continuously being made about patients' diagnosis and management. Arguably, decision making is the most important aspect of a patient's care and the most likely to affect their safety, yet physicians generally do not receive comprehensive training in this basic skill. In this chapter, dual process theory, the dominant model of clinical decision making, is reviewed. The two basic modes of decision making are *intuitive* and *analytical*. The properties of the two systems are discussed, as is their dynamic relationship with each other in the operating characteristics of the model.

Many of the requirements for improving decision making can be found in the burgeoning literature on critical thinking. Significant gains in decision making skills can be made by teaching the basics of decision making within a critical-thinking framework and by thoroughly understanding the nature and extent of cognitive and affective biases and how to mitigate them. There remains an overarching need for research in clinical decision making that is relevant to the clinical settings and conditions under which decisions are made.

Keywords

Clinical decision making • Dual process theory • Cognitive and affective bias • Cognitive de-biasing • Critical thinking

Imagine that your family has just moved to a new town, and one of your children has a previously diagnosed heart problem. You need a new doctor and are concerned that both you and your family members will receive the best care. What qualities in that doctor would you look for: likeable personality, good listener, knowledgeable, good

P. Croskerry, MD, PhD, FRCP (Edin)
Critical Thinking Program, Division of Medical Education, Faculty of Medicine, Department of Emergency Medicine, QE – Health Sciences Centre, Halifax Infirmary, Dalhousie University, Suite 355, 1796 Summer Street, Halifax, NS B3H 2Y9, Canada
e-mail: croskerry@eastlink.ca

P.R. Barach, J.P. Jacobs, S.E. Lipshultz, P.C. Laussen (eds.),
Pediatric and Congenital Cardiac Care: Volume 2: Quality Improvement and Patient Safety,
DOI 10.1007/978-1-4471-6566-8_33, © Springer-Verlag London 2015

communicator, team-player, empathic, good decision maker, professional manner, strong ethical values? Imagine again that if you can only select two, which would they be? Although the qualities listed are all important, most of us would probably opt for someone who was both knowledgeable and a good decision maker. These two seem to provide the absolute basic requirements for someone who is going to give you the best chance of having your family members correctly diagnosed and appropriately managed.

For graduates of accredited medical schools, we can reasonably assume that their knowledge base is sufficient. Most schools cover the fundamentals and examine their graduates for competence at stages along the way. Graduates will have been required to pass National and Board examinations that exhaustively test their knowledge. Further, they will have access to various online resources that provide access to the best, up-to-date medical evidence. But what guarantees would you have that you have also selected a good decision maker, someone who has been trained to reason effectively and make best decisions? The answer, unfortunately, is that you would have none.

Few, if any, medical schools offer a comprehensive course in decision making. Excellent material for rational decision making is usually available [1], but basic instruction about intuitive decision making is virtually non-existent. This lack is worrying because psychologists tell us that we make most of our decisions intuitively [2, 3]. Unless something about the medical mind is different, the sad truth is that we are not explicitly teaching doctors the properties of intuitive thinking and the decision making that goes with it. To put it bluntly, we are seriously short-changing trainees in, arguably, their most critical skill—how to make safe and reliable decisions.

Decision Making

Historically, doctors have been largely responsible for generating their own approaches to clinical decision making. The teachings of renowned clinicians, such as William Osler, Zachary Cope, Ernest Codman, and others have been followed, and their principles, aphorisms, caveats, and maxims have been passed down through successive generations of mentors and teachers and remain influential today. However, this tradition spans only a few generations. Of necessity, these teachings were based on the brutal lessons of clinical trial and error and, until recently, no specific effort was made to explicitly teach decision making. Instead, it was acquired more tacitly through observation, mimicry, osmosis, or some other means but not deliberately or systematically. It now seems odd that clinical skill in decision making—clinical acumen as it was known—was such a highly prized skill but attracted so little research interest.

In recent years, decision making has been approached scientifically, largely through the efforts of cognitive psychologists. Cognitive psychology deals with human thinking, reasoning, and decision making. It is defined by the American Psychological Association as: "the study of higher mental processes such as attention, language use, memory, perception, problem solving, and thinking" [4]. However, the theoretical basis of much of what cognitive psychologists do lies outside the remit (and interest) of most practicing clinicians; nevertheless, we can at least borrow from the major findings of the field. One of these theories, a basic model of decision making termed "dual process theory," has emerged as the dominant model for decision making. However, it is more than a model. Professional consensus and converging lines of evidence from neuroanataomy, neurology, neurophysiology, genetics, cognitive psychology, sociology, and philosophy support the view that the human brain has two distinct types of processes [5]. Through functional magnetic resonance imaging studies, the anatomical loci for the two processes in the brain are now known [6].

Dual Process Decision Making

The two principal modes of decision making, *automatic* and *controlled*, were originally described by Schneider and Shiffrin over 35 years ago [7] and are now commonly referred

Table 33.1 Properties of Types 1 and 2 decision making processes

Property	Type 1 processes	Type 2 processes
Decision making	Intuitive Heuristic Associative Concrete	Analytical Normative Deductive Abstract
Proportion of cognitive time	High	Low
Awareness	Low	High
Automaticity, reflexivity	High	Low
Speed of response	Fast	Slow
Effort required	Minimal	Considerable
Resource cost	Low	High
Vulnerability to bias	Yes	Less so
Errors	Common	Few
Affective involvement	Often	Less so
Importance of context	High	Low
Hard-wired	Sometimes	No
Able to be overridden	Yes Metacognition Mindfulness Decoupling	Yes Impulsivity Mindlessness Dysrationalia

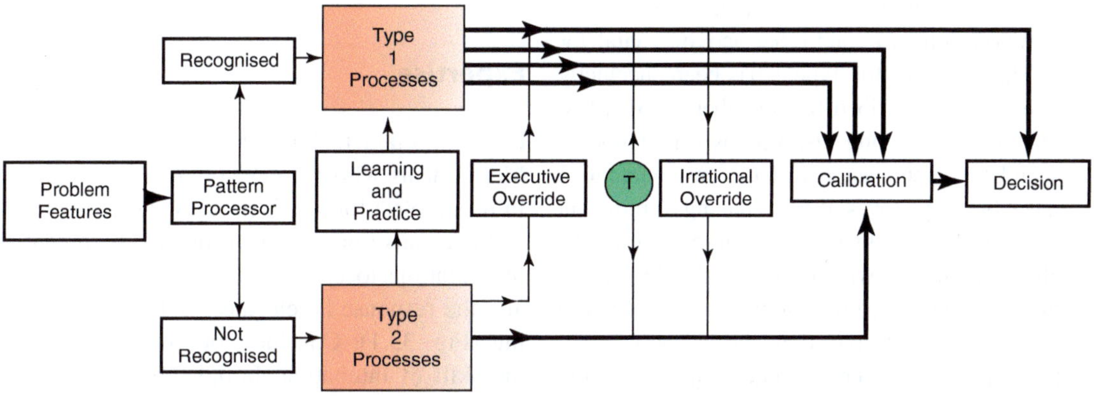

Fig. 33.1 The dual process model of decision making. The multiple *arrows* shown for Type I processing indicate different subgroups. Many Type 1 decisions will be acted upon without calibration

to as *intuitive* and *analytical*, respectively. Psychologists see intuitive decision making driven by "Type 1" or "System 1" processes and analytical reasoning by "Type 2" or "System 2" processes (Table 33.1).

A variety of approaches to decision making and reasoning have been proposed, but most are compatible with this dual process model [5]. The first application of the model in medicine appears to have been made by Dawson [8], and has since been adopted as a universal approach to clinical decision making (CDM) [9] (Fig. 33.1). The model is relatively straightforward and can be easily taught.

Type 1 Decision Making

As soon as one sees, smells, hears, tastes, or feels anything, the brain's automatic and initial response is to try to match it to a familiar pattern. These patterns may be hard-wired or acquired through experience. If a matching pattern can be found, an automatic response results, and Type 1 processing occurs. Importantly, it is reflexive and subconscious. We can make decisions and act on Type 1 output, but we do not deliberately reason in Type 1. Stanovich refers to these processes as The Autonomous Set of Systems [10]. In medicine, it is the system that delivers the *augenblick* ("moment of an eye") response—when a pattern of symptoms or signs presents itself and the clinician reflexively makes the diagnosis [11]. Often, the diagnosis is correct, especially for highly pathognomonic cases, but trusting completely in such spot diagnoses can be dangerous. The eminent surgeon, Cope, observed: "Spot diagnosis may be magnificent, but it is not sound diagnosis. It is impressive but unsafe" [12].

Most of our decision making occurs in Type 1. Psychologists say that we spend about 95 % of our waking lives there [2], and mostly it serves us well. Type 1 processing includes creativity, imagination, inspiration, romance, and other activities vital for life. The necessity for Type 1 has been succinctly and elegantly described by Smallberg [13]. Most importantly, prevailing dispositions (or biases) to respond to salient features of the environment in predictable ways saves us from having to re-invent every wheel in our lives. These biases give us the ability to perform a wide variety of simple to complex acts automatically, allowing us to achieve much of what needs to be done through serial associations [14]. However, as Denes-Raj and Epstein note (referring to Type 1 as the experiential system): "Although experiential processing is highly efficient and adaptive in most circumstances, in other circumstances it is error-prone and a source of maladaptive biases" [15]. Such bias, notes Smallberg, "is the thumb that experience puts on the scale" [13]. In short, we cannot live without Type 1 processing, but we must be vigilant when we use it.

Type 2 Thinking

If the sensory input is not matched with any existing pattern, we default to Type 2 thinking. Now, we seek to understand the stimulus in a conscious, deliberate, rational manner, generating and testing hypotheses. This is a more reliable way of making decisions and generally results in fewer errors. It is rational and therefore follows the laws of logic and science but it can still be seen as a form of pattern matching. Fundamentally, scientific enquiry represents an effort to make sense of and find patterns in data. Clinicians who follow the rules of science, logic, rationality, and critical thinking get the most out of Type 2 processing. Clinicians who do not may expose themselves—and their patients—to peril. Importantly, cognitive debiasing depends upon Type 2 thinking—the means by which we can mitigate bias in decision making. However, Type 2 thinking is time-consuming and resource-intensive; neither is it completely error free. Healthcare leaders, for example, may rationally deliberate and decide on policies that turn out to be fundamentally flawed. When error does occur in Type 2 thinking, the consequences may be far-reaching.

Expertise

It is important to know how the Dual Process Model deals with the development of expertise. In its simplest form, this process can be depicted as the acquisition of a habit or skill by repeated presentations to Type 2 processing where eventually the response is relegated to Type 1 processing (Fig. 33.1). Consider for example learning the skill of intubation. Initial efforts at intubation, usually on a mannequin, require holding a strange instrument in the non-dominant hand and attempting to visualize an anatomically indistinct area to which an endotracheal tube needs to be directed with the dominant hand. It is a complex, visual-motor-haptic skill that takes many repetitions to accomplish smoothly and become what is often a life-saving maneuver in real patients. With experience comes expertise, depicted in pathway A of Fig. 33.2. However, as with many skills, some become better than others, and experience does not always lead to expertise. Pathway B represents someone who has become experienced through multiple repetitions of the behavior but who has not become expert, perhaps from poor instruction, a poor learning environment,

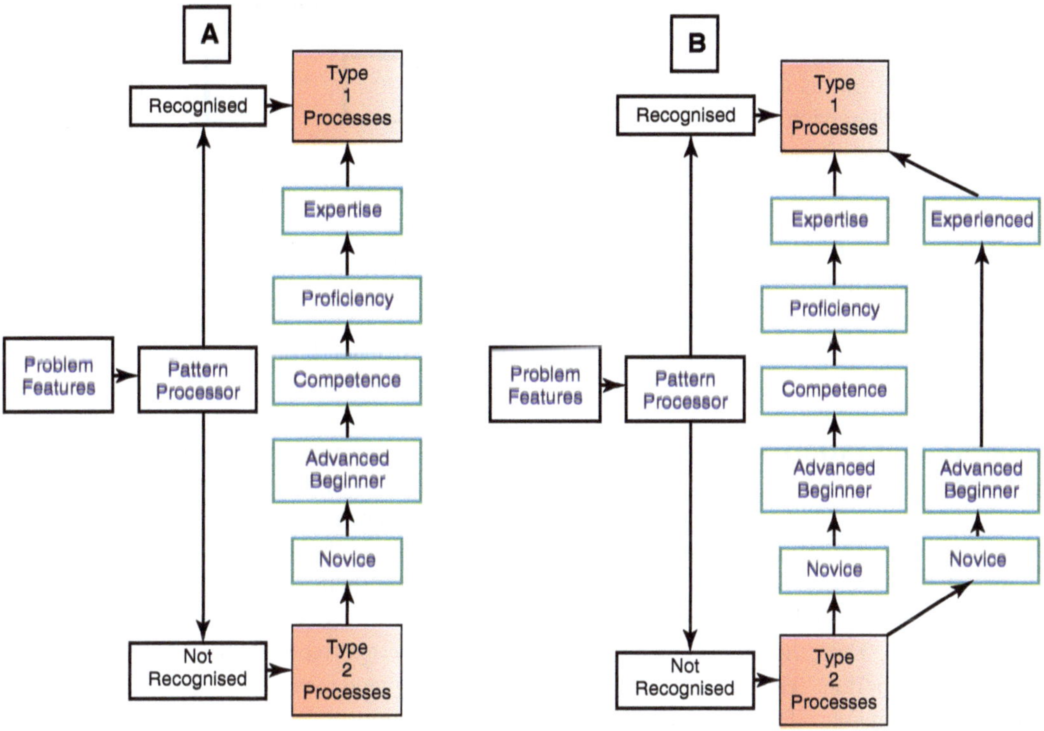

Fig. 33.2 Acquisition of expertise (**a**) versus becoming an experienced non-expert (**b**)

or through other factors [16]. In the longer term, there is some evidence that as physicians age, they will spend less time in Type 2 and more in Type 1 thinking.

The Executive Override Ability

Several more properties of the model need to be explained. Although Type 1 processes are reflexive, this does not mean that the decision maker is unaware of them or that they cannot be changed. Say, for example, a middle-aged patient presents to an emergency department with flank pain, vomiting, and hematuria. The physician's immediate response may be that the patient has a kidney stone; an *augenblick* diagnosis based on an extremely familiar pattern. But the physician does not need to commit to it. He can observe his own response and may be reminded that he saw a case presented at morbidity and mortality rounds recently where a patient had similar signs and symptoms but was undergoing abdominal aortic dissection. His Type 2 thinking therefore overrides the initial Type 1 response, resulting in purposeful thinking to exclude other diagnoses. This check is referred to as *executive override*, also known as reflective thinking, mindful practice, and metacognition; it is also the basis for cognitive debiasing discussed below. After the override, the clinician may return to Type 1 thinking for more inspiration or might establish a differential diagnosis and systematically work through the options.

Irrational Decision Making

Type 1 processing can also override Type 2 thinking. Despite knowing the most rational thing to do in a particular situation, the clinician may do something else, often following his or her intuition. For example, if a clinician assesses a patient with a neck injury and finds that the physical examination and mechanism of injury do not warrant a cervical radiograph according to published decision rules but orders a radiograph anyway, he or she is overriding a well researched rule with usually high sensitivities that would probably outperform his or her decision making on most days. Stanovich refers to this Type 1 override of Type 2 as *dysrationalia* [17]. Historically, it is also known as *akrasia* [18], *irrational* behavior, *dysfunctional* decision making, or *weakness of will* [19, 20]. Road rage, binge eating, drinking to excess, gambling, and a variety of other human behaviors are vivid examples in everyday life.

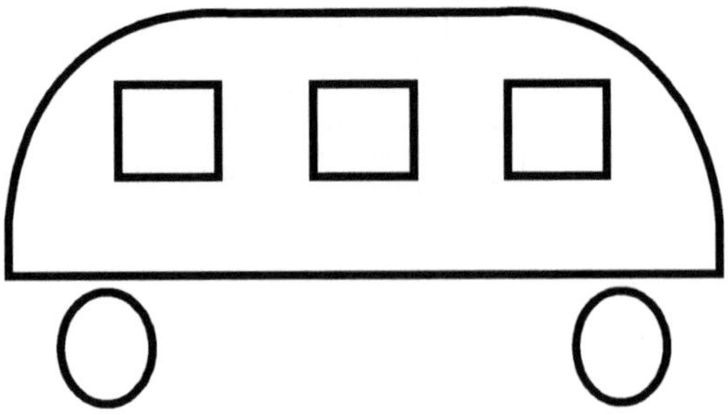

Fig. 33.3 Cognitive miser function. In which direction is the bus travelling? There are two possible answers: left or right

Dynamic Calibration of the Two Systems

In many schematic presentations of the dual process model, there is a start point at which the initial stimulus is presented and an end point at which a decision is made. Thus, the model appears linear. However, an important feature is that the model is inherently dynamic. The first point, already mentioned, is the executive override junction. A transition from Type 1 to 2 processing is accomplished, which may then result in a return to Type 1 and perhaps reactivation of Type 2. This exchange can be thought of as a "toggle function" that allows for dynamic oscillation between the two types. There has been debate about whether Type 1 and Type 2 processing are on a continuum or whether they toggle back and forth [21], but the consensus is that the two types are parallel and distinct from each other.

The final part of the model is a calibration junction. The mark of a well calibrated thinker is the ability to balance the right blend of intuition and analytical reasoning in decision making for a particular situation.

The Cognitive Miser Function

The brain generally seeks to conserve energy. It can do so by defaulting to Type 1 processing where very little effort is required to keep the cognitive wheels turning. The evolutionary imperative for this conservation is related to the brain's metabolic demand for 20 % of resting metabolic energy, despite comprising only 2 % of total body weight. In our ancient past, when calories were hard to come by, those who conserved energy had a selective advantage and were more likely to get their genes into the next generation. In modern times, several phenomena are associated with cognitive miserliness. For example, the prevailing tendency is to resist change, preserve the status quo, and avoid the uptake of new information, all of which require Type 2 thinking. One of the reasons for not dealing with decisions in Type 2 thinking, notes Kahneman, is that it requires cognitive effort [14].

There is an overwhelming tendency to revert to Type 1 decision making, becoming what Pink Floyd called "comfortably numb," or as the Foundation for Critical thinking describes it, "living an unexamined life … in a more or less automated, uncritical way" [22]. An example is given in Fig. 33.3, which shows a side-view of a school bus, and the question is: Which direction is the bus travelling? Most people, seeing the symmetrical figure, conclude that it is impossible to say which direction the bus is travelling, yet preschoolers usually get it right and say the bus is going left. Their reason, which escapes most adults, is they cannot see the entry door (if they live in a country where you drive on the left side of the road, the direction of the bus is to the right). For the preschooler, the door is extremely important for getting on the bus, but adults who are too far removed from the problem and reluctant to make the cognitive effort to solve the problem will fail. Under various conditions (fatigue, sleep deprivation, cognitive overload, and negative moods) there is an increased tendency to default into Type 1 processing [23] and take the path of least resistance.

Individual Differences in Decision Making

Medical educators assume, perhaps naively, that there is a greater consistency among decision makers than probably exists and, given some basic variance, there is a reasonable degree of rational, logical, and intellectual homogeneity in a medical class. Thus, if a particular topic is adequately covered, the decision making performance of the class should be reasonably predictable. However, in practice, things may turn out a little differently. We tend not to acknowledge that sex, age, intellectual ability, rationality, personality, and other individual characteristics may all substantially influence people's decisions [24]. Further, individual decision making is influenced by discipline-specific training; a process that may result in a predictable distortion of the way in which clinicians will see the world.

The Importance of Context and Ambient Conditions

Decisions are not made in isolation; each has some sort of context [25]. Decision making typically involves detecting a signal and distinguishing it from interference or noise; signals rarely arise without some noise attached to them. Noise is not simply acoustic, it may occur in any of the five senses and influence perception. Hogarth's "wicked" environments [15] typically have marked amounts of noise that interfere with the ability to accurately interpret particular signals. This concept must be considered in any process that examines decision making out of context. A good example is morbidity and mortality rounds. Although they provide some of the best clinical learning opportunities, the signal is typically separated from the context in which it was originally perceived, and most of the surrounding context is usually lost. A further complication is that the outcome is usually known and, through hindsight bias, may distort our perception of the original decision making. Further, the impact of fatigue, sleep deprivation, sleep debt, dysphoria, cognitive overloading, interruptions, distractions, and other factors that influence decision making are rarely considered and difficult to assess, once the original environment is left. Critical incident reviews and root-cause analyses, always performed after the fact, suffer similar shortcomings as well as memory failures.

Cognitive Failure

A variety of factors lead to cognitive failure in the individual decision maker: cognitive and affective biases, reasoning failures, knowledge deficits, and others. Cognitive laziness is uncommon in medicine, but certain conditions may lend themselves to slipping into the cognitive miser mode. Mindlessly adopting various strategies to conserve thinking effort can lead to problems: failure to do a thorough history and physical exam, accepting biased or gratuitous comments from others, accepting verbatim the information given at handover, cutting and pasting someone else's history and physical, deferring to authority without question, adopting a non-skeptical attitude, and many others. Healthcare providers cannot afford to be comfortably numb when patient care is at stake. By far the most important problem, however, appears to be the influence of cognitive and affective bias on decision making.

The Bias Problem

A universal feature of human decision making is its vulnerability to bias. Over a 100 cognitive, affective, and social biases have been described [26–30]. According to the Foundation for Critical Thinking: "Everyone thinks; it is our nature to do so. But much of our thinking, left to itself, is biased, distorted, partial, uninformed, or down-right prejudiced. Yet the quality of our life and that of what we produce, make or build depends precisely on the quality of our thought…

Table 33.2 Impediments to the awareness and understanding of cognitive biases in clinical judgment

Impediment	Effect
Lack of perceived clinical relevance	Medical undergraduates are not explicitly exposed to cognitive training in decision making. Historically, this area has not been seen as relevant to clinical performance and calibration
Lack of awareness	Although the lay press has heavily promoted the impact of cognitive and affective biases on everyday decision making, clinicians are generally unaware of their potential impact on medical decision making
Invulnerability	Even where awareness does exist, physician hubris, overconfidence, and lack of intellectual humility may deter them from accepting that they are just as vulnerable as others to biased judgments
Status quo bias	It is always easier for clinicians to continue to make decisions as they have done in the past. There is a prevailing tendency against learning de-biasing strategies and executing them, given the additional required cognitive effort and time
Vivid-pallid dimension	Cognitive and affective processes are mostly invisible and, at present, can only be inferred from outcomes or the clinician's behavior. Descriptions of them are invariably abstract and uninteresting. They typically lack the vividness and concrete nature of clinical disease presentations that are far more meaningful and appealing to the medically trained mind

Excellence in thought, however, must be systematically cultivated" [31]. These problems in thinking are compounded by clinicians being unaware of the many biases that affect their decision making, a condition known as "blind spot" bias. Several other biases may impede optimal decision making (Table 33.2). Bias should be considered a normal operating characteristic of the human brain – biases are everywhere and have the potential to influence almost every decision we make [32].

As noted earlier, two major issues in medical decision making affect outcome: the knowledge base of the decision maker and how critically the decision maker thinks. Again, most medical school curricula cover the rational aspects of decision making well—specificities, sensitivities, likelihood ratios, probability theory, and so forth are reasonably well covered [1]. However, physicians spend most of their cognitive time in Type 1 processing and are, therefore, vulnerable to the biases and other distortions that reside there. For physicians to believe that they are not vulnerable to bias is blind optimism at best and sheer arrogance at worst. Within the last decade, however, several disciplines have acknowledged the importance of cognitive biases and their impact on clinical reasoning: Anesthesia [33], Dermatology [34], Emergency Medicine [35], Medicine [26, 36], Neurology [37], Obstetrics [38], Ophthalmology [39], Pathology [40, 41], Pediatrics [42], Psychiatry [43], Radiology [44], Surgery [45], as well as specialty environments such as Intensive Care Units [46], and also Dentistry [47].

De-biasing in Decision Making

Given that bias has been repeatedly identified as a major problem in decision making, the obvious answer would be to find ways to debias clinicians. Cognitive psychologists began work on debiasing over 30 years ago with Fischoff's classic work [48]. His conclusion—that debiasing is not easy—has been the prevailing experience with researchers since; it does appear to be extraordinarily difficult. Given that intuition works reasonably well most of the time, and given the general inertia against doing the additional work in Type 2 required to overcome bias, the conclusion is not altogether surprising. Not only are we hard-wired to react to things in set ways, but cognitive habits, once established, are difficult to change. When effective strategies did not immediately present themselves, a general mood of pessimism appears to have settled in.

More recently, renewed efforts may be leading to more positive results. Besides the publication of numerous articles in major journals, several books have appeared by notable cognitive scientists, neurologists, and others on the working of the human brain, its fallibility, and suggestions for improving it [14, 16, 49–55]. There is widespread interest in the popular literature; more than 30 books have appeared on the subject in the past decade [56–67]. These books have not only drawn attention to the fallibility of decision making, they have also suggested various strategies for overcoming bias.

Cognitive psychologist Keith Stanovich has examined the theoretical basis of de-biasing in considerable depth [68]. First, he proposes that Type 2 (analytical) processing occurs on two levels: the *algorithmic* mind and the *reflective* mind. The algorithmic mind is associated with "fluid intelligence," known as Gf, which is that feature of general intelligence that provides the capacity to think logically and to solve problems in novel situations without necessarily having specialized learning about the topic. A critical feature of such thinking is the ability to suppress automatic responses in the intuitive mode by decoupling from it; this is the executive override function. It is what makes possible both inductive reasoning (the logic of experience) and deductive reasoning and is especially applicable to scientific and technical reasoning.

However, Stanovich proposes further that overall monitoring of the need to decouple resides at the second level of Type 2 processing, the reflective mind. Measurable thinking dispositions at this level use situational cues to detect the need to override the biased response and to sustain its inhibition (cognitive decoupling) while looking for and testing alternative solutions. These solutions must of course have been learned and stored in memory as declarative knowledge and strategic rules that are referred to as *mindware*; these require "crystallized intelligence," or Gc. De-biasing involves having both the correct mindware to substitute for a biased response and the thinking dispositions that are able to trigger overrides of Type 1 processing.

Stanovich has also provided insight into Type 1 processes by deconstructing them into four subgroups: (1) those that are hard-wired and derived from our ancient evolutionary past; (2) those based in our emotions; (3) those that originate from implicit learning; and (4) those that are over-learned. These subgroups are important in that future research might show that each may be matched to different debiasing strategies.

Three recent articles in the medical literature provide a foundation for tackling debiasing head on. The first is an extensive review of the psychological factors that underpin diagnostic error [69], which has an estimated rate of about 15 % in medicine [70], much of which is attributed to psychological factors underlying flawed decision making, as opposed to knowledge deficits. The other two are companion papers that first describe the theoretical basis of cognitive debiasing and then outline a range of strategies with the potential to achieve it [71, 72]. Hopefully, these papers will ignite further interest in debiasing in medical decision making and stimulate much-needed clinically relevant research.

Thus far, several broad conclusions can be drawn from these reviews: (1) the overall level of awareness about bias and the need for debiasing needs to be raised; (2) debiasing is not easy; (3) different strategies are likely needed for particular biases;(4) multiple debiasing interventions will probably be required; and (5) lifelong maintenance of skills will be necessary.

Critical Thinking

An important question all clinicians should ask themselves is: how do I become a better decision maker? From the foregoing discussion, it seems clear that a knowledge of the decision making process and an understanding of the contextual conditions that may compromise it, the personal variables that may influence it, the inevitable biases that influence it, and the imperative for debiasing are all important considerations. Given our overall goal to improve reasoning, problem solving, and decision making, it would make sense to embed them within an overall cognitive framework. The appropriate choice is critical thinking. It has been defined as: "the ability to be in control of one's thinking. It includes the ability to consciously examine the elements of one's reasoning, or that of another, and evaluate that reasoning against universal intellectual standards— clarity, accuracy, precision, relevance, depth, breadth, and logic. It also involves the structured examination of sources of information" [73].

Some believe that critical thinking requires exceptional intelligence and that one needs to be an Einstein to accomplish it. This is a misconception. Critical thinking skills can be taught across the intellectual continuum and are easily shown to improve reasoning and problem solving. Like other skills, they can be coached and will improve with practice. In several studies, different groups of students showed marked gains in critical thinking after specific training in the topic [74–77]. These results reinforce the widely held view that many of us do not use our full capacity for critical thinking; that the prevailing tendency is to do enough to get by. The cognitive miser function will suffice for most routine decisions of everyday life, and there is often little incentive to invest more cognitive effort than appears necessary. Because many clinicians are unaware of their biases and prejudices, they blissfully continue in a state of cognitive mindlessness or "comfortable numbness" [3]. Even when this decision mode fails them, they may still lack the insight to understand why.

Much interest has developed in critical thinking in recent years. The conclusion from a 2006 meta-analysis of 29 studies in secondary education found that teaching thinking skills was the single most effective intervention in improving reasoning and problem solving skills in children between 5 and 16 years old [78]. The overall effect size of the intervention was impressive: the equivalent of moving an average student (at the 50th percentile) up to the 26th percentile. The age range studied covers a period when critical thinking ability is rapidly increasing in a linear fashion [79]. From Denney's data [80], the ability appears to plateau between ages 20 and 50 years and to slowly decline over the next 30 years. Thus, there is no basis for believing that that it is too late to teach critical thinking in medical school, or in postgraduate training, because the opportunity has passed; that is, there does not appear to be a window or critical period for the acquisition of critical thinking skills. In healthy people, the acquisition and maintenance of critical thinking can be a lifelong habit. This is an issue that medical educationists and faculty should address in the design of curricula for the future.

Studying Clinical Decision Making

Science typically improves our understanding of processes by breaking them down into their component parts and subjecting them to experimental scrutiny. Such reductionism usually improves control of both dependent and independent variables and may minimize or eliminate the influence of extraneous variables. This situation often is achieved, perforce, in laboratory settings. Historically, the experimental study of critical decision making (CDM) has taken insufficient account of the inherent complexity of the process [81]. Isolating the dependent variable, that is, CDM, to study one or two independent variables essentially strips away the context, much like the study of the structure of a molecule of cholera toxin during a cholera epidemic [82]. It seems that, in the process of studying CDM, the baby sometimes gets thrown out with the bathwater.

Although experimental psychology methods have thrown considerable light on the study of affective and cognitive biases, they have lent themselves less well to the study of CDM. What typically remains of CDM after most of the independent and extraneous variables are removed may bear little relation to the actual process itself. Oncologists faced with making the best treatment decision will consider the patient's stage of illness, age, co morbidities, and other factors for selecting an option. This procedure is how many see the decision making process; a quantified, carefully considered decision in the cold light of day. However, this idealized decision procedure is far removed from that of a fatigued pediatric intensivist who has just dealt with the difficult death of a patient in the early hours of the morning and is now confronted with a new emergent situation in which other patients and priorities may be involved. Ultimately, what is needed is a combined approach in which reductionist methods are used to generate data and hypotheses that have testable ecological validity and can be meaningfully applied in the clinical setting.

At the end of the day, ways and means to effectively study how to improve the judgment of medical professionals will be found. However, with the number of deaths annually in the US due to diagnostic failure estimated at 40,000 – 80,000, this goal is no longer an option for medical educators, it is an imperative [83].

Conclusions

In recent years, clinicians have come to appreciate the importance of CDM, and much has been learned about it. The dual process model has been helpful in understanding the multiple and complex processes of CDM. Awareness is also increasing of the importance of individual factors, context, and ambient conditions in decision making, as well as of the need to consider these factors when devising experimental methods so that findings have clinical relevance and meaning. Critical thinking appears to provide the most appropriate cognitive scaffold on which CDM can go forward.

References

1. Rao G. Rational medical decision making: a case based approach. New York: McGraw-Hill Medical; 2007.
2. Lakoff G, Johnson M. Philosophy in the flesh: the embodied mind and its challenge to western thought. New York: Basic Books; 1999.
3. Croskerry P. From mindless to mindful practice: cognitive bias and clinical decision making. N Engl J Med. 2013;368(26):2445–8.
4. American Psychological Association. Glossary of psychological terms. From: http://www.apa.org/research/action/glossary.aspx. Retrieved 30 May 2013.
5. Croskerry P. Clinical cognition and diagnostic error: applications of a dual process model of reasoning. Adv Health Sci Educ Theory Pract. 2009;14:27–35.
6. Lieberman MD, Jarcho JM, Satpute AB. Evidence-based and intuition-based self-knowledge: an FMRI study. J Pers Soc Psychol. 2004;87(4):421–35.
7. Schneider W, Shiffrin RM. Controlled and automatic human information processing: 1. Detection, search, and attention. Psychol Rev. 1977;84:1–66.
8. Dawson NV. Physician judgment in clinical settings: methodological influences and cognitive performance. Clin Chem. 1993;39:1468–80.
9. Croskerry P. A universal model for diagnostic reasoning. Acad Med. 2009;84:1022–8.
10. Stanovich KE. The robot's rebellion: finding meaning in the age of Darwin. Chicago: The University of Chicago Press; 2004.
11. Campbell WW. Augenblickdiagnose. Semin Neurol. 1998;18:169–76.
12. Silen W. Cope's early diagnosis of the acute abdomen. 15th ed. New York: Oxford University Press; 1979.
13. Smallberg G. Bias is the nose for the story. In: Brockman J, editor. This will make you smarter. New York: Harper Perennial; 2012. p. 43–5.
14. Kahneman D. Thinking, fast and slow. 7th ed. Toronto: Doubleday Canada; 2011.
15. Denes-Raj V, Epstein S. Conflict between intuitive and rational processing: when people behave against their better judgment. J Pers Soc Psychol. 1994;66: 819–29.
16. Hogarth RM. Educating intuition. Chicago: The University of Chicago Press; 2001.
17. Stanovich KE. Dysrationalia: a new specific learning disability. J Learn Disabil. 1993;26:501–15.
18. Rorty AO. Self-deception, akrasia and irrationality. In: Elster J, editor. The multiple self. Cambridge: Cambridge University Press; 1985. p. 115–31.
19. Kalis A, Mojzisch A, Schweizer TS, Kaiser S. Weakness of will, akrasia, and the neuropsychiatry of decision making: an interdisciplinary perspective. Cogn Affect Behav Neurosci. 2008;8:402–17.
20. Stroud S, Tappolet C. Weakness of will and practical irrationality. New York: Oxford University Press; 2008.
21. Hammond KR. Intuitive and analytic cognition: information models. In: Sage A, editor. Concise encyclopedia of information processing in systems and organizations. Oxford: Pergamon Press; 1990. p. 306–12.
22. Critical Thinking Community. Our concept and definition of critical thinking. From: http://www.criticalthinking.org/pages/our-concept-of-critical-thinking/411. Accessed 20 May 2013.
23. Croskerry P. ED cognition: any decision by anyone at any time. ED administration series. CJEM. 2014;16(1): 13–9.
24. Croskerry P, Musson D. Individual factors in patient safety. In: Croskerry P, Cosby KS, Schenkel S, Wears R, editors. Patient safety in emergency medicine. Philadelphia: Lippincott Williams & Wilkins; 2008. p. 269–76.
25. Croskerry P. Context is everything or how could I have been that stupid? Healthc Q. 2009;12(Suppl):e171–s1763. doi:10.12927/hcq.2009.20945.
26. Croskerry P. The importance of cognitive errors in diagnosis and strategies to prevent them. Acad Med. 2003;78:1–6.
27. Croskerry P. Cognitive and affective dispositions to respond. In: Croskerry P, Cosby KS, Schenkel S, Wears R, editors. Patient safety in emergency medicine. Philadelphia: Lippincott Williams & Wilkins; 2008. p. 219–27.
28. Jenicek M. Medical error and harm: understanding, prevention and control. New York: Productivity Press, Taylor and Francis Group; 2011.
29. Wikipedia, the Free Encyclopedia. List of cognitive biases. From: http://en.wikipedia.org/wiki/List_of_cognitive_biases. Accessed 31 May 2013.

30. Dobelli R. The art of thinking clearly. New York: HarperCollins; 2013.
31. The Critical Thinking Community: Critical Thinking: Where to Begin. From: http://www.criticalthinking.org/pages/critical-thinking-where-to-begin/796. Accessed 1 May 2013.
32. Croskerry P. Bias: a normal operating characteristic of the diagnosing brain. Diagnosis. 2014;1:23–7.
33. Stiegler MP, Neelankavil JP, Canales C, Dhillon A. Cognitive errors detected in anaesthesiology. Br J Anaesth. 2012;108:229–35.
34. David CV, Chira S, Eells SJ, Ladrigan M, Papier A, Miller LG, Craft N. Diagnostic accuracy in patients admitted to hospital with cellulitis. Dermatol Online J. 2011;17:1.
35. Croskerry P. Achieving quality in clinical decision making: cognitive strategies and detection of bias. Acad Emerg Med. 2002;9:1184–204.
36. Hershberger PJ, Markert RJ, Part HM, Cohen SM, Finger WW. Understanding and addressing cognitive bias in medical education. Adv Health Sci Educ Theory Pract. 1997;1:221–6.
37. Vickrey BG, Samuels MA, Ropper AH. How neurologists think: a cognitive psychology perspective on missed diagnoses. Ann Neurol. 2010;67(4):425–33.
38. Dunphy BC, Cantwell R, Bourke S, Fleming M, Smith B, Joseph KS, Dunphy SL. Cognitive elements in clinical decision-making. Toward a cognitive model for medical education and understanding clinical reasoning. Adv Health Sci Educ Theory Pract. 2010;15:229–50.
39. Margo CE. A pilot study in ophthalmology of inter-rater reliability in classifying diagnostic errors: an under investigated area of medical error. Qual Saf Health Care. 2003;12:416–20.
40. Foucar E. Error in anatomic pathology. Am J Clin Pathol. 2001;116:S34–46.
41. Crowley RS, Legowski E, Medvedeva O, Reitmeyer K, Tseytlin E, Castine M, Jukic D, Mello-Thoms C. Automated detection of heuristics and biases among pathologists in a computer-based system. Adv Health Sci Educ Theory Pract. 2013;18(3):343–63. doi:10.1007/s10459-012-9374-z. Published online: 23 May 2012.
42. Singh H, Thomas EJ, Wilson L, Kelly PA, Pietz K, Elkeeb D, Singhal G. Errors of diagnosis in pediatric practice: a multisite survey. Pediatrics. 2010;126:70–9.
43. Crumlish N, Kelly BD. How psychiatrists think. Adv Psychiatr Treat. 2009;15:72–9.
44. Sabih D, Sabih A, Sabih Q, Khan AN. Image perception and interpretation of abnormalities; can we believe our eyes? Can we do something about it? Insights Imaging. 2011;2:47–55.
45. Shiralkar U. Smart surgeons, sharp decisions: cognitive skills to avoid errors and achieve results. Shropshire: TFM Publishing; 2010.
46. Gillon SA, Radford ST. Zebra in the intensive care unit: a metacognitive reflection on misdiagnosis. Crit Care Resusc. 2012;14:216–21.
47. Hicks EP, Kluemper GT. Heuristic reasoning and cognitive biases: are they hindrances to judgments and decision making in orthodontics? Am J Orthod Dentofacial Orthop. 2011;139:297–304.
48. Fischoff B. Debiasing. In: Kahneman D, Slovic P, Tversky A, editors. Judgment under uncertainty; heuristics and biases. Cambridge: Cambridge University Press; 1982. p. 422–44.
49. Kahneman D, Slovic P, Tversky A, editors. Judgment under uncertainty; heuristics and biases. Cambridge: Cambridge University Press; 1982.
50. Plous S. The psychology of judgment and decision making. New York: McGraw-Hill; 1993.
51. Baron J. Thinking and deciding. 3rd ed. New York: Cambridge University Press; 2000.
52. Gilovich T, Griffin D, Kahneman D. Heuristics and biases: the psychology of intuitive judgment. New York: Cambridge University Press; 2002.
53. Bishop MA, Trout JD. Epistemology and the psychology of human judgment. New York: Oxford University Press; 2005.
54. Vohs KD, Baumeister RE, Loewenstein G. Do emotions help or hurt decision making? A hedgefoxian perspective. New York: Russell Sage; 2007.
55. Damasio A. Self comes to mind: constructing the conscious brain. New York: Pantheon Books; 2010.
56. Konnikova M. Mastermind: how to think like Sherlock Holmes. New York: Viking; 2013.
57. Markman A. Smart thinking; three essential keys to solve problems, innovate, and get things done. New York: Perigree; 2012.
58. Chabris C, Simons D. The invisible gorilla. New York: Crown; 2010.
59. Lehrer J. How we decide. New York: Houghton Mifflin Harcourt; 2009.
60. Hallinan JT. Why we make mistakes: how we look without seeing, forget things in seconds, and are all pretty sure we are way above average. New York: Broadway Books; 2009.
61. Thaler RH, Sunstein CR. Nudge: improving decisions about health, wealth, and happiness. New York: Penguin; 2008.
62. Brafman O, Brafman R. Sway: the irresistible pull of irrational behavior. New York: Broadway Books; 2008.
63. Ariely D. Predictably irrational: the hidden forces that shape our decisions. New York: HarperCollins; 2008.
64. Wolpert L. Six impossible things before breakfast: the evolutionary origins of belief. New York: W.W. Norton; 2007.
65. Tavris C, Aronson E. Mistakes were made (but not by me): why we justify foolish beliefs, bad decisions and hurtful acts. Orlando: Harcourt Inc.; 2007.
66. Myers DG. Intuition: its powers and perils. New Haven: Yale University Press; 2002.
67. Piattelli-Palmarini M. Inevitable illusions: how mistakes of reason rule our minds. New York: Wiley; 1994.
68. Stanovich KE. Rationality and the reflective mind. New York: Oxford University Press; 2011.
69. Graber ML, Kissam S, Payne VL, Meyer D, Sorensen A, Lenfestey N, et al. Cognitive interventions to

reduce diagnostic error: a narrative review. BMJ Qual Saf. 2012;21:535–57.
70. Berner ES, Graber ML. Overconfidence as a cause of diagnostic error in medicine. Am J Med. 2008;121(5, Suppl 1):S2–23.
71. Croskerry P, Singhal G, Mamede S. Cognitive debiasing 1: origins of bias and theory of de-biasing. BMJ Qual Saf. 2013;22 Suppl 2:ii58–64.
72. Croskerry P, Singhal G, Mamede S. Cognitive debiasing 2: impediments to and strategies for change. BMJ Qual Saf. 2013;22 Suppl 2:ii65–72.
73. Eichhorn R. Developing thinking skills: critical thinking at the army management staff college. Strategic Systems Department Army Management Staff College. 2013. From: http://www.au.af.mil/au/awc/awcgate/army/critical/roy.htm. Accessed 15 May 2013.
74. Miller DR. Longitudinal assessment of critical thinking in pharmacy students. Am J Pharm Educ. 2003; 67:1–8.
75. Solon T. Generic critical thinking infusion and course content learning in introductory psychology. J Instr Psychol. 2007;34:95–109.
76. Twardy CR. Argument maps improve critical thinking. Teach Philos. 2004;27:2.
77. Butler HA, Dwyer CP, Hogan MJ, Franco A, Riva SF, Saiz C, Almeida LS. The halpern critical thinking assessment and real-world outcomes: cross-national applications. Thinking Skills Creativity. 2012;7:112–21.
78. Higgins S, Hall E, Baumfield V, Moseley D. A meta-analysis of the impact of the implementation of thinking skills approaches on pupils. In: Research evidence in education library. London: EPPI-Centre, Social Science Research Unit, Institute of Education, University of London; 2005. From: http://eppi.ioe.ac.uk/cms/Default.aspx?tabid=338. Accessed 30 May 2013.
79. Friend CM, Zubek JP. The effects of age on critical thinking ability. J Gerontol. 1958;13:407–13.
80. Denney NW. Critical thinking during the adult years: has the developmental function changed over the last four decades? Exp Aging Res. 1995;21:191–207.
81. Croskerry P, Petrie D, Reilly J, Tait G. Deciding about fast and slow decisions. Acad Med. 2014;2:197–200.
82. Fang FC, Casadevall A. Reductionistic and holistic science. Infect Immun. 2011;79:1401–4.
83. Stark M, Fins JJ. The ethical imperative to think about thinking. Cambridge Quarterly of Healthcare Ethics. 2014;23:386–96.

Design of Cardiac Surgery Operating Rooms and the Impact of the Built Environment

34

Paul R. Barach and Bill Rostenberg

Abstract

This chapter is intended to provide a common language to enable both medical and design professionals to improve their dialog and collaborative work processes when designing pediatric cardiac care settings. This approach will help provide knowledge that can be applied to new construction or renovation of cardiovascular operating rooms and cardiac catherisation laboratories. It is not uncommon during the course of healthcare facility design for numerous people to use common terms that have different meanings for each person and community, and then be surprised to later discover that their conversations were about different meanings that led to a different understanding and mindset.

Within the context of this chapter, the term "hybrid (surgical) room" is used to describe a procedure room designed and intended for either "open" or "closed" procedures, or both. They may be built for use by specific sub-specialists, or they may be shared by diverse users. This is a prime example of the necessity to clarify the operational, technological, cultural and political strategies explicitly prior to design inception and master planning.

This chapter is not only about architectural design and planning, although that is its primary focus. Its underlying message is that the design of cardiovascular surgical procedure rooms or suites – regardless of how innovative they are or how much advanced medical technology they contain – will likely only be successful if they are closely aligned with the evolving changes in models of care, medical practices, local culture, politics and a concern for safety and high reliability of care. Cardiovascular spaces must also be designed with strategies that enable them to constantly evolve and be

P.R. Barach, BSc, MD, MPH
Department of Health Management
and Health Economics, University of Oslo,
Oslo 1074, Norway
e-mail: pbarach@gmail.com

B. Rostenberg (✉)
Architecture for Advanced Medicine,
115 Corte Anita, Greenbrae, CA 94904, USA
e-mail: brostenberg@gmail.com

P.R. Barach, J.P. Jacobs, S.E. Lipshultz, P.C. Laussen (eds.),
Pediatric and Congenital Cardiac Care: Volume 2: Quality Improvement and Patient Safety,
DOI 10.1007/978-1-4471-6566-8_34, © Springer-Verlag London 2015

prepared for future changes in care models and technology requirements. Traditional boundaries – both physical and virtual – between surgical and non-surgical specialists, as well as within surgical and interventional subspecialties are eroding with the emergence of hybrid interventionalists.

The chapter encourages the development of a new design ethos and practice to be considered: one in which the commonalities – instead of the differences – of traditional surgical and interventional environments form the building blocks of facility design for tomorrow's cardiovascular procedures.

Keywords
Operating Room (OR) • OR design • Healthcare architecture • Evidence based design • Surgical work flow • Safety • Hybrid OR • Surgical suite • Catherisation laboratories

The Impact of the Built Environment

The surgical space, by its nature, is a high-risk environment where hazards lurk around every corner and for every patient. The patients who come to surgery are generally among the sickest and at more advanced stages of disease. The very act of treatment involves interventions that are often considerably invasive with vigorous and unpredictable physiologic responses. The level of complexity, both in task-oriented and cognitive demands, results in a dynamic, unforgiving environment that can magnify the consequences of even small lapses and errors [1].

Surgical processes and safety are influenced by numerous factors including surgical workflow, clinical competence, cultures of teamwork, organizational structure and attributes of the built environment. Together, these variables interact in an an highly coupled system in which variations in any one will influence the entire system. While this chapter focuses explicitly on the built environment – design and construction of surgical suites and operating rooms (ORs) – one should consider that design alone cannot overcome insufficiencies of the other essential variables. Improper design, however, can detrimentally compromise clinical excellence. It can complicate work flow that might otherwise be optimal and it can introduce additional risk into an otherwise safe culture [2].

Another consideration of the built environment is its relatively static nature. Compared to medicine with its continuous rapid evolution and transformation, the walls, floors and ceilings of the surgical suite are stationary. Surgical processes change in parallel as best practices evolve. New clinical techniques can be implemented by decision; by establishing new protocols and subsequent behaviors. In contrast, changing the physical environment is more challenging; it requires capital investment, disruptive renovation and adequate space (an often rare commodity). Thus, an initially well-designed surgical environment can quickly become outdated. As such, work flow can erode and safe practices can become compromised. As time goes by in which clinical practices continue to evolve but the physical environment does not, the detrimental impact of this discrepancy can become increasingly significant. For this reason, the design of surgical environments requires strategies for long-term flexibility, including setting aside undifferentiated spaces in addition to strategies for efficient work flow and improved safety.

Risk Management of Cardiovascular Surgical Procedure Rooms

Safe outcomes in cardiovascular surgical procedure rooms have been linked to several variables including institutional and surgeon-specific volumes, complexity of cases, and systems design [3]. Interventions and change risk strategies however, have had some impact but not enough has been done to accommodate the necessary impact on cardiovascular surgery outcomes. This may be attributable to a lack of appreciation of the evidence about human factors in cardiovascular surgery, including a poor understanding of the complexity of interactions between physical design, technical task, stressful cardiovascular settings especially in the pediatric setting, rigid staff hierarchies, lack of time to brief and debrief, and resistance to change [4].

Technical skills [5] are fundamental to good outcomes but non- technical factors also impact significantly on individual and team performance and patient outcomes [6]. The nature of these interactions has only been recently studied, and these lessons have yet to be applied to the design of cardiovascular procedure rooms [7]. Understanding the impact of design and its relationship between recognized human factors, such as teamwork (e.g., cooperation, collaboration, etc.), fatigue, organizational dynamics, authority gradients, shift work and task performance, that influence the effectiveness of surgical teams in charge of pediatric cardiac surgery is needed [8].

High reliability – or consistent performance at high levels of safety over long periods of time – is a hallmark for non-health, high-risk industries such as aviation and nuclear power [9]. In the face of health reform and increased market competition moving to high reliability requires adopting and supporting a 'culture of mindfulness' in understanding the relationship and synergy of a variety of organizational risk factors and their effect on producing patient harm and inefficiency.

In addition to the overarching atmosphere of collective mindfulness, high-reliability organizations have two other features in common. First, after organizations identify potential deficiencies in safety processes, they eliminate these deficiencies through the use of robust process improvement methodologies to improve their processes. Second, the organizations rely on a particular organizational culture to ensure the performance of improved safety processes over long periods of time and to remain constantly aware of the possibility of failure. This is often referred to as a safety culture [10].

Surgical Work Flow Considerations

Surgical work flow throughout the surgical suite (intra-departmental work flow) and within the surgical operating room (intra-room work flow) is uniquely influenced by the surrounding physical environment. Often, two potentially opposing goals are in play: one is to maximize throughput and increase financial benefits, by increasing the number of procedures per operating/procedure room per day or per year; the other, is to perform all activities with minimal risk and at the highest standard of care with excellent clinical outcomes. A well designed facility should support both goals without compromising the other goals.

Intra-departmental Work Flow

Intra-departmental work flow is influenced by key adjacencies, such as travel distances between preoperative beds, operating rooms and the post anesthesia recovery unit (PACU) or intensive care unit (ICU); whether the entire surgical suite is on one contiguous floor of the building or on separate floors; and, the distance and physical relationship (e.g. horizontal versus vertical) between operating rooms and central sterile processing functions. Work flow to and from the ICU and central sterile processing may be considered inter-departmental if those areas are run as departments separate from surgery.

One operational concept that varies considerably across both geographic locations and clinical cultures is OR-adjacent induction versus in-room induction [11]. OR-adjacent induction (Fig. 34.1) is common in Europe, the United Kingdom and many Commonwealth Nations. This approach enables the patient to be anesthetized immediately outside the operating room and then transported into the adjoining operating room, thus potentially increasing throughput through simultaneous parallel processing of related activities, such as patient induction and room set-up. Dedicated induction

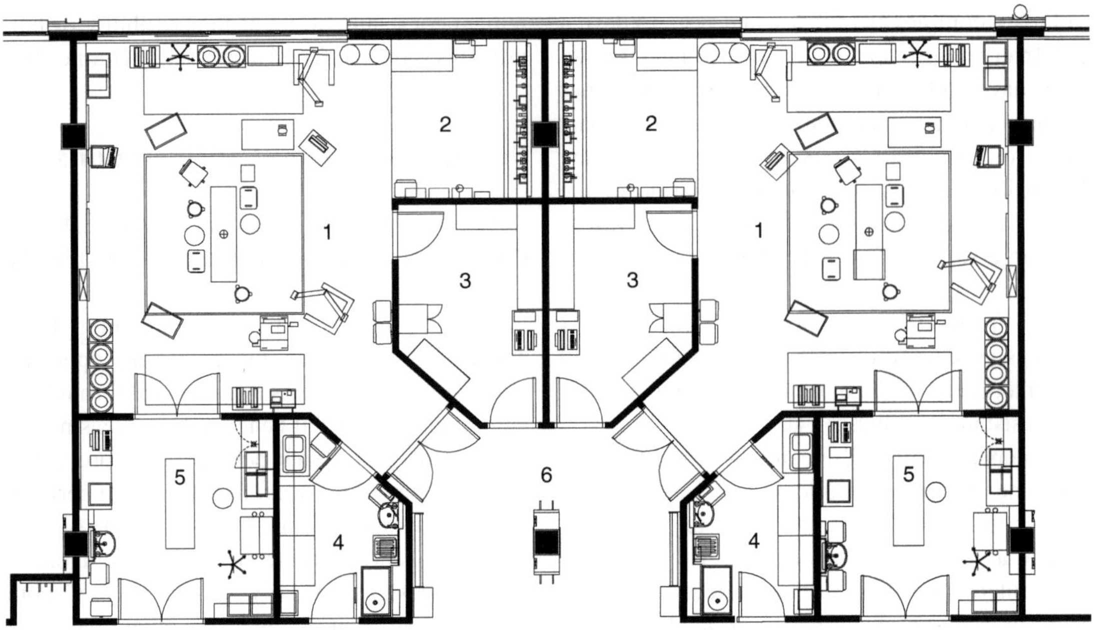

Fig. 34.1 OR-adjacent Induction Room: Layout illustrating OR-adjacent induction rooms (often referred to as "anaesthesia rooms" (Used with permission from Stantec Architecture, Inc. ©2013 Stantec)

rooms also have the potential benefit of providing privacy and relaxing ambience that may increase patient satisfaction and comfort [12]. This is particularly important for pediatric surgery where parents can accompany their children into the induction room, a concept known as parent-present induction. Some critics however, suggest that transporting an anesthetized patient including disconnecting from stable monitors, even a short distance, may introduce otherwise unnecessary risk factors.

In contrast, in-room induction – common throughout much of North America and Scandinavia – is designed for serial processing in which the patient is anesthetized in the operating room, after (rather than while) the operating room is being set-up. Compared to OR-adjacent induction, in-room induction generally requires less overall space because dedicated induction rooms are not needed, but case turn-over time is potentially increased because induction cannot take place concurrently while the operating room is being set up. Some facilities designed for in-room induction for adult surgery, however, are designed for OR-adjacent induction for pediatric surgery.

What remains unclear is the impact of an induction room model on the whole surgical process, its phases and delays between the phases, and the number of cases performed. Torkki et al., found that the mean non-operative time was reduced by 45.6 %, whereas the surgery time remained unchanged [13]. The time savings contributed to the concurrent anesthesia induction and the cut down in delays between the phases. The new model allowed one additional case to be performed during a 7-h working day. The daily raw utilization of the surgical procedure room increased by 8.9 %.

The decision to choose one of the parallel workflow models that could be economically favorable will depend on several physical and organizational variables, such as:

- The cost of the additional space and equipment required to allow the parallel processing to occur;
- The utilization of the procedure room and induction room;
- The cost of each additional person, whether it be physician, nurse, or technician; and,

- The duration of cases: short procedures benefit the most from individual induction rooms.

In contrast, if a surgery suite has longer cases with fewer turnovers, a single centralized induction room serving several multiple procedure rooms may be the way to go.

The revenues gained by parallel processing would need to offset any increased costs of personnel and loss of revenue producing procedure room spaces. Success for such parallel processes may be best achievable with a select patient population and a limited number of types of cases.

Intra-room Workflow

In contrast to intra-departmental workflow which is influenced by traffic to and from the operating room, intra-room workflow considers various types of flow possibilities and limitations within the operating room. Variations to the built environment that most greatly influence intra-room work flow include the number and location of doors into the operating room, how the flow of clean and soiled goods are (or are not) separated as they enter and exit the space, how the surgical table is placed within the room, and the position and configuration of medical and information technology (IT) devices. Related, Lynch et al have showed that the number of OR door openings increases in direct proportion to case length, compromising the sterile environment of the operating room and increasing risk of mediastinal infections [14]. Young and O'Regan demonstrated that in 46 cases analyzed, there were 4,273 door openings recorded. The mean frequency of door openings per case was 92.9 (45–205), with 19.2 (6.4–38.2) openings per hour. The theatre door was open for 10.7 % of each hour of operating. Door opening disturbs theatre airflow and results in increased air and wound contamination and may be a contributor to surgical mistakes [15].

Functional zones within the operating room should be clearly delineated and the design team must understand the various processes (such as room set-up, patient transport, pre-operative preparation, surgical procedures, post-operative activities, room turn-over, and so forth) as well as the numerous personnel types (such as surgeons, nurses, anesthesiologists, perfusionists, imaging technologists, students fellow, residents, and so forth) that participate in the many procedures that the room will accommodate. In general, a room that has clear separation and delineation of sterile, circulating and anesthesia zones within the operating room (Fig. 34.2) should yield efficient and effective intra-room work flow and accommodate a greater variety of procedure types. Specifically, consideration should be given to the ease of transporting the patient into the room and loading them onto the surgical table without intruding into the sterile or anesthesia zones; ease of bringing clean and sterile supplies into the room and placing them where they are needed without disrupting other activities; and, the ease of emergency access and egress during critical events.

While numerous studies have examined causes of surgical errors, few focus on causation related to the built environment. One pilot study conducted at the Medical University of South Carolina [16] examines how the design of a cardiothoracic operating room can influence flow disruptions. While studying disruptions related to communications, environmental hazards, equipment failures, general interruptions, room layout and usability across pre-operative, peri-operative and post-operative phases, the most frequent flow disruptions were related to room layout. These occurred most often in the peri-operative phase and least often in the post-operative phase. Room design recommendations for the specific operating room that was studied include, "expand the anesthesia work space at the head of the table, expand space for perfusion between table and wall and/or eliminate travel through area, swing entry doors out and/or relocate closer to the footwall of the room".

While these recommendations apply to the particular design features of the specific room studied, one can apply general considerations of overall room size and configuration, size and configuration of internal room zoning, door placement and direction of swing, and placement and movement of equipment and devices to the design of most operating rooms. Careful consideration should be given to the placement of

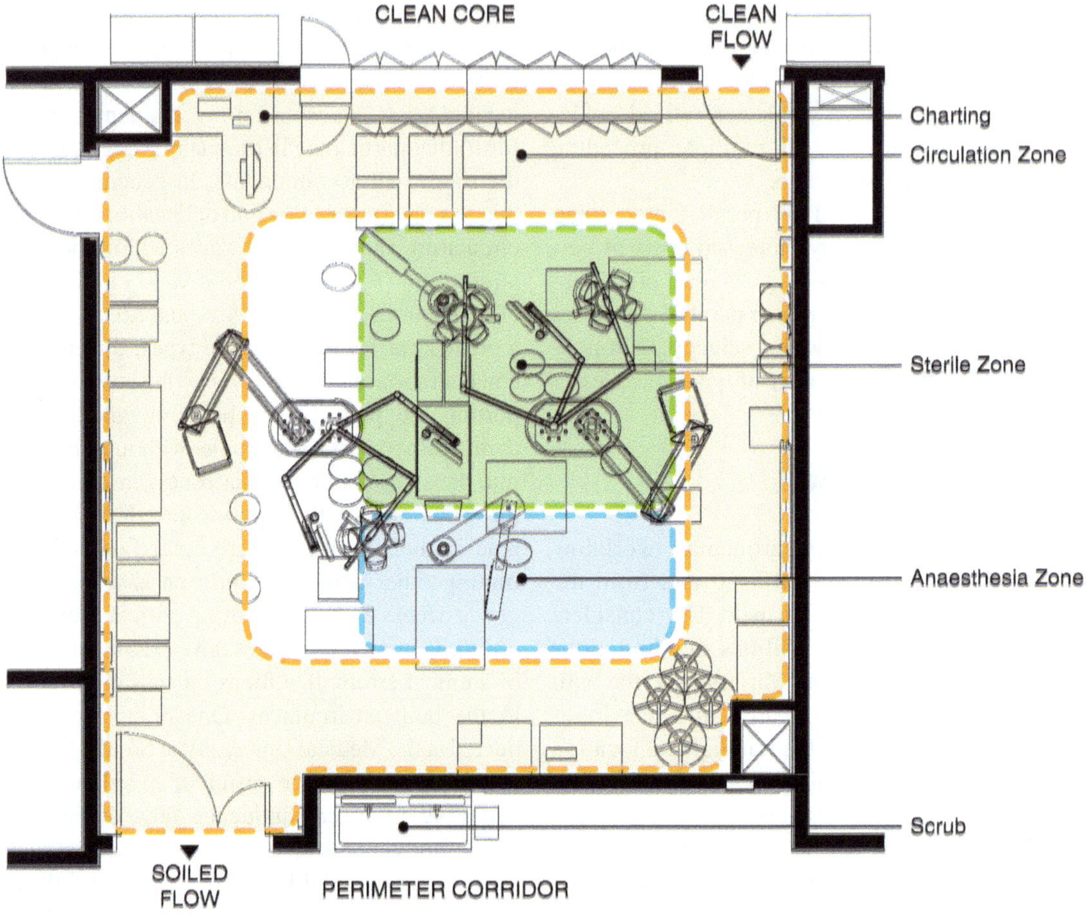

Fig. 34.2 Operating Room Zoning Diagram: Diagram illustrating the various functional zones within a typical operating room (OR) (Used with permission from Stantec Architecture, Inc. ©2013 Stantec)

patient entry doors so that patient transport does not conflict with anesthesia and sterile set-up. Similarly, circulating traffic should enable supplies to be brought directly to their primary places of use without passing through unrelated zones. Where possible, door leaves should not swing directly into areas of congestion or where disruption is most detrimental. The use of bypass or sliding doors in jurisdictions where they are permitted may further reduce spatial conflicts and collisions.

Another suggested design feature is to orient nurse charting stations so the person doing the charting faces the area where the surgery is being conducted rather than facing the opposite wall. The charting station, however, should not adversely protrude into the room or circulation zones and corners of the workstation should be rounded.

Design for proper intra-room work flow can become increasingly complex for hybrid operating rooms or other surgical rooms where the often opposing requirements of both surgical and imaging equipment and personnel must be considered. Design considerations for hybrid operating rooms are discussed later in this chapter.

Work Flow Typologies

Design strategies for separating clean and soiled goods influence both intra-room work flow and intra-department work flow. Three key surgical

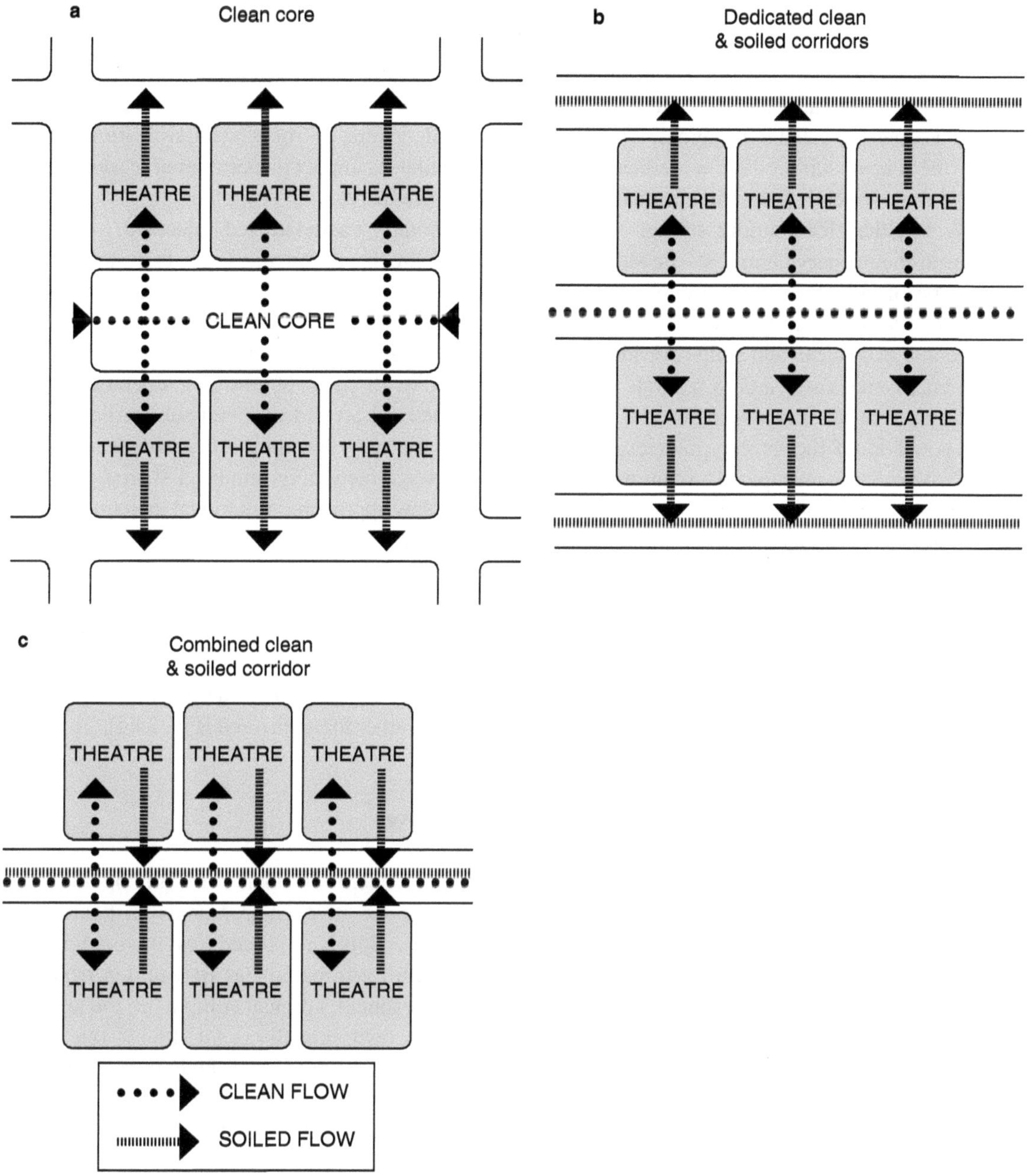

Fig. 34.3 Surgical Suite Typologies: Three surgical suite layout typologies: (**a**) clean core; (**b**) dedicated clean and soiled corridors and (**c**) combined clean and soiled corridor; (Used with permission from Stantec Architecture, Inc. ©2013 Stantec)

suite typologies are common (Fig. 34.3). A "clean core" layout places several operating rooms around a common clean core, from which clean and wrapped sterile goods flow "one way" into a dedicated "clean" side of each operating room and exit through a dedicated "soiled" side of the room. A clean core often includes dedicated clean and soiled lifts connecting the core to a central sterile supply area on a different floor but directly above or below the core, enabling a dedicated vertical connection via the lifts. A clean core layout often requires more space than the other typologies.

Dedicated "clean and soiled corridors" layouts provide similar flow of soiled and clean goods as does the clean core layout, but does not store the clean supplies in a dedicated core. Instead they typically travel in case carts from a nearby satellite clean supply storage area or to and from the primary central sterile supply area. This type of layout usually requires less overall space than a clean core layout.

A combined "clean and soiled corridor" layout relies on covered case carts to separate clean and soiled goods as both types of material share the same corridor. Of the three typologies, the combined corridor layout typically requires the least amount of space, but requires a well-managed transport system to maintain appropriate infection control. This also requires more oversight to ensure effective infection control.

Standardization

Adopting standardized processes from non-healthcare industries, such as aerospace and manufacturing has long been applied to healthcare in an effort to improve safety and communications [17]. A well-known example is incorporating aeronautical flight-ready checklists into operating room protocol to reduce the risk of wrong-patient and wrong site procedures as well as to invoke other safe practices.

Standardization can also be applied to room design. For example, standardized inpatient nursing units – with 'handed' instead of 'mirrored' patient rooms – have been designed and built for decades. A handed nursing unit configures all patient rooms identically, for example all with the entrance door on the right side and the headwall on the left side of the room. In contrast, a mirrored layout configures each pair of rooms identically, but the rooms within each room pair are mirror opposites of each other, often sharing a common plumbing wall between the pair. The assumed benefit of same-handed rooms is that staff will intuitively know exactly where essential supplies are at critical times and all process will be standardized due to the unvarying built environment, thus improving safety by eliminating physical variation. While this logic may appear to be sound, definitive evidence of the overall benefit of room standardization, and in particular its impact on perioperative room design remains elusive.

Similarly, standardized "handed" operating rooms are based on the logic that standardized work process and consistent placement of critical supplies and devices improve work flow and safety. Historically, surgical suites have been configured with pairs of mirrored operating rooms symmetrical around a shared sub-sterile room in much the way that mirrored inpatient rooms are placed symmetrically around a shared plumbing wall. New approaches to surgical infection control, including recommendations against routine use of flash sterilization [18] , have resulted in surgical suite layouts that either eliminate sub-sterile rooms or incorporate a satellite instrument processing station adjacent to a shared clean core. Such layouts easily accommodate all operating rooms to be handed rather than mirrored (Fig. 34.4).

Air Flow

Hospital operating rooms are among the most infection-sensitive environments in health care facilities. Surgical procedures increase patient vulnerability to pathogens transmitted from surgical personnel, surgical equipment, the air and a patient's own skin flora. Air flow is one of the most important aspects of the built surgical environment with regard to infection control, human comfort and clinical outcomes. Surgical site infections account for roughly 15 % of all nosocomial infections among hospitalized patients [19] and of those, 80–90 % of surgical wound bacterial contamination comes from the ambient air. In the United States alone, approximately 700,000 patients a year are affected by surgical site infections [20]. Recent evidence shows that IV poles, anesthesia workstations and OR personnel are teeming with antimicrobial bugs and serve as a significant source of patient environmental contamination in the operating room [21].

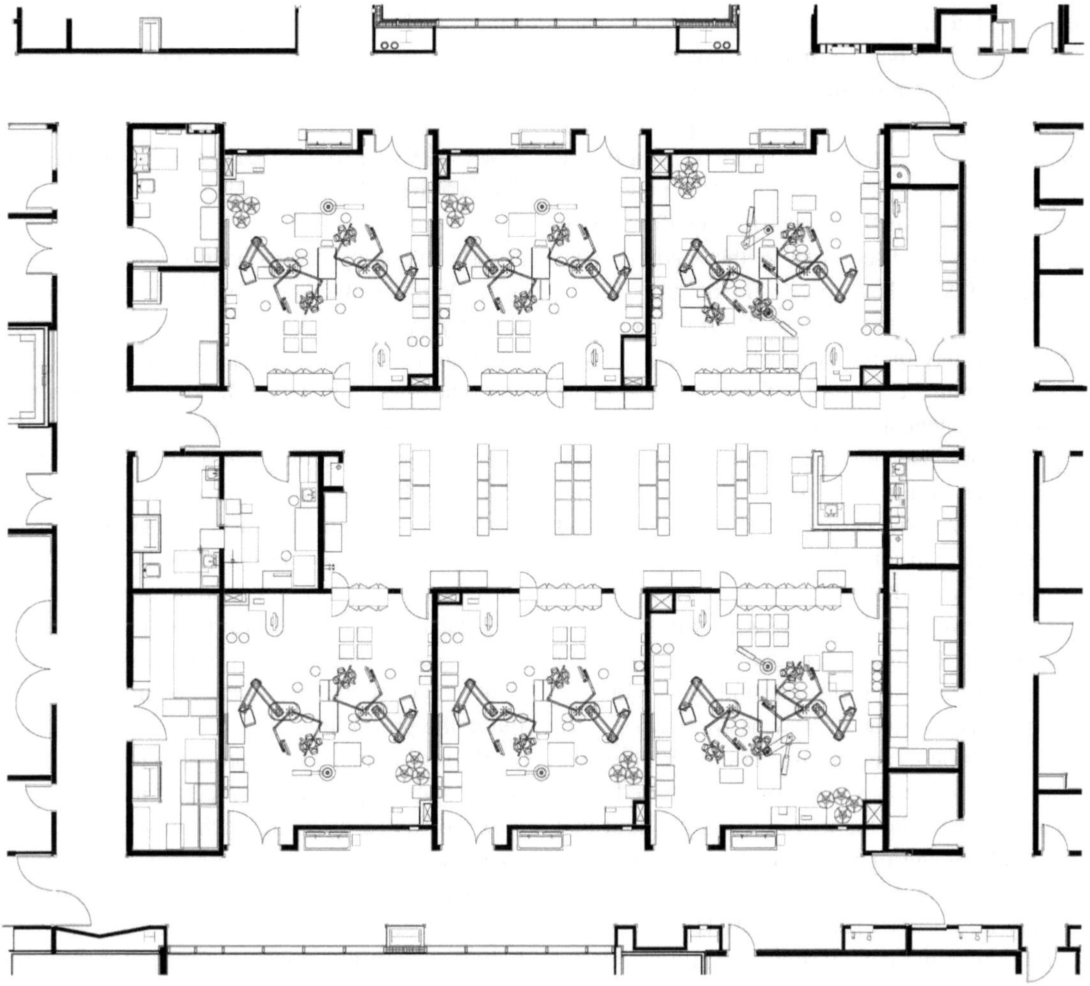

Fig. 34.4 Clean Core Surgical Suite: Six operating rooms organized around a central clean supply core. Architect of Record: Co Architects; Associate Architect: Stantec. (Used with permission from Palomar Pomerado Health. ©2013 PPH)

Surgical air handling system design requires the knowledge of qualified mechanical engineers experienced in the development of state-of-the-art surgical facilities. Basic design considerations include air system types, air change rates and filtration levels. Regulatory requirements are written for both architectural and engineering surgical facility design, but the specific requirements of these building codes vary by jurisdiction and sometimes differ for various types of operating rooms.

Numerous air flow strategies – cross flow, displacement, air curtains and laminar flow – are commonly used in healthcare facilities; however, only the last two are appropriate for the surgical suite with laminar flow often being preferred, and specifically required for certain types of operating rooms in some jurisdictions. Laminar air flow – a system similar to that used in clean room environments – provides unidirectional supply air flow. The air typically enters the operating room through a ceiling-mounted diffuser array (large enough to cover the entire surgical site) and exits through several low level exhaust registers, creating a downward flow of particles away from the surgical site. Ideally, exhaust registers are placed at all four corners of the room at approximately eight inches above the floor surface, but many appropriately designed operating rooms have only two low exhaust registers. The registers should not be blocked by furniture, equipment or other devices that could compromise air flow. Since most anesthetic gasses are heavier then air, low level returns are also positive for removal of these gases which may be released into the space and bypass the local anesthetic gas scavenging systems. Anesthetic gases must be removed because they may cause health problems such as induce fetal malformations or abortions or discomfort to the medical team inside the OR, and may pose a fire hazard [20].

Laminar flow has been found to result in low concentrations of airborne contaminants, especially within the vicinity of the surgical table [20]. Placement and installation of laminar air flow assemblies must be carefully coordinated with other equipment in the operating room, especially nearby ceiling-mounted booms and assemblies. Structural support of proximate equipment can interfere with that of the laminar system above the ceiling, and nearby items below the ceiling (including lights, booms, imaging equipment, and so forth) can interfere with and compromise laminar air flow performance.

In addition to specifying certain air flow systems, building codes also specify required rates of air changes (the number of times per hour that the total amount of air in the operating room is replenished). Most regulations require at least twenty air changes per hour (ACH) and do not permit recirculation of room air. While higher ACH rates are sometimes implemented, evidence does not suggest that they improve the system's ability to limit the number of colony-forming units of contaminants, which are measured in particles per square meter of room volume.

Air filtration – applied in conjunction with appropriate air change quantities and air flow systems – removes airborne particles (sources of contamination and infection). HEPA filters installed within ducts at the location where air enters the room are effective but tend to be difficult to maintain and replace. Alternately, HEPA filters placed at the room side of the laminar flow ceiling assembly are both effective and accessible for maintenance and replacement. HEPA filters, which remove up to 99.7 % of particles as small as 0.3 μm are effective in removing bacteria colonies, but are ineffective in controlling smaller virus-laden contaminants. For removal of these smaller viruses, ultra violet (UV) lamps can be employed, but care must be taken to prevent harmful exposure to UV radiation.

Special Considerations for Hybrid Operating Rooms [12]

Hybrid operating rooms have become prevalent in academic medical centers (Fig. 34.5) and more recently even in smaller general hospitals and in community hospitals. Hybrid operating rooms combine the often contradictory environmental needs of surgery and interventional radiology and interventional cardiology and thus, pose unique design challenges. For the purpose of this chapter the hybrid operating room is defined as an invasive treatment space designed for both open and closed surgical procedures; configured for sterile surgical infection control precautions; designed for the use of general anesthesia; and, equipped with integrated image guidance equipment essential to the procedure.

Hybrid rooms, when compared to more traditional operating rooms, typically integrate complex advanced imaging technologies, such as rotational fluoroscopy, computed tomography, magnetic resonance, ultrasound or combinations of each. Currently, the majority of cardiothoracic hybrid operating rooms employ fluoroscopic imaging systems. Because both surgical and imaging equipment are integrated within the same space, physical conflicts between the movement ranges of equipment movement can occur unless the placement of every item is carefully coordinated in all three spatial dimensions. Equipment conflicts are most likely to occur along the ceiling plane since it is common to mount both imaging and surgical equipment from the ceiling in order to leave the floor plane clear, clean and flexible.

A typical example of a hybrid operating room "real estate conflict" occurs when ceiling-mounted surgical lights, booms and monitors are proximate to a laminar air flow assembly and a ceiling-mounted C-arm assembly with intensifiers, flat panel detectors, and additional monitors needed to traverse the same space. One coordination strategy is to use extended boom arms so the vertical boom and light connections can be placed away from the

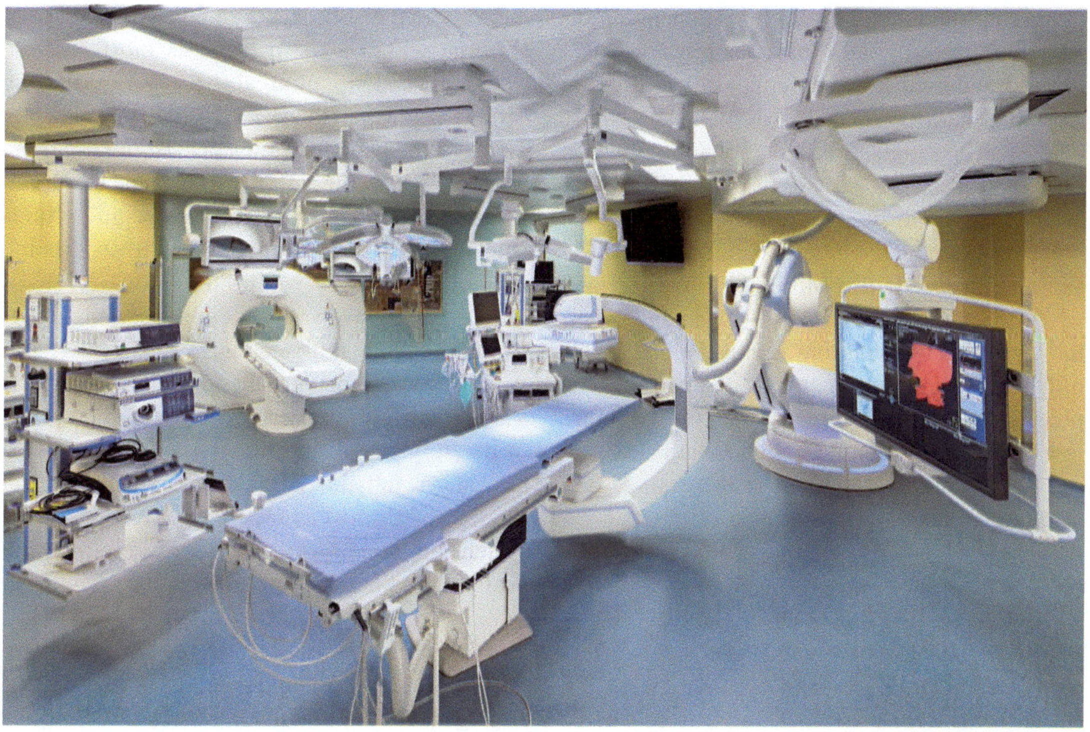

Fig. 34.5 Hybrid Operating Room: A state-of-the-art hybrid operating room (Used with permission from the photographer and Stantec Architecture, Inc. ©2013 Ed Massery)

sterile field and the movement of the imaging assembly but the devices themselves can be placed wherever they are needed. This demands meticulous three-dimensional coordination and may require special boom construction to control vibration and to manage integrative wiring of various independent devices that need to function intraoperably. The services of a surgical technology integrator can be invaluable for coordinating the movement of the numerous assemblies and to assure they work together as clinically necessary. Most of the major imaging equipment manufacturers now offer imaging systems specifically designed for hybrid operating rooms.

Selecting an optimal table for hybrid operating rooms can be challenging as table characteristics necessary for surgery and image-guided interventional procedures respectively vary considerably. Surgical tables are often portable, highly cleanable and capable of assuming myriad positions that correspond to variations in body or extremity placement necessary for different surgical procedures, such as tilting (Trendelenburg), head-to-foot pivoting and left-to-right rotating. Conversely, the table components of most image-guided equipment assemblies are permanently affixed to the floor, difficult to clean and restricted in their precise configuration and positioning options. Imaging equipment manufacturers have begun to partner with surgical table manufacturers to offer competitively compatible assemblies that combine the positional flexibility of surgical tables with the performance and durability of image-guided table assemblies. In addition to positional flexibility, most have high weight-bearing capacities and are radio-translucent to accommodate radiation-emitting imaging. Where non-radiating imaging techniques (such as magnetic resonance imaging [MRI]) are employed, significantly different devices and assemblies (and room design) are required.

Lighting requirements for hybrid procedure rooms similarly require unique and often conflicting luminance requirements of both surgical and interventional procedure rooms. Three types of lighting should be provided: (1) general ambient lighting appropriate during the procedure; (2) focused and precise procedural surgical lighting that illuminates areas of incision and the sterile field; and, (3) high levels of room illumination for cleaning activities between procedures.

Luminance level requirements for surgical procedures tend to be higher than those for interventional procedures. Minimally-invasive and vascular access procedures utilize image monitors and thus benefit from relatively low levels of general room illumination as do open surgical procedures. However, open procedures require less intense use of monitors than do closed procedures. Monitor brightness is increasing, thus enabling ambient room illumination.

Environmental Factors — Noise and Alarm Fatigue

Much evidence shows that surgical procedure rooms are too noisy, and that actual levels for continuous background noise are far higher than guideline values established by the World Health Organization. A review of 35 studies by Busch-Vishniac and colleagues concluded that noise levels in hospitals internationally have been steadily rising since the 1960s [22]. For example, continuous background noise in the procedure room typically ranges from 75 to 90 dB, and can increase to almost 120 dB (e.g., during high-speed gas-turbine drill use) [23].

In the procedure room noise may be generated by multiple conversations, mechanical ventilation, suction, overhead pages, use of medical equipment, and uncoordinated alarms. High noise levels create a positive feedback situation, where noisy rooms require louder voices and louder alarms leading to increased noise levels, missed clinical events, and patient harm. There is a growing literature on how hospitals can incorporate noise mitigation, avoid overhead paging, and more. For example, by focusing on user input — clinicians and patients, intensive care units have been incorporating elements of creating less noise [24].

Noise mitigation is important and not always given as high a priority as it should. In general there are two distinct types of noise transmission: airborne within a room (such as most of these examples) and vibration- al (i.e. vibrational noise carried from one space to another through elements of the built environment). Things are often done to reduce the noise of mechanical ventilation systems and more recently to "begin" to mitigate noise emitting from MRIs. Most airborne noise transmission within the room (such as alarms and conversations), construction details would not likely mitigate this noise.

Acoustic dampening surface materials (such as acoustic ceilings and carpet) are not appropriate in the surgical space. Infection control protocol typically results in "hard" surfaces which reflect (instead of absorb) ambient noise. A white noise system might add to the noise; more effectively design modification of the noise producing devices (alarms) themselves might help.

High noise levels interfere with effective verbal and handover communications in cardiac care settings (called sound intelligibility or the degree to which *speech* can be understood). Patient handovers are always important in the operating room, but may be critical during certain events such as resuscitations when it is vital for team members to hear clearly other members of the team. High noise levels in operating rooms can also detrimentally affect short-term memory tasks, mask task-related cues, impair auditory vigilance (e.g., the ability to detect and identify alarms), and cause distractions during critical periods [25].

Exposure to loud noise activates the sympathetic nervous system affecting mood and performance [26]. The resulting stress response has been suggested to interact with other performance-shaping factors resulting in impaired decision making during critical clinical incidents [27].

Finally, the current international standard for alarms, IEC 60601- 1-8, stipulates that medical device audible alarms should be priority-encoded and validated for efficacy. Evidence suggests that the melodic alarms described in the standard do not function as originally intended. Urgency information can be encoded via modulation of the physical characteristics of sounds and should become a standard for all companies [28].

Summary and Recommendations

Surgical and interventional imaging suites are both areas where medical errors can occur commonly and where the built environment has a profound impact on injuries to patients and to medical outcomes and overall safety and well-being. Exceptional design of pediatric cardiac care spaces will provide an environment of patient safety as well as a safety-oriented organizational culture for staff. It will require a constant focus on safety and reliability by the perioperative leadership, physicians, and staff. This can only be accomplished through a continuous cycle of evaluation and improvement of the facility, equipment, technology, and processes. Designers of integrated surgical facilities need to prioritize the importance of safety in addition to efficiency as an essential concern in their designs. Design of advanced medical facilities is an interactive process that requires intense collaboration among both medical and design professionals. The medical professional must describe current and future clinical models of care, financial boundaries and operational practices, while the design professional, explores and advises how the built environment might best be shaped to accommodate these needs and constraints.

The first challenge is for each of these professional groups to understand the language of the other. The second challenge is to think – not only based on one's past experiences – but at the same time think anew, based on how clinical practice, finance and operations will likely differ in the future. The third challenge is how to judiciously determine how to best accommodate tomorrow's uncertain needs before the future arrives. Often we know generally how the future will differ from the present. We are usually challenged, however, to predict specifically what and how much to invest in order to assure that we accommodate the needs of tomorrow in a way that will do so within clear financial constraints.

Cardiovascular surgery is in the midst of enormous changes in models of care, medical technology, and financial reimbursement. The greatest changes in models of care that are influencing architectural design include the transition from open to closed procedures and the convergence of surgery and medical imaging. Cardiovascular surgical procedure rooms of the future therefore, will differ significantly from those in use today. Most likely they will be hybrids blending elements of today's surgical suite and catheterization laboratory heavily influenced by ways to mitigate the detrimental impact of the human factors that are key to maximizing performance. They will provide more surgical-like (sterile) environments than today's catheterization labs and more advanced imaging technology than today's typical surgical procedure rooms. Successful design solutions will be those that not only provide more space and equipment, but those that also consider new patterns of work flow, multi-disciplinary collaboration and increased building systems capacities. This new approach requires close cooperation between the design and clinical community while using a robust social-technical approach to create optimal conditions for providing safe and high valued care [29].

References

1. Debajyoti P, Harvey T, Barach P. Quality improvement of care through the built environment. Continuous quality improvement in health care. In: McLaughlin C, Johnson J, Sollecito W, editors. Implementing continuous quality improvement in health care: A global casebook. 4th edition. Jones and Bartlett; 2011. p. 349–62. ISBN 978-0-7637-9536-8.
2. Debajyoti P, Barach P. Application of environment psychology theories and frameworks in evidence-based healthcare design In: Valentin J, Gamez L, editors. Environmental psychology: new developments. Nova Publishers; 2010. p. 1–36, ISBN 978-1-60876-911-7.
3. Elbardissi AW, Wiegmann DA, Dearani JA, Sundt TM. Application of the human factors analysis and classification system methodology to the cardiovascular surgery operating room. Ann Thorac Surg. 2007;83(4): 1412–9.
4. Catchpole KR, Giddings AE, de Leval MR, et al. Identification of systems failures in successful paediatric cardiac surgery. Ergonomics. 2006;49(5–6): 567–88.
5. Karamichalis J, Barach P, Henaine R, Nido del P. Bacha E. Assessment of Surgical Competency in Pediatric cardiac surgery. Progress in Pediatric Cardiology – January 2012;Vol. 33; 1 15-20, DOI: 20110.1016/j.ppedcard.2011.12.003.

6. Schraagen JM, Schouten A, Smit M, vander Beek D, vande Ven J, Barach P. A prospective study of paediatric cardiac surgical microsystems: assessing the relationships between non-routine events, teamwork and patient outcomes. BMJ Qual Saf. 2011;20(7):599–603.
7. Barach P, Johnson JK, Ahmed A, et al. A prospective observational study of human factors, adverse events, and patient outcomes in surgery for pediatric cardiac disease. J Thorac Cardiovasc Surg. 2008;136(6):1422–8.
8. Schraagen JM, Schouten T, Smit M, et al. Assessing and improving teamwork in cardiac surgery. Qual Saf Health Care. 2010;19:1–6.
9. Weick K, Quinn R. Organizational change and development. Annu Rev Psychol. 1999;50:361–86.
10. Bognar A, Barach P, Johnson JK, et al. Errors and the burden of errors: attitudes, perceptions, and the culture of safety in pediatric cardiac surgical teams. Ann Thorac Surg. 2008;85:1374–81.
11. The Advisory Board Company. OR-Adjacent Induction Rooms – Practice # 18 – hardwiring a culture of efficiency. 2007: 161–5.
12. Rostenberg B, Barach P. Design of cardiovascular operating rooms for tomorrow's technology and clinical practice – part 2. Prog Pediatr Cardiol. 2012; 33(1):57–65.
13. Torkki Paulus M, Marjamaa A, Torkki M, Kallio Pentti E, Kirvelä A. Use of anesthesia induction rooms can increase the number of urgent orthopedic cases completed within 7 hours. Anesthesiology. 2005;103(2):401–5.
14. Lynch RJ, Englesbe MJ, Sturm L, et al. Measurement of foot traffic in the operating room: implications for infection control. Am J Med Qual. 2009;24(1):45–52. doi:10.1177/1062860608326419.
15. Young RS, O'Regan DJ. Cardiac surgical theatre traffic: time for traffic calming measures? Interact Cardiovasc Thorac Surg. 2010;10(4):526–9. doi:10.1510/icvts.2009.227116. Epub 2010 Jan 25.
16. Allison D, Abernathy J, Shappell S, Swinton G. Mapping and graphically analyzing tasks disruptions to understand and inform operating room design for improved safety, outcomes, and operational efficiency – a presentation at Healthcare Design'12. The Center for Health Design Phoenix. 6 Nov 2012.
17. Reiling J. Safe by design: designing safety in health care facilities, processes, and culture. Oakbrook Terrace: Joint Commission Resources; 2007.
18. Virgo Publishing. A quick guide to flash sterilization considerations. 2013. http://infectioncontroltoday.com/posted 04/16/2008; downloaded 05/11/2013.
19. Rui Z, Guangbei T, Jihong L. Study on biological contaminant control strategies under different ventilation models in hospital operating room. Build Environ. 2008;43:793–803.
20. Balaras CA, Dascalaki EG, Gaglia A. HVAC and indoor thermal conditions in hospital operating room. Energy Build. 2007;39:454–70.
21. Loftus RW, Muffly MK, Brown JR, Beach ML, Koff MD, Corwin HL, Surgenor SD, Kirkland KB, Yeager MP. Hand contamination of anesthesia providers is an important risk factor for intraoperative bacterial transmission. Anesth Analg. 2011;112(1):98–105. doi:10.1213/ANE.0b013e3181e7ce18. Epub 2010 Aug 4.
22. Busch-Vishniac IJ, West JE, Barnhill C, Hunter T, Orellana D, Chivukula R. Noise levels in Johns Hopkins Hospital. J Acoust Soc Am. 2005;118(6):3629–45. 17 pages.
23. Weinger MB, Smith NT. Vigilance, alarms, and integrated monitoring systems. In: Ehrenwerth J, Eisenkraft JB, editors. Anesthesia equipment: principles and applications. Malvern: Mosby Year Book; 2005.
24. Barach P, Potter-Forbes M, Forbes I. Designing safe intensive care units of the future, intensive and critical care medicine. In: World Federation of Societies of Intensive and Critical Care Medicine. Dordrecht: Springer; 2009. p. 525–41.
25. Weinger MB, Smith NT. Vigilance, alarms, and integrated monitoring systems. In: Ehrenwerth J, Eisenkraft JB, editors. Anesthesia equipment: principles and applications. Malvern: Mosby Year Book; 1993. p. 350–84.
26. Weinger M, Englund C. Ergonomic and human factors affecting anesthetic vigilance and monitoring performance in the operating room environment. Anesthesiology. 1990;73:995–1021.
27. Selye H. Forty years of stress research: principal remaining problems and misconceptions. Canadian Medical Association. CMAJ. 1976;115:53–6.
28. McNeer R, Bohorquez J, Varon A, Ozdamar O, Barach P. Human factors engineering of urgency-encoded audible alarm signals, Journal of Clinical Monitoring and Computing. J Clin Monit Comput. 2007;21(6):353–63.
29. Barach P. Designing reliable and safe hospitals. In: Samsom M, editor. International Academy of Design press; 2013. pp. 32–7.

Simulation-Based Training to Enhance Patient Safety in Pediatric Cardiovascular Care

35

Catherine K. Allan and Peter Weinstock

Abstract

Pediatric cardiovascular care is delivered within clinical microsystems (operating room, catheterization laboratory, intensive care unit) characterized by complex teams and environments, high technical and cognitive demands, and need for frequent handovers. These features, also present in other high risk industries such as aviation and nuclear power, increase susceptibility to adverse events related to human error. In acute care areas of medicine broadly, and increasingly in pediatric cardiovascular care, simulation has emerged as an important tool to train individuals and teams in a structured environment far from patient harm to accelerate acquisition of technical skills, identify systems hazards, and reduce the risk of error due to human factors. Such simulation-based training programs are maximally effective when they are developed and delivered using rigorous, structured processes based on the principles of adult learning theory. Fundamental components of this process include formal needs assessment, development of scenarios that address specific learning objectives appropriately targeted to the level of the learner, and structured debriefing to aid learners in processing the simulation event. Recent innovations in simulation technology, such as development of high fidelity infant and pediatric-specific task trainers, are expanding the role of simulation in pediatric cardiovascular care.

Keywords

Simulation • Patient safety • Human factors • Curriculum design • Needs assessment • Latent safety threats

C.K. Allan, MD (✉)
Division of Cardiac Intensive Care, Department of Cardiology, Boston Children's Hospital, 300 Longwood Ave., Boston, MA 02115, USA
e-mail: catherine.allan@cardio.chboston.org

P. Weinstock
Division of Critical Care Medicine, Department of Anesthesia, Perioperative and Pain Medicine, Boston Children's Hospital, Harvard Medical School, Boston, MA, USA
e-mail: peter.weinstock@childrens.harvard.edu

P.R. Barach, J.P. Jacobs, S.E. Lipshultz, P.C. Laussen (eds.),
Pediatric and Congenital Cardiac Care: Volume 2: Quality Improvement and Patient Safety,
DOI 10.1007/978-1-4471-6566-8_35, © Springer-Verlag London 2015

Adverse Events and Medical Errors in Pediatric Cardiovascular Care: The Need for Strong Training Models

The acute care of children with congenital heart defects spans clinical microsystems, including the operating room, intensive care unit, and cardiac catheterization laboratory. These microsystems are characterized by the need for multiple care providers to function as a team while performing complex procedures at a very high technical and cognitive level within a sophisticated organizational structure [1, 2] (Table 35.1). These characteristics, along with periods of vulnerability during patient handoffs between clinical microsystems [3], predispose to a high risk of error related to human factors for pediatric cardiac patients.

The Bristol Royal Infirmary Inquiry and the Manitoba Pediatric Cardiac Surgery Inquest, two highly publicized investigations of mortality in pediatric cardiac surgery, provided strong evidence that the deaths were related not only to surgical errors but to systems failures and poor communication as well [4, 5]. Subsequent rigorous human factors research has shown that errors are common in the realm of pediatric cardiac surgery. Direct observation of 102 pediatric cardiac surgery cases found a median of 1.1 major (potential to cause serious consequences) safety events and 18.3 minor events per case [6]. A multicenter study using direct observation of arterial switch operations reported that mortality and "near misses" were linked most strongly to major events but that minor events also increased the odds of death and that the impact of minor events was additive [7]. In the study by Barach et al., minor events most commonly represented communication errors [6]. Likewise, cardiac surgery teams with more effective teamwork strategies, including better communication, had fewer minor

Table 35.1 Clinical microsystems in pediatric cardiovascular care

Component	Catheterization laboratory	Intensive care unit/ECMO Care	Cardiac operating room
Personnel	Catheterizer	Intensivist	Surgeon
	Catheter technician	Surgeon	Assistant surgeon
	Anesthesiologist	Nurse	Anesthesiologist
	Nurse	Respiratory therapist	Scrub nurse
	Trainees	ECMO specialist/perfusionist	Circulating nurse
	Surgeon (for hybrid procedures)	Trainees	Perfusionist
		Consultants	Trainees
			Echocardiographer
Equipment	Fluoroscopy equipment	ECMO circuit	CPB Circuit
	Fixed catheterization table	Resuscitation carts	Anesthesia machine
	Instrument table	Surgical instrument table	Minimally invasive equipment
	Surgical instruments (for hybrid procedures)	Surgical equipment (cautery, headlamp, etc.)	Echocardiography machine
Clinical/systems	Rapidly changing physiology	Multiple patients	Time pressures on CPB
	Radiation exposure	Bed-availability issues	High level technical skills
	Multiple equipment changes (catheters)	Blended teams	Hierarchy of personnel
	Communication between control room and lab	Hierarchy of personnel	
	High level technical skills		
	Hierarchy of personnel		

Children with cardiac disease move between clinical microsystems, which are defined by complex team structures, equipment needs, and systems concerns about latent safety threats and the potential for patient harm
ECMO extracorporeal membrane oxygenation, *CPB* cardiopulmonary bypass

intraoperative events, improved intraoperative performance, and reduced operative times [3].

The literature also supports the pervasive nature of medical errors in the intensive care unit—an environment comprised of a multitude of technologies, large interdisciplinary provider teams, critically ill patients, high emotionality, and fatiguing work schedules—and the relevance of human error and systems failures [8, 9]. In around-the-clock direct patient and provider observations in an ICU, Donchin et al. identified an average of 1.7 errors per patient per day, 30 % of which could have led to marked deterioration in patient status or death without prompt recognition and management [10]. In pediatrics, a multicenter chart review of 15 ICUs documented 1,488 adverse events among 734 patients, with 62 % of patients suffering at least one adverse event, 45 % of which were classified as preventable [11]. Furthermore, analysis of errors and adverse events in the ICU showed lack of teamwork and communication to be major contributors to nearly half of critical incidents [12, 13].

Both in and out of the operating room, effective teamwork behaviors have been linked to positive outcomes. For instance, during both simulated and real resuscitations, factors such as effective leadership have a positive impact [14–16]. The ability of the leader to organize a team, avoid "task fixation," and articulate a global assessment of the patient's status and plans for management was associated with improved performance measures, such as hands-on time when providing chest compressions and time to defibrillation after recognizing ventricular fibrillation. These performance measures are clinically important, given that early defibrillation and increased CPR fraction are associated with improved survival after cardiac arrest [17–19]. The importance of specific teamwork skills has been acknowledged in recent resuscitation guidelines from the American Heart Association, including the Pediatric Advanced Life Support Guidelines [20]. Thus, incorporating multidisciplinary teamwork training across the cardiovascular care environment may help decrease preventable non-technical errors and improve patient outcomes.

The contribution of human factors to catastrophic accidents and failures in non-medical high-risk industries, including nuclear power and aviation, has long been recognized, and substantial efforts have gone towards training staff in principles of teamwork to mitigate the effects of human error in non-technical skills. After analyzing a series of catastrophic accidents, the aviation industry turned to simulation-based teamwork training, in the form of "Crew Resource Management" Training, to overcome non-technical errors and improve teamwork. Crew Resource Management Training has now become a mandatory component of initial pilot licensure and maintenance of certification. In this training, highly realistic flight simulators are utilized to recreate emergency scenarios that the crew might encounter in flight, and post-simulation debriefings led by trained facilitators focus on teamwork principles.

Given the parallels between aviation and medicine in terms of the contribution of human factors to errors and accidents, the lessons from the aviation industry were transferred to medical training through the introduction of simulation-based Crisis Resource Management (CRM) Training. Indeed, since the introduction of immersive simulation in medicine in the 1980s [21], simulation has been applied broadly throughout acute care areas [22–24], not only for teamwork training but also for clinical skills training, competency assessment, and systems evaluation to identify latent safety threats at the point of care delivery.

Simulation training is particularly important in pediatric subspecialties, where high-risk events, such as cardiopulmonary arrest, are relatively rare, creating a "pediatric training paradox" [25]. Low numbers of training opportunities can result in an unfavorable "volume-outcome relationship" that may render providers ill-prepared to conduct pediatric resuscitation [26–28]. This effect is magnified in the field of pediatric cardiovascular care, where specific resuscitation skills, such as emergent chest re-opening, temporary epicardial pacing, and ECMO cannulation, fall outside the scope of traditional pediatric advanced life support training [29–32]. Additionally, work hour restrictions and societal expectations that senior physicians be involved at the bedside limit trainees' clinical experience and opportunities and may delay acquisition of full proficiency before training is completed. Simulation offers unique solutions to this challenge in pediatric cardiovascular training through authentic on-demand, structured experiences combined with opportunities for summative and formative feedback. As a result, simulation is beginning to be applied across the spectrum of cardiovascular care—from the intensive care unit [29], to the catheterization laboratory [33], to the operating room [34].

Simulation for Team Training in Cardiovascular Care: Principles and Evidence

In the early 1980s, an early precursor to today's high fidelity, whole-body mannequin simulators was developed by David Gaba and colleagues at Stanford University. The simulator interacted with monitors and anesthesia equipment to realistically replicate patient physiology as part of an immersive simulation environment (CASE, Comprehensive Anesthesia Simulator Environment) in which participants were able to engage in real-time clinical problem solving [35]. Gaba's early work in anesthesia was unique in medicine in its recognition of the importance of human factors in the operating room [36]. He and others [37] defined standards of leadership and team behavior now described as the principles of Crisis Resource Management (CRM). These principles have since been widely adopted in training programs across acute care, including the emergency department [38], intensive care unit [29, 39], and operating room [40]. Likewise, a growing number of simulation-based CRM training programs applied to pediatric cardiac critical care have been shown to improve the comfort level of providers in navigating critical incidents [29, 30, 33].

Principles of Crisis Resource Management address issues related to event leadership, followership, communication, and team coordination (Table 35.2).

1. *Role Clarity.* Team members are assigned to specific tasks and responsibilities. Key to these are the "Event Manager" who organizes the team by assigning tasks, controlling communication, creating a shared mental model through frequent updates and maintaining global perspective on the evolving crisis. Effective Event Managers support an environment of psychological safety to promote free and effective communication [41].

Table 35.2 Fundamental principles of crisis resource management training

Principle	Key components
Role clarity	Event manager is explicitly identified
	Task assignments are clear
Communication	Names and eye contact are used between speaker and listener
	Closed loop (receiver confirms understanding sender)
	Communication is explicit (no "hints")
	Communication is channeled through the event manager
	Updates on task progress are given often
	Communication is respectful
Personnel support	Support personnel/consultants are mobilized appropriately
Resource utilization	Equipment and resources are mobilized appropriately
	Hospital emergency protocols and procedures are followed
Global assessment	The "50,000-foot view" is maintained by event manager throughout
	Fixation on one aspect of the task at the expense of other aspects avoided
	Event manager frequently updates team on progress
	An environment of psychological safety is maintained
	Input from the team is invited

2. *Communication.* Effective communication strategies emphasize clear and explicit statements directed to specific individuals combined with consistent "closed-loop" communication (in which the listener confirms an understanding of the speaker's message) and in which team members provide updates on assigned tasks as well as offering information and suggestions to the event manager—all of which occur across authority gradients.
3. *Global Assessment.* The "50,000-foot view," or situational awareness, of the entire event and environment is maintained to avoid "fixation errors," in which participants focus on one aspect of the event at the expense of other relevant events. Strategies include provision of frequent updates by the Event Manager and team-based review of clinical status.
4. *Personnel Support.* Proactively identifying and mobilizing additional resources, including expert consultants (i.e., "Calling for help early").
5. *Resource Utilization.* The use of systematic and institutional resources for critical event management is optimized. This issue includes understanding human and technical resource availability and operations and is supported by a working knowledge of current hospital policy and procedure.

Crisis Resource Management courses, once exclusively delivered at stand-alone centers, are now more frequently being applied directly to the point at which clinical care is delivered. Such in-situ or point-of-care simulations allow full native teams to train within their own complex care environments [42]. In the cardiac operating room and catheterization laboratory in particular, in situ training programs can optimize authenticity, realism, and engagement by including inherent environmental nuances that might otherwise be difficult to recreate (Fig. 35.1). In the catheterization laboratory, for instance, resuscitation efforts may be hampered by the dark environment and bulky fluoroscopy equipment that may obstruct access to the patient and challenge communication between team members. In addition, the ongoing need for fluoroscopy during resuscitation poses the threat of exposure to ionizing radiation to caregivers, underscoring team member safety during the resuscitation process.

Crisis Resource Management training holds both the intuitive appeal of a practice-makes-perfect model, as well as a rapidly growing literature of effectiveness at multiple levels, including (1) knowledge acquisition, (2) team-based elements, (3) behavioral processes (measures of communication, self-correction, etc.), (4) performance outcomes, and (5) translation to patient care. Applied to pediatric cardiac ICU, CRM training can increase self-efficacy, preparedness, and comfort for participants [29, 30, 32].

Although data specific to patient outcomes in pediatric cardiovascular care may be lacking, a growing literature base from other pediatric acute-care specialties suggests that CRM training substantially improves patient outcomes. In neonatology, trainees exposed to Neonatal Resuscitation Program training supplemented with high fidelity simulation practice, demonstrated more effective teamwork behavior, including information-sharing, updating the team on the patient's status, and inquiry of other team members [39]. In the Emergency Room, team training reduces error rates [43]. A study from the Veterans Administration health care system found an 18 % reduction in annual mortality rates among centers in which formal team training programs were implemented compared to 7 % among those where team training was not introduced [44, 45]. Morbidity was likewise reduced in centers with formal team training programs [45]. In obstetrics, a field similar to pediatric cardiovascular care in that it relies heavily on resuscitation practices and skills outside of pediatric or advanced cardiac life support algorithms, Draycott et al. found clear links between effective utilization of teamwork principles and improved, more efficient care delivery, as well as patient outcomes. Particular team skills that correlated positively with outcomes included verbal declaration of a crisis, closed-loop communication, and effective resource utilization[45], whereas clinical knowledge of management of obstetric emergencies, clinical skills in a simulator setting, or attitudes towards teamwork and patient safety were not correlated [46], suggesting that these factors alone are not

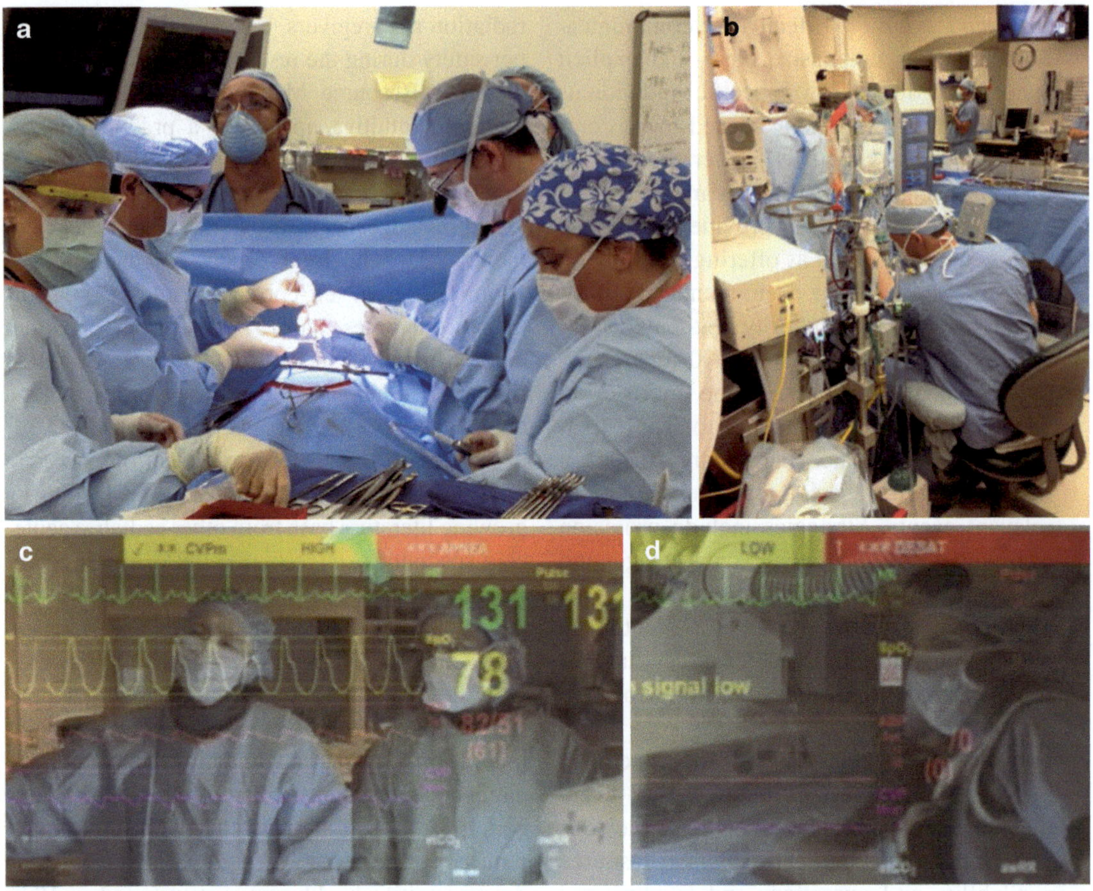

Fig. 35.1 Team Training at the Point of Delivery in Pediatric Cardiovascular Care. Native team training within native environments incorporates preparedness training into the daily workflow. Participation of complete complement of care providers during high-fidelity simulation courses in the highly nuanced environments, such as the cardiothoracic operating room (**a**, **b**) and the catheterization Laboratory (**c**, **d**)

sufficient for effective team performance. A decrease in the interval between diagnosis of cord prolapse and emergency cesarean delivery from 25 to 14.5 min ($P<0.001$) after team training in a large UK maternity center further supports the value of CRM in improving care [47].

Simulation-Based Technical Skills Training in Pediatric Cardiovascular Care

Early applications of medical simulation focused on technical or clinical skills, and included trainers for endotracheal intubation [21], as well as the Harvey Cardiology Patient Simulator, developed in the late 1960s to teach cardiovascular examination skills [48, 49]. The efficacy of simulation-based procedural skills training has been established in several lines of inquiry related to acute care medicine. In one medical intensive care unit, simulation-based curricula regarding safe placement of central venous lines reduced the mean number of attempts (1.70 vs. 2.78, $P=0.04$), failure rates (22.8–16.0 %, $P=0.02$) and overall complication rates (32.9–22.9 %, $P<0.01$) among trainees [50]. The curricula also reduced catheter-associated blood stream infections by 70 % and saved money [51].

Work hour restrictions, increased public scrutiny of clinical outcomes, and pressures to reduce operative times all threaten procedural "hands-on" time for trainees and, as a result, impact the quality of experiences to learn complex procedures [52]. Simulation-based skills training, both through analog and virtual reality models, has the ability to overcome these threats by providing dedicated hands-on practice time without harming patients. Simulation-based surgical training, such as virtual reality laparoscopic training, can improve skill acquisition through repetitive, deliberate practice combined with rigorous assessment and feedback [53, 54]. Additionally, a sole focus on teaching skills apart from actual patient care may create a less-threatening environment for the trainee and thereby enhance quality of teaching at the level of skills acquisition [55].

The pathway to procedural competency begins with acquisition of technical skills followed by the associated cognitive skills, including complex intraoperative decision making, communication, and the ability to adapt based on changing circumstances during a procedure. By deliberatively focusing on each element in order through well -designed curricula, simulation stands to accelerate the learning curve from novice to expert, and thus make the greatest educational use of real intraoperative time when ready [56]. These factors, combined with the development of integrated 6-year cardiothoracic surgery training programs [57] increasingly focused on competency-based training [58], have lead the field of adult cardiothoracic surgery to invest heavily in simulation-based curricula, relevant models, and assessment tools to teach technical skills [59, 60] that range from coronary anastomosis [61, 62], to mitral valve repair [63], to cardiopulmonary bypass management [64, 65].

Virtual reality simulators are also being used increasingly in invasive cardiology and electrophysiology, where they have accelerated learning among novices performing trans-septal puncture and diagnostic catheterization [33, 55] with associated reductions in fluoroscopy time [66]. Given the heterogeneous nature of congenital cardiac defects, the development of high fidelity simulation-based models for skills training has been slower than in adult cardiovascular fields, although our group has recently reported on the development of a highly realistic infant ECMO cannulation trainer (Fig. 35.2). Use of this trainer within the context of a full cannulation training curriculum improved cannulation time and a composite technical score that evaluates both the individual steps of cannulation, and patient management [67]. Engineering advances, such as three-dimensional ("rapid prototyping") printers, have the potential to speed the development of pediatric-specific trainers by translating individual patient imaging data into highly realistic trainers that accurately replicate complex pediatric anatomy.

Point-of-Care Simulation to Enhance Systems Safety in Pediatric Cardiovascular Care

Simulation applied at the point of care offers opportunities not only to improve individual and team performance but also to study and improve the care system itself. Both in situ multidisciplinary team training programs [42, 68] and formalized simulation-based programs using rigorous human factors methodologies, such as "Lean [69]" or "Plan-Do-Study-Act (PDSA)," are now being employed as rapid-cycle-improvement methods to identify patient safety threats and to guide the design and implementation of system improvements [70]. Common factors among successful latent safety threat-analysis programs include (1) using expertise from multiple areas, including multidisciplinary clinical providers, simulation experts, risk management or systems safety experts, and equipment experts during planning, simulation, and debriefing; (2) a preparation phase to identify possible areas of vulnerability and key areas for testing and to clearly define steps in clinical processes when relevant; (3) iterative simulation events to identify safety threats and test changes implemented in reaction to identified threats; and (4) structured debriefing focusing not on individual performance but rather on identifying system deficiencies and generating solutions to threats [70] (Fig. 35.3).

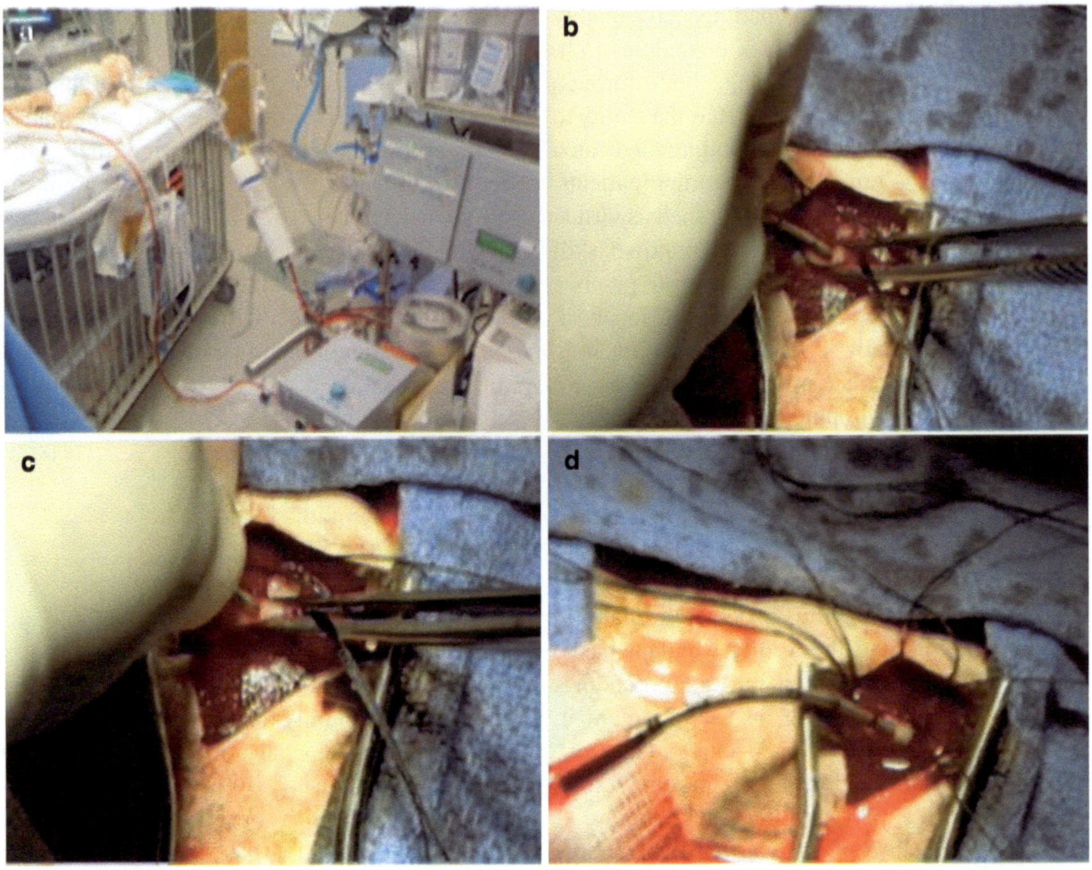

Fig. 35.2 The integrated ECMO cannulation skills trainer allows contextualized skills training for emergent ECMO cannulation during CPR. Contextualized skills training in the native cardiac intensive care unit environment (**a**) uses a highly realistic, embedded surgical skills trainer that allows dissection, vessel cannulation (**b**, **c**), and establishment of ECMO flow, and authentic "bleeding" from the surgical site (**d**) (Reprinted with permission from Allan et al. [67])

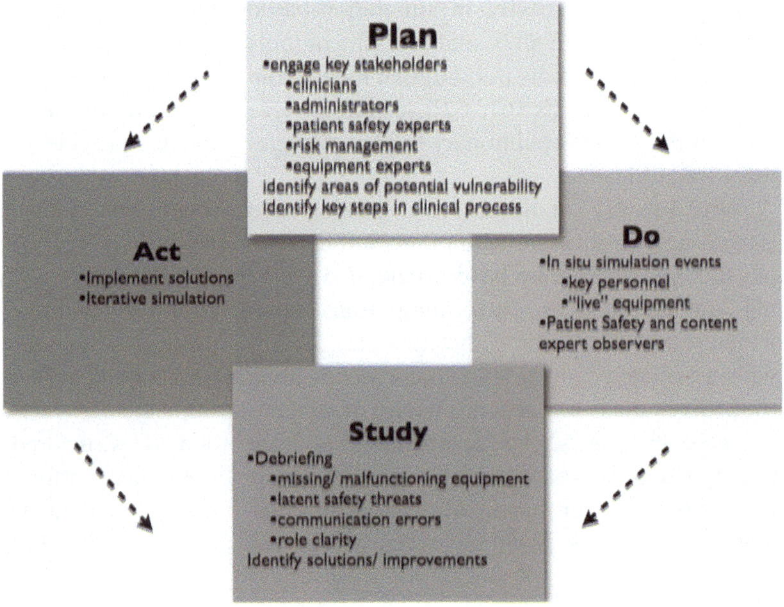

Fig. 35.3 The Plan-Do-Study-Act cycles used in simulations for systems evaluation and improvement

Rodriguez-Paz et al. reported the use of in situ simulation as part of a systematic process to identify hazards before opening of a new intraoperative program for delivery of high-dose radiation therapy. A multidisciplinary group, including stakeholders from all involved disciplines (surgery, radiation therapy, radiation safety, nursing, anesthesia, risk management, etc.) completed multiple simulations and identified 20 latent safety threats related to equipment, supplies, teamwork, and communication. Solutions were then designed and implemented, including pre-operative checklists, which were then followed by the successful opening of the intraoperative program without any adverse event [71]. Similarly, Geis et al. used in situ simulation to safely open a new satellite emergency department by identifying needed environmental improvements (e.g., equipment placement, inadequate oxygen ports), team member roles, and equipment concerns (e.g., inadequate numbers of defibrillators) [72].

Complex pediatric cardiovascular care microsystems and their interactions make the field perfectly suited for such simulation-based approaches to quality improvement and optimization. Examples include magnetic resonance imaging (MRI) suites and hybrid catheterization-surgical suites, both of which include important interplay among specific safety considerations (e.g., magnetic fields, radiation), complex teams, and physical equipment (e.g., fluoroscopy).

Optimizing Delivery of Simulation-Based Training to Enhance Patient Safety

Informing the Design of Simulation-Based Curricula with Principles of Adult Learning Theory

Although technical authenticity is important in simulations, there is a growing appreciation that effectiveness of simulation methodology has less to do with "what" is being delivered and more to do with "how" and by whom. In particular, curricula design, implementation, and ultimately facilitation should be firmly founded on established principles of adult learning theory to create the best experience.

David Kolb describes four types of adult learners based on preferences for *acquiring information*, either through concrete experience or abstract conceptualization, and for *processing new knowledge*, either through reflection or active experimentation [73]. For example, one individual may learns best if material is first presented in an abstract format such as a lecture followed by an opportunity to experiment with new information (such as through a simulation), whereas another individual might learn best when material is presented first as part of a concrete experience (e.g. simulation) with an opportunity for subsequent reflection (e.g. debriefing). Thus, a curriculum which uses only simulation without opportunity for processing (debriefing) or presents only didactic material without opportunity for active engagement and experimentation with the material will not effectively serve all adult learners. Through "cycles of learning"—which incorporate didactics (abstract conceptualization), hands-on experiences (the scenario) followed by structured reflection and conceptualization (debriefing), followed by further experimentation with new learned concepts—a single, simulation-based curricula can effectively and efficiently engage each type of learner [74].

Malcolm Knowles' principles of adult learning (also known as "andragogy") describe that adult learners are typically intrinsically rather than extrinsically motivated, often by a specific "problem" to be solved. They draw extensively on prior knowledge and experiences when faced with new material, and work to incorporate new knowledge into an existing framework. Thus, adult educational experiences should be highly relevant to and draw on the learner's past experiences. To achieve this, formal needs assessment should be used in designing new curricula. Learning in the simulation environment often involves multidisciplinary teams, and, therefore, to ensure value for all learners, the needs assessment process should include representatives from all disciplines and key stakeholders. Learning objectives are then identified, and scenarios and didactic materials are tailored to specifically address these objectives. Awareness and application of these fundamental adult learning principles to curricular design, particularly for the busy acute care practitioner, can optimize participation as well as buy-in for simulation-based training across all levels of expertise.

Scenario Design

Scenario design begins by identifying key learning objectives [75] and then tailoring content and complexity to the learner's level of expertise. In procedural or skills-based simulations for instance, novice learners may benefit from mentored practice, with a focus on acquiring psychomotor skills, perhaps on an isolated skills trainer. Learners already proficient in the technical aspects of the skill may benefit from more immersive and realistic simulations (e.g., those including noise, distractions, and so on) to further refine psychomotor and cognitive skills, such as clinical decision making and managing high-risk, low-frequency events [76, 77].

As described by Rudolph et al., scenario realism itself can be thought of as having three main components—technical, conceptual, and emotional—and should be tailored to the needs and experience of the learner [78]. Technical realism refers to how closely the mannequins, training devices, and equipment resemble those that are part of the actual patient care experience. Technical realism can be enhanced through simulation delivered within the native environment (in situ) using real equipment (e.g., defibrillators, code carts, surgical instruments). The importance of technical realism for learner engagement may be higher with more advanced learners and objectives. Likewise, a high degree of technical realism may be unnecessary for more novice learners [79] and may, in fact, distract from learning objectives for this group.

Particularly germane to procedurally based aspects of cardiovascular care (cardiac surgery and catheterization), requirements for technical realism in skills-training models must be carefully considered in the context of both the learner's level of technical expertise and the nature of learning objectives. For example, expert analysis suggests that low-fidelity bench models for adult cardiac surgical training may be sufficient for novice trainees to learn basic psychomotor skills, but higher, fully contextualized training experiences may be important for more advanced trainees [67].

Conceptual realism refers to clinical or physiologic relevancy (e.g., how the scenario story and stages unfold) and is as important as technical realism in learner engagement [78, 80]. That is, the clinical context of a case must make sense, the physiology must be presented realistically, and responses to interventions must be consistent with real life. Conceptual reality is particularly relevant in pediatric cardiovascular care, where patient physiology is highly nuanced, so much so that conceptual realism may be as or even more relevant than technical realism for the most advanced participants [80].

Emotional realism refers to the overall experience of the simulation and how the participant feels and responds to the environment as well as to the team [80]. Emotional reality can be optimized though involvement of native teams in native environments, with participation reflecting the natural compliment of caregivers for a particular event.

Debriefing

Critically important in effective simulation methodology is well-executed, focused and structured feedback or debriefing, optimally given by trained debriefers [81, 82, 83, 84, 85]. The fundamental purpose and goal of effective debriefing is to foster reflection, and encourages learners to compare new and prior experiences to help them incorporate new and improved approaches to thinking about clinical problems [86]. In so doing, the debriefer helps individuals and teams identify and close specific performance gaps. To encourage reflection, the debriefer must create a structured and psychologically safe environment. This environment is achieved with specific strategies, such as maintaining transparency (e.g., explicit ground rules, outlining the structure of the debriefing process), honesty, mutual respect, and confidentiality and approaching debriefing from a stance of curiosity (e.g., problem solving) rather than certainty [87].

Although many debriefing methodologies have been described [87–89], no one method has proven most effective. Rather, specific debriefing strategies should be matched to the level of the learner, the learning objectives of the simulation, and time available for debriefing. For instance, team debriefings focused on human factors should focus on open-ended "why" questions, as opposed to the "what" and "how" questions of clinical skills training.

The role of the debriefer in a human factors course is to moderate the discussion using open-ended questions with participants who typically have high technical expertise and who are prepared to be self-reflective [90]. One purpose of a human factors debriefing is to use specific examples from a simulation to explore generalizable concepts related to team performance, rather than to discuss nuances of clinical medicine. Robust methodologies for human factors debriefings in health care have been developed [87, 88], and require rigorous facilitator training.

On the other end of the spectrum are facilitation techniques for novice learners in highly focused simulation-based curricula designed to teach procedural skills or algorithmic care. In these sessions, facilitators may integrate debriefing within the simulation itself, pausing mid-scenario to redirect or lead participants with focused questions. At the extreme of this approach is frank instruction, in which side-by side mentoring is used to teach fundamental procedural skills to novice learners (e.g., suturing). The critical importance of high-quality debriefing is further emphasized by the requirement among accrediting organizations for formal simulator faculty development [91].

Summary

The use of medical simulations has grown rapidly over the past decade, prompted by changes in healthcare delivery and education, and is now broadly applied across acute care specialties and all members of the healthcare team. The field of pediatric cardiovascular care, with all its complexity of patients, teams, and systems, is perfectly suited for simulation to be applied at multiple levels, from skills training to team training to systems safety analysis, as a major patient safety initiative.

For maximum efficacy, simulation science requires that simulation be used in the context of rigorous curriculum development or safety testing methodology. In particular, curricula must be aligned with the level of the learner to keep all practitioners on the "edge of their learning curve," independently of their level of expertise. Appropriate technical, conceptual, and emotional realism will optimize engagement. Simulation training and curricula should be delivered by trained facilitators in a realistic, respectful, psychologically safe manner. By adhering to these principles, simulation can greatly improve the care of infants and children with cardiovascular disease.

References

1. Bacha EA. Patient safety and human factors in pediatric cardiac surgery. Pediatr Cardiol. 2007;28(2): 116–21 [Review].
2. Mohr J, Barach P, Cravero J, Blike G, Godfrey M, Batalden P, and Nelson E. Microsystems in Health Care. Joint Commission Journal on Quality and Safety 2003;29:401–8.
3. Catchpole KR, Giddings AE, Wilkinson M, Hirst G, Dale T, de Leval MR. Improving patient safety by identifying latent failures in successful operations. Surgery. 2007;142(1):102–10 [Research Support, Non-U.S. Gov't].
4. Sinclaire M. Report of the Manitoba Pediatric Cardiac Surgery Inquest. cited 7 July 2013. Available from: http://www.pediatriccardiacinquest.mb.ca/.
5. Kennedy I. Learning from Bristol: the report of the public inquiry into children's heart surgery at the Bristol Royal Infirmary 1984–1995 2001. Cited 7 July 2013; Available from: http://webarchive.nationalarchives.gov.uk/20090811143745/http://www.bristol-inquiry.org.uk.
6. Barach P, Johnson JK, Ahmad A, Galvan C, Bognar A, Duncan R, et al. A prospective observational study of human factors, adverse events, and patient outcomes in surgery for pediatric cardiac disease. J Thorac Cardiovasc Surg. 2008;136(6):1422–8 [Research Support, Non-U.S. Gov't].
7. de Leval MR, Carthey J, Wright DJ, Farewell VT, Reason JT. Human factors and cardiac surgery: a mul-

ticenter study. J Thorac Cardiovasc Surg. 2000;119(4 Pt 1):661–72 [Multicenter Study Research Support, Non-U.S. Gov't].

8. Donchin Y, Seagull FJ. The hostile environment of the intensive care unit. Curr Opin Crit Care. 2002;8(4): 316–20.
9. Michael St. Pierre GH, Cornelius Buerschaper. Crisis management in acute care settings. Berlin: Springer; 2008.
10. Donchin Y, Gopher D, Olin M, Badihi Y, Biesky M, Sprung CL, et al. A look into the nature and causes of human errors in the intensive care unit. Crit Care Med. 1995;23(2):294–300 [Research Support, Non-U.S. Gov't].
11. Agarwal S, Classen D, Larsen G, Tofil NM, Hayes LW, Sullivan JE, et al. Prevalence of adverse events in pediatric intensive care units in the United States. Pediatr Crit Care Med. 2010;11(5):568–78 [Multicenter Study].
12. Reader T, Flin R, Lauche K, Cuthbertson BH. Non-technical skills in the intensive care unit. Br J Anaesth. 2006;96(5):551–9 [Review].
13. Reader TW, Flin R, Cuthbertson BH. Communication skills and error in the intensive care unit. Curr Opin Crit Care. 2007;13(6):732–6.
14. Cooper S, Wakelam A. Leadership of resuscitation teams: "Lighthouse Leadership". Resuscitation. 1999;42(1):27–45.
15. Hunziker S, Tschan F, Semmer NK, Zobrist R, Spychiger M, Breuer M, et al. Hands-on time during cardiopulmonary resuscitation is affected by the process of teambuilding: a prospective randomised simulator-based trial. BMC Emerg Med. 2009;9:3 [Randomized Controlled Trial Research Support, Non-U.S. Gov't].
16. Marsch SC, Muller C, Marquardt K, Conrad G, Tschan F, Hunziker PR. Human factors affect the quality of cardiopulmonary resuscitation in simulated cardiac arrests. Resuscitation. 2004;60(1):51–6.
17. Christenson J, Andrusiek D, Everson-Stewart S, Kudenchuk P, Hostler D, Powell J, et al. Chest compression fraction determines survival in patients with out-of-hospital ventricular fibrillation. Circulation. 2009;120(13):1241–7 [Multicenter Study Research Support, N.I.H., Extramural Research Support, Non-U.S. Gov't].
18. Chan PS, Krumholz HM, Nichol G, Nallamothu BK. Delayed time to defibrillation after in-hospital cardiac arrest. N Engl J Med. 2008;358(1):9–17 [Research Support, N.I.H., Extramural Research Support, Non-U.S. Gov't].
19. Ali B, Zafari AM. Narrative review: cardiopulmonary resuscitation and emergency cardiovascular care: review of the current guidelines. Ann Intern Med. 2007;147(3):171–9 [Practice Guideline Research Support, N.I.H., Extramural Review].
20. Kleinman ME, Chameides L, Schexnayder SM, Samson RA, Hazinski MF, Atkins DL, et al. Part 14: pediatric advanced life support: 2010 American Heart Association Guidelines for Cardiopulmonary Resuscitation and Emergency Cardiovascular Care. Circulation. 2010;122(18 Suppl 3):S876–908.
21. Cooper JB, Taqueti VR. A brief history of the development of mannequin simulators for clinical education and training. Postgrad Med J. 2008;84(997): 563–70 [Review].
22. Eppich WJ, Adler MD, McGaghie WC. Emergency and critical care pediatrics: use of medical simulation for training in acute pediatric emergencies. Curr Opin Pediatr. 2006;18(3):266–71 [Review].
23. Yager PH, Lok J, Klig JE. Advances in simulation for pediatric critical care and emergency medicine. Curr Opin Pediatr. 2011;23(3):293–7 [Review].
24. Dull KE, Bachur RG. Simulation in the pediatric emergency department. Clin Pediatr (Phila). 2012; 51(8):711–7.
25. Weinstock PH, Kappus LJ, Kleinman ME, Grenier B, Hickey P, Burns JP. Toward a new paradigm in hospital-based pediatric education: the development of an onsite simulator program. Pediatr Crit Care Med. 2005;6(6):635–41 [Comment].
26. Hannan EL, Popp AJ, Tranmer B, Fuestel P, Waldman J, Shah D. Relationship between provider volume and mortality for carotid endarterectomies in New York state. Stroke. 1998;29(11):2292–7 [Research Support, Non-U.S. Gov't].
27. Hannan EL, Racz M, Kavey RE, Quaegebeur JM, Williams R. Pediatric cardiac surgery: the effect of hospital and surgeon volume on in-hospital mortality. Pediatrics. 1998;101(6):963–9.
28. Marx WH, Simon R, O'Neill P, Shapiro MJ, Cooper AC, Farrell LS, et al. The relationship between annual hospital volume of trauma patients and in-hospital mortality in New York State. J Trauma. 2011;71(2): 339–46.
29. Allan CK, Thiagarajan RR, Beke D, Imprescia A, Kappus LJ, Garden A, et al. Simulation-based training delivered directly to the pediatric cardiac intensive care unit engenders preparedness, comfort, and decreased anxiety among multidisciplinary resuscitation teams. J Thorac Cardiovasc Surg. 2010;140(3):646–52 [Research Support, Non-U.S. Gov't].
30. Figueroa MI, Sepanski R, Goldberg SP, Shah S. Improving teamwork, confidence, and collaboration among members of a pediatric cardiovascular intensive care unit multidisciplinary team using simulation-based team training. Pediatr Cardiol. 2013;34(3):612–9.
31. Chan SY, Figueroa M, Spentzas T, Powell A, Holloway R, Shah S. Prospective assessment of novice learners in a simulation-based extracorporeal membrane oxygenation (ECMO) education program. Pediatr Cardiol. 2013;34(3):543–52.
32. Lo TY, Morrison R, Atkins K, Reynolds F. Effective performance of a new post-operative cardiac resuscitation simulation training scheme in the Paediatric Intensive Care Unit. Intensive Care Med. 2009;35(4):725–9.
33. De Ponti R, Marazzi R, Ghiringhelli S, Salerno-Uriarte JA, Calkins H, Cheng A. Superiority of simulator-based training compared with conventional

training methodologies in the performance of transseptal catheterization. J Am Coll Cardiol. 2011;58(4): 359–63 [Randomized Controlled Trial Research Support, Non-U.S. Gov't].
34. Fann JI, Feins RH, Hicks Jr GL, Nesbitt JC, Hammon JW, Crawford Jr FA. Evaluation of simulation training in cardiothoracic surgery: the Senior Tour perspective. J Thorac Cardiovasc Surg. 2012;143(2):264–72 [Evaluation Studies Research Support, Non-U.S. Gov't].
35. Gaba DM, DeAnda A. A comprehensive anesthesia simulation environment: re-creating the operating room for research and training. Anesthesiology. 1988;69(3):387–94 [Research Support, Non-U.S. Gov't Research Support, U.S. Gov't, Non-P.H.S.].
36. Howard S, Gaba D, Fish K, Yang G, Sarnquist F. Anesthesia crisis resource management training: teaching anesthesiologists to handle critical incidents. Aviat Space Environ Med. 1992;63(9):763–70.
37. Salas E, Sims DE, Burke CS. Is there a "Big Five" in teamwork? Small Group Res. 2005;36:555–99.
38. Reznek M, Smith-Coggins R, Howard S, Kiran K, Harter P, Sowb Y, et al. Emergency medicine crisis resource management (EMCRM): pilot study of a simulation-based crisis management course for emergency medicine. Acad Emerg Med. 2003;10(4): 386–9.
39. Thomas EJ, Taggart B, Crandell S, Lasky RE, Williams AL, Love LJ, et al. Teaching teamwork during the Neonatal Resuscitation Program: a randomized trial. J Perinatol. 2007;27(7):409–14 [Randomized Controlled Trial Research Support, U.S. Gov't, P.H.S.].
40. Volk MS, Ward J, Irias N, Navedo A, Pollart J, Weinstock PH. Using medical simulation to teach crisis resource management and decision-making skills to otolaryngology housestaff. Otolaryngol Head Neck Surg. 2011;145(1):35–42 [Research Support, Non-U.S. Gov't].
41. Edmondson A. Psychological safety and learning behavior in work teams. Adm Sci Q. 1999;44:350–83.
42. Weinstock PH, Kappus LJ, Garden A, Burns JP. Simulation at the point of care: reduced-cost, in situ training via a mobile cart. Pediatr Crit Care Med. 2009;10(2):176–81 [Research Support, Non-U.S. Gov't].
43. Morey JC, Simon R, Jay GD, Wears RL, Salisbury M, Dukes KA, et al. Error reduction and performance improvement in the emergency department through formal teamwork training: evaluation results of the MedTeams project. Health Serv Res. 2002;37(6):1553–81 [Multicenter Study Research Support, U.S. Gov't, Non-P.H.S.].
44. Neily J, Mills PD, Young-Xu Y, Carney BT, West P, Berger DH, et al. Association between implementation of a medical team training program and surgical mortality. JAMA. 2010;304(15):1693–700 [Multicenter Study].
45. Young-Xu Y, Neily J, Mills PD, Carney BT, West P, Berger DH, et al. Association between implementation of a medical team training program and surgical morbidity. Arch Surg. 2011;146(12):1368–73.
46. Siassakos D, Draycott TJ, Crofts JF, Hunt LP, Winter C, Fox R. More to teamwork than knowledge, skill and attitude. BJOG. 2010;117(10):1262–9 [Multicenter Study Randomized Controlled Trial Research Support, Non-U.S. Gov't].
47. Siassakos D, Hasafa Z, Sibanda T, Fox R, Donald F, Winter C, et al. Retrospective cohort study of diagnosis-delivery interval with umbilical cord prolapse: the effect of team training. BJOG. 2009;116(8): 1089–96.
48. Gordon MS, Ewy GA, DeLeon Jr AC, Waugh RA, Felner JM, Forker AD, et al. "Harvey," the cardiology patient simulator: pilot studies on teaching effectiveness. Am J Cardiol. 1980;45(4):791–6 [Research Support, U.S. Gov't, P.H.S.].
49. Sajid AW, Ewy GA, Felner JM, Gessner I, Gordon MS, Mayer JW, et al. Cardiology patient simulator and computer-assisted instruction technologies in bedside teaching. Med Educ. 1990;24(6):512–7.
50. Sekiguchi H, Tokita JE, Minami T, Eisen LA, Mayo PH, Narasimhan M. A pre-rotational simulation-based workshop improves the safety of central venous catheter insertion: results of a successful internal medicine house staff training program. Chest. 2011;140(3):652–8. Epub 2011 Jun 9.
51. Khouli H, Jahnes K, Shapiro J, Rose K, Mathew J, Gohil A, et al. Performance of medical residents in sterile techniques during central vein catheterization: randomized trial of efficacy of simulation-based training. Chest. 2011;139(1):80–7 [Comparative Study Randomized Controlled Trial Research Support, Non-U.S. Gov't].
52. Marshall MB. Simulation for technical skills. J Thorac Cardiovasc Surg. 2012;144(3):S43–7.
53. Larsen CR, Oestergaard J, Ottesen BS, Soerensen JL. The efficacy of virtual reality simulation training in laparoscopy: a systematic review of randomized trials. Acta Obstet Gynecol Scand. 2012;91(9):1015–28 [Review].
54. Vassiliou MC, Dunkin BJ, Marks JM, Fried GM. FLS and FES: comprehensive models of training and assessment. Surg Clin North Am. 2010;90(3):535–58 [Review].
55. Bagai A, O'Brien S, Al Lawati H, Goyal P, Ball W, Grantcharov T, et al. Mentored simulation training improves procedural skills in cardiac catheterization: a randomized, controlled pilot study. Circ Cardiovasc Interv. 2012;5(5):672–9 [Randomized Controlled Trial].
56. Nesbitt JC, St Julien J, Absi TS, Ahmad RM, Grogan EL, Balaguer JM, et al. Tissue-based coronary surgery simulation: medical student deliberate practice can achieve equivalency to senior surgery residents. J Thorac Cardiovasc Surg. 2013;145(6):1453–8. discussion 8–9.
57. Crawford Jr FA. Thoracic surgery education–past, present, and future. Ann Thorac Surg. 2005;79(6): S2232–7 [Historical Article].

58. Collins JP. International consensus statement on surgical education and training in an era of reduced working hours. Surgeon. 2011;9 Suppl 1:S3–5 [Consensus Development Conference].
59. Carpenter AJ, Yang SC, Uhlig PN, Colson YL. Envisioning simulation in the future of thoracic surgical education. J Thorac Cardiovasc Surg. 2008;135(3):477–84 [Congresses Editorial].
60. Baker CJ, Sinha R, Sullivan ME. Development of a cardiac surgery simulation curriculum: from needs assessment results to practical implementation. J Thorac Cardiovasc Surg. 2012;144(1):7–16 [Research Support, Non-U.S. Gov't].
61. Fann JI, Calhoon JH, Carpenter AJ, Merrill WH, Brown JW, Poston RS, et al. Simulation in coronary artery anastomosis early in cardiothoracic surgical residency training: the Boot Camp experience. J Thorac Cardiovasc Surg. 2010;139(5):1275–81 [Evaluation Studies Research Support, Non-U.S. Gov't].
62. Lee R, Enter D, Lou X, Feins RH, Hicks GL, Gasparri M, et al. The Joint Council on Thoracic Surgery Education coronary artery assessment tool has high interrater reliability. Ann Thorac Surg. 2013;95(6): 2064–9. discussion 9–70.
63. Joyce DL, Dhillon TS, Caffarelli AD, Joyce DD, Tsirigotis DN, Burdon TA, et al. Simulation and skills training in mitral valve surgery. J Thorac Cardiovasc Surg. 2011;141(1):107–12 [Research Support, Non-U.S. Gov't].
64. Schiralli MP, Hicks GL, Angona RE, Gangemi JJ. An inexpensive cardiac bypass cannulation simulator: facing challenges of modern training. Ann Thorac Surg. 2010;89(6):2056–7.
65. Hicks Jr GL, Gangemi J, Angona Jr RE, Ramphal PS, Feins RH, Fann JI. Cardiopulmonary bypass simulation at the Boot Camp. J Thorac Cardiovasc Surg. 2011;141(1):284–92 [Research Support, Non-U.S. Gov't].
66. De Ponti R, Marazzi R, Doni LA, Tamborini C, Ghiringhelli S, Salerno-Uriarte JA. Simulator training reduces radiation exposure and improves trainees' performance in placing electrophysiologic catheters during patient-based procedures. Heart Rhythm. 2012;9(8):1280–5 [Research Support, Non-U.S. Gov't].
67. Allan CK, Pigula F, Bacha E, Emani S, Fynn-Thompson F, Thiagarajan RR, et al. An extracorporeal membrane oxygenation cannulation curriculum featuring a novel integrated skills trainer leads to improved performance among pediatric cardiac surgery trainees. Simul Healthc. 2013;8(4):221–8.
68. Patterson MD, Geis GL, Falcone RA, Lemaster T, Wears RL. In situ simulation: detection of safety threats and teamwork training in a high risk emergency department. BMJ Qual Saf. 2013;22(6): 468–77.
69. Going Lean in Health Care. IHI Innovation Series white paper. 2005: Available from: http://www.ihi.org/knowledge/Pages/IHIWhitePapers/GoingLeaninHealthCare.aspx.
70. Kobayashi L, Overly FL, Fairbanks RJ, Patterson M, Kaji AH, Bruno EC, et al. Advanced medical simulation applications for emergency medicine microsystems evaluation and training. Acad Emerg Med. 2008;15(11):1058–70 [Research Support, Non-U.S. Gov't].
71. Rodriguez-Paz JM, Mark LJ, Herzer KR, Michelson JD, Grogan KL, Herman J, et al. A novel process for introducing a new intraoperative program: a multidisciplinary paradigm for mitigating hazards and improving patient safety. Anesth Analg. 2009;108(1): 202–10.
72. Geis GL, Pio B, Pendergrass TL, Moyer MR, Patterson MD. Simulation to assess the safety of new healthcare teams and new facilities. Simul Healthc. 2011;6(3):125–33.
73. Kolb DA. Experience as the source of learning and development. Englewood Cliffs: Prentice Hall; 1984.
74. Armstrong E, Parsa-Parsi R. How can physicians' learning styles drive educational planning? Acad Med. 2005;80(7):680–4.
75. Rosen MA, Salas E, Wu TS, Silvestri S, Lazzara EH, Lyons R, et al. Promoting teamwork: an event-based approach to simulation-based teamwork training for emergency medicine residents. Acad Emerg Med. 2008;15(11):1190–8 [Research Support, U.S. Gov't, Non-P.H.S.].
76. Kopta JA. An approach to the evaluation of operative skills. Surgery. 1971;70(2):297–303.
77. Lippert 3rd FG, Spolek GA, Kirkpatrick GS, Briggs KA, Clawson DK. A psychomotor skills course for orthopaedic residents. J Med Educ. 1975;50(10):982–3.
77. Rudolph JW, Simon R, Raemer DB. Which reality matters? Questions on the path to high engagement in healthcare simulation. Simul Healthc. 2007;2(3): 161–3 [Comment].
79. Palter VN, Grantcharov T, Harvey A, Macrae HM. Ex vivo technical skills training transfers to the operating room and enhances cognitive learning: a randomized controlled trial. Ann Surg. 2011;253(5):886–9 [Comparative Study Randomized Controlled Trial Research Support, Non-U.S. Gov't].
80. Dieckmann P, Gaba D, Rall M. Deepening the theoretical foundations of patient simulation as social practice. Simul Healthc. 2007;2(3):183–93 [Comparative Study].
81. Ericsson KA. Deliberate practice and acquisition of expert performance: a general overview. Acad Emerg Med. 2008;15(11):988–94.
82. Mahmood T, Darzi A. The learning curve for a colonoscopy simulator in the absence of any feedback: no feedback, no learning. Surg Endosc. 2004;18(8):1224–30 [Clinical Trial Randomized Controlled Trial].
83. Savoldelli GL, Naik VN, Park J, Joo HS, Chow R, Hamstra SJ. Value of debriefing during simulated crisis management: oral versus video-assisted oral

feedback. Anesthesiology. 2006;105(2):279–85 [Comparative Study Randomized Controlled Trial Research Support, Non-U.S. Gov't].
84. Rall M, Manser T, Howard S. Key elements of debriefing for simulator training. Eur J Anaesthesiol. 2000;17:516–7.
85. Issenberg SB, McGaghie WC, Petrusa ER, Lee Gordon D, Scalese RJ. Features and uses of high-fidelity medical simulations that lead to effective learning: a BEME systematic review. Med Teach. 2005;27(1):10–28 [Research Support, Non-U.S. Gov't Research Support, U.S. Gov't, Non-P.H.S. Review].
86. Christansen U, Heffener L, Barach P, Simulation in Anesthesia. In: Anesthesia General Special, Principles Procedures and Techniques, Romano (ed.), 2nd edition, 2005, pp. 687–98.
87. Rudolph JW, Simon R, Rivard P, Dufresne RL, Raemer DB. Debriefing with good judgment: combining rigorous feedback with genuine inquiry. Anesthesiol Clin. 2007;25(2):361–76 [Review].
88. Rudolph JW, Simon R, Dufresne RL, Raemer DB. There's no such thing as "nonjudgmental" debriefing: a theory and method for debriefing with good judgment. Simul Healthc. 2006;1(1):49–55 [Research Support, Non-U.S. Gov't Research Support, U.S. Gov't, Non-P.H.S.].
89. Zigmont JJ, Kappus LJ, Sudikoff SN. The 3D model of debriefing: defusing, discovering, and deepening. Semin Perinatol. 2011;35(2):52–8 [Review].
90. McDonnell LK, Jobe KK, Dismukes RK. Facilitating LOS debriefings: synopsis of a training manual. In: Dismukes RK, Smith GM, editors. Facilitation and debriefing in aviation training operations. Aldershot: Ashgate Publishing Ltd; 2000. p. 26–49.
91. Certified Healthcare Simulation Educator Information. Available from: http://www.ssih.org/certification.

Epilogue – A Vision for the Future 36

Paul R. Barach, Jeffrey P. Jacobs, Peter C. Laussen, and Steven E. Lipshultz

Keywords

Patient safety • quality improvement • high reliability organizations • culture

Pediatric and congenital cardiac care and the associated outcomes have improved radically over the past generation. However, despite this improvement, treatments continue to be misused, underused, and overused, and preventable harm continues to occur. By highlighting the best practices for measuring outcomes, this book proposes a framework to help map out and support the next leap in improving pediatric and congenital cardiac care.

Major changes are needed in the current model of care delivery. Given the pressures on healthcare, in order to thrive, institutions must focus on quality of care, including cost-efficiency, through innovations that align the incentives of payers, patients, and providers. Engaging clinical staff is critical to accomplishing this realignment.

With the changes in the medical and social care of children have come an uneasy and increased scrutiny and public oversight of medical practice. Improving the reliability of care will require accepting this forced transparency and embracing the opportunities inherent in this new and hyper connected and social medical driven world. In 2014, the thirst of the public for more information and

P.R. Barach, BSc, MD, MPH (✉)
Department of Health Management and Health Economics, University of Oslo, Oslo, Norway
e-mail: pbarach@gmail.com

J.P. Jacobs, MD, FACS, FACC, FCCP
Division of Cardiac Surgery, Department of Surgery, Johns Hopkins All Children's Heart Institute, All Children's Hospital and Florida Hospital for Children, Johns Hopkins University, Saint Petersburg, Tampa and Orlando, FL, USA

Division of Cardiac Surgery, Department of Surgery, Johns Hopkins University, Baltimore, MD, USA
e-mail: jeffjacobs@msn.com; jeffjacobs@jhmi.edu

P.C. Laussen, MBBS, FCICM
Department of Critical Care Medicine, The Hospital for Sick Children, Toronto, ON, Canada

Department of Anaesthesia, University of Toronto, Toronto, ON, Canada
e-mail: peter.laussen@sickkids.ca

S.E. Lipshultz, MD, FAAP, FAHA
Department of Pediatrics, Wayne State University School of Medicine, Children's Hospital of Michigan, Detroit, MI 48201-2196, USA
e-mail: slipshultz@med.wayne.edu

P.R. Barach, J.P. Jacobs, S.E. Lipshultz, P.C. Laussen (eds.),
Pediatric and Congenital Cardiac Care: Volume 2: Quality Improvement and Patient Safety,
DOI 10.1007/978-1-4471-6566-8_36, © Springer-Verlag London 2015

transparency, coupled with payers and regulators seeking safer and higher-value care, led both the UK and the US to expand programs of public reporting of cardiac surgical outcomes. The release of such data is just the beginning of a major international revolution to make data about the outcomes of patients and the cost of healthcare publically available and available for more effective decisions about care.

Pediatric and congenital cardiac care is a model for medicine because of its success in fostering cross-disciplinary and multi-disciplinary collaboration and has pioneered the collection and sharing of risk-adjusted data. At the heart of a sustainable, generative, and continuously improving organizational culture of healthcare is a system with three interlinked aims [1]:

- better outcomes (e.g., for individuals and populations),
- better performance of the system (e.g., higher quality, safety, value), and
- better professional development (e.g., improved work-related competence, joy, and pride).

How does the present culture and style of management of hospitals providing pediatric and congenital cardiac care support these three interlinked aims?

Organizations and communities, including those in healthcare, respond to positive and affirmative thoughts and information: "Energy flows where attention goes." Real quality improvement requires bringing multiple systems of knowledge together. If done effectively, this combination could guide other fields in healthcare down a bold path on "how to" think different, be transparent, and emotionally and intellectually engage all stakeholders.

Mistrust in healthcare systems and among providers has contributed to cynicism, burn out, and the disengagement by clinicians. The growing pressures of an expensive and laborious system of medical liability can ultimately harm patients; the system of medical liability focuses on blame and shame, and drives defensive and sometimes perverse actions by providers and institutions. Meaningful change through learning happens at the level of discourse, and not through the courts of law. The best clues to changing the culture of healthcare will come from listening to how clinicians and staff talk about their work, organizations, colleagues, and the joy in continuing to work and prosper as pediatric cardiovascular providers future.

If we are to receive a continuous flow of information about possible hazards, near misses, or unsafe conditions in healthcare, trust has to be (re)built and maintained in two areas. In the first, all front-line clinical and administrative staff must feel that it is *safe to identify a specific problem that may involve or uncover errors made by others* [2]. No-fault models could detoxify the present situation while compensating patients for preventable harm. This process must also include committing to full disclosure when things go awry, and establishing peer-support programs, both for clinicians as well as for patients, families, and providers involved in cases of adverse care or events. Recent evidence confirms that programs of open-disclosure based on peer support, and guided by senior clinicians who mentor and support caregivers before and during an adverse event, can improve the outcomes of patients, providers, and organizations.

In the second area, trust must be built around efforts to *ensure hierarchical and organizational transparency*. When clinicians do not feel safe or it they feel unsupported and threatened, they do not speak up about ongoing and emerging threats and consequences that undermine safe practices [3]. Avoiding difficult conversations keeps us from becoming more reliable. Without trust, clinicians tend to resist intentional change, partly because competing commitments and assumptions effectively hold the "status quo" in place. Moreover, the inability to implement change can be exacerbated by patters of work flow that incorporate "normalized deviance," in which some processes of care have evolved over time to fit established work flow and systems, even though these practices may be viewed as "unsafe" and not sanctioned [4]. Further, if a culture of fear is contributing to normalized deviance, this will keep clinicians from doing the right thing the joy in continuing to work and prosper as pediatric cardiovascular providers [5]. The cognitive dissonance that clinicians and executives feel when confronted by organizational opaqueness is predictable and can lead to a lack of sharing of information, lack of learning, and ultimately disruptive behaviors, frustration, burnout, and high churn rates [6].

In this book, we have synthesized many of the leading theories from the clinical sciences, organizational communication, medical sociology, change management, process improvement, and public policy. We have described how these theories will advance pediatric and congenital cardiac care. Developing an inclusive and pragmatic conceptual framework of the factors that shape sharing of knowledge may help improve learning, team building, system resilience, and quality outcomes in cardiac care. This new framework is consistent with the resilience engineering model around the importance of occupational and organizational structure [7]. There are three compatibility factors in this model that can be applied to cardiac care:

- **knowledge factors** related to the epistemological differences between groups and "silos" in care; for example, how groups make sense of their work; how they understand the role of other professionals; and how meaning is articulated by managers versus by staff;
- **cultural factors** related to the shared meanings and values that shape communication; for example, when knowledge should be shared and with whom and how institutional norms, identities, and trust reinforce boundaries and hoarding of knowledge; and
- **organizational factors** related to the influence of departmental, regulatory, and institutional factors that shape sharing of knowledge, such as socio-legal rules, professional jurisdictions, organizational priorities, and constraints of resource.

Complexity theory [8] points to three types of problems:

1. **simple**, in which the relationship between cause and effect is obvious to all (e.g., placing a chest tube; an antibiotic cures a bacterial infection);
2. **complicated** (e.g., putting a patient on extracorporeal membrane oxygenation [ECMO]; diagnosing a bacterial infection); and
3. **complex** (e.g., tracing the bacterial infection to contaminated water; repairing the defective heart of a child, designing new software).

In complex settings where all the elements and interactions are not knowable, and even with a shared aim and relationships among the members of the team, adverse events may still occur.

The systems approach many authors evoke in our book draws attention to the wider organization, management, and culture of healthcare. Research has revealed, for example, that threats to safety in the acute phase (i.e., in the operating theater), subacute phase, and hospital discharge phase are shaped by inter-departmental relationships, attitudinal differences, and cultures that normalize risk. To date, however, this research has tended to focus on systems of care within confined areas and single clinical environments or organizational settings, such as settings of primary or secondary care, the operating room, the intensive care unit, and the emergency department. Little attention however has been paid to the threats to patient safety that arise when patients and information move between and across systems (microsystems) of care.

It is important to appreciate both the barriers and drivers leading to safe and reliable outcomes. These barriers and drivers are usually a complex and meshed "constellation" of factors found within and between organizational processes [9]. These barriers and drivers include:

- regulatory and media pressures;
- organizational boundaries;
- perverse financial incentives; and,
- shifting of professional responsibility.

Continuous quality improvement in healthcare requires bringing multiple systems of knowledge together and being open to constant refinement and reflection. "Good" science involves more than evidence of effect; it requires innovative methods of research, including "action research," "expansive learning," and other "ethno-methodologies." These new methods can help shed light on the relationships and interactions between providers, patients, and the technologies that support and mediate this interaction. The shared benefit of these methods can lead to the active engagement of patients, providers, and the research community, working together to engender respect, trust, and collaborative relationships. This engagement will also help maintain the joy of working, nurture the passion that originally drew providers to healthcare, and reinforce the commitment of dedicated clinicians, allowing them to be courageous and compassionate.

High-reliability organizational approaches—those capable of prolonged, consistent, and

safe performance—are a hallmark of high-risk industries, outside of healthcare [10]. In the face of the growing forces of healthcare reform and increased market competition in for-profit systems, moving to high reliability requires adopting and supporting a culture of mindfulness, engagement and transparency. Such a culture will shed light on the relationship and synergy of a variety of organizational risk factors and their effect on producing harm and inefficiency. This culture strives to understand how to support mindful technologies and learning that are embedded in routine practice, and encourages norms and values that characterize high-reliability organizations, including a:

- preoccupation with preventing failure;
- reluctance to simplify operations;
- commitment to resilience; and,
- deference to sharp-end, front-line clinicians.

The engagement of clinicians occurs when it makes sense and clinicians can see that it adds value to patient care. Strategies to promote clinician engagement must [11]:

- mobilize clinicians to move and experiment within their own systems;
- provide permission, space, and time to find purpose and set directions in partnership with their patients and consumers;
- direct attention to what is happening at the level of delivery of service; and,
- facilitate respectful interaction between clinicians and managers.

Ackoff et. al. wrote about "power over" versus "power to" in regards to getting things done [12]. "Power over" is the use of authority to punish or reward. "Power to" is the use of ideas to inspire, engage, and transform front-line workers into champions of new ideas. The success of health organizations shifts from "power over" workers and patients, to "power to" from top-down management to a partnership with patients, families, and communities. Although there is little question that quality improvement and patient safety lie at the heart of a major shift in how people think about and deliver pediatric and congenital cardiac care, the shift itself will require a full generation to fully mature [13]. The foundation of this evolution in pediatric and congenital cardiac care requires an depth appreciation of the inter-relationships of the domains of outcomes analysis, quality improvement, and patient safety (Fig. 36.1) [14].

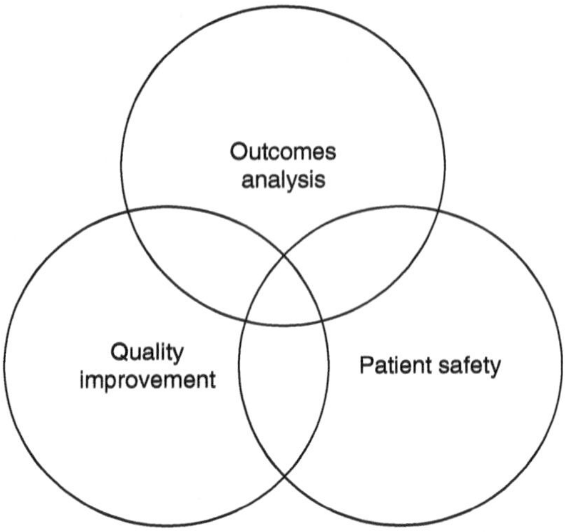

Fig. 36.1 The foundation of this evolution in pediatric and congenital cardiac care is a solid understanding of the inter-relationships of the domains of outcomes analysis, quality improvement, and patient safety

The Venn diagram (Fig. 36.1) demonstrates the close and overlapping relationships between the three domains of this textbook: outcomes analysis, quality improvement, and patient safety.

The editors feel that the ideas in this book could not be timelier, and we therefore appreciate the thoughts and wisdom from the community of experts we have assembled. These ideas present a road map: how to "think different" and how to better engage patients, clinicians, and providers emotionally and intellectually in transforming health care—the core work of this generation of committed professionals. We hope you will find this book helpful and trust you will enjoy reading it as much as we have enjoyed preparing it.

References

1. West E. Organisational sources of safety and danger: sociological contributions to the study of adverse events. Qual Health Care. 2000;9(2):120–6.
2. Phelps G, Barach P. Why the safety and quality movement has been slow to improve care? Int J Clin Pract. 2014: 68(8);932–5.
3. Edmonson A. Psychological safety and learning behavior in work teams. Admin Sci Quar. 1999;44(2): 350–83.

4. Vaughan D. The dark side of organizations: mistake, misconduct, and disaster. Annu Rev Sociol. 1999;25: 271–305.
5. Barach P, Phelps G. Clinical sensemaking: a systematic approach to reduce the impact of normalised deviance in the medical profession. J R Soc Med. 2013; 106(10):387–90. doi: 10.1177/0141076813505045.
6. Amalberti R, Auroy Y, Berwick DM, Barach P. Five system barriers to achieving ultrasafe health care. Ann Intern Med. 2005;142(9):756–64.
7. Sanchez J, Barach P. High reliability organizations and surgical microsystems: re-engineering surgical care. Surg Clin North Am. 2012;92(1). doi. 10.1016/j.suc.2011.12.005.
8. Glouberman S, Zimmerman B. Complicated and complex systems: what would successful reform of Medicare look like? Discussion paper no. 8. Saskatoon: Commission on the Future of Health Care in Canada; 2002.
9. Carroll JS. Organizational learning activities in high-hazard industries: the logics underlying self-analysis. J Management Stud. 1998;35(6):699–717.
10. Weick K, Sutcliffe K, Obstfeld D. Organizing for high reliability: processes of collective mindfulness. In: Boin RA, editor. Crisis management, vol. 3. Thousand Oaks: Sage Publications Ltd; 2008. p. 31–67.
11. Hesselink G, Zegers M, Vernooij-Dassen M, Barach P, Kalkman C, Flink M, Öhlen G, Olsson M, Bergenbrant S, Orrego C, Suñol R, Toccafondi G, Venneri F, Dudzik-Urbaniak E, Kutryba B, Schoonhoven L, Wollersheim H; European HANDOVER Research Collaborative. Improving patient discharge and reducing hospital readmissions by using Intervention Mapping. BMC Health Serv Res. 2014;14:389. doi: 10.1186/1472-6963-14-389.
12. Ackoff RL, Magidison J, Addison HJ. Idealized design: how to dissolve tomorrow's crisis…today. Upper Saddle River: Prentice Hall; 2006.
13. Barach P, Moss, F. Delivering safe health care: Safety is a patient's right. BMJ. 2001;323:585–6.
14. Barach P. The end of the beginning. J Leg Med. 2003;24:7–27.

Index

P.R. Barach, J.P. Jacobs, S.E. Lipshultz, P.C. Laussen (eds.),
Pediatric and Congenital Cardiac Care: Volume 2: Quality Improvement and Patient Safety,
DOI 10.1007/978-1-4471-6566-8, © Springer-Verlag London 2015

T

MIX
Papier aus verantwortungsvollen Quellen
Paper from responsible sources
FSC® C105338

If you have any concerns about our products,
you can contact us on
ProductSafety@springernature.com

In case Publisher is established outside the EU,
the EU authorized representative is:
Springer Nature Customer Service Center GmbH
Europaplatz 3, 69115 Heidelberg, Germany

Printed by Libri Plureos GmbH
in Hamburg, Germany